Essentials of
MEDICAL PARASITOLOGY

SECOND EDITION

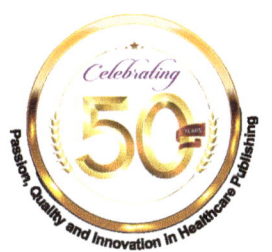

Essentials of
MEDICAL PARASITOLOGY

SECOND EDITION

Apurba S Sastry MD DNB MNAMS PDCR
*Hospital Infection Control Officer
Officer in-charge HICC
Antimicrobial Stewardship Lead
Associate Professor*
Department of Microbiology
Jawaharlal Institute of Postgraduate Medical Education and Research (JIPMER), Puducherry, India

Sandhya Bhat MD DNB MNAMS PDCR
Professor
Department of Microbiology
Pondicherry Institute of Medical Sciences (PIMS)
(A Unit of Madras Medical Mission)
Puducherry, India

Co-Editor
Debadutta Mishra MD, Fellow (Parasitology)
Ex Senior Resident
Department of Microbiology
JIPMER, Puducherry, India

Forewords
Lynne S Garcia MS CLS FAAM
Author of the famous book 'Textbook of Diagnostic Parasitology'
Sujatha Sistla MD
Professor and *Head*, Department of Microbiology, JIPMER, Puducherry, India

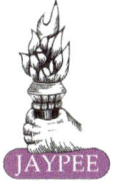

JAYPEE BROTHERS MEDICAL PUBLISHERS
The Health Sciences Publisher
New Delhi | London | Panama

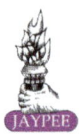 **Jaypee Brothers Medical Publishers (P) Ltd**

Headquarters

Jaypee Brothers Medical Publishers (P) Ltd
4838/24, Ansari Road, Daryaganj
New Delhi 110 002, India
Phone: +91-11-43574357
Fax: +91-11-43574314
Email: jaypee@jaypeebrothers.com

Overseas Offices

J.P. Medical Ltd
83 Victoria Street, London
SW1H 0HW (UK)
Phone: +44 20 3170 8910
Fax: +44 (0)20 3008 6180
Email: info@jpmedpub.com

Jaypee Brothers Medical Publishers (P) Ltd
17/1-B Babar Road, Block-B, Shaymali
Mohammadpur, Dhaka-1207
Bangladesh
Mobile: +08801912003485
Email: jaypeedhaka@gmail.com

Jaypee-Highlights Medical Publishers Inc
City of Knowledge, Bld. 235, 2nd Floor, Clayton
Panama City, Panama
Phone: +1 507-301-0496
Fax: +1 507-301-0499
Email: cservice@jphmedical.com

Jaypee Brothers Medical Publishers (P) Ltd
Bhotahity, Kathmandu
Nepal
Phone: +977-9741283608
Email: kathmandu@jaypeebrothers.com

Website: www.jaypeebrothers.com
Website: www.jaypeedigital.com

© 2019, Jaypee Brothers Medical Publishers

The views and opinions expressed in this book are solely those of the original contributor(s)/author(s) and do not necessarily represent those of editor(s) of the book.

All rights reserved. No part of this publication may be reproduced, stored or transmitted in any form or by any means, electronic, mechanical, photocopying, recording or otherwise, without the prior permission in writing of the publishers.

All brand names and product names used in this book are trade names, service marks, trademarks or registered trademarks of their respective owners. The publisher is not associated with any product or vendor mentioned in this book.

Medical knowledge and practice change constantly. This book is designed to provide accurate, authoritative information about the subject matter in question. However, readers are advised to check the most current information available on procedures included and check information from the manufacturer of each product to be administered, to verify the recommended dose, formula, method and duration of administration, adverse effects and contraindications. It is the responsibility of the practitioner to take all appropriate safety precautions. Neither the publisher nor the author(s)/editor(s) assume any liability for any injury and/or damage to persons or property arising from or related to use of material in this book.

This book is sold on the understanding that the publisher is not engaged in providing professional medical services. If such advice or services are required, the services of a competent medical professional should be sought.

Every effort has been made where necessary to contact holders of copyright to obtain permission to reproduce copyright material. If any have been inadvertently overlooked, the publisher will be pleased to make the necessary arrangements at the first opportunity. The **CD/ DVD-ROM** (if any) provided in the sealed envelope with this book is complimentary and free of cost. **Not meant for sale.**

Inquiries for bulk sales may be solicited at: jaypee@jaypeebrothers.com

Essentials of Medical Parasitology

First Edition: 2016

Second Edition: **2019**

ISBN: 978-93-5270-480-4

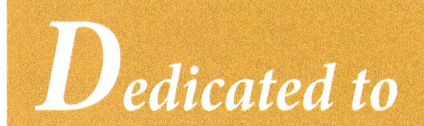

Our Beloved Parents, Family Members
And, above all, the Almighty

"Life is the most difficult exam. Many fail because they tend to copy others, not realizing that everyone has a different question paper."

Gold medalists are not made up of gold. They are made up of determination and hard work and ready to kill themselves to achieve their goal.

Forewords

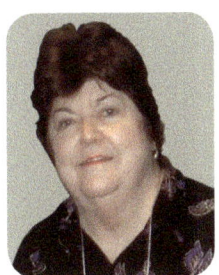

Essentials of Medical Parasitology has been released at a time when there is strong demand for a parasitology textbook for Indian medical school students. This book is fully updated with a simple lucid presentation style. It contains the latest information including recent advances in laboratory diagnosis, treatment, prophylaxis, and epidemiology of each parasitic disease. The life cycles are simple and easy to reproduce. The book is written in a concise and bulleted format for easy understanding.

I congratulate Dr Apurba S Sastry and his wife Dr Sandhya Bhat for this comprehensive work.

Lynne S Garcia MS CLS FAAM
Director, LSG and Associates
Santa Monica
California
United States

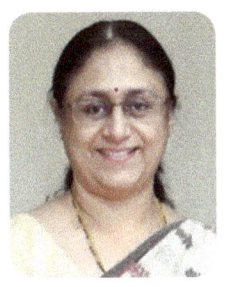

I am happy to know that the second edition of *Essentials of Medical Parasitology* is released. The first edition was widely appreciated among faculty and students. This edition comprises of a complete update on various parasitic diseases.

The life cycles are simple and easy to reproduce. Many controversial and debatable topics have been clarified with updated and corrected information such as presence of pseudocyst stage for *Trichomonas vaginalis* and precyst and cyst stages for *Dientamoeba fragilis* and non-existence of *Sarcocystis lindemanni*.

Epidemiology is the most striking feature of this book. It precisely represents the current geographical distribution; adapted from standard references such as World Health Organization (WHO) and Indian government health programs such as National Vector Borne Disease Control Program (NVBDCP).

Laboratory diagnosis of the different parasitic diseases include the latest molecular, serological methods and automation available. Treatment has been adapted from the standard national and international guidelines. The update in the treatment, drug resistance and ongoing vaccine trials for various parasitic diseases, of note, malaria and leishmaniasis is praiseworthy. Recent changes in nomenclature have also been incorporated such as *Isospora* to *Cystoisospora* and *Balantidium* to *Neobalantidium*.

The information in the book is reliable, modernized and in accordance with the current need of medical school students; written in a concise and bulleted format for easy understanding.

I must admit that the authors have done an outstanding work.

Dr Sujatha Sistla MD
Professor and Head
Department of Microbiology
Jawaharlal Institute of Postgraduate
Medical Education and Research (JIPMER)
Puducherry, India

Preface to the Second Edition

It is a proud moment to announce the release of the second edition of *Essentials of Medical Parasitology*. The first edition was widely appreciated among faculty and students. The second edition has also been designed in a similar fashion taking all your feedback and suggestions into consideration. The newer concepts and recent advances incorporated are as follows:

- **Chapter 1 (General Introduction to Parasitology):** Updates on newer antiparasitic drugs with their mechanism of action have been added in this chapter.
- **Chapter 2 (Introduction to protozoa):** Taxonomic classification of protozoa has been updated. Changes in nomenclature of parasites have been included.
- **Chapter 3 (Amoeba):** Updates such as *Entamoeba bangladeshi*, latest diagnostic methods for *E. histolytica*, update on pathogenesis of *E. histolytica*, and recent advances in laboratory diagnosis and treatment of free-living amoebae have been incorporated. Newer free-living amoebae such as *Sappinia pedata*, *Vahlkampfia*, *Hartmannella* and *Paravahlkamfia* have been included. Many controversies have been resolved such as possible role of immature cyst of *E. histolytica* in transmission of infection and possible association of *E. bangladeshi* and *E. moshkovskii* with intestinal amoebiasis.
- **Chapter 4 (Intestinal and genital flagellates):** In giardiasis, recent updates in genotyping, pathogenesis, epidemiology, laboratory diagnosis, treatment and drug resistance have been included. Many interesting changes have been incorporated such as existence of pseudocyst in *Trichomonas vaginalis*, InPouch TV diagnostic system for culturing *T. vaginalis*, virulence factors of *T. vaginalis*, existence of cyst in *Dientamoeba fragilis*, updates in laboratory diagnosis and treatment in *T. vaginalis* and *D. fragilis*.
- **Chapter 5 (Hemoflagellates):** Leishmaniasis underwent a major update. Epidemiology has been thoroughly updated. Clinical Features and laboratory diagnosis of visceral leishmaniasis have been revised. Treatment regimens of all types of leishmaniasis have been updated according to WHO guideline. Note on leishmaniasis elimination program and vaccination strategies has been incorporated. Trypanosomiasis has been updated with recent advances in laboratory diagnosis, epidemiology and clinical manifestations.
- **Chapter 6 (Malaria parasite and Babesia):** Updates have been made in topics such as *Plasmodium knowlesi*, epidemiology of malaria, malaria elimination in India, advances in laboratory diagnosis such as quantification of malaria parasites, RDT under NVBDCP, molecular methods, automated systems, advances in treatment of vivax and falciparum malaria according to NVBDCP guideline, antimalarial drug resistance and its mechanism, and geographical distribution, prophylaxis against malaria including malaria vaccine strategies and trials (WHO, 2018) with a special note on RTS, S/AS01 vaccine. Babesiosis has been revised with incorporation of updates in laboratory diagnosis and treatment.
- **Chapter 7 (Opportunistic Coccidian parasites):** *Toxoplasma gondii* has been thoroughly updated in pathogenesis including *Toxoplasma* encephalitis, life cycle, laboratory diagnosis with a special emphasis on diagnosis of congenital toxoplasmosis and update on IgG avidity test. *Cryptosporidium* has been revised with interesting facts such as *C. hominis* as human pathogen rather than *C. parvum*, recent advances in pathogenesis and laboratory diagnosis. The recent change of nomenclature of *Isospora* to *Cystoisospora* has been incorporated. *Sarcocystis* also underwent a major change. The controversy about non-existence of *Sarcocystis* "lindemanni" has been clarified and accordingly the life cycle has been revised.
- **Chapter 8 (Miscellaneous protozoa):** Microsporidia has been updated with recent advances in laboratory diagnosis, inclusion of new species such as *Tubulinosema*. The proposal of change in nomenclature of *Balantidium* to *Neobalantidium* has been mentioned. *Blastocystis* species needs a special mention, as recently it has been increasingly reported to be associated with human disease. This topic is thoroughly revised in all aspects from life cycle to its pathogenic potential and laboratory diagnosis and treatment.

- ❖ **Chapter 9 (Introduction to helminths):** Typographical errors are rectified; differences between cestodes, trematodes and nematodes have been updated.
- ❖ **Chapter 10 (Cestodes):** *Diphyllobothrium latum* has been updated in its epidemiology, pathogenesis and laboratory diagnosis. Epidemiology of *Spirometra* has been revised. Taeniasis has been thoroughly updated in its laboratory diagnosis with incorporation of revised DelBrutto's diagnostic criteria and epidemiology. Update has been made in echinococcosis in the areas of genotyping, advances in laboratory diagnosis with special mention on USG and other imaging methods, and treatment modalities.
- ❖ **Chapter 11 (Trematodes or Flukes):** General outline of life cycle of all trematodes has been described which will help students to understand and memorize the life cycles easily. Recent advances in laboratory diagnosis and recent updates in geographical distribution of all trematodes have been incorporated. Less common liver flukes such as *Dicrocoelium* and *Eurytrema* and less common intestinal flukes such as *Nanophyetus salmincola* have been incorporated.
- ❖ **Chapter 12 (Intestinal nematodes):** Flowcharts depicting life cycles of all intestinal nematodes have been included which will help for better understanding and memorizing. Latest update in laboratory diagnosis has been incorporated. Newer nematodes infecting man such as *A. ceylanicum* has been included. A detailed note on soil-transmitted helminths and WHO's deworming strategy for prevention and global elimination has been discussed.
- ❖ **Chapter 13 (Nematodes of lower animals that rarely infect man):** All the parasites under this chapter have been thoroughly revised in their laboratory diagnosis, epidemiology and life cycle. *Thelazia* species needs a special mention, as it has been discussed in detail.
- ❖ **Chapter 14 (Somatic nematodes):** Recent advances in laboratory diagnosis, treatment and epidemiological distribution of lymphatic filariasis, onchocerciasis and loiasis have been incorporated. A special note on filariasis elimination program and its strategies have been discussed. The current status of global dracunculiasis elimination has been discussed. Trichinellosis has been revised in its laboratory diagnosis and pathogenesis.
- ❖ **Chapter 15 (Laboratory diagnosis of parasitic diseases):** This chapter definitely needs a special mention. It is thoroughly updated with latest advancement in methods of stool examination, blood examination methods, serological, molecular, imaging and other techniques for the diagnosis of parasitic diseases.
- ❖ **Chapter 16 (Medical entomology):** Vectors and their role in disease transmission have been updated.
- ❖ **Appendices:** All the appendices have been thoroughly updated. A new annexure comprising morphology of stool parasites according to their relative size has been incorporated.
- ❖ Inclusion of more tables, flowcharts, real images and schematic diagrams was made for better understanding.
- ❖ **Clinical case-based essay questions** have been incorporated at the end of each chapter.
- ❖ **Most features of the first edition have been maintained:** Such as concept of more content-less pages, concise, bulleted format and to-the-point text, simple and lucid language, and separate boxes for summary of laboratory diagnosis and treatment for quick review.

As you know, human errors are inevitable; and no book is immune from it. We would request all the readers to provide any errata found and also valuable suggestions and updates via e-mail.

We are confident and hoping that you all will fall in love with the book.

Apurba S Sastry
drapurbasastry@gmail.com

Sandhya Bhat
sandhyabhatk@gmail.com

Preface to the First Edition

Medical parasitology is an interdisciplinary science that deals with the study of animal parasites which infect and produce diseases in human beings. This book is designed specifically for undergraduate medical and paramedical students as well as for postgraduate students.

Medical students always complain that there is no standard Indian textbook on parasitology at present which can fulfil the need of the examination and for the management of the parasitic diseases.

Currently available Indian medical parasitology books are neither updated with recent advances nor presented in a student-friendly manner. Day-to-day developments in the field of parasitology and the unavailability of a standard textbook fulfilling the needs and expectation of the students, motivated us to write a book in an updated format with recent epidemiological data, laboratory techniques, treatment strategies, etc. in such a way that students can grasp it easily.

The whole content of the book has been arranged in a bulleted format and use of subheads has increased the readability. Entire book is divided into four sections—General introduction, Protozoology, Helminthology and Miscellaneous. At the end, six appendices have been incorporated which will be of immense use and initiate interest among the students. Expected questions including MCQs have been added at the end of each chapter which will help to reinforce and understand the related topic in a better way. Life cycles are drawn in lucid and easy-to-grasp manner, exactly according to the text. Real microscopic images of parasites and specimens from various sources are being incorporated to correlate their impressions with the related parasitic diseases. Laboratory diagnosis and treatment boxes are introduced as a different entity for a quick review for students as well as for physicians.

Our endeavor will be successful, if the book is found to be useful for students as well as for the faculty.

Apurba S Sastry
drapurbasastry@gmail.com

Sandhya Bhat
sandhyabhatk@gmail.com

Acknowledgments

The release of second edition of *Essentials of Medical Parasitology* would not have been possible without our close association with many people. We take this opportunity to extend our sincere gratitude and appreciation to all those who made this book possible.

Hearty acknowledgments to our teachers, departmental staff, family members and others for their blessings and support

1. We would like to sincerely thank **Dr Lynne S Garcia**, author of "Textbook of Diagnostic Parasitology" and Director, LSG and Associates, California, United States, for her willingness to write an encouraging foreword.
2. We express heart-felt gratitude to **Dr Sujatha Sistla**, Professor and Head, Department of Microbiology, JIPMER, for giving the foreword, for her guidance during manuscript preparation and giving permission to reproduce photographs from the department. She is an extremely friendly and knowledgeful person. She has been our '**Google Search**'; clarifying all our doubts all the time. I (Dr Apurba) am greatly indebted to you mam for your timely support and guidance.
3. We are extremely thankful to **Dr S Vivekanandam**, Director, JIPMER, Puducherry and also the previous Director **Dr Vishnu Bhat**, for giving the permission to revise this textbook.
4. We are grateful to **Dr Renu G Boy Varghese**, Director-Principal, Pondicherry Institute of Medical Sciences (PIMS), Puducherry, for giving permission to revise this textbook.
5. We would like to express our special word of thanks to **Dr Reba Kanungo**, Dean Research, Professor and Head, Department of Microbiology, Pondicherry Institute of Medical Sciences (PIMS), for giving permission to reproduce photographs from the department. I (Dr Sandhya) am truly grateful to you mam for your wholehearted support.
6. **Other Faculty of Department of Microbiology, JIPMER**— Dr Jharna Mandal (Additional Professor), Dr Rakesh Singh (Additional Professor), Dr Rahul Dhodapkar (Additional Professor), Dr Noyal M Joseph (Associate Professor), Dr Rakhi Biswas (Associate Professor) and Dr Nonika Rajkumari (Assistant Professor).
7. **Other Faculty of Department of Microbiology, PIMS**— Dr Shashikala (Professor); Dr Sheela Devi (Professor); Dr Johny Asir (Associate Professor); Dr Vivian Joseph P (Associate Professor), Dr Sujitha E (Associate Professor); Dr Anandhalakshmi (Associate Professor), Dr Arthi E (Associate Professor), Mrs Patricia Anita (Assistant Professor), Dr Ramya SR (Assistant Professor), Dr Meghna (Assistant Professor) and Mrs Desdemona Rasitha (Tutor).
8. **Residents and postgraduates, JIPMER**— Dr Deepashree, Dr Ramya, Dr Suman, Dr Prasanna, Dr Kavita, Dr Sunil, Dr Radha, Dr Rachna, Dr Sushmita, Dr Sneha, Dr Akshatha, Dr Sruthi, Dr Subhashree, Dr Dhanalakshmi, Dr Sarumathi, Dr Anitha, Dr Kalpana, Dr Debdutta, Ms Amritha, Ms Manisha, Ms Kavipriya and Ms Sugalya. I (Dr Apurba) would like to keep in record the immense help provided by all my residents. I must say that you guys are highly talented, will be the bright future of Indian Microbiology.
9. **HICC, JIPMER**— Infection control nurses and other office staff such as Ilaveni and Venkat.
10. **Special thanks to our teachers**— Dr SC Parija (JIPMER), Dr BN Harish (JIPMER), Dr ER Nagaraj (SSMC, Tumkur), Dr Sharadadevi Mannur (SSMC, Tumkur) and Dr Renushree (SSMC, Tumkur).
11. **For providing photographs**—We are extremely thankful to all people/institutes/companies, who have agreed to provide valuable photographs.
12. **Microbiology Faculty from our previous working places—**
    - Meenakshi Medical College, Chennai—Dr Senthamarai, Dr Sivasankari, Dr Kumudavathi, Dr Somasundar and others
    - ESIC Medical College and PGIMSR, Chennai—Dr Manisha S Mane and others
    - Sri Siddhartha Medical College, Tumkur, Karnataka, India (all faculty members)
13. **Our friends**—Dr Godfred, Dr Sadia, Dr Sreeja, Dr Wajid, Dr Ramakrishna, Dr Mridula, Dr Srinivas Acharya, Dr Chaya, Dr Manisha, Dr Ira and others.
14. **Family**— Parents, brother, sister and other family members, maternal and paternal cousins and all other well-wishers.

Sincere acknowledgments for helping in manuscript preparation and providing photographs

Name of the person/institute	Contribution(s)
DPDx Image Library, Centers for Disease Control and Prevention (CDC), Atlanta	For giving permission to reproduce photographs of public domain
Public Health Image Library, Centers for Disease Control and Prevention (CDC), Atlanta	For giving permission to reproduce photographs of public domain
Swierczynski G, Milanesi B. Atlas of human intestinal protozoa microscopic diagnosis	For giving permission to reproduce photographs of public domain
Dr Debadutta Mishra, Fellow (Parasitology), JIPMER, Puducherry	For your timely support and inputs during edition of the book
Dr Anand B Janagond, Associate Professor, S Nijalingappa Medical College, Bagalkot, Karnataka	For providing photographs
Dr Subhadra, Associate Professor, Radiology, JIPMER, Puducherry	For providing radiology photographs
Dr Ravikumar K, National Vector Borne Disease Control Program (NVBDCP), Karnataka	For giving inputs during manuscript preparation of national health programs of filariasis and other vector-borne diseases
Dr Mahalakshmy T, Associate Professor, P & SM, JIPMER, Puducherry	For giving inputs regarding filariasis control program
Dr Sherly Antony, Faculty, Pushpagiri Medical College, Kerala	For providing photographs and giving inputs in the correction of content error of first edition
Ex-residents from JIPMER: Dr Raja S, Dr Deepika, Dr Udhaya Sankar and Dr Meenatchi	For giving inputs in the correction of content errors of first edition
Each and every reader (faculty and students) from various parts of the country	For communicating to us by email and other electronic media about the content correction and updates from time to time

Special acknowledgments to my publishers

Jaypee Brothers Medical Publishers (P) Ltd., New Delhi, India

- Shri Jitendar P Vij (Group Chairman)
- Mr Ankit Vij (Managing Director)
- Mr MS Mani (Group President)
- Ms Ritu Sharma (Director–Content Strategy): She is extremely sweet, and dynamic. She has been the backbone behind publishing this book. We are glad to work with you mam.
- Ms Pooja Bhandari (Production Head)
- Ms Seema Dogra (Cover Visualizer)
- Ms Nidhi Sinha (Development Editor)
- **The Development Team:** Mr Vakil Khan, Mr Deepak Saxena, Mr Manoj Pahuja, Mr Rajesh Ghurkundi, Mr Deep Kumar, Mr Laxmidhar Padhiary, Ms Geeta Barik. These guys are simply outstanding in their work. A special mention for Mr Deepak Saxena, we must say that he is the best operator of India in medical publishing. The way Rajesh Ghurkundi and Manoj Pahuja do the designing of photographs is extraordinary. It is a treat for us to work with all of you. You guys are extremely workaholic and have a very good team spirit. We salute them for their professionalism.
- **Staff from other branch office:** Mr Venugopal, Mr Palani A and Mr Venkatesh E (Bengaluru Branch), Mr Parimal, Mr Sharma and Mr Rajesh Malothu (Hyderabad Branch), Mr Senthil Kumar, Mr TM Bhaskar, Mr Dharani Kumar P and Mr RK Dharani (Chennai Branch), Mr Muralidharan (Puducherry Branch), Mr CS Gawde (Mumbai Branch), Mr Sandip Gupta and Mr Sanjoy Chakraborty (Kolkata Branch), Mr Vasudev H (Mangaluru Branch), Mr Arun Kumar (SSPO Thiruvananthapuram Branch), Mr Sujeesh (Kochi Branch) and Mr Dinesh Waghade (Ahmedabad Branch).

Lastly, we would like to keep in record that without the support of our son, parents (of both Dr Sandhya and Dr Apurba) and other family members, it would have been impossible to continue the spirit on, during the journey of the current edition. A special mention to our son (Master Adarsh), who really helped us in giving cooperation. In fact, he was encouraging us to work for the book. We deeply apologize to you as we could not give enough time and care to you during the manuscript preparation.

Apurba S Sastry
Sandhya Bhat

Contents

Section 1: Introduction

1. General Introduction: Parasitology — 3

Section 2: Protozoology

2. Introduction to Protozoa — 15
3. **Amoeba**: *Entamoeba histolytica*, nonpathogenic intestinal amoeba and free-living amoeba — 17
4. **Flagellates—I (Intestinal and Genital)**: *Giardia* and *Trichomonas* — 37
5. **Flagellates—II (Hemoflagellates)**: *Leishmania* and *Trypanosoma* — 49
6. **Apicomplexa—I (Malaria Parasite and Babesia)** — 71
7. **Apicomplexa—II (Opportunistic Coccidian Parasites)**: *Toxoplasma, Cryptosporidium, Cyclospora, Cystoisospora* and *Sarcocystis* — 93
8. **Miscellaneous Protozoa**: Microsporidia, *Balantidium coli* and *Blastocystis* — 111

Section 3: Helminthology

9. Introduction to Helminths — 123
10. **Cestodes**: *Diphyllobothrium, Taenia, Echinococcus, Hymenolepis, Dipylidium* and others — 125
11. **Trematodes or Flukes**: *Schistosoma, Fasciola, Clonorchis, Opisthorchis, Fasciolopsis, Paragonimus* and others — 152
12. **Nematodes—I (Intestinal Nematodes)**: *Trichuris, Enterobius,* Hookworm, *Strongyloides* and *Ascaris* — 174
13. **Nematodes—II (Nematodes of Lower Animals that Rarely Infect Man)** — 198
14. **Nematodes—III (Somatic Nematodes)**: Filarial nematodes, *Dracunculus* and *Trichinella* — 209

Section 4: Miscellaneous

15. Laboratory Diagnosis of Parasitic Diseases — 233
16. Medical Entomology — 257

Appendices
- Appendix 1: Clinical syndromes in parasitology — 265
- Appendix 2: Relative size of morphological forms of parasites — 267

Index — *269*

Further Reading

1. Centers for Disease Control and Prevention, Atlanta, USA.
2. Garcia's Diagnostic Medical Parasitology, 6th edition.
3. Gillespie's Medical Parasitology at a Glance, 4th Edition.
4. Harrison's Principles of Internal Medicine, 19th Edition.
5. Mandell, Douglas, and Bennett's Principles and Practice of Infectious Diseases, 8th Edition.
6. Manson's Tropical Diseases, 23rd Edition.
7. National Vector Borne Disease Control Program (NVBDCP), India.
8. Plotkin's Vaccines, 7th Edition.
9. Topley and Wilson's Microbiology and Microbial Infections, 10th Edition.
10. World Health Organization (WHO).
11. Various national and international journals and other internet sources.

SECTION 1

INTRODUCTION

Section Outline

1. General Introduction: Parasitology *3*

General Introduction: Parasitology

CHAPTER 1

CHAPTER OUTLINE

- Taxonomy of parasites
- Parasite
- Host
- Host-parasite relationship
- Transmission of parasites
- Life cycle of the parasites
- Pathogenesis of parasitic diseases
- Immunology of parasitic diseases
- Laboratory diagnosis of parasitic diseases
- Treatment of parasitic diseases

Medical Parasitology deals with the study of animal parasites, which infect and produce diseases in human beings.

TAXONOMY OF PARASITES

According to the binomial nomenclature as suggested by Linnaeus, each parasite has two names—a genus and a species name.

These names are either derived from: names of their discoverers, Greek or Latin words of the geographical area where they are found, habitat of the parasite, or hosts in which parasites are found and its size and shape.

All parasites are classified under the following taxonomic units—the kingdom, subkingdom, phylum, subphylum, superclass, class, subclass, order, suborder, superfamily, family, genus and species.

The generic name of the parasite always begins with an initial capital letter and species name with an initial small letter, e.g. *Entamoeba histolytica*.

PARASITE

Parasite is a living organism, which lives in or upon another organism (host) and derives nutrients directly from it, without giving any benefit to the host.

Protozoa and helminths (animal parasites) are studied in Medical Parasitology.

Parasites may be classified as:
- **Ectoparasite:** They inhabit the surface of the body of the host without penetrating into the tissues. They are important vectors transmitting the pathogenic microbes. The infection by these parasites is called as **infestation**, e.g. *Sarcoptes scabiei* causing scabies
- **Endoparasite:** They live within the body of the host (e.g. *Leishmania*). Invasion by the endoparasite is called as **infection**.

The endoparasites are of following types:
- **Obligate parasite:** They cannot exist without a parasitic life in the host (e.g. *Plasmodium* species)
- **Facultative parasite:** They can live a parasitic life or free-living life, when the opportunity arises (e.g. *Acanthamoeba*)
- **Accidental parasite:** They infect an unusual host (e.g. *Echinococcus granulosus* infect humans accidentally)
- **Aberrant parasite or wandering parasite:** They infect a host where they cannot live or develop further (e.g. *Toxocara* in humans).

HOST

Host is defined as an organism, which harbors the parasite and provides nourishment and shelter.

Hosts may be of the following types:
- **Definitive host:** The host in which the adult parasites replicate sexually (e.g. *Anopheles* species), is called as definitive host. The definitive hosts may be human or nonhuman living things
- **Intermediate host:** The host in which the parasite undergoes asexual multiplication is called as intermediate host. (e.g. in malaria parasite life cycle, humans are the intermediate hosts)
  - Intermediate hosts are essential for the completion of the life cycle for some parasites
  - Some parasites require two intermediate hosts to complete their different larval stages. These are known as the first and second intermediate hosts

respectively (e.g. Amphibian snails are the first intermediate host and aquatic plants are the second intermediate host for *Fasciola hepatica*).

Hosts can also be:
- **Reservoir host:** It is a host, which harbors the parasites and serves as an important source of infection to other susceptible hosts. (e.g. dog is the reservoir host for echinococcosis)
- **Paratenic host:** It is the host, in which the parasite lives but it cannot develop further and not essential for its life cycle (e.g. fresh water prawn and crab for *Angiostrongylus cantonensis,* big suitable fish for plerocercoid larva of *Diphyllobothrium latum* and freshwater fishes for *Gnathostoma spinigerum*). It functions as a transport or carrier host
- **Amplifier host:** It is the host, in which the parasite lives and multiplies exponentially.

HOST-PARASITE RELATIONSHIP

The relationship between the parasite and the host, may be divided into the following types:

- **Symbiosis:** It is the close association between the host and the parasite. Both are interdependent upon each other that one cannot live without the help of the other. None of them suffer any harm from each other
- **Commensalism:** It is an association in which the parasite only derives the benefit without causing any injury to the host. A commensal is capable of living an independent life
- **Parasitism:** It is an association in which the parasite derives benefit from the host and always causes some injury to the host. The host gets no benefit in return.

Disease: The disease is the clinical manifestation of the infection, which shows the active presence, and replication of the parasite causing damage to the host. It may be mild, severe and fulminant and in some cases may even cause death of the host.

Carrier: The person who is infected with the parasite without any clinical or subclinical disease is referred to as a **carrier**. He can transmit the parasites to others.

TRANSMISSION OF PARASITES

It depends upon:
- Source or reservoir of infection
- Mode of transmission.

Sources of Infection

- **Man:** Man is the source or reservoir for a majority of parasitic infections (e.g. amoebiasis, enterobiasis, etc.) The infection transmitted from one infected man to another man is called as **anthroponoses**
- **Animal:** The infection which is transmitted from infected animals to humans is called as **zoonoses**. The infection can be transmitted to humans either directly or indirectly via vectors. (e.g. echinococcosis from dogs and toxoplasmosis from cats)
- **Vectors:** Vector is an agent, usually an arthropod that transmits the infection from one infected human being to another. Vector can be biological or mechanical. An infected blood sucking insect can transmit the parasite directly into the blood during its blood meal.
  Note: Vectors have been dealt in detail in Chapter 16 (Medical Entomology)
- **Contaminated soil and water:** Soil polluted with human excreta containing eggs of the parasites can act as an important source of infection, e.g. hookworm, *Ascaris* species, *Strongyloides* species and *Trichuris* species.
  Water contaminated with human excreta containing cysts of *E. histolytica* or *Giardia lamblia,* can act as source of infection
- **Raw or under cooked meat:** Raw beef containing the larvae of *Cysticercus bovis* and pork containing *Cysticercus cellulosae* are some of the examples where undercooked meat acts as source of infection
- **Other sources of infection:** Fish, crab or aquatic plants, etc.

Modes of Transmission

The infective stages of various parasites may be transmitted from one host to another in the following ways:
- **Oral or feco-oral route:** It is the most common mode of transmission of the parasites. Infection is transmitted orally by ingestion of food, water or vegetables contaminated with feces containing the infective stages of the parasite. (e.g. cysts of *E. histolytica,* and ova of *Ascaris lumbricoides*)
- **Penetration of the skin and mucous membranes:** Infection is transmitted by the penetration of the larval forms of the parasite through unbroken skin (e.g. filariform larva of *Strongyloides stercoralis* and hookworm can penetrate through the skin of an individual walking bare-footed over fecally contaminated soil), or by introduction of the parasites through blood-sucking insect vectors. (e.g. *Plasmodium* species, *Leishmania* species and *Wuchereria bancrofti*)
- **Sexual contact:** *Trichomonas vaginalis* is the most frequent parasite to be transmitted by sexual contact. However, *Entamoeba, Giardia* and *Enterobius* are also transmitted rarely by sexual contact among homosexuals
- **Bite of vectors:** Many parasitic diseases are transmitted by insect bite (Table 16.2 in Chapter 16) such as—

malaria (female *Anopheles* mosquito), filariasis (*Culex*), leishmaniasis (sandfly), Chagas' disease (reduviid bug) and African sleeping sickness (tsetse fly)
- ❖ **Vertical transmission:** Mother to fetus transmission is important for few parasitic infections like *Toxoplasma gondii*, *Plasmodium* species and *Trypanosoma cruzi*
- ❖ **Blood transfusion:** Certain parasites like *Plasmodium* species, *Babesia* species, *Toxoplasma* species, *Leishmania* species and *Trypanosoma* species can be transmitted through transfusion of blood or blood products
- ❖ **Autoinfection:** Few intestinal parasites may be transmitted to the same person by contaminated hand (external autoinfection) or by reverse peristalsis (internal autoinfection). It is observed in *Cryptosporidium parvum*, *Taenia solium*, *Enterobius vermicularis*, *Strongyloides stercoralis* and *Hymenolepis nana*.

LIFE CYCLE OF THE PARASITES

The life cycle of the parasite may be direct (simple) or indirect (complex).
- ❖ **Direct/simple life cycle:** When a parasite requires only one host to complete its development, it is referred as direct/simple life cycle (Table 1.1)
- ❖ **Indirect/complex life cycle:** When a parasite requires two hosts (one definitive host and another intermediate host) to complete its development, it is referred as indirect/complex life cycle (Table 1.2). Some of the helminths require three hosts (one definitive host and two intermediate hosts) (Table 1.3).

PATHOGENESIS OF PARASITIC DISEASES

The parasites can cause damage to humans in various ways.
- ❖ **Mechanical trauma:**
  - **Eggs:** Trematode eggs being large in size, can be deposited inside the intestinal mucosa (*Schistosoma mansoni*), bladder (*Schistosoma haematobium*), lungs (*Paragonimus*), liver (*Fasciola hepatica*) and can cause mechanical irritation
  - **Larvae:** Migration of several helminthic larvae (hookworms, *Strongyloides* or *Ascaris*) in the lungs produce traumatic damage of the pulmonary capillaries leading to pneumonitis

Table 1.1: Direct/simple life cycle—parasites that need only one host (man)

Protozoa	Helminths
• Entamoeba histolytica	• Cestodes
• Giardia lamblia	• Hymenolepis nana
• Trichomonas vaginalis	• Nematodes
• Balantidium coli	• Ascaris lumbricoides
• Cryptosporidium parvum	• Hookworm
• Cyclospora cayetanensis	• Enterobius species
• Cystoisospora belli	• Trichuris trichiura
• Microsporidia	• Strongyloides species

Table 1.2: Indirect/complex life cycle—parasites requiring one definitive host and one intermediate host

Man acts as definitive host		
Parasites	Definitive host (man)	Intermediate host
Leishmania species*	Man	Sandfly
*Trypanosoma cruzi**	Man	Reduviid bugs
*Trypanosoma brucei**	Man	Tsetse fly
Taenia solium (intestinal taeniasis)	Man	Pig
Taenia saginata	Man	Cattle
Hymenolepis diminuta	Man	Rat flea
Schistosoma species	Man	Snail
Trichinella spiralis	Man	Pig
Filarial worms	Man	Mosquito (*Culex, Aedes, Anopheles*) and flies (blackflies and deerflies)
Dracunculus medinensis	Man	Cyclops
Man acts as intermediate host		
Parasites	Definitive host	Intermediate host
Plasmodium species	Female *Anopheles* mosquito	Man
Babesia species	Tick	Man
Sarcocystis lindemanni	Cat and dog	Man
Toxoplasma gondii	Cat	Man
Echinococcus granulosus	Dog	Man
Taenia solium (Cysticercosis)	Man	Man

*Note: In *Leishmania* and *Trypanosoma*, the definitive and intermediate host terminologies are not applicable as there is no sexual cycle. The better terminologies used are vertebrate host (man) and the invertebrate host (insect vectors)

Table 1.3: Indirect/complex life cycle—parasites requiring one definitive host and two intermediate hosts

Parasites	Definitive host	First intermediate host	Second intermediate host
Diphyllobothrium species	Man	Cyclops	Fish
Fasciola hepatica	Man	Snail	Aquatic plant
Fasciolopsis buski	Man	Snail	Aquatic plant
Paragonimus species	Man	Snail	Crab and fish
Clonorchis species	Man	Snail	Fish
Opisthorchis species	Man	Snail	Fish
Gnathostoma spinigerum	Cat, dog and man	Cyclops	Fish

- **Adult worms:** Adult worms of hookworm, *Strongyloides*, *Ascaris* or *Taenia* get adhere to the intestinal wall and cause mechanical trauma.
- ❖ **Space-occupying lesions:** Certain parasites produce characteristic cystic lesion that may compress the surrounding tissues or organs, e.g. hydatid cysts and neurocysticercosis
- ❖ **Inflammatory reactions:** Most of the parasites induce cellular proliferation and infiltration at the site of their multiplication, e.g. *E. histolytica* provokes inflammation of the large intestine leading to the formation of amoebic granuloma. Adult worm of *W. bancrofti* causes mechanical blockage and chronic inflammation of the lymphatics and lymph vessels. Trematode eggs can induce inflammatory changes (granuloma formation) surrounding the area of egg deposition
- ❖ **Enzyme production and lytic necrosis:** Obligate intracellular parasites of man (*Plasmodium, Leishmania* and *Trypanosoma*), produce several enzymes, which cause digestion and necrosis of host cells. *E. histolytica* produces various enzymes like cysteine proteinases, hydrolytic enzymes and amoebic pore forming protein that lead to destruction of the target tissue
- ❖ **Toxins:** Some of the parasites produce toxins, which may be responsible for pathogenesis of the disease, e.g. *E. histolytica*. However, in contrast to bacterial toxin, parasitic toxins have minimal role in pathogenesis
- ❖ **Allergic manifestations:** Many metabolic and excretory products of the parasites get absorbed in the circulation and produce a variety of allergic manifestations in the sensitized hosts.
  Examples include schistosomes causing cercarial dermatitis, rupture of hydatid cyst producing anaphylactic reactions and occult filariasis (tropical pulmonary eosinophilia)
- ❖ **Neoplasia:** Some of the parasitic infections can contribute to the development of neoplasia (e.g. *S. haematobium* causes bladder carcinoma, *Clonorchis* and *Opisthorchis* cause cholangiocarcinoma)
- ❖ **Secondary bacterial infections:** Seen in some helminthic diseases (schistosomiasis and strongyloidiasis).

IMMUNOLOGY OF PARASITIC DISEASES

The immune response against the parasitic infections depends on two factors:
1. **Host factors:** Immune status, age, underlying disease, nutritional status, genetic constitution and various defense mechanisms of the host
2. **Parasitic factors:** Size, route of entry, frequency of infection, parasitic load and various immune evasion mechanisms of the parasites.

Broadly, the host immunity against the parasitic diseases may be of two types:
1. Protective immune response
   i. Innate immunity
   ii. Adaptive/acquired immunity.
2. Unwanted or harmful immune response (hypersensitive reactions).

Protective Immune Response

Both innate and acquired immunity play an important role in protecting the hosts against parasites. Some of the parasitic infections can be eliminated completely by the host immune responses (complete immunity) while few are difficult to eliminate. In some infections, the immune defense of the host is sufficient to resist further infection but insufficient to destroy the parasite. Immunity lasts till the original infection remains active and prevents further infection. This is called as *infection immunity* or *premunition* or *concomitant immunity* or *incomplete immunity*. This is observed in malaria, schistosomiasis, trichinellosis, toxoplasmosis and Chagas' disease.

(i) Innate Immunity

Innate immunity is the resistance which an individual possesses by birth, due to genetic and constitutional makeup.

Factors influencing innate immunity

- ❖ **Age of the host:** Both the extremes of age are more vulnerable to parasitic infections. Certain diseases are common in children like giardiasis and enterobiasis while certain infections occur more commonly in adults like hookworm infection. Congenital infection occurs commonly with *Toxoplasma gondii*; whereas newborns are protected from falciparum malaria because of high concentration of fetal hemoglobin
- ❖ **Sex:** Certain diseases are more common in males like amoebiasis, whereas females are more vulnerable to develop anemia due to hookworm infection
- ❖ **Nutritional status:** Both humoral and cellular mediated immunity are lowered and neutrophil activity is reduced in malnutrition
- ❖ **Genetic constitution of the individuals:** People with hemoglobin S (sickle cell disease), fetal hemoglobin and thalassemia hemoglobin are resistant to falciparum malaria, whereas Duffy blood group negative red blood cells (RBCs) are resistant to vivax malaria.

Components of innate immunity

- ❖ **Anatomic barriers (skin and mucosa):** Skin is an important barrier for the parasites that enter by cutaneous routes like schistosomes, hookworm and *Strongyloides*

- **Physiologic barriers:** It includes temperature, pH, and various soluble molecules like lysozyme, interferon and complement. Gastric acidity acts as a physiologic barrier to *Giardia* and *Dracunculus*
- **Phagocytosis:** Phagocytes like macrophages and microphages (neutrophils, basophils and eosinophils) act as first line of defense against the parasites
- **Complements:** They play an important role for killing the extracellular parasites by forming membrane attack complexes; which leads to the formation of holes in the parasite membrane
- **Natural killer cells:** Natural killer (NK) cells are another important mediator of innate immunity. They play a central role in killing few of the helminthic parasites.

(ii) Acquired/Adaptive Immunity

This is the resistance acquired by an individual during life following exposure to an agent. It is mediated by antibody produced by B lymphocytes (humoral immune response) or by T cells (cell mediated immune response).

Cell mediated immune response

- When a parasite enters, the parasitic antigens are processed by the antigen presenting cells, (e.g. macrophages) which present the antigenic peptides to T helper (T_H) cells. The antigen presenting cells also secrete interleukin-1 (IL-1) that activates the resting T_H cells. Activated T helper cells differentiate into $T_H 1$ and $T_H 2$ cells
- $T_H 1$ secrete interleukin-2 (IL-2) and interferon gamma.
  - Interleukin-2 activates the cytotoxic T cells (T_C) and NKs, which are cytotoxic to the target parasitic cells. They produce perforin and granzyme that form pores and lyse the target cells
  - IFN-γ activates the resting macrophages which in turn become more phagocytic and release free radicals like reactive oxygen intermediate (ROI) and nitric oxide (NO) that kill the intracellular parasites.
- $T_H 2$ release IL-4, IL-5, IL-6 and IL-10 which are involved in activation of B cells to produce antibodies [immunoglobin E (IgE) by IL-4]. IL-5 also acts as chemoattractant for the eosinophils. Eosinophilia is common finding in various helminthic infections.

Humoral immune response

$T_H 2$ response activates the B cells to produce antibodies which in turn have various roles against the parasitic infections. They are:
- **Neutralization** of parasitic toxins (mediated by IgA and IgG)
- **Preventing** attachment to the gastrointestinal tract (GIT) mucosa (mediated by secretory IgA)
- **Agglutinating** the parasitic antigens thus preventing invasion (mediated by IgM)
- **Complement activation (by IgM and IgG):** Complements bind to the Fc portion of the antibody coated to the parasitic cells. Activation of the complements leads to membrane damage and cell lysis
- **Antibody dependent cell-mediated cytotoxicity (ADCC)** is important for killing of the helminths. NK cells bind to the Fc portion of the IgG antibody coated to the helminths. Activation of NKs leads to release of perforin and granzyme that in turn cause membrane damage and cell lysis
- **Mast cell degranulation:** IgE antibodies coated on mast cells when get bound to parasitic antigens, the mast cells become activated and release a number of mediators like serotonin and histamine.

The Unwanted or Harmful Immune Responses

Sometimes immune responses may be exaggerated or inappropriate in the sensitized individuals on re-exposure to the same antigen. Such type of immunopathologic reactions are called as hypersensitivity reactions that may be harmful to the hosts causing tissue damage. These are of four types (Table 1.4).

Parasitic Factors that Evade the Host Immune Response

Sometimes, the hosts find it difficult to contain the parasitic infections mainly because of the following reasons:
- Large size of the parasites
- Complicated life cycles
- Antigenic complexity.

There are a number of mechanisms by which the parasites evade the host immune responses (Table 1.5).

LABORATORY DIAGNOSIS OF PARASITIC DISEASES

It plays an important role in establishing the specific diagnosis of various parasitic infections. Following techniques are used in diagnosis of parasitic infections (discussed in detail in Chapter 15):
- Parasitic diagnosis—either microscopically or macroscopically
- Culture methods
- Immunodiagnostic methods (antigen and antibody detection)
- Intradermal skin tests
- Molecular methods
- Xenodiagnostic techniques
- Animal inoculation
- Imaging techniques.

Table 1.4: Hypersensitivity reactions seen in parasitic diseases

Hypersensitive reactions	Parasitic diseases
Type I hypersensitivity reactions These are allergic or anaphylactic reactions, occurring within minutes of exposure to parasitic antigens due to IgE mediated degranulation of mast cells	• Cercarial dermatitis (Swimmer's Itch) in schistosomiasis • Loeffler's syndrome in ascariasis • Ground itch (Hookworm infection) • Anaphylaxis due to leakage of hydatid fluid (*Echinococcus granulosus*) • Casoni's test (hydatid disease) • Tropical pulmonary eosinophilia (occult filariasis)
Type II hypersensitivity reactions These are mediated by IgG or rarely IgM antibodies produced against the antigens on surfaces of the parasitic cells causing antibody mediated destruction of the cells by i) the complement activation or ii) by the NK cell activation (ADCC -antibody dependent cell mediated cytotoxicity)	• Anemia in malaria • Black water fever in malaria following quinine therapy • Myocarditis in Chagas' disease • Killing of the helminths by NK cells
Type III hypersensitivity reactions Immune complexes are formed by the combination of parasitic antigens with the circulating antibodies (IgG) which get deposited in various tissues	• Nephrotic syndrome in *Plasmodium malariae* • Katayama fever in schistosomiasis • African trypanosomiasis • Onchocerciasis
Type IV hypersensitivity reactions This is T-cell mediated delayed type of hypersensitivity reaction. Previously sensitized T helper cells secrete a variety of cytokines, on subsequent exposure to the parasitic antigens. Usually, the pathogen is cleared rapidly with little tissue damage. However, in some cases, it may be destructive to the host resulting in granulomatous reaction	• Elephantiasis (in filariasis) • Granulomatous disease in schistosomiasis and other helminthic infections • Leishmaniasis

Abbreviations: IgE, immunoglobulin E; IgG, immunoglobulin G; IgM, immunoglobulin M; NKs, natural killer cells.

Table 1.5: Immune evasion mechanisms of the parasites

Immune evasion mechanisms	Parasites involved
By intracellular location	*Plasmodium* species, *Babesia* species, *Trypanosoma* species, *Toxoplasma* species, *Leishmania* species and Microsporidia
Enters an immunologically protected site soon after infection	*Plasmodium* species entering into hepatocytes
Leave the site where the immune response is already established	*Ascaris* undergoes intestinal phase and migratory lung phase during its life cycle
Survives in macrophages by preventing phagolysosome fusion	*Leishmania, Trypanosoma* and *Toxoplasma*
Antigenic shedding (capping): Surface membrane antigens of the parasites bound to the antibodies undergo redistribution so that the parasite is covered by a folded membrane that later extrude as a cap containing most of the antibodies that were originally bound to the membrane	*Entamoeba histolytica, Trypanosoma brucei* and *Ancylostoma caninum*
Antigenic variation: By change of antigenic composition, the parasites can be protected from the antibodies which are formed against the original antigens	*P. falciparum* (pf-EMP protein), *Giardia* and *Trypanosoma brucei*
Antigenic mimicry: The adult flukes of *Schistosoma* get coated with the host red cell antigens and histocompatibility antigens, so that they are not recognized as foreign and live free from host attack	*Schistosoma* species
Inhibit antibody binding	*Schistosoma mansoni*
Lymphocyte suppression	*Schistosoma mansoni*
Polyclonal stimulation of lymphocytes	*P. falciparum, Trypanosoma brucei, Babesia, Trichinella* and *E. histolytica*
Suppression of immune system	*Trypanosoma, Plasmodium* and *Leishmania*

TREATMENT OF PARASITIC DISEASES

Treatment of parasitic disease is primarily based on chemotherapy and in some cases by surgery.

Antiparasitic Drugs

Various chemotherapeutic agents are used for the treatment and prophylaxis of parasitic infections (Table 1.6).

Surgical Management

For management of parasitic diseases like echinococcosis (or hydatid disease) and neurocysticercosis surgery is indicated. Semi-conservetive surgery is followed wherever possible; for example, PAIR (percutaneous aspiration, injection and reaspiration) is done for treatment of hydatid disease.

Table 1.6: Common antiparasitic drugs, their mechanism of action and clinical indications

Drugs for amoebiasis	Mechanism of action	Clinical indications
Metronidazole, tinidazole and ornidazole	Bioactivated to form reduced cytotoxic products which damage DNA	DOC for the amoebic colitis, amoebic liver abscess, and other extraintestinal amoebiasis
Dehydroemetine	Inhibits protein synthesis	Parenterally used for severe hepatic amoebiasis
Chloroquine	Probably by concentrating in parasite food vacuoles	Used for extraintestinal amoebiasis
Paromomycin (Aminoglycoside)	Inhibits protein synthesis by binding to 16S ribosomal RNA	Effective luminal agent
Diloxanide furoate (Acetanilide compound)	Unknown; it is thought to interfere with protein synthesis	Effective luminal agent
Iodoquinol (8-hydroxyquinoline compound)	Unknown	Luminal agent
Amphotericin B	Complex and multifaceted	DOC for *Naegleria fowleri*
Drugs for flagellates	**Mechanism of action**	**Clinical indications**
Intestinal/Genital Flagellates		
Giardiasis		
Metronidazole and tinidazole	Bioactivated to form reduced cytotoxic products which damage DNA	DOC for giardiasis
Nitazoxanide	Interference with the PFOR enzyme dependent electron transfer reaction which is essential for anaerobic energy metabolism	
Furazolidone	Cross linking of DNA	Given to children
Paromomycin	Protein synthesis inhibitor in nonresistant cells by binding to 16S ribosomal RNA	Can be given in pregnancy
Trichomoniasis		
Metronidazole or tinidazole	Bioactivated to form reduced cytotoxic products having nitro groups which damage DNA	DOC for trichomoniasis, given to both the partners
Drugs for hemoflagellates		
Chagas' disease (American trypanosomiasis)		
Nifurtimox	Forms nitro-anion radical metabolite, which reacts with the nucleic acids of the parasite, causing a significant breakage in the DNA	Chagas' disease
Benznidazole	Production of free radicals, to which *Trypanosoma cruzi* is particularly sensitive	Effective in the treatment of reactivated *T. cruzi* infections caused by immunosuppression (AIDS patients or patients of organ transplants)
Sleeping sickness (African trypanosomiasis)		
Pentamidine	Accumulates to micromolar concentrations within the parasite to kill it by inhibiting enzymes and interacting with DNA	DOC for East African sleeping sickness
Suramin	Trypanocidal activity; inhibits enzymes involved with the oxidation of reduced NADH	DOC for West African sleeping sickness

Contd...

Contd...

Leishmaniasis	Mechanism of action	Clinical indications
Sodium stibogluconate Meglumine antimoniate	Inhibition of the parasite's glycolytic and fatty acid oxidative activity resulting in decreased reducing equivalents for antioxidant defense and decreased synthesis of ATP	Leishmaniasis
Amphotericin B	Bind to ergosterol and disrupts cell membranes	Leishmaniasis
Paromomycin	Discussed earlier under giardiasis	Leishmaniasis
Miltefosine	Can trigger programmed cell death (apoptosis)	Leishmaniasis
Drugs for malaria	**Mechanism of action**	**Clinical indications**
Chloroquine	Probably, concentrating in parasite food vacuoles, preventing the polymerization of the hemoglobin into the toxic product hemozoin	DOC for uncomplicated benign malaria
Artemisinin derivative (Artemisinin or artemether or arte-ether)	Generate highly active free radicals that damage parasite membrane	DOC for complicated or falciparum malaria
Quinine	Probably similar to chloroquine; still not clear	DOC for complicated or falciparum malaria
Mefloquine	Same as chloroquine	DOC for complicated or falciparum malaria
Primaquine	Generating reactive oxygen species	DOC for relapse of vivax and ovale malaria
Sulfadoxine-pyrimethamine	Inhibits the production of enzymes involved in the synthesis of folic acid within the parasites	DOC for complicated or falciparum malaria
Lumefantrine	Accumulation of heme and free radicals	Complicated or falciparum malaria
Drugs for babesiosis	**Mechanism of action**	**Clinical indication**
Clindamycin plus quinine	Clindamycin: inhibits protein synthesis Quinine: discussed earlier	DOC for severe babesiosis
Atovaquone plus azithromycin	Azithromycin: inhibits protein synthesis Atovaquone: inhibits mitochondrial transport in protozoa by targeting the cytochrome bc_1 complex	DOC for mild babesiosis
Drugs for toxoplasmosis	**Mechanism of action**	**Clinical indications**
Cotrimoxazole (Trimethoprim-sulfamethoxazole)	Inhibiting folate synthesis from PABA (para-aminobenzoic acid), thus inhibiting purine metabolism	DOC for prophylaxis in HIV-infected people
Spiramycin	Inhibition of protein synthesis in the cell during translocation	DOC in pregnancy
Drugs for Cryptosporidium	**Mechanism of action**	**Clinical indications**
Nitazoxanide	Interferes with the PFOR enzyme-dependent electron-transfer reaction, which is essential to anaerobic metabolism in protozoan and bacterial species	DOC for *Cryptosporidium* infection
Drugs for Cystoisospora and Cyclospora	**Mechanism of action**	**Clinical indications**
Cotrimoxazole (Trimethoprim-sulfamethoxazole)	Inhibiting folate synthesis from PABA (Para aminobenzoic acid), thus inhibiting purine metabolism	DOC for *Cystoisospora* and *Cyclospora* infection
Drugs for cestodes	**Mechanism of action**	**Clinical indication**
Praziquantel	Increases the permeability of the membranes of parasite cells toward calcium ions which induces contraction of the parasites, resulting in paralysis in the contracted state	DOC for all cestode infections
Niclosamide	Niclosamide uncouples oxidative phosphorylation	Alternative drug for cestode infections
Albendazole	Causes loss of the cytoplasmic microtubules leading to impaired uptake of glucose by the larval and adult stages of the susceptible parasites, and depleting their glycogen stores	Given for cysticercosis and hydatid disease
Drugs for trematodes	**Mechanism of action**	**Clinical indication**
Praziquantel	Discussed earlier under cestodes	DOC for most of the trematode infections
Triclabendazole	Binds to beta-tubulin and prevent the polymerization of the microtubules	DOC for *Fasciola hepatica* and *F. gigantica*

Contd...

Contd...

Drugs for nematodes	Mechanism of action	Clinical indication
Intestinal nematodes		
Mebendazole or albendazole	Discussed earlier under cestodes	DOC for most of the intestinal nematodes
Pyrantel pamoate	Acts as a depolarizing neuromuscular blocking agent, thereby causing sudden contraction, followed by spastic paralysis of the helminths	Alternative drug for intestinal nematodes
Ivermectin	Kills by interfering with nervous system and muscle function, in particular by enhancing inhibitory neurotransmission resulting in flaccid paralysis	DOC for strongyloidiasis. Alternative drug for *Trichuris* infections
Filarial nematodes		
Diethylcarbamazine (DEC)	An inhibitor of arachidonic acid metabolism in microfilaria. This makes the microfilaria more susceptible to phagocytosis	DOC for lymphatic filariasis, *Loa loa* and *Mansonella* infections
Albendazole	Discussed earlier under cestodes	Alternative drug for lymphatic filariasis, *Loa loa* and *Mansonella* infections
Ivermectin	Discussed earlier under intestinal nematodes	Used for lymphatic filariasis in Africa. DOC for onchocerciasis. Alternative drug for *Loa loa* and *Mansonella* infections
Doxycycline	Targets the intracellular *Wolbachia* present inside the Microfilaria	Alternative drug for lymphatic filariasis

Abbreviations: DNA, deoxyribonucleic acid; DOC, drug of choice; RNA, ribonucleic acid; PFOR, pyruvate ferredoxin oxidoreductase enzyme; ATP, adenosine triphosphate; NADH, nicotinamide adenine dinucleotide.

EXPECTED QUESTIONS

I. Write short notes on:
  a. Paratenic host.
  b. Reservoir host.
  c. Indirect/complex life cycle.
  d. Immune evasion mechanisms of the parasites.
  e. Antiparasitic drugs.

II. Differentiate between:
  a. Definitive host and intermediate host.
  b. Direct and indirect life cycle.

III. Multiple choice questions (MCQs):
  1. A host harboring adult or sexual stage of a parasite is called:
     a. Definitive host
     b. Intermediate host
     c. Reservoir host
     d. None of the above
  2. Parasite which may be transmitted by sexual contact is:
     a. *Trypanosoma cruzi*
     b. *Trichomonas vaginalis*
     c. *Trypanosoma brucei*
     d. *Ascaris*
  3. Cholangiocarcinoma is associated with chronic infection of:
     a. *Paragonimus westermani*
     b. *Fasciola hepatica*
     c. *Clonorchis sinensis*
     d. *Schistosoma haematobium*
  4. Which of the following parasite is transmitted by dog:
     a. *Taenia saginata*
     b. *Hymenolepis nana*
     c. *Echinococcus granulosus*
     d. *Diphyllobothrium latum*
  5. Blood-sucking vector may transmit:
     a. *Ascaris lumbricoides*
     b. *Ancylostoma duodenale*
     c. *Strongyloides stercoralis*
     d. *Plasmodium*

Answers
1. a 2. b 3. c 4. c 5. d

SECTION 2

PROTOZOOLOGY

Section Outline

2. Introduction to Protozoa *15*
3. Amoeba *17*
4. Flagellates—I (Intestinal and Genital) *37*
5. Flagellates—II (Hemoflagellates) *49*
6. Apicomplexa—I (Malaria parasite and Babesia) *71*
7. Apicomplexa—II (Opportunistic Coccidian Parasites) *93*
8. Miscellaneous Protozoa *111*

Introduction to Protozoa

CHAPTER 2

CHAPTER OUTLINE
- General features of protozoa
- Classification of protozoa

GENERAL FEATURES OF PROTOZOA

The protozoa are though unicellular, they belong to lower eukaryotes as they possess cellular organelles and have metabolic pathways similar to that of eukaryotes.
- More than two lakhs protozoa are named, but only about 80 species belonging to nearly 30 genera infect human beings
- Many of these protozoa are relatively harmless but few may cause some of the important diseases of tropical countries like malaria, kala azar, sleeping sickness and Chagas' disease, etc.
- With the advent of HIV/AIDS, some of them are increasingly being recognized as opportunistic pathogens like toxoplasmosis, cryptosporidiosis, etc.

CLASSIFICATION OF PROTOZOA

The Traditional 1980s Classification

This classification of protozoan parasites was based on the recommendation of the committee on Systematics and Evolution of the Society of Protozoologists conducted by Levine et al. (1980). It was widely used before; now obsolete and replaced by molecular classification.

Corliss's Interim User-Friendly Classification (1994)

Corliss proposed a user-friendly classification trying to meet the requirements of both protozoologists and medical parasitologists.

He divided the living creatures into six kingdoms. Unicellular parasites (generally accepted as protozoa) are categorized into two phylum—Archezoa and Protozoa.

Molecular Classification (2000)

The hierarchical system can be accurately represented by the ribonucleic acid (RNA) and protein sequences of the organisms. With advance of molecular techniques, the ribosomal RNA and protein sequences are studied, and a new classification has been devised.

- Cavalier and Smith's six kingdoms classification, also called as molecular classification is based on the six kingdom theory proposed by Cavalier and Smith (1998). They are bacteria, protozoa, animalia, fungi, plantae and chromista
- Kingdom Protozoa constitutes 11-13 phyla, of which six contain parasites that infect man
- The present classification differs from traditional (1980) classification in two aspects: (i) Microsporidia, are now classified under the Kingdom Fungi, (ii) *Blastocystis*, is now placed under Kingdom Chromista. However for the sake of familiarity, this book describes both the organisms under Protozoa (Table 2.1)
- The description in the individual chapters of this book will be according to this classification.

Kingdom Protozoa

They are unicellular eukaryotic, phagotrophic, non-photosynthetic organism without a cell wall.

Subkingdom Archezoa

They are unicellular eukaryotic organisms, exhibiting various prokaryotic features in ribosomes and transfer ribonucleic acid (tRNA) and lacking mitochondria and other organelles. It has one Phylum Metamonada; which comprises of intracellular intestinal and genital flagellates.

Subkingdom Neozoa

Unicellular eukaryotic organisms typically possessing mitochondria and other organelles.
- **Phylum Amoebozoa:** They are unicellular eukaryotic organisms with pseudopodia, which is used for locomotion and feeding
  - **Class Amoebaea:** Free living amoeba with mitochondria
  - **Class Archamoebea:** Obligate amoeba with secondary loss of mitochondria.

Table 2.1: Molecular classification (2000)

Kingdom	Subkingdom	Phylum	Class	Order	Genus
Protozoa	Archezoa	Metamonada (intestinal and genital flagellates)	Trepomonadea	Diplomonadida	*Giardia, Enteromonas*
			Retortamonadea	Retortamonadida	*Retortamonas, Chilomastix*
			Trichomonadea	Trichomonadida	*Trichomonas, Pentatrichomonas, Dientamoeba*
	Neozoa	Amoebozoa (amoebae)	Archamoebea	Euamoebida	*Entamoeba, Endolimax, Iodamoeba*
			Amoebaea	Acanthopodida	*Acanthamoeba, Balamuthia*
		Percolozoa (flagellated amoeba)	Heterolobosea	Schizopyrenida	*Naegleria*
		Euglenozoa (blood and tissue flagellates)	Kinetoplastidea	Trypanosomatida	*Leishmania* *Trypanosoma*
		Apicomplexa (sporozoan parasites)	Coccidea	Eimeriida	*Eimeria, Toxoplasma, Cryptosporidium Cyclospora, Cystoisospora, Sarcocystis*
				Haemosporida	*Plasmodium*
				Piroplasmida	*Babesia*
		Ciliophora (ciliates)	Litostomatea	Trichostomatia	*Balantidium*
Fungi		Microspora	Microsporea	Microsporida	*Enterocytozoon, Encephalitozoon, Pleistophora, Trachipleistophora, Brachiola, Nosema, Vittaforma, Microsporidium, Tubulinosema*
Chromista	Chromobiota	Bigyra	Blastocystea		*Blastocystis*

Adapted from: Topley and Wilson's Microbiology and Microbial Infections, 10th edition and Patrick Murray's Manual of Clinical Microbiology, 11th Edition, ASM Press.

- ❖ **Phylum Apicomplexa:** Unicellular organisms having 1–4 temporary flagella and mitochondria but lacking Golgi bodies
- ❖ **Phylum Euglenozoa:** Unicellular organisms having 1–4 flagella, mitochondria and Golgi bodies
- ❖ **Phylum Apicomplexa:** Unicellular eukaryotic organisms possessing apical complex made up of polar rings, rhoptries, micronemes and conoid
- ❖ **Phylum Ciliophora:** Unicellular organisms having cilia as locomotor organ and two nuclei of different size and ploidy—(1) macronucleus and (2) micronucleus.

Kingdom Fungi

Eukaryotic heterotrophic organisms lacking plastids but possessing cell wall containing chitin and β-glucan.

Kingdom Chromista

Unicellular eukaryotic, photosynthetic filamentous or colonial, organisms (in part "algae"); some with secondary loss of plastids.

EXPECTED QUESTIONS

I. Write short notes on:
  a. Molecular classification (2000) of parasites.
  b. Subkingdom Neozoa.

II. Multiple choice questions (MCQs):
  1. Which of the following protozoa belongs to phylum Euglenozoa?
     a. *Leishmania* species
     b. *Entamoeba* species
     c. *Cryptosporidium* species
     d. *Plasmodium* species
  2. Which of the following protozoa belongs to kingdom Chromista?
     a. *Cystoisospora* species
     b. *Babesia* species
     c. *Giardia* species
     d. *Blastocystis* species
  3. Which of the following protozoa belongs to order Schizopyrenida?
     a. *Plasmodium* species
     b. *Naegleria* species
     c. *Acanthamoeba* species
     d. *Entamoeba* species
  4. Which of the following protozoa belongs to phylum Apicomplexa?
     a. *Giardia* species
     b. *Trichomonas* species
     c. *Plasmodium* species
     d. *Entamoeba* species

Answers
1. a   2. d   3. b   4. c

Amoeba

CHAPTER 3

CHAPTER OUTLINE

- Introduction
- Intestinal amoeba
- Pathogenic intestinal amoebae
- Nonpathogenic intestinal amoebae
- Free-living amoebae

INTRODUCTION

Amoeba is a single-celled protozoa that constantly changes its shape. The word **"amoeba"** is derived from the Greek word **"amoibe"** meaning **"change"**. They constantly change their shape due to presence of an organ of locomotion called as "pseudopodium".

Amoebae can be classified in two ways.

- Based on habitat: Amoebae are classified as:
  1. Intestinal amoebae (reside in large intestine): They comprise of both pathogenic (e.g. *E. histolytica*) and nonpathogenic amoebae.
  2. Free living amoebae: They are widely distributed in soil and water. (Table 3.1).
- Taxonomical classification: Amoebae are classified taxonomically based on molecular structure (ribosomal RNA) (Table 3.2).

PATHOGENIC INTESTINAL AMOEBAE

Entamoeba histolytica

Introduction

E. histolytica is worldwide in distribution but more common in tropical and subtropical countries. *E. histolytica* causes amoebic dysentery and a wide range of other invasive diseases, including amoebic liver abscess.

There are three other species of *Entamoeba* such as *E. dispar*, *E. moshkovskii* and *E. bangladeshi* which are morphologically similar to *E. histolytica*; can be differentiated from each other by molecular and other methods described later. All of them are found as commensal in human intestine; *E. moshkovskii* and *E. bangladeshi* are reported to be associated with infants with diarrhea.

Table 3.1: Classification of amoebae based on habitat

Intestinal amoebae (large intestine)		Free living amoebae (in soil and water)
Pathogenic	**Nonpathogenic**	**Opportunistic pathogen**
• Entamoeba histolytica • E. moshkovskii (infants) • E. bangladeshi (infants) (unknown virulence)	• E. dispar • E. coli • E. polecki • E. hartmanni • Endolimax nana • Iodamoeba butschlii • E. gingivalis* (mouth)	• Acanthamoeba species • Naegleria fowleri • Balamuthia mandrillaris • Sappinia species

The habitat of *E. gingivalis** is oral cavity, not large intestine.
Note: *E. moshkovskii* and *E. bangladeshi* are occasionally reported to be associated with infants with diarrhea.

Table 3.2: Taxonomic classification of amoebae

Class	Order	Genus
Phylum: Amoebozoa		
Archamoebea	Euamoebida	Entamoeba Endolimax Iodamoeba
Amoebaea	Acanthopodida	Acanthamoeba Balamuthia
Phylum: Percolozoa		
Heterolobosea [flagellated amoeba]	Schizopyrenida	Naegleria

Note: All amoebae belong to Kingdom Protozoa and Subkingdom Neozoa.

History

E. histolytica was first described by Fedor Losch (1875) from Russia. The species name was coined by Fritz Schaudinn in 1903.

Epidemiology

Amoebiasis is a major health problem worldwide.

- The largest burden of the disease occurs in tropics of China, Central and South America, and Indian subcontinents affecting 10% of the world's population (500 million)
- It is the third most common parasitic cause of death in the world (after malaria and schistosomiasis)
- Globally, approximately 50 million cases and 110, 000 deaths have been reported annually by World Health Organization (WHO)
- The incidence of invasive disease is considerably higher in urban areas of Mexico city; Medellin (Colombia) and Durban (South Africa) than in the rest of the world. Contributing factors though not well delineated, it may be attributed to poor nutrition, tropical climate, stress, altered bacterial flora in the colon, traumatic injuries to the intestinal mucosa, decreased immunity, alcoholism, and genetic factors
- In India, the prevalence rate is around 15% (ranges from 3.6% to 47.4%). It has been reported throughout India.

Morphology

E. histolytica has three stages—(1) trophozoite, (2) precyst and (3) cyst (immature and mature).

Trophozoite

It is the invasive form as well as the feeding and replicating form of the parasite found in the feces of patients with active disease.
- It measures 12–60 μm (average 15–20 μm) in diameter.
- Cytoplasm of trophozoite is divided into a clear ectoplasm and a granular endoplasm
- Granular endoplasm looks as **ground glass** appearance and contains red blood cells (RBCs), white blood cells (WBCs) and food vacuoles containing tissue debris and bacteria. RBCs are found only in the stage of invasion
- **Pseudopodia:** Ectoplasm has long finger like projections called as pseudopodia (organ of locomotion); which exhibits active, unidirectional rapid progressive and purposeful movement
- Nucleus is single, spherical, 4–6 μm size, contains central dot like compact karyosome surrounded by a clear halo. Nuclear membrane is thin and delicate and is lined by a layer of fine chromatin granules. The number of chromosomes varies between 30 and 50
- The space between the karyosome and the nuclear membrane is traversed by spoke like radial arrangement of achromatic fibrils (cart wheel appearance)
- Amoebic trophozoites are anaerobic parasites. They lack mitochondria, endoplasmic reticulum and Golgi apparatus (Fig. 3.1A).

Precyst

It is the intermediate stage between trophozoite and cyst.
- It is smaller to trophozoite but larger to cyst (10–20 μm)
- It is oval with a blunt pseudopodia. Food vacuoles and RBCs disappear. Nuclear structures are same as that of trophozoite (Fig. 3.1B).

Cyst

It is the infective form as well as the diagnostic form of the parasite found in the feces of carriers as well as patients with active disease (Fig. 3.1C).
- It measures 10–20 μm (average 12–15 μm) in diameter
- Nuclear structures are same as in trophozoites. First, the cyst is uninucleated; later the nucleus divides to form binucleated and finally becomes quadrinucleated cyst
- Cytoplasm of uninucleated cyst contains 1–4 numbers refractile bars with smooth rounded edges called as **chromatoid bodies** (aggregation of ribosome) and a large **glycogen mass** (stains brown with iodine)

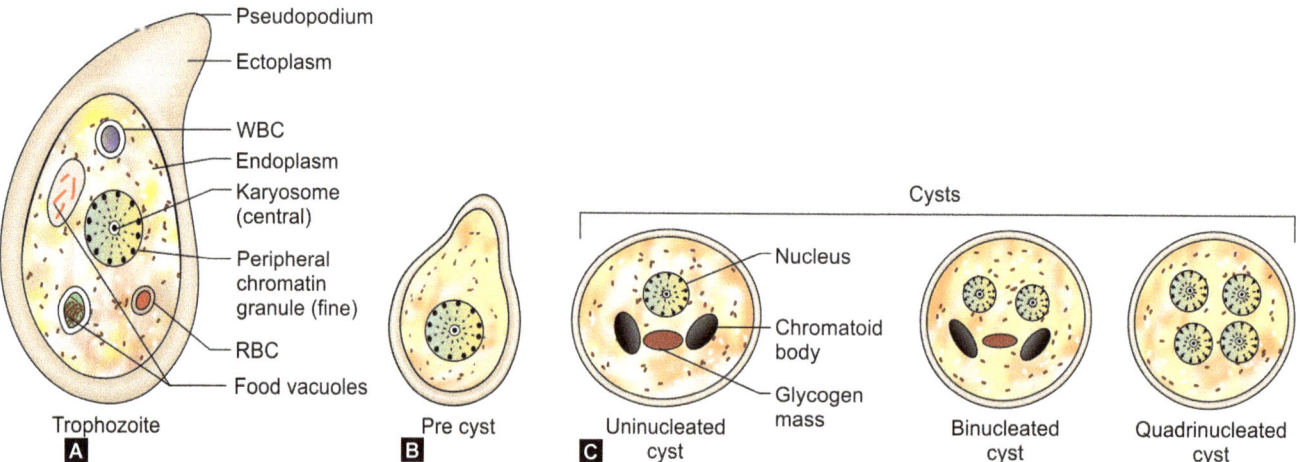

Figs 3.1A to C: *Entamoeba histolytica* (schematic diagram): (A) Trophozoite; (B) Precyst; (C) Cysts

CHAPTER 3 ◆ Amoeba

- Both chromatoid body and glycogen mass gradually disappear, and they are not found in mature quadrinucleated cyst
- Cysts are present only in the gut lumen; they never invade the intestinal wall.

"Minuta" form of *Entamoeba histolytica*: They are the commensal phase of *E. histolytica*, living in the lumen of gut. They are usually smaller in size (trophozoite 12–14 μm and cyst <10 μm) and often mistaken as *E. hartmanni*.

Life Cycle (Fig. 3.2)

Host: *E. histolytica* completes its life cycle in single host, i.e. man.

Infective form: Mature quadrinucleated cyst is the infective form. However, uni or binucleated cysts can also be infective. Cysts can resist chlorination, gastric acidity and desiccation and can survive in a moist environment for several weeks.

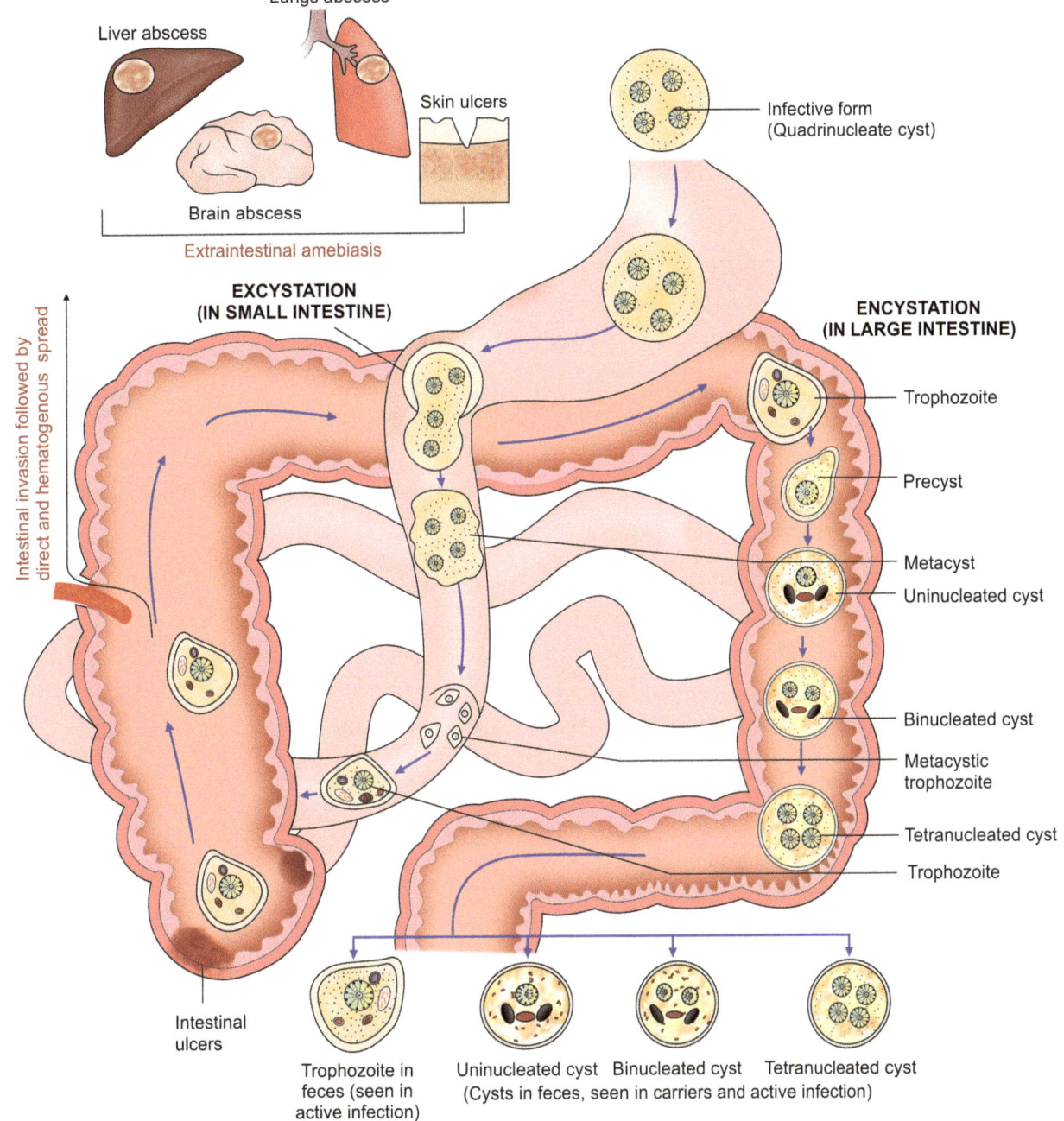

Fig. 3.2: Life cycle of *Entamoeba histolytica*

Mode of transmission

- **Feco-oral route (most common):** By ingestion of contaminated food or water with mature quadrinucleated cysts
- **Sexual contact:** Rare, either by anogenital or orogenital contact (especially in developed countries among homosexual males)
- **Vector:** Very rarely, flies and cockroaches may mechanically transmit the cysts from feces, and contaminate food and water.

Development in man (small intestine)

- **Excystation:** In small intestine (neutral or slightly alkaline pH), the cyst wall gets lysed by trypsin and a single tetranucleated trophozoite (metacyst) is liberated, which eventually transforms into four small **metacystic trophozoites**
- Metacystic trophozoites are carried by the peristalsis to ileocecal region of large intestine and multiply by binary fission, and then colonize on the mucosal surfaces and crypts of the large intestine
- After colonization, trophozoites show different courses depending on various factors like host susceptibility, age, sex, nutritional status, host immunity, intestinal motility, transit time and intestinal flora
- **Asymptomatic cyst passers:** In majority of individuals, trophozoites do not cause any lesion, transform into cysts and are excreted in feces
- **Amoebic dysentery:** Trophozoites of *E. histolytica* secrete proteolytic enzymes that cause destruction and necrosis of tissue, and produces flask shaped ulcers on the intestinal mucosa. At this stage, large numbers of trophozoites are liberated along with blood and mucus in stool producing amoebic dysentery. Trophozoites usually degenerate within minutes
- **Amoebic liver abscess:** In few cases, erosion and necrosis of small intestine are so extensive that the trophozoites gain entrance into the radicals of portal veins and are carried away to the liver where they multiply causing amoebic liver abscess.

Development in man (large intestine)

- **Encystation:** After some days, when the intestinal lesion starts healing and patient improves, the trophozoites transform into precysts then into quadrinucleated cysts which are liberated in feces
- Encystation occurs only in the large gut. Cysts are never formed once the trophozoites are excreted in stool
- Factors that induce cyst formation include food deprivation, overcrowding, desiccation, accumulation of waste products, and cold temperatures
- Cysts released in feces can survive in the environment and become the infective form. Trophozoites are also excreted, but get disintegrated in the environment or by gastric juice when ingested (Fig. 3.2).

Pathogenesis

Trophozoite of *E. histolytica* is the invasive form and possesses many virulence factors that play role in the pathogenesis of intestinal as well as extraintestinal amoebiasis (Table 3.3).

Pathogenesis of intestinal amoebiasis

The pathogenesis of intestinal amoebiasis occurs through the following steps:

- **Colonization:** Trophozoites first colonize the intestinal mucosa; facilitated by the bacterial flora which lower the oxygen tension
- **Adhesion:** Then the trophozites penetrate the mucus layer and adhere to the host cells by means of Gal/GalNAc lectin and other adhesion molecules (Table 3.3)
- **Invasion:** Amoebae then invade the host cells; helped by cysteine proteases, hydrolytic enzymes, neuraminidase and metallocollagenases
- **Host cell death:** This is mediated through contact dependent cell lysis, calcium influx, tyrosine dephosphorylation, cell lysis due to pore formation (mediated by amoeba pores) and finally apoptosis via caspase 3 activation.

Table 3.3: Virulence factors of *Entamoeba histolytica*

Adhesins

Amoebic lectin antigen:
- It is a 260 kDa galactose and N-acetylgalactosamine inhabitable surface protein (Gal/NAG lectin)
- It has two subunits—heavy (170 kDa) and—light (35 kDa) subunits linked by disulfide bridge
- Lectin antigen is the principle virulence factor, present on the surface of trophozoites of pathogenic *E. histolytica* but not on nonpathogenic *E. dispar*. Its various pathogenic mechanisms are:
  - *Adhesion:* By binding to glycoprotein receptors on intestinal epithelium and vascular endothelium
  - *Cytotoxicity:* By contact dependent cytolysis of the target cells by increasing the calcium level
  - *Complement resistance:* 170kDa subunit resembles CD59 (a human complement blocker) that prevent membrane attack complex (C5-C9) formation

Other adhesins include: 220-kDa lectin, a 112-kDa adhesins and a surface lipophosphoglycan.

Other virulence factors

- **Amoebapore:** It is a 5 kDa pore forming protein, inserts ion channels in the target cell membrane causing leakage of ions. Its equivalent found in *E. dispar* is called as dispar pores
- **Cysteine proteases:** They are responsible for invasion, secreted only by trophozoites of pathogenic *E. histolytica*. They degrade extracellular matrix, IgA, IgG, anaphylotoxins such as C3a and C5a. Examples include histolysin, amoebapain and cathepsin B like proteases
- **Hydrolytic enzymes** such as RNAse, neutral protease and phosphatases—help in the destruction of the target tissue
- **Neuraminidase and metallocollagenase:** Help in invasion
- **Thioredoxin reductase system:** It prevents and repairs the damage caused by oxidative stress.

Host factors

- **Genetic factor:** People with Q223R mutation in the leptin receptor gene are at four times increased risk of contracting amoebiasis
- **Role of zinc:** Zinc alters the functionality of amoebae causing a decrease in replication and adhesion; there by inhibiting amoebic pathogenicity
- **Role of IgA:** IgA response to Gal/GalNAc lectin attachment appears to be protective (provides local immunity). Serum IgG antibodies are not protective; the titre correlates with the duration of illness rather than the severity of the disease.

Trophozoites produce characteristic ulcerative lesions and profuse bloody diarrhea (described as amoebic dysentery). Males and females are affected equally with a ratio of 1:1.

Pathology (Amoebic ulcer)

The classical ulcer is **flask-shaped** (broad base with a narrow neck).

- Amoebic ulcers most often develop in cecum; other areas being appendix, sigmoidorectal area and rarely throughout the colon, (affecting flexure regions of colon)
- Ulcers are usually scattered with intervening normal mucosa
- It may be superficial (confined to muscularis mucosa and heal without scar) or deep ulcer (beyond muscularis mucosa and heals with scar formation)
- Size ranging from pin head to inches
- Shape round to oval
- Margin ragged and undermined
- Base is formed on muscle coat.

Complications of intestinal amoebiasis (Fig. 3.3)

There are following types of complications:

- **Fulminant amoebic colitis:** Resulting from generalized necrotic involvement of entire large intestine, occurs more commonly in immunocompromised patients and in pregnancy
- **Amoebic appendicitis:** Results when the infection involves appendix
- **Intestinal perforation and amoebic peritonitis:** Occurs when the ulcer progresses beyond the serosa
- **Toxic megacolon and intussusception** (segment of intestine invaginates into the adjoining intestinal lumen, causing bowel obstruction)
- **Amoebiasis cutis or cutaneous amoebiasis:** It is a virulent form of amoebiasis, presents as perianal skin ulcers as extension of amoebic colitis; may also be seen following anal intercourse (males > females)
- **Amoeboma (amoebic granuloma):** A diffuse pseudotumor like mass of granulomatous tissue found in rectosigmoid region
- **Chronic amoebiasis:** It is characterized by thickening, fibrosis, stricture formation with scarring and amoeboma formation.

Pathogenesis of extraintestinal amoebiasis

Following 1–3 months of intestinal amoebiasis, about 2–8% of patients develop extraintestinal amoebiasis.

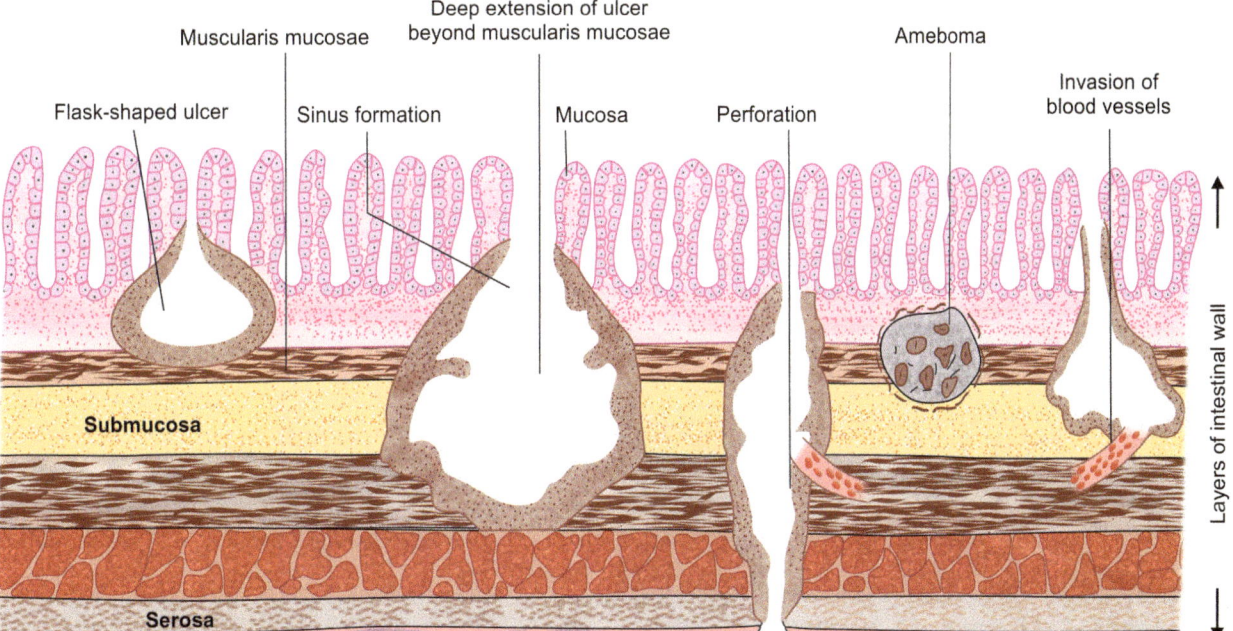

Fig. 3.3: Complications of intestinal amoebiasis (cross-section of intestinal wall)

- Liver is the most common site (because of the carriage of trophozoites through the portal vein) followed by lungs, brain, genitourinary tract and spleen
- Resistance to complement-mediated lysis is a crucial property of *E. histolytica* (lacks in *E. dispar*), critical for its survival in the bloodstream.

Amoebic liver abscess

The most common group affected: Young adult males (male and female ratio is 9:1).

- The most common affected site is the posterior-superior surface of the right lobe of liver. Abscess is usually single or rarely multiple (Fig. 3.4A)
- Amoebic trophozoites occlude the hepatic venules; which leads to anoxic necrosis of the hepatocytes. Inflammatory response surrounding the hepatocytes leads to the formation of abscesses
- Neutrophils recruited to the site are lysed by amoebae, leading to release of mediators that contribute to hepatic necrosis
- Microscopically, the abscess wall is comprised of:
  - Inner central zone of necrotic hepatocytes without amoeba
  - Middle zone of degenerative hepatocytes, RBC, few leukocytes and occasionally amoebic trophozoites
  - Outer zone: comprised of healthy hepatocytes invaded with amoebic trophozoites.
- **Anchovy sauce pus:** Liver abscess pus is thick chocolate brown in color. The fluid is acidic and pH 5.2–6.7 and is comprised of necrotic hepatocytes without any pus cells and occasional amoebic trophozoites (mainly found in last few drops of pus) as amoebae multiply in the wall of abscess (Fig. 3.4B).

Complications of amoebic liver abscess

With continuous hepatic necrosis, abscess may grow in various direction of liver discharging the contents into the neighboring organs.

- Right sided liver abscess may rupture externally to skin causing skin lesions on abdominal wall called as **granuloma cutis (amoebiasis cutis)** or rupture into lungs (pulmonary amoebiasis with trophozoites in sputum) or into the right pleura (**amoebic pleuritis**, the most common complication)
- Rupture of liver abscess below the diaphragm leads to subphrenic abscess and generalized peritonitis
- Left sided liver abscess may rupture into stomach or left pleura or pericardial cavity (**amoebic pericarditis**)
- Hematogenous spread can occur from liver affecting brain (causing brain abscess and secondary amoebic encephalitis), lungs, spleen and genitourinary organs (causing painful genital ulcers).

Clinical Manifestations of Amoebiasis

Asymptomatic amoebiasis

About 90% of infected persons are asymptomatic carriers and excrete cysts in their feces. Now it is confirmed that many of these carriers harbor *E. dispar*.

The remaining 10% of people (who are truly infected by pathogenic *E. histolytica*) produces a spectrum of diseases varying from intestinal amoebiasis to amoebic liver abscess.

Intestinal amoebiasis

Incubation period varies from one to four weeks. Intestinal amoebiasis is characterized by four clinical forms:

1. **Amoebic dysentery:** Symptoms include bloody diarrhea (up to 10 times per day) with mucus and pus cells, colicky abdominal pain, fever, prostration, and weight loss. Amoebic dysentery should be differentiated from bacillary dysentery (Table 3.4)
2. **Amoebic appendicitis:** Presented with acute right lower abdominal pain
3. **Amoeboma:** It presents as palpable abdominal mass
4. **Fulminant colitis:** Presents as intense colicky pain, rectal tenesmus, more than 20 motions/day, fever, nausea, anorexia and hypotension.

Amoebic liver abscess

Presents with tender hepatomegaly and fever (most consistent features) along with weight loss, sweating and weakness, very rarely jaundice, and cough.

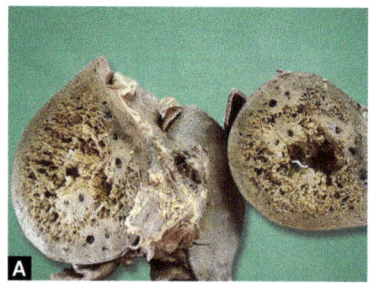
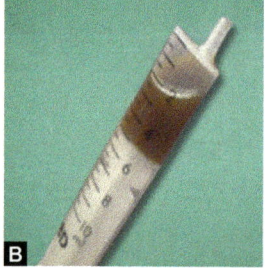

Figs 3.4A and B: (A) Cross section of liver showing amoebic liver abscess (right side); (B) Anchovy sauce pus aspirated from amoebic liver abscess

Source: Head, Department of Pathology, Meenakshi Medical College, Chennai.

Laboratory Diagnosis — **Intestinal amoebiasis**

- **Stool microscopy** by wet mount, permanent stains, etc.—detects cysts (round, 1–4 nuclei) and trophozoites (with finger like pseudopodia)
- **Histology**—intestinal biopsies stained with PAS or H&E stains reveal trophozoites
- **Stool culture**—Polyxenic and axenic culture
- **Stool antigen detection** (copro-antigen)— ELISA (detecting 170-kDa of lectin Ag) and ICT (detecting 29-kDa surface Ag)
- **Serology**
  - Amoebic antigen—ELISA (170-kDa of lectin Ag)
  - Amoebic antibody—IHA, ELISA and IFA
- **Isoenzyme** (zymodeme) analysis
- **Molecular diagnosis**—Nested multiplex PCR and real time PCR (18S rRNA) and Biofire FilmArray

CHAPTER 3 — Amoeba

Laboratory Diagnosis of Intestinal Amoebiasis

Sample collection

Stool is the specimen of choice. Minimum of three stool samples should be collected on alternate day (within 10 days) as amoebae are shed intermittently.

- Other samples include rectal exudates and rectal ulcer tissues collected by colonoscopy
- Stool specimen should be collected in wide mouthed clean container before administration of interfering substances like kaolin, bismuth, barium sulfate, antiamoebic drugs
- It should be examined immediately within 1–2 hours of collection or can be preserved in merthiolate iodine or formalin. However, refrigeration is not recommended.

Stool macroscopy

Stool is foul smelling, copious in amount, dark red in color mixed with blood and mucus and not adherent to the container.

Stool microscopy

Direct examination of stool (from the blood streaked area) by saline and iodine mount is done to demonstrate:

- Trophozoites (Figs 3.5A to D)
- Quadrinucleated cysts (Figs 3.6A to C).

On saline mount, motility of the trophozoites can be appreciated, while iodine mount clearly demonstrates the internal structures of the cyst (Table 3.5).

- Microscopy is poorly sensitive (25–60% with single sample) but the sensitivity increases to ~90% when six stool samples are examined. However due to cost effectiveness, three specimens can be examined
- When the amoeba load in stool is less (as in chronic amoebiasis or convalescent stage), stool samples can be examined after concentration by formalin ether sedimentation method

Table 3.4: Differences in stool characters between amoebic dysentery and bacillary dysentery

Character	Amoebic dysentery	Bacillary dysentery
Pathology		
Ulcer	Deep	Shallow
Margin	Ragged and undermined	Uniform
Intervening mucosa	Normal	Inflamed
Necrosis type	Pyknosis (pyknotic bodies)	Karyolysis (ghost cells)
Cellular response	Mononuclear	Polymorphonuclear
Stool macroscopic feature		
Number of motion	6–10/day	> 10/day
Amount	Copious amount	Small quantity
Color	Dark red	Bright red
Odor	Offensive	Odorless
Reaction	Acidic	Alkaline
Consistency	Not adherent to the container	Adherent to the container
Stool microscopic feature		
Red blood cells (RBCs)	In clumps	Discrete or in rouleaux
Pus cells	Few	Numerous
Macrophages	Few	Numerous*
Eosinophils	Present	Absent or rare
Charcot Leyden crystal	Present	Absent
Pyknotic body**	Present	Absent
Ghost cell	Absent	Present
Organism detected	*E. histolytica* cyst or trophozoite	Bacteria (e.g. *Shigella*)

*Macrophage may contain RBCs, so can be mistaken as trophozoite of *E. histolytica*
**Pyknotic body: nuclear remains of tissue cells and leukocytes

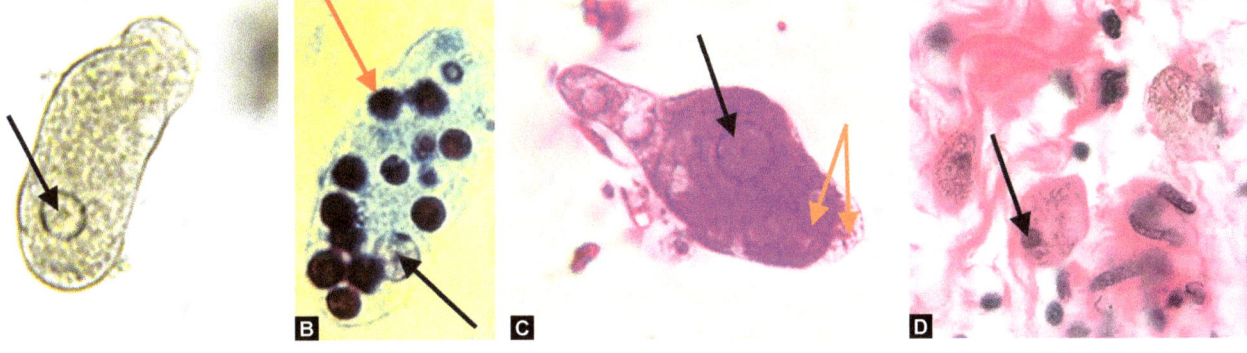

Figs 3.5A to D: *Entamoeba histolytica* trophozoites: (A) Saline mount; (B and C) Trichrome stain, note the single nucleus (black arrow), RBCs (red arrow) and ectoplasm and endoplasm (orange arrows); (D) Trophozoites in colon tissue stained with H&E
Source: Swierczynski G, Milanesi B. Atlas of human intestinal protozoa microscopic diagnosis (*with permission*).

Table 3.5: Trophozoite and cyst of E.histolytica in saline mount and iodine mount

E.histolytica	Saline mount	Iodine mount
Trophozoites	Demonstration of hematophagous trophozoite in freshly-passed stool is considered as **gold standard** microscopic test. • Measures 15–20 µm, actively motile, with finger-like pseudopodia • Presence of ingested RBCs (**erythrophagocytosis**) differentiates it from *E. dispar* • Single nucleus, not visible clearly but a faint outline may be detected	Though trophozoites can be stained, one should not report trophozoite based on iodine mount as iodine kills the trophozoite and motility cannot be appreciated
Cyst	Cyst has a smooth and thin cyst wall. Immature cyst contains round refractile chromatoid bars	**Useful to study the nuclear characteristics** • Cysts appear round, 12–15 µm in size containing 1–4 nuclei • Nucleus has a central karyosome and fine peripheral chromatins lining the nuclear membrane; both appear bright yellow • Cytoplasm appears smooth and hyaline • Glycogen masses stain golden brown • Chromatoid bars are not stained in iodine mount; but stained can be stained with Burrow's stain, Sargeaunt's stain and acridine orange stain

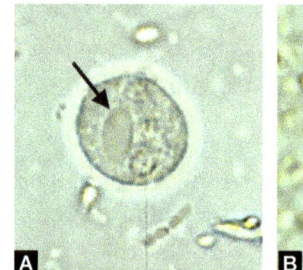
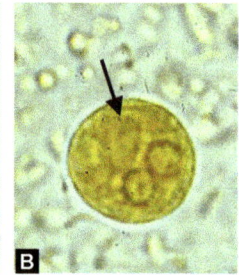
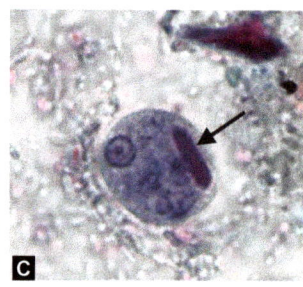
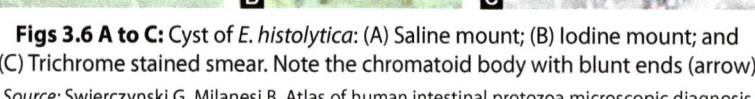

Figs 3.6 A to C: Cyst of *E. histolytica*: (A) Saline mount; (B) Iodine mount; and (C) Trichrome stained smear. Note the chromatoid body with blunt ends (arrow)
Source: Swierczynski G, Milanesi B. Atlas of human intestinal protozoa microscopic diagnosis

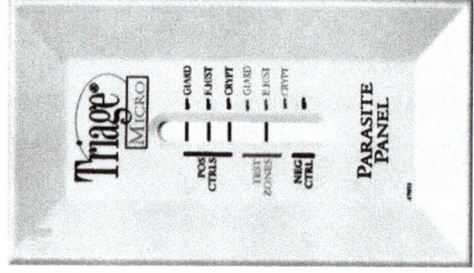

Fig. 3.7: Triage parasite panel, positive for *E. histolytica/E. dispar* antigen
Source: Alere Diagnostics.

- Stool can also be examined by staining with permanent stains like trichrome stain and iron hematoxylin stain. Internal structures of cysts and trophozoites are well demonstrated by permanent stains (Figs 3.5B, C and 3.6C)
- **Reporting:** Cyst and trophozoites of *E. histolytica* are indistinguishable from that of *E. dispar* or *E. moshkovskii* or *E. bangladeshi* except the presence of RBCs in trophozoites of *E. histolytica* (which might not be there after dysentery episode is over). So, the report should always be sent as "cyst or trophozoite of *E. histolytica/dispar/moshkovskii/E. bangladeshi* found in the stool microscopy."

Histology

Trophozoites can be detected in sigmoidoscopy guided biopsies collected from at least six areas of colonic mucosa and stained with PAS or H&E stains or ideally with peroxidase staining with anti-*E. histolytica* antibodies (Fig. 3.5D).

Stool culture

Culture methods are not routinely used for diagnosis. They are useful in research and teaching purpose. Culture methods are discussed in detail in Chapter 15.

Polyxenic culture: Culture media contains bacterial supplement, starch and serum providing nourishment to amoeba.

- Polyxenic media are used for cultivation of amoeba from stool samples of chronic and asymptomatic carriers passing less number of cysts
- Stool culture shows 50–70% sensitivity and 100% specificity
- Various culture media used are:
    - National Institute of Health (NIH) media
    - Boeck and Drbohlav egg serum medium containing Locke's solution
    - Balamuth's medium
    - Nelson's medium
    - Robinson's medium.

Axenic culture: It lacks bacterial supplement, e.g. diamond's medium. Axenic culture is useful when the bacterial flora interferes with the test results such as:
- Studying pathogenicity of amoeba
- Testing antiamoebic drug susceptibility
- Preparation of amoebic antigen in mass for serological tests
- For harvesting the parasite to determine the zymodeme pattern.

Stool antigen detection (coproantigen)

Various tests used to demonstrate amoebic coproantigen in stool are:
- Enzyme-linked immunosorbent assay (ELISA)
- Immunochromatographic test (ICT)

Since, the antigens get denatured by stool preservatives, only fresh or frozen stool sample should be used.
- **ELISA detecting 170 kDa of lectin antigen** (e.g. TechLab *E. histolytica* II, Alere) in stool shows more than 95% sensitivity and specificity. It can also differentiate pathogenic *E. histolytica* (lectin antigen positive) and nonpathogenic *E. dispar* (lectin antigen negative)
- **Immunochromatographic test** is available for the simultaneous detection of antigens specific for *Giardia lamblia* (alpha-1 giardin antigen), *E. histolytica/ E. dispar* (29 kDa surface antigen), and *Cryptosporidium parvum* (protein disulfide isomerase) from stool
  - It is cartridge based, commercially available as the Triage parasite panel (Fig. 3.7)
  - It shows sensitivity (83–96%) and specificity (99–100%).

Serology

Amoebic antigen: Amoebic antigen in serum is found only in patients with active infection and disappears after clinical cure. So its presence in serum indicates recent and active infection.
- ELISA is done using monoclonal antibody specific for 170-kDa of lectin antigen—usually positive in early stage of the disease (sensitivity of 65%)
- ELISA is also available using monoclonal antibody specific for various other antigens like—serine rich *E. histolytica* protein (SREHP), lysine rich surface antigen.

Amoebic antibody: Serum antibodies (IgG) appear only in the later stages of intestinal amoebiasis.
- Various tests include:
  - ELISA
  - Indirect fluorescent antibody (IFA) test
  - Indirect hemagglutination (IHA) test.
- IHA using crude antigens shows 10% sensitivity in asymptomatic cysts passers and 50–60% sensitivity in acute infection. It is less commonly used nowadays.
- ELISA detecting antibody against lectin antigen shows 90% sensitivity in convalescent stage and 75–85% in early stage.

Isoenzyme (zymodeme) analysis

E. histolytica possesses several isoenzymes like malate dehydrogenase, hexokinase, glucophosphate isomerase, and phosphoglucomutase.
- When these isoenzymes are subjected to electrophoresis, based on the electrophoretic mobility of the isoenzymes, 23 zymodeme patterns of *Entamoeba* have been reported, out of which 13 are pathogenic (*E. histolytica*); can be differentiated from the rest (10), which are non-pathogenic (e.g. *E. dispar*)
- However, zymodeme analysis has a number of disadvantages such as: difficulty of performing the test, time-consuming and difficulty in preparing the antigens by culture.

Molecular diagnosis

Molecular methods have emerged as the gold standard diagnosis for amoebiasis.
- Nested multiplex polymerase chain reaction (PCR) is available targeting small subunit rRNA genes that can differentiate *E.histolytica* (439 bp), *E.dispar* (174 bp) and *E.moshkovskii* (553 bp) with a sensitivity nearing 90% and specificity of 90–100%
- Real-time PCR (TaqMan) targeting 18S rRNA gene can be used as an alternative to the conventional PCR. It is more sensitive, quantitates the parasite load and takes less time with less contamination rates
- **BioFire FilmArray:** It is a fully automated commercial PCR system from bioMérieux. Its gastrointestinal panel is used to detect common bacterial, viral, parasitic (*Cryptosporidium, Cyclospora, E. histolytica, Giardia*) diarrheal pathogens.

Imaging method

Colonoscopy can be performed to detect collar button or flask shaped amoebic ulcers.

Other nonspecific findings

- Charcot Leyden crystals in stool: They are diamond-shaped, eosinophilic breakdown products found in stool of some cases
- Moderate leucokytosis in blood.

Laboratory Diagnosis — **Amoebic liver abscess**

- **Microscopy**—detects trophozoites (<25% sensitive)
- **Antigen detection** (in serum, liver pus and saliva)—by ELISA (170–kDA of lectin Ag)
- **Antibody detection**—IHA, IFA, ELISA (Ab to 170-kDA lectin Ag)
- **Molecular diagnosis**—Nested multiplex PCR and real time PCR (detecting 18S rRNA)
- **Ultrasonography**—detects the site of abscess and its extension

Laboratory Diagnosis of Amoebic Liver Abscess

Microscopy

Microscopy of liver pus can detect trophozoites (but never cyst) with less than 25% sensitivity. However, it confirms the diagnosis. Trophozoites may be found only in the last portion of the aspirated material from the abscess wall, not in the necrotic debris obtained from the center of the abscess. Stool microscopy is not useful.

Antigen detection

Lectin antigen is usually absent in stool but can be demonstrated in serum (70% sensitive in late stage, 100% sensitive when tested before treatment), liver pus (100% sensitive when tested before treatment) and saliva (70% sensitive).

Antibody detection

Antibody detection in serum is much more useful in extra-intestinal than intestinal amoebiasis. The currently used methods are ELISA, IHA and IFA.

- However, antibody persists even after the cure, so it cannot differentiate recent and old infection
- IHA (using crude antigenic extract) and IFA with titer of ≥1:256 and 1:200 respectively are considered as significant
- ELISA detecting antibody against 170-kDa lectin antigen is now replacing IHA and has reported sensitivity of 90% and specificity of 85%. ELISA does not give false-negative results and usually becomes negative within 6-12 months of cure, whereas IHA may remain positive for >10 years.

Molecular diagnosis

PCR done on amoebic liver pus approaches sensitivity of 100% and specificity of 90–100%. Nested multiplex PCR and real-time PCR can also be done detecting 18S rRNA.

Imaging methods

Ultrasonography (USG) of liver shows the site of the abscess and its extension. CT and MRI scan can be done alternatively.

Treatment	Amoebiasis
☐ Metronidazole or tinidazole is the drug of choice for intestinal amoebiasis and amoebic liver abscess (Table 3.6) ☐ Other measures include fluid and electrolyte replacement and symptomatic treatment.	

Drug Resistance

- Metronidazole resistance has been reported in *E. histolytica*; mainly in patient with liver abscess. The

Table 3.6: Drug therapy for amebiasis

Class	Agents
Luminal agents	Act on amoeba present in gut lumen. Examples include: • Iodoquinol • Paromomycin • Diloxanide furoate
Tissue agents	Effective on intestinal wall, liver and other tissues. Examples include: • Metronidazole, tinidazole, ornidazole, benzimidazole • Emetine • Chloroquine (hepatic)

Indication	Therapy
Asymptomatic carriage	**Luminal agents:** Iodoquinol (650 mg tid for 20 days) or Paromomycin (500 mg tid for 10 days)
Acute colitis	**Tissue agents:** Metronidazole (750 mg PO or IV tid for 5–10 days) or Tinidazole, 2 g/d PO for 3 days plus **Luminal agents** as above
Amoebic liver abscess	**Tissue agents:** Metronidazole, 750 mg PO or IV for 5–10 days; or Tinidazole, 2 g PO once; or ornidazole, 2 g PO once; plus **Luminal agents** as above

genes involved are *SOD* (superoxide dismutase) gene and *PFOR* (pyruvate ferredoxin oxidoreductase) gene
- Multidrug resistance has also been reported against iodoquinol, diloxanide furoate and emetine; mediated by *EhPgp* gene.

Prevention

Preventive measures are as follows:
- Avoidance of ingestion of food and water contaminated with human feces
- Treatment of asymptomatic persons who pass *E. histolytica* cysts in the stool may help to reduce opportunities for disease transmission.

Vaccination

Till now, there is no effective vaccine licensed for human use. However, colonization blocking vaccines are under trial targeting three *E. histolytica* specific antigens such as: SREHP, 170 kDa subunit of lectin antigen and 29kDa cysteine rich protein.

AMOEBAE MORPHOLOGICALLY RESEMBLING WITH E. HISTOLYTICA

E. dispar, *E. moshkovskii* and *E. bangladeshi* are the amoebae which are morphologically (both cyst and trophozoite) similar to that of *E. histolytica*.

- *E. dispar* is a non-pathogenic commensal in intestine.
- *E. moshkovskii* and *E. bangladeshi* may cause occasionally non-invasive diarrhea in infants.

Entamoeba dispar

- *E. dispar* though morphologically similar to *E. histolytica*, it can be differentiated from the later by:
  - Zymodeme study
  - Molecular methods such as PCR amplifying small subunit rRNA gene)
  - Detection of lectin antigen in stool
  - RBC inside trophozoites—present only in *E. histolytica*.
- It was described by Brumpt in 1993
- It is nonpathogenic, usually colonizes in the large intestine (10 times more than *E. histolytica*) but doesn't invade intestinal mucosa
- It grows well in polyxenic media, however, poorly grows on axenic media
- *E. dispar* does not induce antibody production.

Entamoeba moshkovskii

E. moshkovskii is also morphologically indistinguishable from *E. histolytica* and *E. dispar*.

- This species was first described from Moscow sewage by Tshalaia in 1941
- It can be distinguished from *E. histolytica* by molecular methods such as PCR
- It is primarily a free-living amoeba, found in polluted water. However various studies worldwide have shown that, it is associated with non-invasive diarrhea in infants
- It has been reported from North America, Italy, South Africa, India and Bangladesh.

Entamoeba bangladeshi

E. bangladeshi was first isolated from Mirpur, Bangladesh in 2010-11.

- Human isolates have been recovered from asymptomatic individuals, as well as those with diarrhea
- It is microscopically indistinguishable from *E. histolytica* in cyst and trophozoite stages
- In xenic culture, *E. bangladeshi* is similar to *E. moshkovskii*; has the ability to grow at both 37°C and room temperature, a property which distinguishes it from *E. histolytica* and *E. dispar*, which grow only at 37°C
- Currently, *E. bangladeshi* is only identifiable by PCR targeting small subunit rRNA gene sequence.

NONPATHOGENIC AMOEBAE

Entamoeba coli

E. coli is a nonpathogenic amoeba that colonizes the large intestine.

- The life cycle is similar to *E. histolytica*
- It also has three forms—(1) trophozoites, (2) precyst and (3) cyst (Table 3.7, Figs 3.8 and 3.9)
- It is frequently found in the stool samples of healthy individuals and should be differentiated from that of *E. histolytica* (Table 3.7).

Entamoeba hartmanni

It is also known as small race variant of *E. histolytica*, i.e. morphologically it is similar to *E. histolytica* but of smaller size; trophozoite is 8–10 μm and cyst is 6–8 μm.

Table 3.7: Differences between *Entamoeba histolytica* and *Entamoeba coli*

	Entamoeba histolytica	Entamoeba coli
Trophozoite		
Size	15–20 μm	20–25 μm
Motility	Very active and unidirectional purposeful motility Pseudopodia with finger-like projection	Sluggish, nonpurposeful and aimless motility in any direction Blunt pseudopodia
Cytoplasm	Clearly differentiated to ectoplasm and endoplasm	Not differentiated
Cytoplasmic inclusions	RBC, leukocytes, tissue debris and bacteria	Same except it does not contain RBC
Nucleus	Karyosome is small and central Nuclear membrane is thin and lined by fine chromatin granules	Karyosome is large and eccentric Nuclear membrane is thick and lined by coarse chromatin granules
Precyst		
	10–20 μm size, oval with blunt pseudopodium, no food vacuoles and nucleus same as trophozoite	Same as *E. histolytica* except size is 20 μm
Cyst		
Size	12–15 μm	15–25 μm
Nucleus	Same as trophozoite	Same as trophozoite
Nuclei	1–4 in number	1–8 in number
Chromatoid body	Thick bars with rounded ends	Filamentous and thread like ends

Abbreviation: RBC, red blood cells.

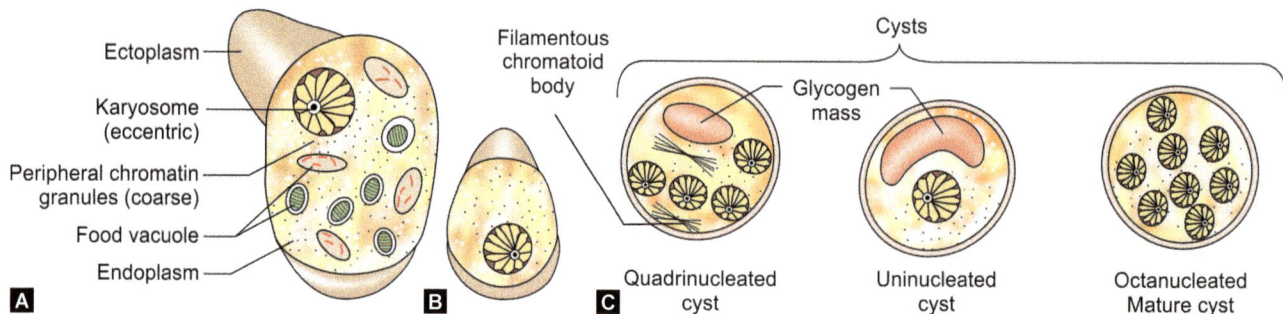

Figs 3.8A to C: *Entamoeba coli* (schematic diagram): (A) Trophozoite, (B) Precyst; and (C) Cyst
Source: Swierczynski G, Milanesi B. Atlas of human intestinal protozoa microscopic diagnosis (*with permission*).

❖ It is nonpathogenic and colonizes the large intestine
❖ Its life cycle is similar to *E. histolytica*.

Entamoeba gingivalis

It is the first parasitic amoeba of humans to be described; recovered from the soft tarter between the teeth.
❖ It is unusual in two respects:
  1. It inhabits in the mouth rather than large intestine
  2. Only trophozoite stage exists; no cystic stage
❖ Trophozoite is similar to that of *E. histolytica* trophozoite except (Figs 3.10A and B):
  ▪ Smaller in size (5–15 μm)
  ▪ Larger food vacuoles containing WBCs (only *Entamoeba* species that contains WBCs)
  ▪ Nucleus similar to that of *E. histolytica*.
❖ It is recovered from:
  ▪ Vaginal secretions of women who use intrauterine devices
  ▪ Oral cavities of patients on radiation therapy and human immunodeficiency virus (HIV) infection
  ▪ Patients with pyorrhea alveolaris.
❖ Though it is considered nonpathogen, but still needs further study to determine its pathogenicity.

Entamoeba polecki

It is a nonpathogenic amoeba usually found in the intestine of pigs and monkeys.
❖ However, human infection is rare, mainly restricted to Papua New Guinea where it is the most common intestinal amoeba in humans
❖ The trophozoites measure 10–12 μm size, motility nonprogressive and sluggish (like *E. coli*) and contain one nucleus having central karyosome and fine peripheral chromatin (like *E. histolytica*)
❖ Cyst is of 5–11 μm size and has one nucleus with features similar to that of trophozoite. It has many chromatoid bodies with thread-like ends (like *E. coli*) and cytoplasm has a large nonglycogen inclusion mass (Figs 3.11A and B).

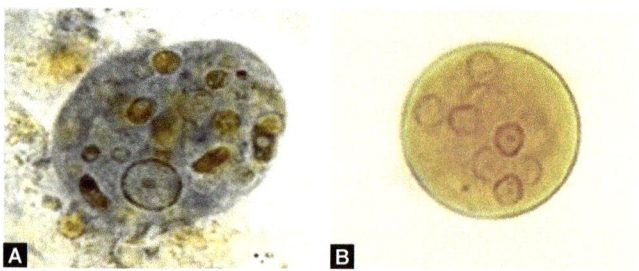

Figs 3.9A and B: *Entamoeba coli*: (A) Trophozoite (iron hematoxylin stain) shows nucleus with coarse peripheral chromatin and abundant food vacuoles in the cytoplasm containing fecal debris; (B) cyst (iodine mount) containing several nuclei
Source: Swierczynski G, Milanesi B. Atlas of human intestinal protozoa microscopic diagnosis (*with permission*).

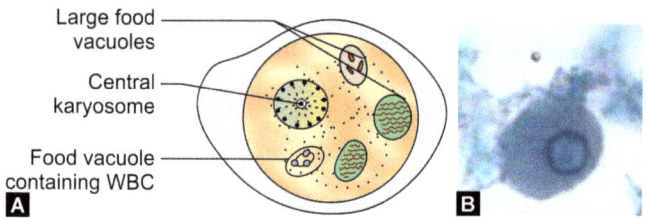

Figs 3.10A and B: Trophozoite of *Entamoeba gingivalis*: (A) schematic diagram; (B) trichrome stain
Source: B—DPDx Image Library, Centers for Disease Control and Prevention (CDC), Atlanta (*with permission*).

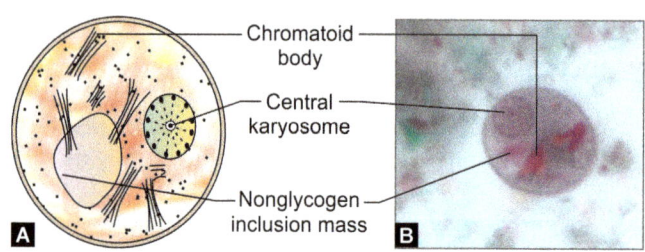

Figs 3.11A and B: *Entamoeba polecki*: (A) Cyst (schematic diagram); (B) Cyst (trichrome stain)
Source: B and C—DPDx Image Library, Center for Disease Control and Prevention (CDC), Atlanta (*with permission*)

Endolimax nana

It is a small (*nana* means small) nonpathogenic amoeba.
- It is worldwide in distribution, frequently resides in the large intestine of humans and other animals
- Trophozoite measures 8–10 µm in size and shows sluggish motility
- Cyst is 6–8 µm in size and contains one to four nuclei. Cytoplasm does not have chromatoid body or glycogen vacuole
- Nucleus (both trophozoite and cyst): Karyosome is eccentric and irregular; from which several achromatic strands extend to the nuclear membrane. There is no peripheral chromatin on nuclear membrane (Figs 3.12A to C).

Iodamoeba butschlii

It is also worldwide in distribution though less common than *E. coli* and *E. nana* (Figs 3.13A to D).
- Trophozoite is 12–15 µm in size. The ectoplasm and endoplasm are not differentiated. Cytoplasm is more vacuolated. Nucleus is similar to that of the cyst
- Cyst measures 10–12 µm in size, round to oval and mostly is uninucleated
  - Nucleus has central karyosome surrounded by refractile chromatin granules (**bull's eye appearance or basket nucleus**). On permanent smear, the nucleus may appear to have a halo surrounding the karyosome
  - Cytoplasm of the cyst contains large iodine stained glycogen mass or iodophilic body (hence named as *Iodamoeba*) and no chromatoid body.

FREE-LIVING AMOEBA

Free-living amoebae are small, freely living, widely distributed in soil and water and can cause opportunistic infections in humans. Among the many genera of free-living amoebae that exist in nature, only four genera have an association with human disease. They are:
1. *Naegleria fowleri* is a causative agent of primary amoebic meningoencephalitis (PAM).
2. *Acanthamoeba* species causes granulomatous amoebic encephalitis (GAE) and amoebic keratitis in contact lens wearers.
3. *Balamuthia mandrillaris* causes GAE.
4. *Sappinia* species: causes encephalitis.

Free-living amoebae differ from intestinal amoebae by:
- Naturally found freely outside the host in the environment (soil and water)
- Possess plenty of mitochondria (intestinal amoebae lack mitochondria)
- Nuclear membrane is distinct, not lined by peripheral chromatin granules and nucleolus is large, deeply stained. (Intestinal amoebae have a delicate nuclear membrane, small pale stained nucleolus)
- Cause opportunistic infection affecting central nervous system (CNS).

Naegleria fowleri

Naegleria is a free-living amoeba, typically found in warm fresh water, such as ponds, lakes, rivers and hot springs. It is also found in soil, near warm-water discharges of industrial plants and swimming pools.
- Only one species, *N. fowleri*, is known to cause infection, although two other species, *N. australiensis* and *N. italica*, can cause infection in mice

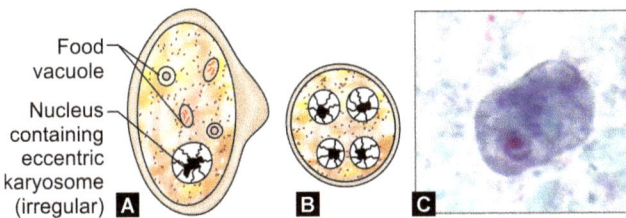

Figs 3.12A to C: *Endolimax nana* (A and B) Trophozoite and cyst (schematic diagram); (C) Trophozoite (trichrome stain)

Source: C—DPDx Image Library, Center for Disease Control and Prevention (CDC), Atlanta (*with permission*).

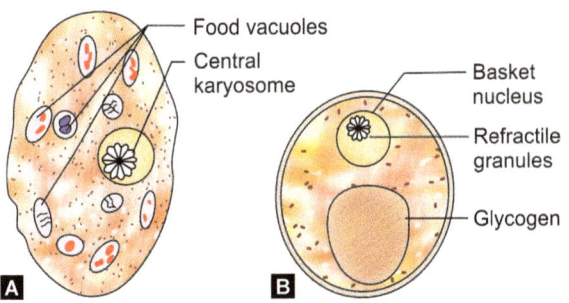 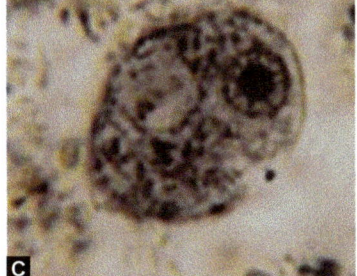 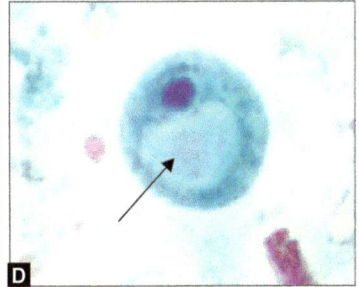

Figs 3.13A to D: *Iodamoeba butschlii:* (A and B) Trophozoite and cyst (schematic diagram); (C) Trophozoite (Iron hematoxylin stain) shows basket nucleus and glycogen vacuole; (D) Cyst (stained)

Source: C—Swierczynski G, Milanesi B—"Atlas of human intestinal protozoa microscopic diagnosis (*with permission*); D—DPDx Image Library, Centers for Disease Control and Prevention (CDC), Atlanta (*with permission*).

- *N. fowleri* (also known as "the brain-eating amoeba") is first described by physicians M. Fowler (hence named as *fowleri*) and R. F. Carter in Australia in 1965.

Morphology

Naegleria fowleri exists in nature as cyst and trophozoite forms (Figs 3.14A to C).

Trophozoite stage

The trophozoites occur in two forms, amoeboid (7–35 μm, average 20 μm) and flagellated form (10–18 μm).

- **Amoeboid form:** It is the only recognizable form in humans. It possesses lobular pseudopodia (called as **lobopodia**). Cytoplasm is granular with food vacuoles; nucleus shows large central karyosome and no peripheral chromatin. It is the only replicating form and it divides by binary fission (Fig. 3.14A)
- **Flagellated form:** When the amoeboid forms are exposed to a change in ionic concentration such as placement in distilled water at 27–37°C, they transform to pear shaped flagellated form that possess two flagella at the broader end. This change occurs very quickly within 20 hours. They show typical jerky or spinning motility. When the flagella are lost, they revert back to amoeboid form (Fig. 3.14B).

Cyst stage

Cysts measure 7–15 μm in size and is surrounded by a thick, smooth double wall. Nucleus is identical to that found in the trophozoite. Cysts are not found in tissue (humans) but can be grown in culture and in nature (Fig. 3.14C and 3.16B).

Life Cycle and Pathogenicity (Fig. 3.15)

Infective form: Amoeboid form is the invasive form and also the usual infective form of the parasite.
Mode of transmission: Man acquires infection by nasal contamination during swimming in fresh hot water bodies like ponds, river, swimming pools or lakes. Rarely, if the flagellated or cyst form enters, soon they revert back to amoeboid form.

- **CNS invasion:** The amoeboid form invades the nasal mucosa, cribriform plate and travels along the olfactory nerve to reach brain. The penetration initially results in significant necrosis and hemorrhages in the nasal mucosa and olfactory bulbs
- The two main mechanisms of pathogenesis are:
  1. Direct ingestion of the brain tissue by producing food cups or **amoebostome** into which the cytopathic enzymes are liberated
  2. Contact dependent cytolysis mediated by hemolytic proteins, cytolysins and phospholipase enzymes.
- Gradually, it produces an acute suppurative meningoencephalitis, known as primary amoebic meningoencephalitis, which becomes hemorrhagic and necrotic later
- Only amoeboid trophozoites are found in cerebrospinal fluid (CSF) and in brain tissue; but not other forms.

Primary Amoebic Meningoencephalitis

N. fowleri causes acute suppurative fulminant infection of CNS known as primary amoebic meningoencephalitis (PAM).

- It is so named because to distinguish it from the secondary invasions of CNS caused by *E. histolytica*
- PAM usually occurs in healthy children or young adults with recent history of swimming in fresh hot water
- **Incubation period:** 1–2 days to 2 weeks after exposure. Clinical course is acute and fulminant
- The initial symptoms include changes in the taste and smell (due to olfactory nerve involvement) followed by headache, anorexia, nausea, vomiting, high fever, and signs of meningeal involvement like stiff neck and a positive Kernig's sign
- Secondary symptoms include confusion, hallucinations, lack of attention, ataxia, and seizures
- The mortality rate is nearly 98%. Death occurs within 7–14 days after exposure.

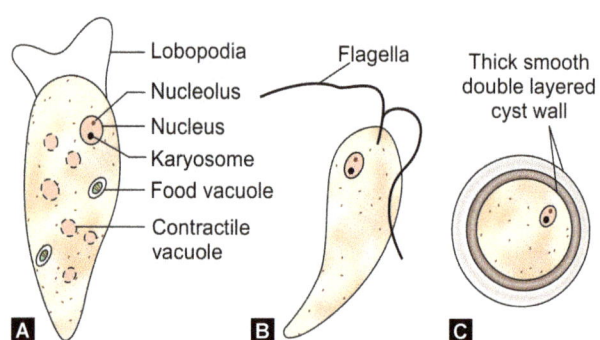

Figs 3.14A to C: *Naegleria fowleri* (schematic diagram): (A) Amoeboid trophozoite; (B) Flagellated trophozoite; (C) Cyst stage

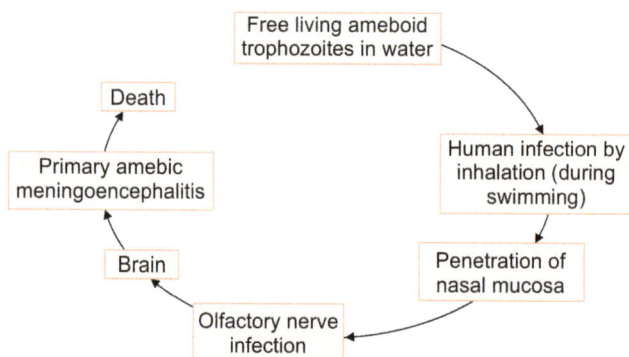

Fig. 3.15: Life cycle of *Naegleria fowleri*

Epidemiology

- The first case was reported from water and soil from Australia and from sewage sludge in India
- Till now more than 300 cases of PAM have been reported mainly from USA (>100 cases) and also from other parts of the world like Czech Republic, Australia, New Zealand and Brazil
- In India, it is reported from Mangalore, Kolkata and Rajasthan (>20 cases reported so far).

> **Laboratory Diagnosis**   *Naegleria fowleri*
>
> - **CSF analysis**—↑neutrophils, proteins, ↑ sugar levels
> - **Microscopy** of CSF—reveals motile amoeboid trophozoite
> - **Histopathology** of brain biopsy tissue—demonstrates trophozoites
> - **Culture** on nonnutrient agar—trail sign observed
> - **Isoenzyme** analysis
> - **Molecular methods**—PCR, multiplex real-time PCR (detecting *Naegleria*, *Acanthamoeba* and *Balamuthia*)
> - **Imaging methods**—CT and MRI

Laboratory Diagnosis

Most cases are diagnosed at autopsy.

Cerebrospinal fluid analysis

CSF is thick purulent, with polymorphonuclear cells more than 20,000/μL, elevated protein and reduced sugar level (mimic bacterial meningitis).

Microscopy

- **Direct microscopy:** Motile amoeboid trophozoites can be demonstrated in wet mount preparation of CSF made with cover slip (counting chamber is not used as trophozites in CSF mimic leukocytes) Other forms are not seen in CSF
- Care should be taken to differentiate the trophozoites from leukocytes. Motile trophozoite containing a spherical nucleus with large karyosome is the clue for identification
- **Phase contrast microscope** yields better result than light microscope
- Refrigeration is not recommended if there is a delay in examining the CSF
- If the parasite load is low then CSF can be centrifuged at low speed (150 g for 5 minutes). Trophozoites won't get damaged, they only lose their pseudopodia
- Trophozoites can also be demonstrated by **direct fluorescence antibody** staining of centrifuged CSF using monoclonal antibody.

Histopathology

Brain biopsied tissue may be stained with Wright's or Giemsa stain to demonstrate trophozoites having sky blue cytoplasm with a pink nucleus (Fig. 3.16A). Other methods used for biopsies include by indirect immunofluorescence and immunoperoxidase.

Culture

CSF sample can be cultivated on **nonnutrient agar (Page's saline and 1.5% agar)**, lawn cultured with bacterial supplement like *E. coli*.

Naegleria feeds on bacteria and crawls over the lawn culture of *E. coli* to produce trails (**Trail sign**).

Enflagellation test

When the scrapping of the nonnutrient agar is transferred to sterile tubes containing distilled water, the amoeboid form undergoes transformation to a pear shaped flagellate form.

Isoenzyme analysis

Isoenzyme analysis has been developed for the specific identification of *N. fowleri* cultured from the CSF and brain specimens of the patients as well as from the environment samples.

Molecular methods

Both conventional PCR and nested PCR assays have been described for the identification of *N. fowleri* targeting specific 5.8s rRNA genes and internal transcribed spacer genes.

A multiplex real-time PCR is available targeting *Acanthamoeba* species, *Balamuthia*, and *N. fowleri*). It is a rapid, sensitive, and specific assay; result can be reported within 4 to 5 hours.

Imaging methods

Computed tomography (CT) scan and magnetic resonance imaging (MRI) show obliteration of cisterns, and diffuse enhancement around midbrain, subarachnoid space and over cerebrum.

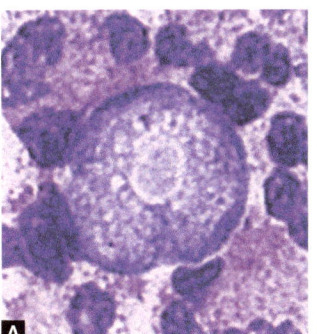 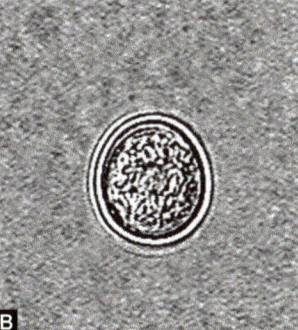

Figs 3.16A and B: *N. fowleri*: (A) Trophozoite in CSF, stained with hematoxylin and eosin (H&E); (B) Cyst grown in culture

Source: DPDx Image Library, Centers for Disease Control and Prevention (CDC), Atlanta (*with permission*).

Treatment	*Naegleria fowleri*
No effective treatment is available for PAM ☐ Amphotericin B has considerable anti-*Naegleria* effect. Four cases were treated successfully with amphotericin B ☐ Other drugs like rifampicin, sulfisoxazole and antifungals like miconazole, fluconazole and miltefosine are also found to be effective.	

Vaccine

Promising vaccine candidate includes *nfa-1* gene which encodes 13 k-Da recombinant protein present on parasite pseduopodia. However, no vaccine has been licensed yet.

Acanthamoeba

Acanthamoeba species is ubiquitous and present worldwide. They have been isolated from soil, fresh and brackish waters.

- Griffin and Sawyer proposed the name in 1975. It is so named because of the spine like pseudopodia present in trophozoite (called as acanthopodia)
- More than 24 species have been identified. Important ones that cause human infection include *Acanthamoeba astronyxis*, *A. castellanii* (type species), *A. culbertsoni* and *A. polyphaga*
- It principally affects CNS, skin and eye
- **Reservoir for bacteria:** Approximately 20–24% of clinical and environmental isolates of *Acanthamoeba* harbor bacterial pathogens such as *Legionella* species *Mycobacterium avium* and *Listeria*, and may serve as a potential reservoir and act as **Trojan horse** of the microbial world.

Morphology

Acanthamoeba species exist in nature as cyst and trophozoite forms. There is no flagellated form (Figs 3.17A and B).

Trophozoite

It is larger than *Naegleria* measuring 25–40 μm size (average 30 μm).

- It bears spine or thorn like pseudopodia (**acanthopodia**)
- Nucleus: Single with central karyosome and no peripheral chromatin

- Organelles of higher eukaryotic cells are present such as Golgi complex, endoplasmic reticulum, ribosomes, mitochondria, etc.

Cyst

It is 10–25 μm, in size and double walled (outer wrinkled ectocyst and inner polyhedral endocyst). The nuclear characteristics are same as trophozoite.

Life Cycle and Pathogenesis (Fig. 3.18)

- **Mode of transmission:** Man acquires infection by inhalation of aerosol contaminated with cyst or trophozoite, or rarely by direct spread through broken skin or infected eye
- Primary sites of infection are sinuses and lungs. From lungs, trophozoites reach CNS by hematogenous route
- It causes **GAE (granulomatous amoebic encephalitis)** in immunocompromised patients like HIV positive patients and **keratitis** in healthy individuals

GAE (granulomatous amoebic encephalitis)

GAE is characterized by:

- **Insidious onset:** Incubation period varies from several weeks to months
- **Subacute to chronic course:** Lasts for months to years
- History of immunosuppression or underlying disease or trauma
- **Pathology:** Focal granulomatous lesions in brain
- **Lymphocytosis** of CSF can be seen. However in patients with AIDS, no cells are seen in CSF
- **Symptoms:** Confusion, dizziness, nausea, headache, stiff neck and sometimes seizure and hemiplegia
- **Epidemiology:** More than 400 cases of GAE due to *Acanthamoeba* have been reported so far, half of those from USA. From India, few cases were reported from Vellore, Chandigarh, Puducherry, Hyderabad and other places.

Amoebic keratitis

Amoebic keratitis is characterized by the following features.

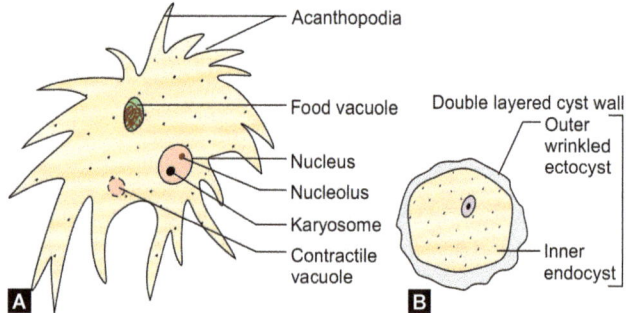

Figs 3.17A and B: *Acanthamoeba* species (schematic diagram): (A) Trophozoite; (B) Cyst

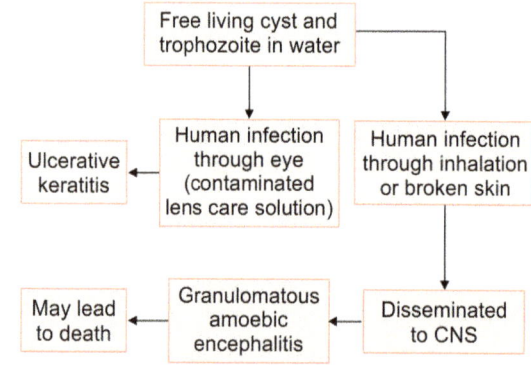

Fig. 3.18: Life cycle of *Acanthamoeba* species
Abbreviation: CNS, central nervous system.

CHAPTER 3 ◆ Amoeba

- **Transmission:** *Acanthamoeba* spreads to cornea either by (i) trauma (onset is rapid) or (ii) contact lens use; especially present in the lens cleaning solution (onset is slow) or (iii) contaminated water (onset is slow)
- **Mechanism of adhesion:** Mannose binding protein on *Acanthamoeba* adheres to glycoprotein receptors on corneal epithelium
- **Manifestations:** Various ocular manifestations can be produced such as ulcerations, iritis, scleritis, hypopyon (pus in anterior chamber), severe pain, and loss of vision
- **From developed countries,** about in 1 to 33 cases of *Acanthamoeba* keratitis occurs per million of contact lens wearers
- **In India,** *Acanthamoeba* accounts for 2% of microbiology-proven cases of keratitis; most of which are associated with contact lens use (80–85%). However, recent data had shown an increase trend of *Acanthamoeba* keratitis in noncontact lens wearers.

In HIV patients

In HIV patients with CD4 T cell <200 /μL, *Acanthamoeba* produces GAE, nasal ulcers, cutaneous ulcers and abscesses, musculoskeletal abscesses.

Laboratory Diagnosis   *Acanthamoeba*

- **Direct microscopy**—Demonstrates both trophozoites (with acanthopodia) and cyst (with outer wrinkled cyst wall)
  - Wet mount examination of CSF or corneal scrapping
  - Permanant staining of brain biopsy
  - Calcofluor stain
- **Culture** on nonnutrient agar with bacterial supplement
- **IFAT** (Indirect fluorescent antibody technique)
- **Molecular methods**—PCR, multiplex real-time PCR (detecting *Naegleria, Acanthamoeba* and *Balamuthia*)
- **CSF examination**—lymphocytosis
- **Imaging method**—CT scan and MRI reveal space occupying ring enhancing lesion.

Laboratory Diagnosis

Direct microscopy

- **Wet mount examination** can be performed on CSF or corneal scraping. Phase contrast microscope gives better results. The following structures can be demonstrated (Fig. 3.19A)
  - Trophozoite is characterized by acanthopodia
  - Cyst has two layers with an outer wrinkled ectocyst; found in corneal scraping, brain biopsy tissues but not in CSF.
- **Permanent staining:** It is done for cytospin cetrifuged CSF and brain biopsy (more reliable than CSF). Hematoxylin and eosin stain, PAS stain are used to visualize characteristic morphology of trophozoite such as prominent nucleolus, contractile vacuole and cytoplasmic vacuole (Fig. 3.19B)
- **Calcofluor stain:** It is recommended to visualize the double walled cyst.

Indirect fluorescent antibody technique

Indirect fluorescent antibody technique (IFAT) with specific antisera can be used for speciation of *Acanthamoeba*. *A. culbertsoni* and *A. castellani* are the most frequently identified species in CSF; whereas *A. polyphaga* and *A. castellanii* from corneal scrapping (Fig. 3.19C).

Culture

Clinical specimens are inoculated onto vaious culture media such as nonnutrient agar with bacterial supplement, tryptic soy agar with 5% horse or rabbit blood, buffer charcoal yeast extract (BCYE) and incubated at 30°C.

- However, unlike *Naegleria*, *Acanthamoeba* is not readily isolated from culture (Table 3.8)
- Bacterial supplement helps in providing nutrition to the parasite. Supplement with most species of live or dead bacteria can be used to recover the trophozoites.

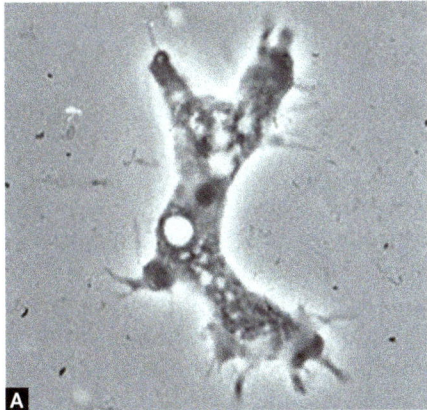
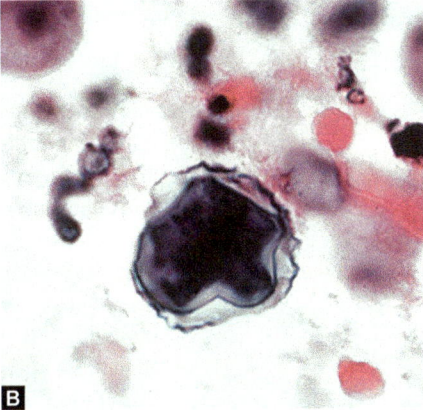
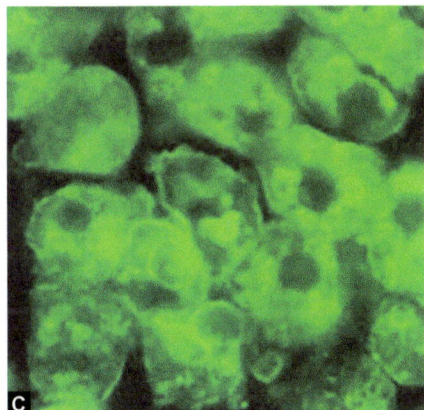

Figs 3.19 A to C: *Acanthamoeba* species: (A) Trophozoite in CSF wet mount; (B) Cyst in brain tissue (hematoxylin and eosin stain); (C) Indirect fluorescent antibody technique of *Acanthamoeba* species viewed under UV microscopy

Source: DPDx Image Library, Centers for Disease Control and Prevention (CDC), Atlanta (*with permission*).

Table 3.8: Differences in the characteristics of *Naegleria* and *Acanthamoeba*

Character	*Naegleria fowleri*	*Acanthamoeba*
Disease	Primary amoebic meningoencephalitis	Granulomatous amoebic encephalitis Ulcerative keratitis, cutaneous lesions, sinusitis
Risk factor	Swimming in contaminated water	Immunodeficiency
Clinical course	Acute	Sub-acute to chronic
Pathology	Diffuse suppurative changes	Focal granulomatous inflammation
Trophozoites	• Two forms, amoeboid and flagellated form • Lobular and blunt pseudopodium (lobopodia) • 8–15 μm size	• One form, no flagellated form • Thorn like pseudopodium (acanthopodia) • 25–40 μm size
Cyst	• Not present in tissue or CSF • Small (7–15 μm), thick and smooth double wall	• Can be found in tissue • Larger (10–25 μm), thin wrinkled double wall
Spread	Direct neural spread	Hematogenous spread
CSF leukocytes	Neutrophils	Lymphocytes
Culture	• Require bacterial supplement • Don't grow with > 0.4% NaCl	• May grow without bacterial supplement • Not affected by NaCl
CT scan	Unremarkable (such as basal arachnoiditis), no specific feature	Space occupying lesion is seen

Abbreviations: CSF, cerebrospinal fluid; NaCl, sodium chloride; CT, computed tomography.

Pseudomonas, *Enterobacter*, or *Stenotrophomonas* give good recovery of cysts
❖ Compared to centrifuation of CSF, parasite detection rate is higher when CSF sample is cultured following filtration through cellulose membrane.

Molecular methods

❖ PCR targeting 18S rRNA gene has been used for investigation of outbreaks and detecting *Acanthamoeba* in reservoirs
❖ A multiplex real-time PCR is available targeting three regions of 18S rRNA of *Acanthamoeba* species, *Balamuthia*, and *N. fowleri* in CSF.

Imaging method

CT scan or MRI reveals space-occupying or ring enhancing lesions in brain.

Treatment	*Acanthamoeba*
Granulomatous amoebic encephalitis ❏ Unfortunately, there are no therapies with proven efficacy against this disease. Only three cases have survived so far ❏ The combination therapy recommended include pentamidine, an azole, sulfonamide (e.g. cotrimoxazole) and possibly flucytosine. **Amoebic keratitis** ❏ Topical antiseptic agents such as a biguanide or chlorhexidine (0.02%) with or without diamidine are used ❏ In early cases confined to epithelium, debridement is sufficient ❏ In severe cases of vision impairment may need penetrating keratoplasty.	

Prevention

Acanthamoeba keratitis can be prevented by: (i) regular cleaning of contact lens case by commercial cleaning solution (avoid homemade saline), (ii) contact lens cases should be allowed to air dry, (iii) changing the case once in 3 month.

Balamuthia mandrillaris

Balamuthia mandrillaris is a free-living, heterotrophic amoeba that also causes GAE.

History

The name goes in the honor of the late Professor William Balamuth and it was first discovered in a pregnant mandrill (an old world monkey) in San Diego in 1986.

Epidemiology

It is distributed in the temperate regions of the world. Till now more than 200 cases have been reported, half of them being from USA and South America. So far, three cases have been reported from India (Delhi and Chandigarh).

Life Cycle

It is similar to *Acanthamoeba*. It has trophozoite and cyst form (no flagellated form).
❖ The trophozoite is approximately 12–60 μm, irregular with extensive branching, single nucleus (occasionally binucleated), centrally located karyosome with no peripheral chromatin (Figs 3.20A and C)
❖ The cyst measures 13–30 μm, surrounded by a three-layered cell wall (outer wrinkled ectocyst, middle mesocyst and inner thin endocyst), and an abnormally large, vesicular nucleus (Figs 3.20B and D).

Clinical Features

It may enter the body through the respiratory tract or through open wounds. In CNS, it causes GAE. It also can

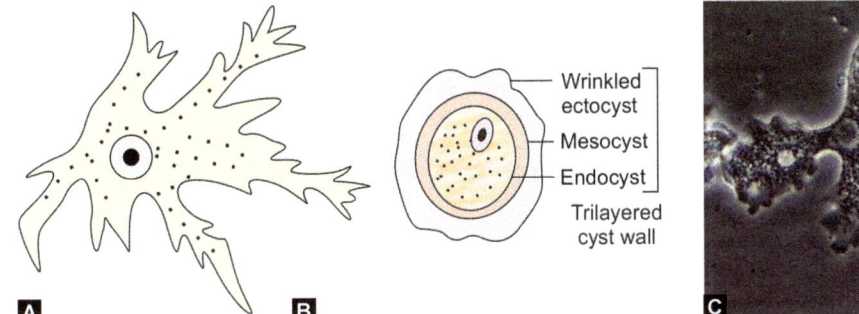
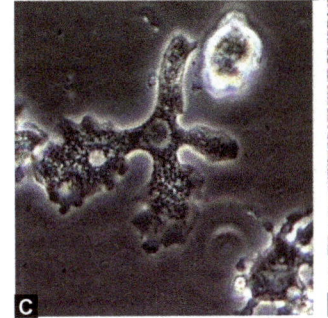
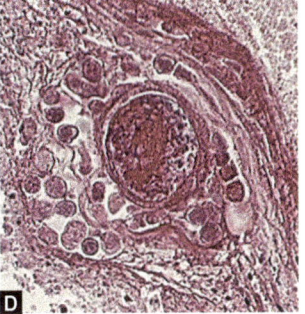

Figs 3.20A to D: *Balamuthia mandrillaris:* (A and B) Trophozoite and cyst (schematic diagram); (C) Trophozoite (saline mount); (D) Cyst (hematoxylin and eosin stain)
Source: C— and D— DPDx Image Library, Centers for Disease Control and Prevention (CDC), Atlanta (*with permission*).

cause skin lesion. Unlike *Acanthamoeba*, *Balamuthia* encephalitis has been found in immunocompetent individuals.

Diagnosis

Microscopy

Both trophozoites and cysts of *Balamuthia* are found in CSF, brain biopsy tissues similar to as seen in *Acanthamoeba* species (Figs 3.20C and D).

Culture

It can be cultured on monkey kidney cell line, MRC, HEp2, Vero and diploid macrophage cell line. It doesn't grow on agar plate culture coated with bacteria.
It can be differentiated from *Acanthamoeba* species by:
- Microscopy: Nucleus contains more than one nucleoli and cyst wall is trilayered
- IFAT using specific antisera
- Culture on cell lines but not in agar plate
- PCR targeting mitochondrial small subunit rRNA gene.

Imaging method

CT scan or MRI reveals space-occupying or ring enhancing lesions in brain.

Treatment	Balamuthia
Multidrug therapy has been recommended. The regimens include some combinations of pentamidine, azithromycin, fluconazole, sulfadiazine, flucytosine, amphotericin, and miltefosine.	

Sappinia

It is a newly recognized pathogenic free-living amoeba found in soil and water.
- Two species have been recognized—*S. diploidea* and *S. pedata*
- One confirmed case of *S. pedata* has been documented so far while the pathogenicity of *S. diploidea* in man is unknown

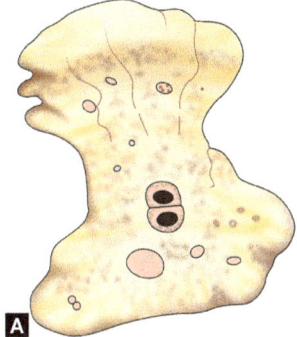
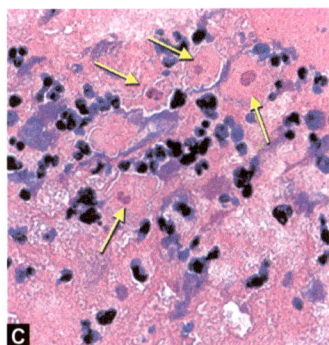

Figs 3.21A and B: *Sappinia pedata:* (A) Trophozoites (schematic); (B) Trophozoites (yellow arrows) in brain tissue, stained with H & E stain
Source: DPDx Image Library, Centers for Disease Control and Prevention (CDC), Atlanta (*with permission*).

- The characteristic feature is both trophozoite and cyst stages are binucleated
- The trophozoite is oval, binucleated (attached), measures 40–70 μm (Fig. 3.21A). The mature cyst is round and measures 15–30 μm, obtained in culture but not found in tissues
- *S. pedata* can be cultivated on nonnutrient agar plate coated with bacteria. Staining of brain biopsy and real-time PCR are the other useful diagnostic tools (Fig. 3.21B).

Other free-living amoebae

There are few other free-living amoebae which have been occasionally associated with human disease include:
- *Vahlkampfia* species, *Hartmannella* species, and *Paravahlkamfia* species have been reported to cause at least one human case of keratitis, often in association with contact lens use or corneal trauma
- *Paravahlkamfia* species has been associated with PAM.

SECTION 2 ◆ Protozoology

EXPECTED QUESTIONS

I. Write essay on:
a. A 17-year-old boy presented with bloody diarrhea with mucus and pus cells, colicky abdominal pain, fever, and prostration. The wet mount examination of the stool sample was performed which showed trophozoites of 5–20 μm, actively motile, with finger-like pseudopodia.
   1. What is the etiological diagnosis?
   2. Write briefly about the life cycle of the etiological agent.
   3. Describe the pathogenesis and clinical manifestations produced.
   4. What are the various diagnostic modalities?
   5. How will you treat this condition?
b. A 42-year-old female patient was brought to the emergency department with complaint of sudden episode of high-grade fever and acute pain in the right hypochondrium. She had a history of dysentery and jaundice for two months Ultrasound scan of the abdomen revealed enlarged liver with acute peritonitis. Pus aspirated from liver was thick chocolate brown in color. Microscopy of liver pus revealed necrotic hepatocytes without any pus cells.
   1. Identify the clinical condition and the most probable causative agent.
   2. What are the various complications seen in this condition?
   3. What are the various diagnostic modalities?
c. List the free-living amoeba. Write in detail about their life cycle, pathogenesis and laboratory diagnosis.

II. Write short notes on:
a. Amoebic liver abscess.
b. *Entamoeba* species morphologically resembling *E. histolytica*.

III. Multiple choice questions (MCQs):
1. What would be the most likely manifestation of extraintestinal amoebiasis?
   a. High periodic fever
   b. Draining skin lesion
   c. Enlarged painful spleen
   d. Tender, enlarged liver
2. A 30-year-old female having habit of keeping her contact lenses in tap water. She noticed deterioration of vision and visited an ophthalmologist who diagnosed her with severe retinitis. Culture of the water as well as vitreous fluid would most likely reveal:
   a. *Naegleria*
   b. *Entamoeba histolytica*
   c. *Acanthamoeba*
   d. *Entamoeba coli*
3. Mature cyst of *Entamoeba histolytica* differs from *Entamoeba coli* by:
   a. Larger and uninucleated
   b. Smaller and binucleated
   c. Smaller and quadrinucleated
   d. Larger and quadrinucleated
4. All nonpathogenic amoebae live in the lumen of large intestine, *except*:
   a. *Entamoeba dispar*
   b. *Entamoeba coli*
   c. *Entamoeba gingivalis*
   d. *Endolimax nana*
5. Lobopodia are seen in trophozoites of:
   a. *Naegleria fowleri*
   b. *Acanthamoeba* species
   c. *Balamuthia mandrillaris*
   d. *Sappinia pedata*
6. *Balamuthia* causes:
   a. Primary amoebic meningoencephalitis
   b. Granulomatous amoebic encephalitis
   c. Keratitis
   d. Liver abscess
7. Infection with *Naegleria* can be acquired by:
   a. Swimming in lakes, ponds or pools containing infective forms
   b. Parenteral route
   c. Orogenital contact
   d. Feco-oral route
8. Which is not a feature of CSF in primary amoebic meningoencephalitis?
   a. Purulent
   b. Lymphocytic leukocytosis
   c. High protein
   d. Low glucose content
9. Cysts of *Entamoeba histolytica* are formed in:
   a. Lumen of the large intestine
   b. Tissues
   c. Lumen of the small intestine
   d. Epithelium of large intestine
10. Infective form and invasive form of *Entamoeba histolytica* are:
    a. Trophozoite and quadrinucleated cyst
    b. Quadrinucleated cyst and trophozoite
    c. Both trophozoite
    d. Both quadrinucleated cyst

Answers
1. d   2. c   3. c   4. c   5. a   6. b   7. a   8. b   9. a   10. b

Flagellates—I (Intestinal and Genital)

CHAPTER 4

CHAPTER OUTLINE
- Classification of flagellates
- *Giardia lamblia*
- *Trichomonas vaginalis*
- Other intestinal flagellates of minor importance

CLASSIFICATION OF FLAGELLATES

This group of parasites bear flagella as the organ of locomotion.
- Flagella are slender, long and thread-like extension of cytoplasm. Its intracellular portion is called as **axoneme**. Flagella arise from kinetoplast (made up of copies of mitochondrial DNA) which in turn consists of:
  - Blepharoplast or basal body or kinetosome from which flagellum arises
  - Parabasal body, through which it passes as axoneme.
- In most of the flagellates, the flagella are external except in *Dientamoeba fragilis* which bears internal flagellum.

Taxonomic Classification
Different flagellates belong to three different phyla (Table 4.1).

Classification Based on Habitat
They are grouped into intestinal, genital and blood flagellates (Table 4.2).

GIARDIA LAMBLIA

History
Giardia lamblia (also called as *G. intestinalis* or *G. duodenalis*) was first observed by AV Leeuwenhoek in 1681 while examining his own stool.

The parasite was described by Dr F Lambl of Prague in 1859 and later was named after him and Professor A Giard of Paris.

Classification
Giardia can be differentiated into various species based on its host.
- *G. lamblia* infects humans and other mammals, *G. muris* in mice, *G. agilis* in amphibians, *G. psittaci* in birds, *G. microti* in voles and *G. ardeae* in herons
- *Giardia* has been classified into two genotypes A and B. Genotype A consists of one assemblage (A) and genotype B comprises of assemblages B to H. Human infections are caused by assemblage A and B. Recently, assemblage E has been associated with human infection.

Epidemiology
G. lamblia is worldwide in distribution, it is considered as one of the most common parasite, causing both endemic and epidemic intestinal disease and diarrhea.
- **Geographical area:** More common in warm climate of tropics and subtropics.
- Assemblage B predominates in most studies from south and southeast Asia including India whereas assemblage A is more common in Africa.

Table 4.1: Taxonomic classification of flagellates

Kingdom	Subkingdom	Phylum	Class	Order	Genus
Protozoa	Archezoa	Metamonada	Trepomonadea	Diplomonadida	Giardia Enteromonas
			Retortamonadea	Retortamonadida	Retortamonas Chilomastix
			Trichomonadea	Trichomonadida	Trichomonas Pentatrichomonas Dientamoeba
	Neozoa	Euglenozoa	Kinetoplastidea	Trypanosomatida	Leishmania Trypanosoma

Table 4.2: Classification of flagellates based on habitat

Intestinal/genital flagellates	Habitat
Giardia lamblia	Duodenum and jejunum
Enteromonas hominis	Large intestine
Retortamonas intestinalis	Large intestine
Chilomastix mesnili	Cecum
Dientamoeba fragilis	Cecum and colon
Trichomonas tenax	Mouth (teeth and gum)
Pentatrichomonas hominis	Ileocecal region
Trichomonas vaginalis	Vagina and urethra
Blood and somatic flagellates	**Habitat**
Leishmania	Blood and tissue
Trypanosoma	Blood and tissue

- **In India:** Prevalence of giardiasis in children ranges from 0.5–70%
- **Zoonotic potential:** *Giardia* has low zoonotic potential although can infect many mammals such as mice, beaver, cattle, dog and cat. Zoonotic water-borne outbreak of giardiasis in humans reported in Canada has been linked to beavers, hence the disease is also called as **beaver fever**.

Habitat

Giardia inhabits in crypts of duodenum and upper part of jejunum in man.

Morphology

It occurs in two forms—(1) trophozoite and (2) cyst (Fig. 4.1).

Trophozoite

The trophozoite has a falling leaf-like motility, usually measures 10–20 µm in length and 5–15 µm in width.
- *Shape*:
  - In front view, it is pear shaped (or tear drop or tennis racket shaped) with rounded anterior end and pointed posterior end
  - Laterally, it appears as a curved portion of a spoon (sickle shaped).
- It is convex dorsally while the ventral surface has a concavity bearing a bilobed adhesive disk. Hence, it appears as sickle shaped in lateral view (FIgs 4.1B and 4.4C)
- Trophozoite is bilaterally symmetrical; bears the following structures. (Figs 4.1A and B):
  - One pair of nuclei
  - Pair of median body
  - Four pairs of basal body or blepharoplast (from which the axoneme arises)
  - Four pairs of flagella—two lateral, one ventral and one caudal pair of flagella
  - Pair of parabasal body (connected to basal bodies through which the axoneme passes)
  - Pair of axonemes (the intracellular portion of the flagella).

Cyst

Giardia cyst is oval shaped, measures 11–14 µm in length and 7–10 µm in width.
- It contains four nuclei, axonemes, and median bodies (Fig. 4.1C)
- It is the infective form as well as the diagnostic form of the parasite.

Life Cycle (Fig. 4.2)

Host: *Giardia* completes its life cycle in one host.
Infective form: Cysts are the infective form.
Mode of transmission: Man acquires infection by ingestion of food and water contaminated with mature cysts or rarely by sexual route (mainly in homosexuals).

Development in Man

- **Excystation:** Two trophozoites are released from each cyst in the duodenum within 30 minutes of entry
- **Multiplication:** Trophozoites multiply by longitudinal binary fission in the duodenum
- **Adhesion:** Trophozoites adhere to the duodenal mucosa by the bilobed adhesive ventral disk
  This is achieved by the microtubules of median bodies, contractile proteins and lectins present on the surface

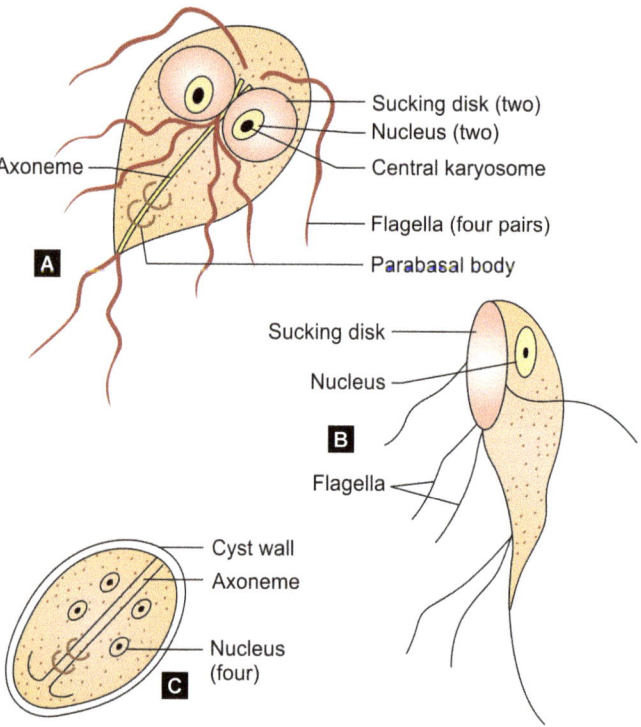

Figs 4.1A to C: *Giardia lamblia* (schematic diagram): (A) Trophozoite front view; (B) Trophozoite lateral view; (C) cyst

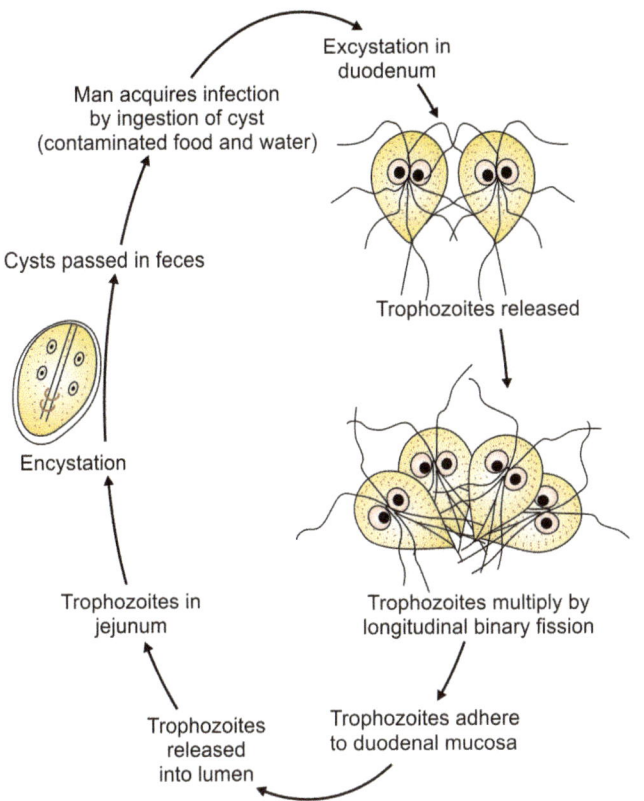

Fig. 4.2: Life cycle of *Giardia lamblia*

of adhesive disk that bind to the intestinal receptors (sugar molecules)
- In active stage of the disease, the trophozoites are excreted in diarrheic stool due to sloughing of intestinal epithelial cells every 72 hours
- **Encystation:** Gradually when the trophozoites pass down to jejunum, encystation begins
  - Promoting factors for encystation are the conjugated bile salts, alkaline pH and cholesterol starvation. DNA topoisomerase II and glucosylceramide transferase activity of the parasite are critical for encystation
  - Encystation begins with retraction of the flagella into axoneme followed by condensation of the cytoplasm and finally formation of the cyst wall
  - **Encystation specific vesicles (ESV)** appear in the cytoplasm that helps in processing and transportation of the cyst wall protein antigens to the exterior of the plasma membrane to synthesize the cyst wall
  - On maturation, nuclei divide to become four. The cysts excreted in feces can survive in the environment and are infective to man.

Pathogenicity

- **Infective dose:** As few as 10–25 cysts can initiate the infection
- **Risk factors:** Children are more commonly affected. Other high-risk groups are elderly debilitated persons and patients with cystic fibrosis, poor hygiene, reduced gastric acidity, prior gastric surgery, and immunodeficiency syndromes such as common variable immunodeficiency and in children with X-linked agammaglobulinemia. However, it does not appear to be associated with HIV/AIDS
- **Human milk and giardiasis:** Human milk appears to be protective against giardiasis as it contains free fatty acid (cytotoxic to trophozoites) and anti-*Giardia* antibodies
- **Several pathogenic mechanisms** have been postulated that include:
  - Trophozoites adhere to the duodenal mucosa and cause disruption of the intestinal epithelial brush border causing villous atrophy that leads to increase permeability and malabsorption. Trophozoites do not invade mucosa, but feed on mucus secretions
  - Very rarely, elaboration of enterotoxin such as cysteine rich surface protein 136 (CRP-136).
- **Malabsorption:** This could be of various types such as:
  - Malabsorption of fat (steatorrhea)— leads to foul smelling profuse frothy diarrhea
  - Disaccharidase deficiencies (lactose, xylose)— leading to lactose intolerance
  - Malabsorption of vitamin A, B12 and iron
  - Protein loosing enteropathy.
- **Antigenic variation:**
  - *Giardia* undergoes frequent antigenic variations due to a cysteine rich protein on its surface called **variant surface protein (VSP)**
  - This helps the parasite in evasion of the host immune system and makes it resistant to intestinal proteases which inturn leads to persistence of infection resulting in chronic and recurrent illness.

Clinical Features

Clinical course of giardiasis can be divided into three stages:
1. **Asymptomatic carriers:** Most infected persons are asymptomatic, harboring the cysts and spreading the infection.
2. **Acute giardiasis:**
   - Incubation period varies from 1 week to 3 weeks (average 12–20 days). Symptoms may develop suddenly or gradually
   - Common symptoms include diarrhea, abdominal pain, bloating, belching, flatus and vomiting
   - Diarrhea is often foul smelling with fat, cellular exudate and mucus but no blood
   - The acute stage lasts for 1 week but usually resolves spontaneously. Very rarely, in some children may last for months
   - *Giardia* is an important cause of traveler's diarrhea.

3. **Chronic giardiasis:**
   - It may present with or without a previous acute symptomatic episode
   - Symptoms are intermittent and recurring
   - Common symptoms include recurrent episodes of foul smelling diarrhea, foul flatus, sulfurous belching with rotten egg taste, and profound weight loss leading to growth retardation
   - Extraintestinal manifestations have been described, such as urticaria, anterior uveitis, salt and pepper retinal changes and arthritis.

Laboratory Diagnosis — *Giardia lamblia*

- **Stool examination** (saline mount)—detects
  - Cysts (oval, 4 nuclei)—indicates carrier/active stage
  - Trophozoites (pear shaped, falling leaf motility)—indicates active infection
  - Other methods—iodine mount, trichrome stain, DFA
- **Entero-test**—duodenal sampling, with the help of gelatin capsule attached to a thread
- **Antigen detection** in stool (coproantigen)—ELISA, ICT (Triage Parasite Panel)
- **Antibody detection** in serum—ELISA, IFA
- **Culture**—for research purpose, not for diagnostics
- **Molecular method**—PCR, BioFire FilmArray, genotyping
- **Radiological findings**—barium meal X-ray.

Laboratory Diagnosis

Stool Examination

Stool microscopy is considered as gold standard for diagnosis of giardiasis.
- *Giardia* cysts can be demonstrated by iodine and saline wet mount preparations but they cannot differentiate active disease from carriers (Figs 4.3A and B)
- Demonstration of the trophozoites with falling leaf like motility by saline mount indicates active stage of the disease (Fig. 4.4A)
- Trophozoites adheres firmly to the duodenal mucosa by adhesive disk leading to intermittent shedding. Hence, repeated stool examination (at least three samples collected on alternate days within 10 days) should be done
- Pus cells or blood (RBCs) will never be seen in stool microscopy in case of giardiasis. If found; suggests alternate diagnosis
- Sensitivity varies from 60% to 80% with one stool and more than 90% after three stools examination
- **Concentration techniques** like zinc sulfate floatation or formalin ether sedimentation methods are employed to increase the chance of detection
- **Duodenal sampling:** If stool examination is negative, then direct duodenal samples like aspirates (obtained by entero-test) or biopsy (done by endoscopy) should be processed
- Permanent stains such as trichrome stain can be used to demonstrate cysts and trophozoites in stool (Figs 4.3C and 4.4B)

Entero-test (or String Test)

It uses a gelatin capsule attached to a thread containing a weight (Fig. 4.5).
- One end of the thread is attached to the outer aspect of the patient's cheek, and then, the capsule is swallowed
- Capsule gets dissolved in stomach releasing the thread which is carried to the duodenum by peristalsis and due to the weight attached to the thread. The thread gets unfolded and takes up duodenal samples
- Four hours later, the thread is withdrawn and shaken in saline to release trophozoites which can be detected microscopically by wet mount or permanent stained smear
- The accuracy of the sample collection from duodenum can be determined by—(i) pH of end of the thread (very low pH indicates that it is in stomach), (ii) end of the thread should be yellow-green in color; indicating that it is bile-stained, hence was in the duodenum
- The entero-test is also useful in the search for other upper intestinal parasites such as *Strongyloides Cryptosporidium* and *Clonorchis*.

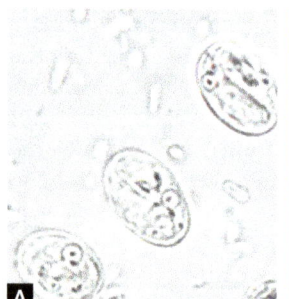 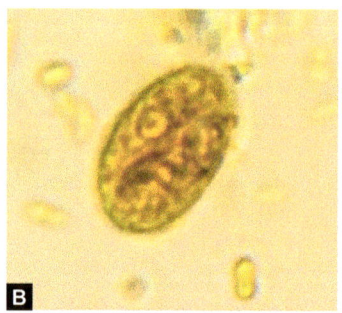 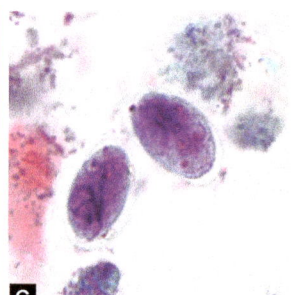 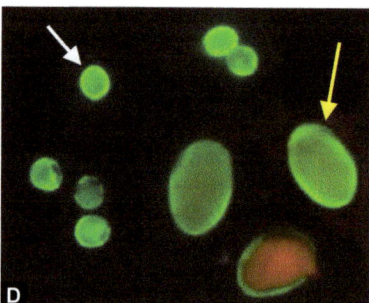

Figs 4.3A to D: Cysts of *Giardia lamblia:* (A) Saline mount; (B) Iodine mount; (C) Trichrome stain; (D) Direct immunofluorescence assay (yellow arrow indicates *Giardia* cyst and white arrow indicate oocyst of *Cryptosporidium*)

Source: A— and B— Giovanni Swierczynski, Bruno Milanesi "Atlas of human intestinal protozoa Microscopic diagnosis" (*with permission*); C and D— DPDx Image Library, Centers for Disease Control and Prevention (CDC), Atlanta (*with permission*).

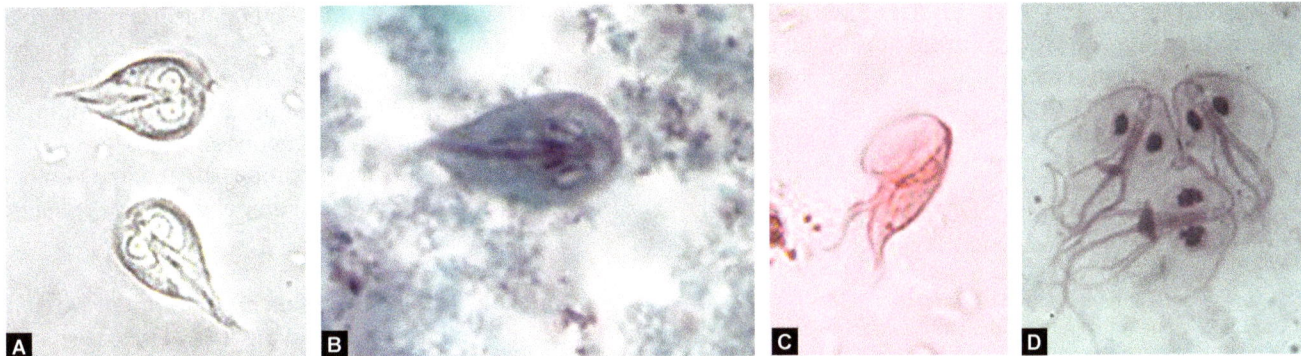

Figs 4.4A to D: Trophozoites of *Giardia lamblia* (A) Saline mount front view; (B) Trichrome stain front view; (C) Merthiolate iodine formalin (MIF) stain lateral view (spoon shaped); (D) Giemsa stained mucosal imprint (front view)
Source: A to C— Giovanni Swierczynski, Bruno Milanesi. "Atlas of human intestinal protozoa Microscopic diagnosis" (*with permission*); D— DPDx Image Library, Centers for Disease Control and Prevention (CDC), Atlanta (*with permission*).

Histopathology

Endoscopy-guided duodenal biopsy tissue can be processed by touch preparation and stained by Giemsa stain to demonstrate the trophozoites (Fig. 4.4D).

Antigen Detection in Stool (Coproantigen)

The enzyme-linked inmunosorbent assay (ELISA) and direct fluorescent antibody tests (DFA, Fig. 4.3D) are available using labeled monoclonal antibodies against cyst wall protein antigens. Both the tests are highly sensitive (90–100%) and specific (99–100%). They are very useful in microscopy negative samples and also in outbreak situations.

Rapid **immunochromatographic test** (commercial name **triage parasite panel**) has been developed that simultaneously detect antigens of *Giardia* (alpha-1 giardin antigen), *Entamoeba histolytica* and *Cryptosporidium* with comparable sensitivity and specificity like ELISA. It is simple, easy to perform, does not require any costly instrument and can be done at peripheral laboratory.

Antibody Detection

Both indirect fluorescent antibody (IFA) and ELISA formats are developed to detect antibodies in serum.
- But unlike microscopy and antigen detection, presence of antibody cannot differentiate recent and past infection
- Hence, serology is only helpful for epidemiological purpose for estimating the prevalence of infection.

Culture

Giardia can be cultivated in axenic media like Diamond's media used for *E. histolytica*. Culture is done for research purpose and to prepare the antigens.

Molecular Methods

Detection of *Giardia* nucleic acid in stool and environmental samples (water) by polymerase chain reaction (PCR) or by gene probes is highly sensitive and specific. PCR can detect as low as 1–2 cyst(s) in sample.
- **BioFire FilmArray**: It is a fully automated commercial PCR system from bioMérieux. The gastrointestinal panel is used to detect common bacterial, viral, parasitic (*Cryptosporidium, Cyclospora, E. histolytica, Giardia*) diarrheal pathogens
- **Molecular typing** (to detect genotype and assemblages) is done by sequencing several genes, such as the glutamate dehydrogenase (*gdh*), β-giardin (*bg*), and triosephosphate isomerase (*tpi*).

Radiological Finding

- Fluoroscopy may reveal hypermotility at the duodenal and jejunal levels
- X-ray after barium meal may reveal non-specific irregular mucosal thickening with large dilated loops of hypotonic bowel (positive in 20% of cases)

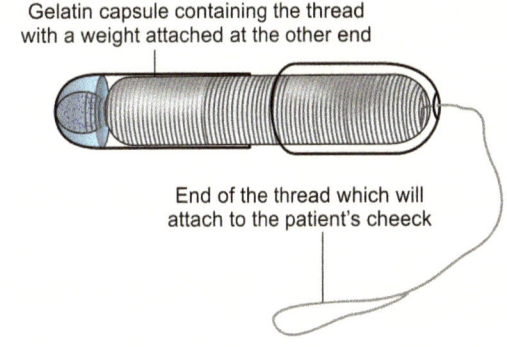

Fig. 4.5: Entero-test equipment showing duodenal capsule attached with thread at other end

- Barium meal may also interfere with the stool examination. So, stool samples should be collected before the barium meal.

Treatment	*Giardia lamblia*
☐ Metronidazole (250 mg thrice daily for 5 days) is usually effective in more than 90% of cases of giardiasis ☐ Tinidazole (2 g once orally) is more effective than metronidazole; considered as the drug of choice ☐ Nitazoxanide (500 mg twice daily for 3 days) is an alternative agent for treatment of giardiasis ☐ Furazolidone is given to children and auranofin, paromomycin can be given in pregnancy ☐ In patients with AIDS and hypogammaglobulinemia, giardiasis is often refractory to treatment. Prolonged therapy with metronidazole (750 mg thrice daily for 21 days) has been successful ☐ Wheat germ agglutinin supplemented diet, albendazole and auranofin can be used for treatment of giardiasis in future; needs further research ☐ Metronidazole resistance has been reported in *Giardia*; linked to pyruvate ferredoxin oxidoreductase (PFOR) gene. Auranofin is shown to be effective against metronidazole-resistant strains of *Giardia*. Cysts are more resistant to metronidazole than trophozoites.	

Prevention

Giardiasis can be prevented by:
- Improved food and personal hygiene
- Boiling or filtering of potentially contaminated water
- Treatment of asymptomatic carriers
- No vaccine is currently available.

TRICHOMONAS

Trichomonas differ from other flagellates as they lack the cyst stage. They exist as only trophozoites although pseudocyst stage may be seen.
- *Trichomonas* belongs to:
  - Class: Trichomonadea
  - Order: Trichomonadida
  - Family: Trichomonadidae.
- Three species of *Trichomonas* are found in man
  1. *Trichomonas vaginalis* is the only pathogen. It resides in the genital tract
  2. *Pentatrichomonas hominis:* Nonpathogen, resides in large intestine
  3. *Trichomonas tenax:* Nonpathogen, resides in mouth (teeth and gum).

TRICHOMONAS VAGINALIS

It is the most common parasitic cause of sexually transmitted infection (STI).
- Females are commonly affected than males
- It was first observed by Donne in 1836 from the purulent genital discharge of a female
- Though it is an eukaryote, its metabolism is similar to a primitive anaerobic bacteria
- Carbohydrate is utilized fermentatively. It is unable to synthesize fatty acid, sterols, purines and pyrimidines and hence depends on exogenous sources
- *T. vaginalis* has the largest protozoan genome known, having six chromosomes encoding about 60,000 proteins.

Habitat

The trophozoites reside in vagina and urethra of women and urethra, seminal vesicle and prostate of men.

Morphology

T. vaginalis exists as trophozoite (flagellate and ameboid form) and the pseudocystic stages. There is no cystic stage.

Trophozoite (flagellated form)

It is pear (pyriform) shaped, measures 7–23 µm and 5–15 µm wide (Fig. 4.6).
- It shows characteristic jerky or twitching motility in saline mount preparation
- It bears five flagella—four anterior flagella and one lateral flagellum called as **recurrent flagellum** as it curves back on the surface of the parasite and traverses as undulating membrane and stops halfway down the side of the trophozoite. It does not come out free posteriorly
- The undulating membrane is supported on to the surface of the parasite by a rod like structure called as **costa**
- The axostyle runs down the middle of the trophozoite and ends in the pointed end of the posterior pole
- It has a single nucleus containing central karyosome with evenly distributed nuclear chromatin and the cytoplasm contains a number of siderophore granules along the axostyle
- The respiratory organelle is called as **hydrogenosome;** which performs respiration through anaerobic

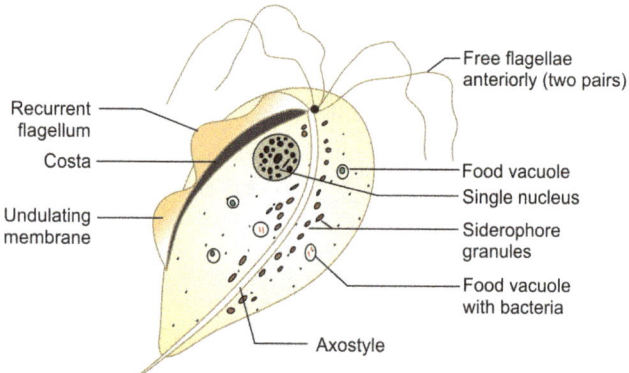

Fig. 4.6: Trophozoite (flagellated) of *Trichomonas vaginalis* (schematic diagram)

fermentation. It differs from mitochondria of higher eukaryotes in lacking cytochromes and respiratory chain enzymes.

Amoeboid Trophozoite

It differs from flagellated form by its variable shape and expressing pseudopodia; but the flagella still remains visible. It is actively replicating, found in the tissue feeding stage of the life cycle.

Pseudocyst

It is round in shape, non-motile, does not possess flagella. There is no true cyst wall. It is recovered in culture, but not during the clinical phase.

Life Cycle

Flagellated trophozoites are the infective stage as well as the diagnostic stage.

- **Transmission:** Asymptomatic females are the reservoir of infection and transmit the disease by sexual route. Though rare, but evidence of non-sexual transmission via fomites and possibly through water has been described
- On exposure to oxygen, the anaerobic flagellated trophozoites undergo cytoskeletal rearrangement and transform into tissue-feeding and actively dividing ameboid trophozoites
- The amoeboid trophozoites divide by longitudinal binary fission and infect urogenital tract
- They again transform back to flagellated trophozoites, which infect other individuals.

Pathogenicity

Trichomoniasis is the most common parasitic cause of sexually transmitted infection (STI).

- It is worldwide in distribution and accounts for 10% of cases of vulvovaginitis
- **Virulence factors:** Pathogenesis is attributed to both virulence factors of the parasite and the environmental factors (Table 4.3)
- Incubation period is variable (4–28 days).

Clinical Feature

The clinical spectrum varies from asymptomatic infection, acute and chronic infection.

- **Asymptomatic infection:** 25–50% of individuals are asymptomatic, harboring the trophozoites and can transmit the infection. One-third of them may become symptomatic within 6 months
- **Acute infection (vulvovaginitis):** Females are commonly affected and are presented as vulvovaginitis, characterized by thin profuse foul smelling purulent vaginal discharge. Discharge may be frothy (10% of cases) and yellowish green color mixed with a number of polymorphonuclear leukocytes
    - Strawberry appearance of vaginal mucosa (**Colpitis macularis**) is observed in 2% of patients. It is characterized by small punctate hemorrhagic spots on vaginal and cervical mucosa
    - Other features include dysuria and lower abdominal pain
    - In males, the common features are nongonococcal urethritis and rarely epididymitis, prostatitis and penile ulcerations
    - Detection of *T. vaginalis* in urine of children raises the suspicion of child abuse or it may be due to possible fecal contamination of urine with *Pentatrichomonas hominis*, which is misidentified as *T. vaginalis*.
- **Chronic infection:** In chronic stage, the disease is mild with pruritus and pain during coitus. Vaginal discharge is scanty, mixed with mucus
- **Complications:** Rarely, it is associated with complications like pyosalpinx, endometritis, infertility, low birth weight and cervical erosions

Table 4.3: Virulence factors of *T. vaginalis* and environmental factors that contribute to pathogenesis

Virulence factors	Role in pathogenesis
Adhesin proteins	Helps in attachment to vaginal epithelium (laminin)
Cysteine proteinases	Degrades IgG, IgA and complements
Cell detaching factor	Causes cytopathic effects in cell culture Associated with severity of clinical illness
Immune system evasion by:	1. Coating the surface with host proteins 2. Epitope phenotypic variation 3. Shedding of immunogenic soluble antigens that neutralize antibodies
Environmental factors	**Role in pathogenesis**
Iron and dsRNA viruses*	Both up regulate virulence
Vaginal pH	Vaginal pH > 4.5 facilitates infection
Vaginal flora	Increased vaginal pH causes concomitant reduction of protective lactobacilli

* Note: *T. vaginalis* can be divided into type 1 and 2, which differ significantly with respect to harboring dsRNA viruses, pathogenesis and susceptibility to metronidazole. Type II parasites usually possess dsRNA viruses which may be associated with higher virulence of the parasite and lower resistance to metronidazole.

Laboratory Diagnosis	Trichomonas vaginalis

- Direct microscopy—detects trophozoites (pears shaped, jerky motility)
  - Wet saline mount
  - Permanent stain
  - Acridine orange fluorescent stain
  - Direct fluorescent antibody test
- Culture (e.g. InPouch TV)— gold standard method
- Antigen detection in vaginal secretion—ELISA, ICT, etc.
- Antibody detection—ELISA using whole cell antigen
- Molecular method—PCR detecting beta tubulin genes
- Other supportive test: Raised vaginal pH, Whiff test

- There is also an association of increased HIV and herpes simplex virus-2 transmission (and vice-versa) and cervical dysplasia
- Respiratory distress may be seen in few cases.

Laboratory Diagnosis

Direct Microscopy

- **Samples:** Vaginal, urethral discharge, urine sediment and prostatic secretions can be examined
- **Wet (saline) mount** of fresh samples (within 10-20 minutes of collection) should be done to demonstrate the jerky motile trophozoites and pus cells. Its sensitivity is variable (40-80%) and specificity is up to 100%
- **Permanent stain:** Giemsa stain and Papanicolaou stain are routinely performed to demonstrate the morphology of trophozoites. Permanent stain is preferred for use if the smear is dry. (Fig. 4.7)
- **Acridine orange fluorescent stain** can be used. It is rapid and sensitive; comparable to wet mount
- **Direct fluorescent antibody test (DFA):** Trophozoites are detected by staining with fluorescent labeled monoclonal antibodies. DFA test is more sensitive (70-90%) than wet-mount examination.

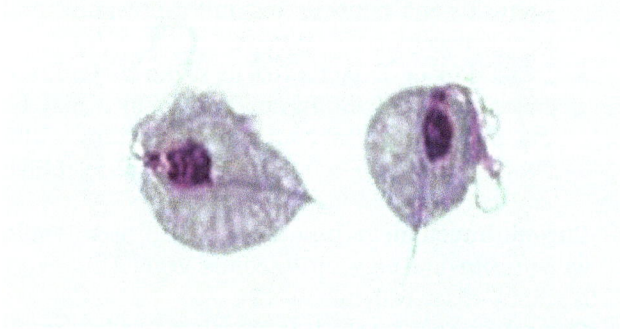

Fig. 4.7: *Trichomonas vaginalis* trophozoite (Giemsa stain)
Source: DPDx Image Library, Centers for Disease Control and prevention (CDC), Atlanta *(with permission)*.

Culture

Culture is the gold standard method for diagnosis. It is highly sensitive 75-96% and specific (100%). It is positive even in microscopy negative samples.

- Specimen should be collected properly and processed immediately (preferably bedside)
- Cultures should be incubated for 3-7 days or longer, followed by mounting of the culture to demonstrate the trophozoites
- If facilities are available, special container like **"InPouch TV"** can be used. It contains a specimen transport container, growth chamber for incubation and a slide for mounting. This is the gold standard culture method. It has sensitivity of 81-94 % and specificity 100% (Fig. 4.8)
- Various culture media can be used like:
  - Lash's cysteine hydrolysate serum media
  - Diamond's trypticase yeast maltose media
  - Cysteine peptone liver maltose media
  - Cell lines like McCoy cell line are highly sensitive, which can detect as low as three trophozoites/mL
  - Modified Columbia agar.

Antigen Detection in Vaginal Secretion

Antigen detection methods are more sensitive than microscopy, easy to perform and indicates recent infection.

- A rapid immunochromatographic test (ICT) (OSOM *Trichomonas* Rapid Test) is available; which shows result within 10 minutes, requires no sophisticated instruments. Compared to culture, it is 83% sensitive

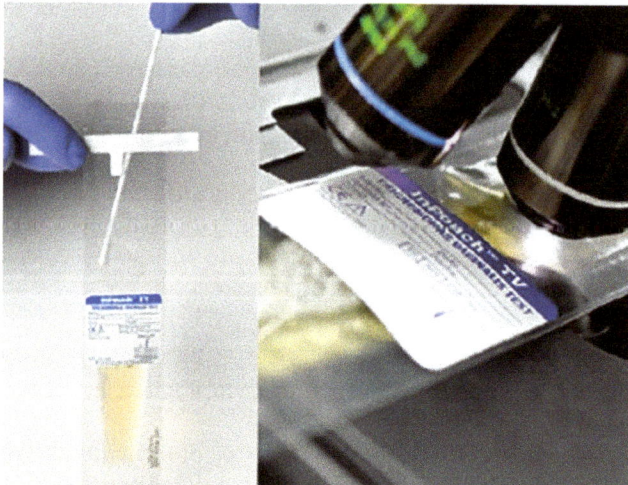

Fig. 4.8: InPouch TV diagnostic system for culturing *T. vaginalis*. The swab containing the specimen is inoculated into the highly selective liquid medium present within the plastic pouch; incubated for 4-7 days at 37°C and then examined under microscope for presence of trophozoites
Source: BIOMED Diagnostics.

and 99% specific. Xenostrip-Tv is another commercial ICT assay available
- ELISA using monoclonal antibodies has been developed; which shows sensitivity of 89% and specificity of 97%.

Antibody Detection

ELISA is available using whole cell antigen preparation and aqueous antigenic extract to detect antitrichomonal antibodies in serum and vaginal secretion of the patients.

However, antibodies persist for longer time, hence cannot differentiate between current infection and past infection. Moreover, its sensitivity is variable.

Molecular Methods

Molecular methods are highly sensitive, replacing culture as gold standard in future.
- PCR detecting *T. vaginalis* specific beta tubulin genes is available with sensitivity and specificity comparable to culture
- PCR-based ELISA format has been developed for urine samples (sensitivity 90% and specificity 93%)
- Recently, transcription-mediated amplification test (GenProbe Aptima *T. vaginalis* assay) has been developed for urine and genital specimens
- Other newer methods are: Strand displacement amplification (BD ProbeTec *T. vaginalis* Qx amplified DNA assay) and nucleic acid probe test (Affirm VPIII assay).

Other Supportive Tests

- **Raised vaginal pH (>4.5):** It is not specific as the vaginal pH is also raised in bacterial vaginosis. However, in vaginal candidiasis, the pH is not raised
- **Positive whiff test:**
    - Fishy odor is accentuated when a drop of 10% KOH is added to vaginal discharge due to production of amine
    - It is positive in more than 75% of cases
    - It is also positive in bacterial vaginosis.
- Increased pus cells on wet mount examination is seen in >75% of cases.

Treatment	*Trichomonas vaginalis*
Metronidazole or tinidazole ☐ **Standard therapy:** 2 g, single dose is usually effective ☐ Both the sexual partners must be treated simultaneously to prevent reinfection, especially asymptomatic males ☐ **Resistance to metronidazole:** ➤ Resistance is rare but has been reported: ♦ 2.5–10% to metronidazole ♦ Less than 1% to tinidazole *Contd...*	
➤ The mechanism of development of resistance to metronidazole is controlled by hydrogenosome ➤ Metronidazole requires hydrogen as an electron acceptor which is provided by hydrogenosome present in *T. vaginalis* ➤ In metronidazole-resistant *T. vaginalis*, the expression levels of the hydrogenosomal enzymes like ferredoxin are reduced dramatically, which probably eliminates the ability of the parasite to activate metronidazole ➤ Resistance is relative and can be overcome with higher doses of oral metronidazole ☐ **If standard therapy fails:** a second dose of metronidazole (2 g) is given ☐ **Refractory cases** (i.e. failure after two doses of standard therapy)—Here, treatment with metronidazole 2 g for 5 days is recommended ☐ **For hypersensitivity to metronidazole:** As there is no other therapy available, desensitization to metronidazole is the only option.	

Prevention

Trichomoniasis can be prevented by:
- Treatment of both the partners
- Safe sex practices like use of condoms
- Avoidance of sex with infected person
- **Vaccine:** There is no effective vaccine licensed so far. However, trials are going on targeting potential immunogenic antigens like 100 kDa protein, adhesin, mucinase and cysteine proteinases.

OTHER INTESTINAL FLAGELLATES OF MINOR IMPORTANCE

Pentatrichomonas hominis

It is worldwide in distribution found both in warm and temperate climates.
- It is a harmless commensal present in large intestine
- Trophozoite is pear shaped, measures 5–15 μm long and 7–10 μm wide, similar to that of *T. vaginalis*, except that the undulating membrane is extended throughout the body and the posterior flagellum extends free beyond the end of the body.

Trichomonas tenax

T. tenax is a harmless commensal in the mouth (gum and tartar of the teeth).
- However, few cases of respiratory infection and thoracic abscesses have been reported from Western Europe particularly in patients with cancer or other underlying lung disease
- The trophozoite is similar to *P. hominis* (except that the posterior flagellum extends only half of the body with

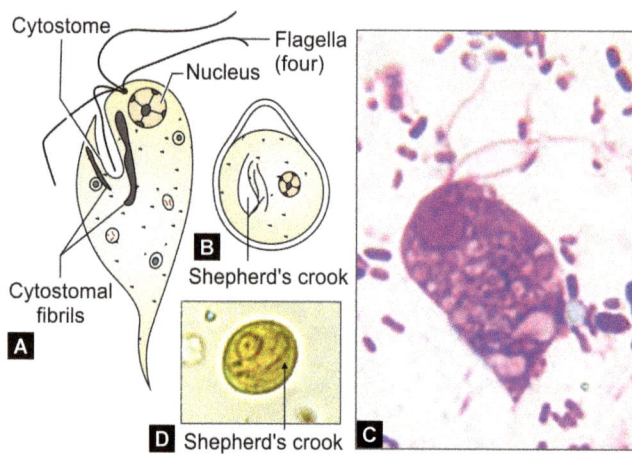

Figs 4.9A to D: *Chilomastix mesnili:* (A and B) Trophozoite and cyst (schematic diagram); (C) Trophozoite (Giemsa stain); (D) Cyst (iodine stain)

Source: C and D— Giovanni Swierczynski, Bruno Milanesi "Atlas of human intestinal protozoa Microscopic diagnosis" (*with permission*).

no free end); and it is smaller (5–12 µm long and 7–9 µm wide) and more slender
- Prevalence may vary from 0% to 0.25% depending on the oral hygiene.

Chilomastix mesnili

Chilomastix mesnili is a harmless commensal of cecum and colon in man.
- It is worldwide in distribution, found more frequently in warm climate
- It has two stages—trophozoite and cyst stages (Fig. 4.9).

Trophozoite

It is pear-shaped, measuring 6–24 µm in length and 4–8 µm in width. If posterior end is not visible, the shape may appear round.
- At the anterior end, there is a single nucleus and a distinct groove present near the nucleus called as cytostome
- It has four flagella—three anterior and one in cytostome
- It shows stiff, rotary movement
- Cytostome is supported by two cytostomal fibrils right one is prominent and curved, left one is straight and less conspicuous (Figs 4.9A and C).

Cyst

It is the infective stage; transmitted by fecal-oral route.
- It is lemon shaped with a narrow anterior hyaline knob, surrounded by a cyst wall
- It measures 6–10 µm in length and 4–6 µm in width
- Bears a single nucleus; cytoplasm is densely granular, separated from the cyst wall at the anterior end
- Remnant of the curved cytostomal fibrils can be seen, called as Shepherd's crook (Figs 4.9B and D).

Laboratory Diagnosis and Treatment

- Both the forms can be demonstrated by permanent staining of the stool samples (Figs 4.9C and D)
- Since, it is a commensal (of cecum) so no treatment is required. However, it should be reported to the physician for additional fecal examination to rule out other fecal pathogens
- Prevention depends on improved personal hygiene.

Enteromonas hominis

Enteromonas hominis is considered as a nonpathogenic commensal that is rarely encountered in human large intestine (cecum).
- It is reported from both tropical (warm) and temperate (cold) climates
- It exists in two forms—(1) trophozoite and (2) cyst.

Trophozoite

It is oval to pear shaped, smaller in size, measuring 4–10 µm long and 5–6 µm wide
- It possesses four flagella—three anterior and one recurrent. The recurrent flagellum extends free posteriorly and supported by a darkly stained fibril
- It shows jerky forward movement
- Nucleus is placed anteriorly and there is no cytostome
- Cytoplasm is vacuolated and contains numerous bacteria (Fig. 4.10A).

Cyst

It is the infective stage
- It is oval, measuring 4–10 µm long and 4–6 µm wide
- Possesses one to four nuclei, binucleated being most common (two nuclei lie at opposite poles) (Fig. 4.10B)
- It resembles like the cyst of *Endolimax nana*
- Infection is transmitted by ingestion of contaminated cyst.

Laboratory Diagnosis and Treatment

- Both the forms can be demonstrated by permanent staining of the stool samples
- Since it is a commensal, no treatment is required
- Prevention depends on improved personal hygiene.

Retortamonas intestinalis

Retortamonas intestinalis is a harmless commensal found less commonly in large intestine of man.
- It is reported from both tropical (warm) and temperate (cold) climate
- It exists in two forms—trophozoite and cyst.

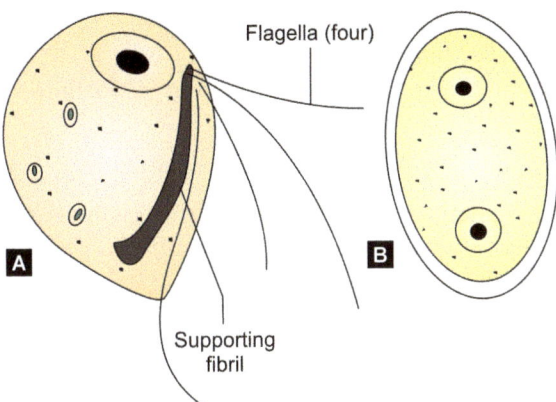

Figs 4.10A and B: *Enteromonas hominis* (schematic diagram): (A) Trophozoite; (B) Cyst

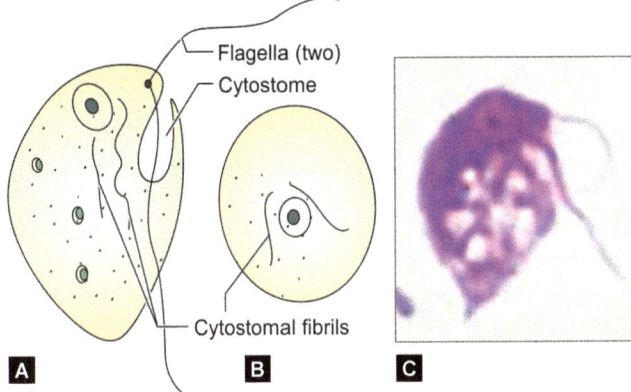

Figs 4.11A to C: *Retortamonas intestinalis*: (A and B) Trophozoite and cyst (schematic diagram); (C) Trophozoite (Giemsa stain)
Source: C— Giovanni Swierczynski, Bruno Milanesi" Atlas of human intestinal protozoa Microscopic diagnosis" (*with permission*).

Trophozoite

- Elongated pyriform or oval shaped, smaller in size, measuring 4–9 μm long and 3–4 μm wide
- It bears two flagella—one anterior and one posterior. It shows jerky movement
- It has a cytostomal groove anteriorly with cytostomal fibrils and a single nucleus (Figs 4.11A and C).

Cyst

- It is the infective stage
- It is pear shaped, measuring 4–9 μm long and 4–6 μm wide
- It resembles like the cyst of *Chilomastix* having single nucleus and cytostome with supporting fibrils extends above nucleus (Bird beak fibril arrangement) (Fig. 4.11B)
- Infection is transmitted by ingestion of contaminated cyst.

Laboratory Diagnosis and Treatment

- Both the forms can be demonstrated by permanent staining of the stool samples (Fig. 4.11C)
- Since it is a commensal, there is no therapy indicated
- Prevention depends on improved personal hygiene.

Dientamoeba fragilis

Dientamoeba fragilis lives in the lumen of the cecum and upper colon of humans.

- It was initially thought to be an amoeba as it bears no external flagella but recently, by electron microscopic studies; it is reclassified as an amoeboflagellate as the flagellum is internal. It closely resembles *Histomonas*, (infecting turkeys) and *Trichomonas* species
- It is cosmopolitan in distribution with incidence rate varies from 1.4% to 19%
- Higher incidence is reported in children.

Morphology

It exists in three forms—trophozoite, precyst and cyst. The precyst and cyst stages have been recently identified.

Trophozoite

- It is irregular in shape (amoeboid), relatively small, varying from 9 μm to 12 μm
- **Nucleus:** One to two number (commonly two nuclei in 60–80% of cases, hence named as *Dientamoeba*) (Figs 4.12A and B)
- The nuclear chromatin is usually fragmented into three to five granules (hence named as **fragilis**), no peripheral chromatin on the nuclear membrane
- The cytoplasm is usually vacuolated and may contain ingested debris as well as some large uniform granules.

Precystic stage

It is spherical; 4–5 μm size with a darkly stained homogenous cytoplasm.

Cyst

Cyst measures 5–8 μm; oval to round with 1 or 2 nuclei (same as trophozoite). It has distinct double-layered cyst wall separated by a peritrophic space (Fig. 4.12C).

Life Cycle

The life cycle is not fully understood. Cysts are the infective forms; transmitted by feco-oral route. Helminth eggs such as *Enterobius* and *Ascaris* are known to carry the parasite. Cysts transform to trophozoites which multiply in the large intestine and excreted in feces. True cysts are rarely seen in feces although precystic forms may be seen rarely (5%).

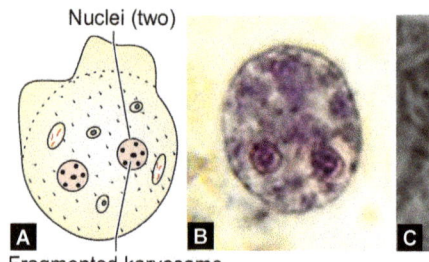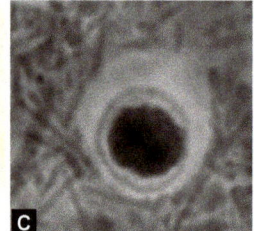

Figs 4.12A to C: *Dientamoeba fragilis*: (A) Schematic diagram of trophozoite; (B) Iron hematoxylin stain showing trophozoite having two nuclei with fragmented karyosome; (C) Cyst (saline mount)

Source: B—Giovanni Swierczynski, Bruno Milanesi "Atlas of human intestinal protozoa microscopic diagnosis" (*with permission*); C—Varuni S. Munasinghe, School of Medical and Molecular Biosciences and the i3 Institute, University of Technology Sydney, Broadway, New South Wales 2007, Australia.

Pathogenesis

This is controversial; the pathogenic status is not well defined.
- Some authors believe that there may be two distinct genotypes one of which may be pathogenic
- The organism has been reported in association with mucous diarrhea, abdominal pain, fatigue, and low-grade fever
- It is associated with inflammatory bowel syndrome
- *D. fragilis* infection is particularly common in Canada.

Laboratory Diagnosis

Stool examination

Trophozoite does not survive for longer time hence the fresh direct wet preparations should be examined immediately or stained by permanent stains.

- The recommended stains are trichrome and iron hematoxylin stain
- Trophozoites are destroyed in a formol-ether concentration technique.

Culture

D. fragilis can be grown in Loeffler's slope medium and modified Earle's balanced salt solution at 42°C under microaerophilic condition (5% oxygen).

Antigen detection in stool

Both immunofluorescence and enzyme immunoassays are available.

Antibody detection in serum

It can be detected by IFA technique and immunoblot method. Immunoblot is more specific, detects antibody to 39 k-Da protein.

Molecular methods

- Multiplex real time PCR and multiplex tandem PCR are available
- EasyScreen PCR assay is recently available commercially for the detection of five common enteric parasites—*Blastocystis* species, *Cryptosporidium* species, *D. fragilis*, *Entamoeba* and *Giardia*. It has shown 92 to 100% sensitivity and 100% specificity.

Treatment	*Dientamoeba fragilis*
Tetracycline or metronidazole is effective. Iodoquinol, paromomycin are the other useful agents.	

EXPECTED QUESTIONS

I. Write essay on:
  a. A 3-year-old boy presented with recurrent episodes of foul smelling diarrhea, foul flatus, sulfurous belching and profound weight loss. The wet mount examination of the stool sample revealed pear-shaped trophozoites of 10–20 μm in length and 5–15 μm in width, showing falling leaf like motility.
    1. What is the etiological diagnosis and life cycle?
    2. What are the various diagnostic modalities?
    3. How will you treat this condition?

II. Write short notes on:
  a. Trichomoniasis.
  b. *Dientamoeba fragilis*.
  c. *Chilomastix mesnili*.

III. Multiple choice questions (MCQs):
  1. How many pairs of flagella are present in the trophozoite of *Giardia lamblia*?
     a. One b. Two
     c. Four d. Eight
  2. *Giardia lamblia* resides in:
     a. Sigmoid colon b. Cossslon
     c. Duodenum d. Vagina
  3. Which is the most common cause of steatorrhea?
     a. *Ascaris lumbricoides* b. *Giardia lamblia*
     c. *Entamoeba histolytica* d. *Enteromonas hominis*
  4. Trophozoites of which of the following bear two nuclei with fragmented karyosome?
     a. *Dientamoeba fragilis* b. *Chilomastix mesnili*
     c. *Retortamonas intestinalis* d. *Enteromonas hominis*
  5. Diagnosis of which of the following parasite uses Entero-Test?
     a. *Cyclospora* species b. *Entamoeba histolytica*
     c. *Giardia lamblia* d. *Dientamoeba fragilis*
  6. Which of the following parasite does not have a cyst stage?
     a. *Enteromonas hominis* b. *Dientamoeba fragilis*
     c. *Pentatrichomonas hominis* d. *Chilomastix mesnili*

Answers
1. c 2. c 3. b 4. a 5. c 6. c

Flagellates—II (Hemoflagellates)

CHAPTER 5

CHAPTER OUTLINE

- Morphology of hemoflagellates
- Leishmania
  - Old world leishmaniasis
  - New world leishmaniasis
- Trypanosoma
  - Trypanosoma cruzi
- Trypanosoma brucei complex

INTRODUCTION

Hemoflagellates are the flagellated protozoa that are found in peripheral blood circulation. They complete their life cycle in two hosts, i.e. vertebrate host and insect vector; therefore, called as **digenetic** or **heteroxenous parasites.** Hemoflagellates of medical importance belongs to:
- Phylum: Euglenozoa
- Class: Kinetoplastidea
- Order: Trypanosomatida
- Family: Trypanosomatidae
- Genera: *Leishmania* and *Trypanosoma*.

MORPHOLOGY OF HEMOFLAGELLATES

Hemoflagellates have an oval to elongated body, nucleus, and a single flagellum arising from kinetoplast.
- **Kinetoplast:** It consists of blepharoplast and parabasal body connected by a delicate fibril (cytoskeleton). It lies tangentially or at right angle to the nucleus. It represents multiple copies of mitochondrial DNA
- **Axoneme:** It extends from blepharoplast to the cell wall. It represents the intracellular portion (root) of flagellum

- Based upon the arrangement of flagellum, they exist in four morphological stages—(1) amastigote, (2) promastigote, (3) epimastigote and (4) trypomastigote. Names are ended with a suffix **"mastigote"** (Greek word Mastix means whip) (Figs 5.1A to D)
  1. **Amastigote form:** Round to oval, lacks flagellum, found in reticuloendothelial cells of man infected with *Leishmania* and *Trypanosoma cruzi.*
  2. **Promastigote form:** Lanceolate shaped; kinetoplast is anterior to nucleus (antinuclear kinetoplast). Flagellum arises from the anterior end. It is found in the mid gut of insect vector. This is the infective stage of *Leishmania* to man.
  3. **Epimastigote form:** Elongated, kinetoplast is placed close to the nucleus (juxtanuclear kinetoplast). Flagellum arises from the lateral side and traverses the body as a short undulating membrane and comes out from the anterior end. This form is seen for *Trypanosoma* in insect vector.
  4. **Trypomastigote form:** Elongated and spindle shaped with central nucleus. Kinetoplast lies near the posterior end. Flagellum arises posteriorly and runs as long undulating membrane. It is the infective

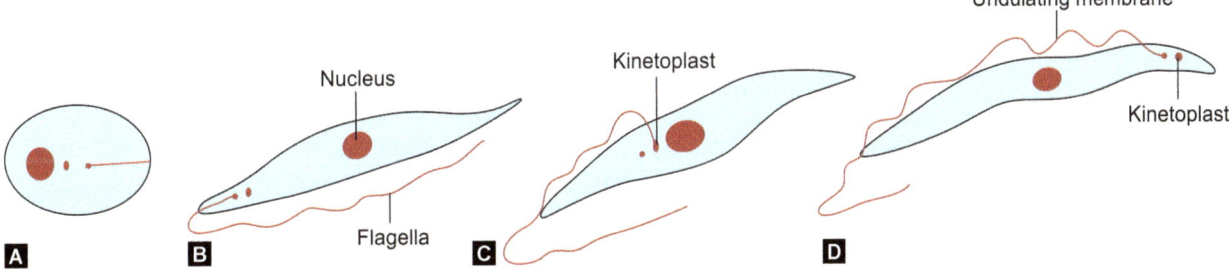

Figs 5.1A to D: Various morphological forms of flagellates (schematic diagrams): (A) Amastigote; (B) Promastigote; (C) Epimastigote; (D) Trypomastigote

stage of *Trypanosoma* found in insect vector and in peripheral blood of humans.

LEISHMANIA

Leishmaniasis is caused by the obligatory intracellular protozoa of the genus *Leishmania*. Primarily, it affects the reticulo-endothelial system of the host.
- *Leishmania* species produce widely varying group of clinical syndromes ranging from self-healing cutaneous ulcers to fatal visceral disease
- Leishmaniasis is mainly a zoonotic disease affecting dogs, foxes, jackals and rodents. Animal reservoir plays a major role for transmission; except in Indian subcontinent where it is anthropophilic affecting only humans
- The parasite is transmitted by bite of the female sandfly vector (refer Fig. 16.5).

Classification of Leishmaniasis

Leishmania has two subgenera *L. Leishmania* and *L. Viannia*.
- The main difference between the two subgenera is that promastigotes of the subgenus *Viannia* develop in the midgut and hindgut of sandfly where as that of subgenus *Leishmania*, develop in the anterior portion of the alimentary tract of sandfly
- Both of the subgenera comprise of nearly 20 species. (Table 5.1)
    - **Old world leishmaniasis:** Affects Asia, Africa and Europe and transmitted by sandfly (Genus *Phlebotomus*)
    - **New World leishmaniasis:** Affects Central and South America and transmitted by sandfly (Genus *Lutzomyia*).
- Clinical syndromes of leishmaniasis include:
    - Visceral leishmaniasis (VL)
    - Post–kala-azar dermal leishmaniasis (PKDL)
    - Cutaneous leishmaniasis (CL)
    - Diffuse cutaneous leishmaniasis (DCL)
    - Leishmaniasis recidivans (LR)
    - Mucocutaneous leishmaniasis (MCL).

Epidemiology

Leishmaniasis is endemic in 97 countries; with four countries have previous reported cases. Most of them are developing countries of tropical and temperate regions.
- More than 616 million people living in the endemic area are at risk

Table 5.1: Classification of *Leishmania*

Species	Geographical distribution	Clinical syndrome	Vector (sandfly)	Reservoir	Transmission
Old World Leishmaniasis					
Leishmania Leishmania (L. L.) donovani complex					
L. L. donovani	South Asia (Indian subcontinent)	VL (Kala-azar), PKDL CL (rare)	*Phlebotomus argentipes*	Humans	Anthroponotic
	Sudan, Ethiopia, Kenya and Uganda	VL, PKDL	*P. orientalis, P. martini*	Humans/ rodents	Anthroponotic/ Zoonotic
	Middle East, Africa and China	VL	*P. perniciosus*		Zoonotic
L. L. infantum	Mediterranean, Middle East, Central Asia and China	VL PKDL (rare, in HIV)	*P. perniciosus*	Dogs, foxes, jackals, etc.	Zoonotic
L. L. tropica Complex					
L. L. tropica (Delhi boil)	Western India, North Africa, Mediterranean littoral, Middle East	CL, LR	*P. sergenti*	Humans	Anthroponotic
L. L. aethiopica	Ethiopia, Uganda, and Kenya	CL, DCL	*P. longipes*	Hyraxes	Zoonotic
L. L major	Middle East, India, China Africa, central and western Asia	CL VL (reported rarely)	*P. papatasi*	Rodents	Zoonotic
New World Leishmaniasis					
L. L. chagasi (new world variant of *L.L. infantum*)	Central and South America	VL, CL PKDL (rare)	*Lutzomyia* species	Dogs, foxes, etc.	Zoonotic
L. L. mexicana complex	Central America and northern parts of South America	CL, DCL VL (rare)	*Lutzomyia* species	Forest rodents	Zoonotic
L. Viannia braziliensis complex	South and Central America	CL, MCL LR (rare)	*Lutzomyia* species	Forest rodents	Zoonotic

Abbreviations: VL, Visceral leishmaniasis; PKDL, post-kala-azar dermal leishmaniasis; CL, cutaneous leishmaniasis; LR, leishmaniasis recidivans DCL, diffuse cutaneous leishmaniasis; MCL, mucocutaneous leishmaniasis.

- **World:** WHO estimated 7,00,000 to 1 million new cases and 20,000 to 30,000 deaths occur annually
  - **VL:** An estimated 50,000 to 90,000 new cases of VL occur worldwide each year. Over 90% of cases of VL come from three regions: (i) South-East Asia: India, Bangladesh, and Nepal; (ii) East Africa: Ethiopia, Sudan, and Kenya; and (iii) Brazil
  - **CL** is the most common form of leishmaniasis with a global annual incidence of 6,00,000 to 1 million new cases. About 95% of CL cases occur in the Americas, the Mediterranean basin, the Middle East and Central Asia
  - **MCL:** Over 90% of mucocutaneous leishmaniasis cases occur in Bolivia, Brazil, Ethiopia and Peru.
- **India:** India is one of the worst affected country. Bihar is affected the most (>70% of cases) followed by Jharkhand, West Bengal and Uttar Pradesh
  - About 57 districts with more than 165 millions of people are at risk.
  - In 2017, about 5,758 cases of VL and 1,949 cases of PKDL have been reported from India with nil death. VL reported maximum from Bihar (71.6%) and PKDL from Jharkhand (62%).

OLD WORLD LEISHMANIASIS

Leishmania donovani

History

Leishmania donovani causes VL or kala azar (a hindi term meaning "black fever")
- It was named after two scientists who discovered the parasite in the same year 1903
  - Sir William Boog Leishman in London observed the amastigotes form of the parasite in the spleen of a British soldier died at Dumdum, Kolkata. (Hence also known as Dum-Dum fever). He thought the parasite may be a trypanosome.
  - Sir Donovan at Madras Medical College, Chennai, suggested that the causative agent was a new parasite.

  Sir Ronald Ross, recognizing the contribution of both, named the parasite as *Leishmania donovani*.
- Charles Nicolle, a 1928 Nobel laureate, at the Pasteur Institute in Tunisia, characterized the new world VL and cultivated the etiologic agent.

Morphology

Leishmania occurs in two forms:

Amastigote form (Fig. 5.2A)

It is an obligate intracellular form and the infective stage to vector, sandfly.
- Found in reticuloendothelial cells like macrophages, neutrophils, endothelial cells of liver, spleen, bone

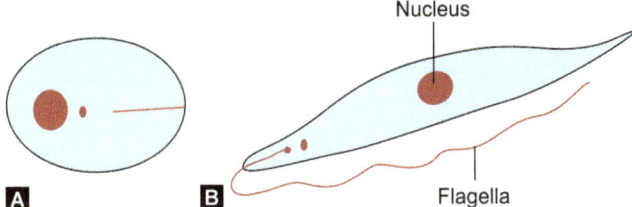

Figs 5.2A and B: *Leishmania* species (schematic diagram): (A) Amastigote form; (B) Promastigote form

marrow, etc. of the vertebrate hosts like humans, dogs and rodents
- Round to oval, 3–5 μm in size
- **Nucleus:** It measures less than 1 μm, oval to round, located in center or side of the cell
- **Kinetoplast:** It consists of mitochondrial DNA. It is made up blepharoplast and parabasal body connected by a delicate fibril (cytoskeleton). It lies at right angle to the nucleus
- **Axoneme:** It extends from blepharoplast to the cell wall. It represents the intracellular portion (root) of flagellum
- There is no external flagellum and it is nonmotile.

Promastigote form (Fig. 5.2B)

This is an extracellular form, infective stage to humans.
- It is mainly found in sandfly and in culture
- It is motile and contains single anterior flagellum of 15–28 μm length
- Pear shaped, 15–20 μm length and 1.5–3.5 μm wide
- Nucleus is situated centrally and kinetoplast is placed near the anterior end transversely
- **Axoneme:** It represents the intracellular portion of flagellum.

Life Cycle (Fig. 5.3)

Host: *Leishmania* completes its life cycle in two hosts:
1. **Vertebrate host** (man, dog, rodents, etc.)
2. **Invertebrate host (female sandfly):** *Phlebotomus argentipes* (see Fig. 16.5).

Vector (Sandfly)

Out of more than 1000 species of sandfly, only 70 are proven vectors. The species specificity is linked to the variability of lipophosphoglycan present on the surface of the parasite.
- Both sexes of sandfly feed on plant sugars, but the females need a blood meal to lay eggs. Therefore, only the females can transmit the infection
- They do not bite during day time; becomes active only at and after the dusk, transmitting the infection
- Sandfly is a very efficient vector; bites are painful as being a pool feeder. It becomes infective after 5–7 days of blood meal. Once infective, it remains infective probably for life.
- Saliva of sandfly secretes **maxadilan**, a potent vasodilator and immunomodulator; which increases the infectivity of promastigotes.

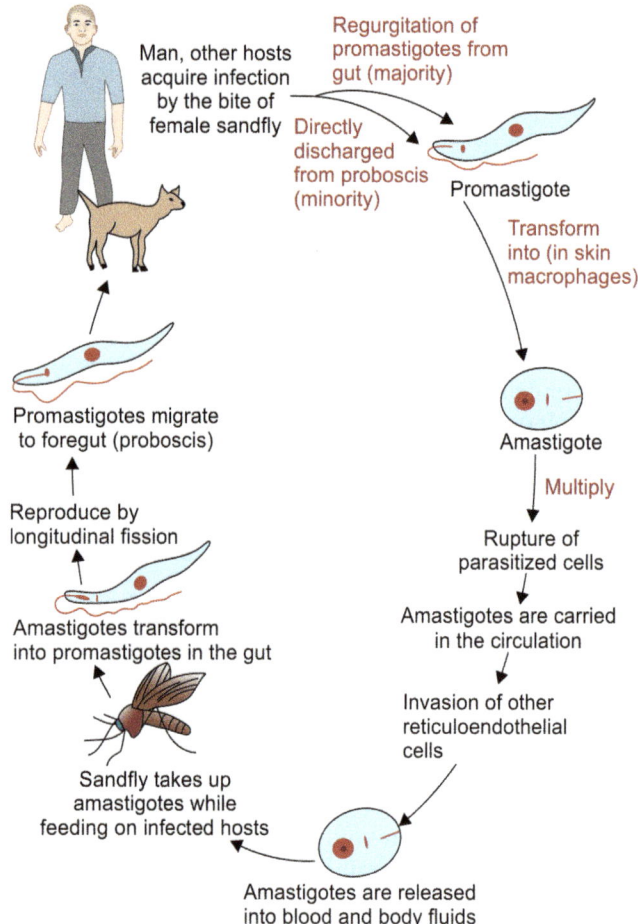

Fig. 5.3: Life cycle of *Leishmania donovani*

Infective form: Promastigote forms found in alimentary canal of female sandfly serve as the infective form.

Mode of transmission: By bite of an infected female sandfly. Minimum 10–1,000 promastigotes per infective bite are required to initiate the infection. Very exceptionally, transmission occurs congenitally, during transfusion, organ transplantation and laboratory accidents.

In vertebrate hosts, including humans:
- Promastigotes are regurgitated from the insect gut rarely or directly discharged from foregut (proboscis) of the female sandfly into the skin of the vertebrate host
- Promastigotes are phagocytosed by the skin macrophages and transform into amastigote forms within 12–24 hours
- The amastigote forms mutiply inside the macrophages, causing cell rupture and releasing into the circulation
- Amastigotes are carried out in the circulation to various organs like liver, spleen and bone marrow and invade the reticuloendothelial cells like macrophages, endothelial cells, etc.

In sandfly:
- During the blood meal, the amastigotes are ingested and transformed into promastigote forms in the insect gut
- Promastigotes multiply in the insect gut by longitudinal fission and a small proportion migrates to the foregut (proboscis). They infect a new host during another blood meal
- The duration of the life cycle in sandfly varies from 5–7 days depending on the species.

Pathogenicity

Various factors contribute to the pathogenesis such as:
- The phagocytosis of the promastigotes is facilitated by binding of the promastigote surface antigens such as 63 kDa glycoprotein (gp-63) and lipophosphoglycan (LPG) to complement receptors (CR3 and Cq1) on macrophages
- The gp-63 antigen also gives protection from proteolytic enzymes secreted from the phagolysosome
- LPG is the principle virulence factor, exhibits variety of functions. It prevents phagosome maturation and protects the parasite against hydrolytic enzymes secreted from the phagolysosome
- The amastigotes multiply within acidic parasitophorous vacuoles
- **Glycosylphosphatidylinositols (GPIs) is a** major surface protein on amastigotes, helps in protecting from phagolysosomal attack inside the macrophage.

Host Immune Response

Depending on the host immune response, the amastigotes are either killed or allowed to multiply inside the macrophages.
- Like leprosy, the immunology of leishmaniasis is complex and bipolar. It has two extreme poles, each which is characterized by one of the two type of T helper (T_H) subset responses, i.e. T_H1 or T_H2 responses.

T helper-1 response

T_H1 response is induced by interleukin-12 (IL-12) which leads to increase production of interferon γ (IFN-γ) and IL-2.
- At the cellular level, IFN-γ activates macrophages which in turn kill amastigotes by induction of nitric oxide synthase and oxidative killing mechanisms
- T_H1 response is observed in:
  - The majority of individuals who mount a successful immune response and control the infection
  - Cutaneous leishmaniasis
  - Patients after recovery/treated for VL
  - Leishmaniasis recidivans.

- These individuals exhibit a delayed-type hypersensitivity (DTH) to leishmanial antigens (positive leishmanin skin test).

T helper-2 response

Stimulation of T_H2 cells results in increased production of IL-10 and IL-4; which in turn causes polyclonal B cell activation leading to hypergammaglobulinemia.
- It is observed in patients developing active VL and in diffuse CL
- IL-10 inhibits macrophages to kill amastigotes by downregulating the production of (TNF-α) and nitric oxide. That helps in enhanced survival and growth of the parasite
- Patients do not show positive leishmanin skin test
- The parasite uses the macrophage much like a Trojan horse. Amastigotes are released periodically by rupture of the macrophages
- They disseminate through the regional lymphatics and the vascular system to infect the reticuloendothelial cells of various organs
- This results in remarkable enlargement of the spleen, liver and bone marrow dysfunction.

Clinical Features

Visceral leishmaniasis

Visceral leishmaniasis is mainly caused by the *L. donovani* and sometimes by *L. infantum*, (designated as *L. chagasi* in the New World) together known as *L. donovani* complex. (Table 5.2).
- Incubation period ranges from 2–6 months
- The hallmark of VL is a pentad of fever, progressive weight loss, hepatosplenomegaly, pancytopenia and hypergammaglobulinemia
- **Fever:** The most common symptom of VL is an abrupt onset of moderate to high-grade fever associated with rigor and chills. Typically, it is described as double or triple rise of fever in 24 hours
- **Splenomegaly:** It is the most consistent sign. The spleen may become hugely enlarged (soft non-tender and friable) and palpable below the umbilicus (Fig. 5.4A)
- Hepatomegaly (non-tender, moderate degree) soon follows splenomegaly
- **Lymphadenopathy:** Common in most of the African endemic regions (rare in Indian subcontinent). Femoral and inguinal nodes are affected commonly
- **Hyperpigmentation:** Earth-gray color skin changes are observed on face, hands, feet, and abdomen; hence the name kala-zar or black fever. This is a characteristic feature of Indian VL
- **Pedal edema and ascites:** Occur due to hypoalbuminemia, may be seen in advanced illness
- Mucosal lesions in mouth and nasopharynx—seen in Sudan, rare in India. This may lead to nasal septum perforation and hoarseness
- **Hematological abnormalities** (bone marrow dysfunction):
    - Pancytopenia: Anemia (normocytic and normochromic), leukopenia and thrombocytopenia
    - Hypergammaglobulinemia (due to polyclonal B cell activation).
- **Leishmanoma:** Nodular skin lesions seen in African cases only
- Weight loss (cachexia) and hair changes (thinning, dryness, hypopigmentation, and loss of curl)
- Secondary infections: Such as measles, pneumonia, tuberculosis, bacillary or amoebic dysentery and gastroenteritis are common
- Death occurs due to superimposed infection, severe anemia and hemorrhages.

Table 5.2: Various forms of visceral leishmaniasis

Characters		Old World VL		New World VL
	Indian VL (kala-azar)	Infantile VL	African VL	Mediterranean VL
Agent	Leishmania donovani	L. infantum	L. donovani	L. chagasi
Vector	Phlebotomus argentipes	P. perniciosus	P. orientalis, P. martini	Lutzomyia longipalpis
Epidemiology	India	Middle East, Central Asia, China and Mediterranean basin	Sudan, Ethiopia, Kenya and Uganda	Central and South America
Age affected	Young adults	Infants and children <5 years of age	Adults	Children
Reservoir	Anthroponotic (human)	Zoonotic (canine)	Anthroponotic, Rarely-Zoonotic (rodents)	Zoonotic (canine)
PKDL	Common	Less common	Common	Less common
Lymph node invovlement	Less common	More common, Aggravated by poor nutrition	Less common	Less common

Abbreviations: VL, visceral leishmaniasis; PKDL, post-kala-azar dermal leishmaniasis.

Post-kala-azar dermal leishmaniasis (PKDL)

PKDL is a nonulcerative lesion of skin occurs in 2–50% of patients of VL following incomplete or inadequate treatment or treatment with antimonials. It is aggravated by exposure to sunlight. PKDL is also seen following *L. infantum* infection, although rare. It was first described by Brahmachari in 1922.

- ❖ Mainly seen in India and East African countries (Table 5.3)
- ❖ It develops as hypopigmented macule (most common feature) near mouth which later on spreads to face and then to arms and trunk (extensor surfaces) and finally becomes nodules resembling leprosy (Figs 5.4B to D)
- ❖ Nodular lesions may serve as reservoir of infection during inter-epidemic period
- ❖ Ocular lesions like conjunctivitis and uveitis are associated in some patients
- ❖ Sometimes, PKDL occurs in subclinical patients without a history of VL
- ❖ In East Africa, the lesions are graded into three types—*Grade-1* involves mainly face, *grade-2* involves face, chest, back, upper arm and upper leg; whereas *grade-3* affects most parts of the body including hands and feet. Crusting and ulceration may be seen
- ❖ **The diagnosis is based on:**
  - Amastigote can be detected in the skin in more than 80% of cases in Sudan. It is more easily detected from nodular lesions than other lesions
  - Serological tests: Direct agglutination test (DAT) and antibodies to rK39 antigen are positive in most of the cases.

Leishmaniasis with HIV co-infection

Co-infection of HIV with VL has been reported from more than 35 countries.

Table 5.3: Post-kala-azar dermal leishmaniasis from Indian Subcontinent and East Africa

Feature	Indian subcontinent	East Africa
Most affected country	Bangladesh, India and Nepal	Sudan, Kenya and Ethiopia
Incidence among patients with VL	2–20%	>50% (rare in other part of Africa)
Interval between VL and PKDL	2–10 years	Can occur during VL within 2 months
Age affected	Any age	Mainly children
History of prior kala-azar	Not necessarily	Yes
PKDL persists for	Long period (20 years)	Few months
Treatment (preferred)	(i) Amphotericin B deoxycholate IV for 4 months or (ii) Miltefosine orally for 12 weeks	(i) Pentavalent antimonials for 30–60 days or (ii) Liposomal amphotericin B for 20 days
Course	Resolve slowly (noncompliance)	Spontaneous cure usually occurs

Abbreviations: VL, visceral leishmaniasis; PKDL, post-kala-azar dermal leishmaniasis.

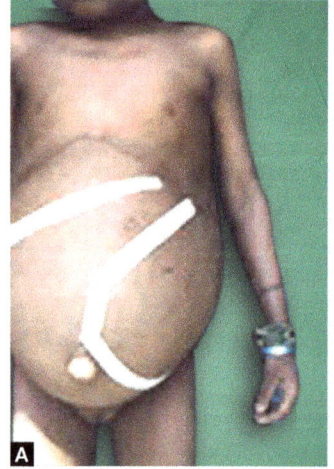
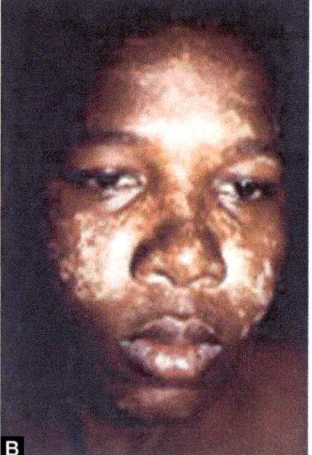
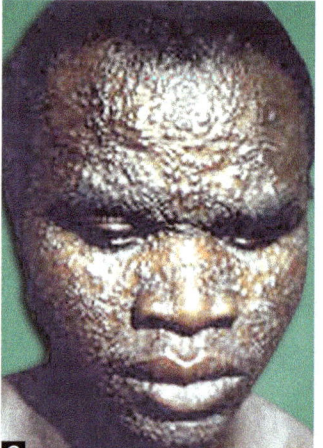
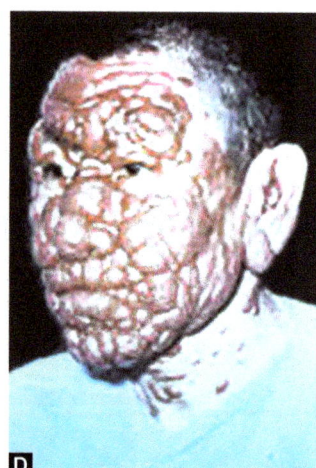

Figs 5.4A to D: Clinical features of leishmaniasis (A) Splenomegaly seen in visceral leishmaniasis; (B) Hypopigmented skin changes in early PKDL; (C and D) Extensive facial nodular lesions in late PKDL

Source: World Health Organization "Manual on visceral leishmaniasis control" Slide1/Desjeux; Slide 4 and 5/ El Hassan; Slide 6/ Bryceson (*with permission*).

- Mainly, it is reported from Southern Europe (France, Italy, Spain and Portugal) where 50–75% of adult cases of VL (usually caused by *L. infantum*) are HIV positive and 7–17% of HIV-infected people with fever have amastigotes
- Also reported from other places like Africa (Ethiopia, Sudan), Brazil and India
- In India, it is reported from Bihar, sub-Himalayan region and other North Indian states. Various studies reported the coinfection prevalence of 5–6%
- Both HIV and *Leishmania* affect each other's pathogenesis
  Effect on HIV:
  - *Leishmania* appears to cause activation of latent HIV
  - It expresses high level of chemokine receptor (CCR5) receptors on macrophages.

  Effect on *Leishmania*:
  - HIV causes activation of T_H2 cells response leading to disease progression
  - *Leishmania* uptake is enhanced by the HIV-infected macrophages
  - Associated with more relapses.
- **Clinical feature:** In HIV co-infected patients, apart from the classical feature of VL, other forms such as CL, MCL, PKDL, etc. may be seen. Atypical presentation such as chronic diarrhea and pleural effusion may be observed if CD4 T cell count is <50/mm^3
- **Relapses are common.** Predictors that favor relapse include CD4 T cell <100 /mm^3, and prior VL relapse. HIV viral load and response to anti-retrovirals do not seem to predict relapse
- There is consideration to include leishmaniasis in CDC clinical category C for the definition of AIDS as an opportunistic pathogen
- **Diagnosis:** Serodiagnostic tests are usually negative. Amastigotes are demonstrated from unusual sites such as bronchoalveolar lavage fluid and buffy coat region of blood.

Treatment	HIV/VL coinfection

Liposomal amphotericin B is the drug of choice for HIV/VL co-infection. But response is poor with frequent relapses.

Laboratory Diagnosis	*Leishmania donovani*

- **Microscopy**—Giemsa staining, detects LD bodies (i.e. macrophage filled with amastigote forms)
  - Splenic aspiration: Most sensitive
  - Bone marrow aspiration: Most commonly preferred
  - Lymph node aspiration (in African patients)
  - Liver biopsy
  - Peripheral blood smear (in HIV-infected people)
  - Biopsy of various organs (in HIV-infected people)

Cotnd...

Laboratory Diagnosis	*Leishmania donovani*

- **Culture** (detects promastigotes)—useful for species identification and drug sensitivity testing
  - NNN medium
  - Schneider's liquid medium
- **Antibody detection** in serum
  - ELISA, IFA and direct agglutination test
  - ICT using rk39 or rKE16 antigens
- **Antigen detection**—carbohydrate antigen in the urine (latex agglutination test)
- Nonspecific tests to detect hypergammaglobulinemia
  - Napier's aldehyde test
  - Chopra's antimony test
- **Molecular method**—PCR, real-time PCR detecting kinetoplast DNA, 18S rRNA, small subunit rRNA
- **Leishmanin test** (montenegro test)—indicates good CMI (DTH reaction); positive in all stages, except active VL and diffuse CL
- **Animal inoculation**—golden hamster
- **Others**—pancytopenia.

Laboratory Diagnosis

Clinical case definition

WHO has stated any case in an endemic area, with fever >2 weeks, splenomegaly and/or weight loss is suspected of having VL and should be subjected to laboratory confirmation.

Microscopy

Demonstration of amastigotes inside the macrophages (also known as **Leishman Donovan bodies** or **LD bodies**) is the gold standard method for the diagnosis of VL (Figs 5.5A and B). Smears should be stained with Leishman, Giemsa or Wright stains. The various samples include:

- **Splenic aspiration:** The sensitivity of splenic smear examination is excellent (>98%) but splenic puncture

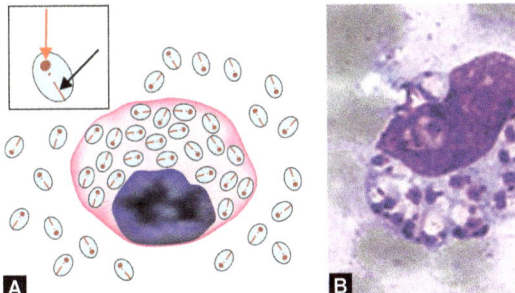

Figs 5.5A and B: *L. donovani* amastigotes: showing a macrophage containing multiple *Leishmania* amastigotes. (A) Schematic; (B) In bone marrow smear stained with Giemsa. Note that each amastigote has a nucleus (red arrow) and a rod-shaped kinetoplast (black arrow)

Source: B—DPDx Image Library, Centers for Disease Control and Prevention (CDC), Atlanta (*with permission*).

Cotnd...

Table 5.4: Grading of splenic smear for detection of *L. donovani* amastigotes

Grades	Density of parasites
6+	>100 parasites/OIF
5+	10–100 parasites/OIF
4+	1–10 parasites/OIF
3+	1–10 parasites/10 OIF
2+	1–10 parasites/100 OIF
1+	1–10 parasites/1000 OIF
Zero	Nil parasites/1000 OIF

Abbreviation: OIF, oil immersion field

is associated with risk of hemorrhage. Grading of LD bodies from splenic smear is useful in determining the parasitic load and monitoring the response to treatment (Table 5.4)

- **Bone marrow aspiration:** Iliac crest aspirate is the most commonly preferred sample though the sensitivity is around 80–85%. If bone marrow findings are negative but the clinical suspicion is strong, then the splenic aspiration is indicated
- **Lymph node aspiration:** It is useful only in African cases of kala-azar and its sensitivity is low (53–65%)
- **Liver biopsy:** Less sensitive and carries the risk of hemorrhage
- **Peripheral blood smear:** Amastigotes within mononuclear cells and neutrophils can be seen in a stained blood smear
    - Sensitivity increases by making thick smears, using centrifuged blood and making smears from buffy coat particularly in HIV patients
    - Amastigotes in blood show periodicity, detected in buffy coat smear more during night (66%) than day time (46%), which reflects the biting habit of the sandfly vector.
- **Biopsy specimens of various organs:** Like oropharynx, stomach, or intestine. This is particularly important in patients with AIDS.

Differentiating from look-alike structures

Leishmania amastigotes may be confused with intracellular round to oval bodies of small 2–6 μm such as *Histoplasma capsulatum*, *Cryptococcus*, *Penicillium marneffei* and granules in normal immature leukocytes in the bone marrow. The presence of nucleus and small rod-shaped kinetoplast with absence of budding characteristically differentiates amastigotes from others.

Culture

- **Sample:** Aspirations from spleen, bone marrow, other tissues and also buffy coat
- **Medium:**
    - **NNN medium** (described by Novy, McNeal–1903 and Nicolle–1908): Novy-MacNeal-Nicolle (NNN) medium is a biphasic medium, composed of two

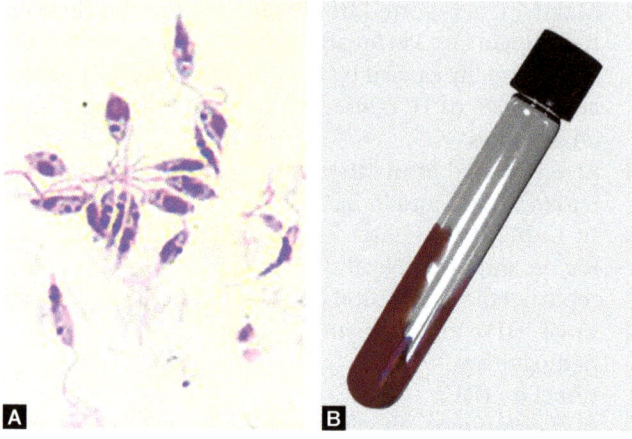

Figs 5.6A and B: (A) Smear made from culture fluid shows promastigote form (Giemsa stain); (B) NNN medium

Source: A—DPDx Image Library, Centers for Disease Control and Prevention (CDC), Atlanta (*with permission*); B—World Health Organization, "Manual on visceral leishmaniasis control" (Slide22/Alvar) (*with permission*).

   parts salt agar and one part defibrinated rabbit blood (Fig. 5.6B)
    - ***Schneider's Liquid medium:*** It contains Schneider's *Drosophila* insect medium supplemented with 30% fetal calf serum. It is found to be more sensitive than NNN media
    - Semisynthetic fetal calf serum free medium
    - Microculture method using microcapillary tubes.
- Culture is useful for species identification and drug sensitivity testing; which is done by isoenzyme electrophoresis, or by using species specific monoclonal antibodies or probe hybridization
- Inoculated specimens are incubated at ambient temperature (24–26°C) and examined weekly for 4 weeks before declared as negative
- Amastigotes transform into promastigotes in the culture fluid which are detected by staining with Giemsa or acridine orange stain (Fig. 5.6A) or by animal inoculation in golden hamster
- Culture is found to be positive in 75% of cases.

Antibody detection in serum

In general, the serological tests are sensitive, but less specific. False-positive results may occur due to cross-reacting antibodies in patients with leprosy, Chagas' disease, CL, and other infections. Antibodies cannot differentiate current and past infection. More so, antibodies may be absent or present in low titer in patients with AIDS

- **Complement fixation test (CFT):** It was used in the past; now obsolete
- **ELISA** and indirect fluorescent antibody **(IFA)** test, are the newer tests found to be more sensitive and have replaced CFT
- **Direct agglutination test (DAT):** Serial dilution of patient serum is added with stained extract of

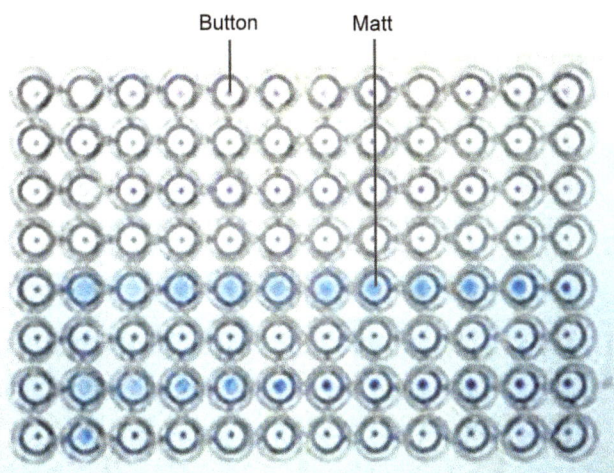

Fig. 5.7: Direct agglutination test
Source: "Manual on visceral leishmaniasis control", World Health Organization (Slide32/Alvar) *(with permission).*

L. donovani axenic amastigote (preferred) or promastigote antigen on microtiter plate and incubated for 18 hours
- If specific antibodies are present, agglutination (matt formation) is visible by naked eyes. Button formation indicates absence of antibodies (Fig. 5.7)
- It is found to be 100% sensitive and specific. It is simple, rapid and does not need any instrument
- It is useful in macular PKDL cases missed by rK39 ICT test
- Disadvantage: However, antibodies persist up to 5 years after the treatment.

❖ **Immunochromatographic test (ICT):** ICT detects leishmanial antibody by using *L. chagasi* recombinant kinesin antigen (rK39)
- It claims 100% sensitivity and 98% specificity, however, the sensitivity is low in East Africa (attributed to extensive diversity of kinesin protein in East African *Leishmania* species) and in HIV patients
- Like DAT, it is also simple, rapid and does not need any instrument (useful in field studies)
- Recently, ICT based on another novel antigen rKE16 (from *L. donovani*) has been developed at AIIMS, New Delhi, India has shown high sensitivity and specificity.

Hypergammaglobulinemia (non-specific tests)
❖ **Napier's Aldehyde test:** Patient's serum (1 mL) is added with a drop of 40% formaldehyde in a test tube. Positive test is indicated by jellification of the serum forming milky white opacity within 3 minutes to 24 hours. Disadvantages include:
- It is negative in the first three months
- False positive results are seen with *Schistosoma japonicum, Trypanosoma cruzi,* multiple myeloma and cirrhosis
- It is negative in CL cases.

❖ **Chopra's antimony test:** Positive test is indicated by formation of profuse flocculation when patient's serum is mixed with 4% urea stibamine solution.

Antigen detection
Recently, latex agglutination test has been available detecting a heat-stable, low-molecular-weight carbohydrate antigen in the urine of VL patients. It has good specificity but variable sensitivity (40–80%). Antigen detection is more useful (i) in HIV-VL co-infection, (ii) as a prognostic marker, (iii) indicating active infection.

Molecular methods
Qualitative detection by PCR, nested PCR and quantitative detection by real-time PCR are available targeting *Leishmania* specific kinetoplast (mitochondrial) DNA. It is mostly confined to the reference laboratories with sensitivity varying from 70% to 93%.
❖ Other targets include 18S-rRNA, small subunit rRNA (more useful in HIV co-infection) and gene encoding cysteine proteinase, β-tubulin and gp63
❖ LAMP assay (loop-mediated isothermal amplification) has recently emerged as a novel molecular method for diagnosis of VL, particularly useful in field setting.

Leishmanin test (Montenegro test)
Introduced by Sir Montenegro in South America.
❖ It is a delayed hypersensitivity skin test to a suspension of killed *L. donovani* promastigote injected intradermally
❖ A positive test is indicated by induration of more than or equal to 5 mm in 72 hours
❖ Positive test indicates prior exposure to *Leishmania* antigens
❖ It is associated with higher false-positive result
❖ It is positive in people with good CMI:
- Asymptomatic individuals: It is used for epidemiological survey to estimate the burden of the disease
- Cutaneous leishmaniasis
- About 6–8 weeks after recovery from VL
- Leishmaniasis recidivans.
❖ However, this test is negative in [when CMI is low]:
- Active visceral leishmaniasis
- Diffuse cutaneous leishmaniasis.

Animal inoculation
Intranasal inoculation of specimens to golden hamsters yields amastigotes after several months. It is not in use nowadays.

Nonspecific tests

- Complete blood count—to detect pancytopenia
- Elevated liver enzymes
- Reversal of albumin globulin ratio (reflects hypergammaglobulinemia).

Treatment: Visceral leishmaniasis

The various drugs used in the treatment of VL are: (i) pentavalent antimonials, (ii) liposomal amphotericin B, (iii) miltefosine (iv) paromomycin. The WHO recommended regimens used for treatment of VL is given in Table 5.5.

Pentavalent antimonials

It has been the drug of choice and widely used in the past for several decades. However as the resistance has been emerged, currently, its use is restricted to regions where resistance has not developed.

- **Dosage:** It is given as 20 mg/kg per day IM or IV for 30 days
- **Mechanism of action:** It is converted to its active trivalent form in body, induces oxidative stress in the parasite and promotes efflux of anti-oxidative factors such as glutathione and other thiols from the parasite
- **Resistance:** Resistance to antimonials has been reported mostly from Bihar, India. Several mechanisms of resistance have been observed
  - Gene deletion in AQP1 (aquaporin): this prevents entry of drug into the parasite
  - Overexpression of gene coding *MRPA*, a transporter: This causes sequestration of the thiol-drug conjugate inside the parasitic vesicles, thus preventing the drug to act on the parasite. This appears to be common in Bihar, India
  - Overexpression of gene coding *MDR-1* (multidrug resistant): This mediates efflux of drug from the macrophage.

Liposomal amphotericin B

It has been the current drug of choice of leishmaniasis, especially in areas where resistance to antimonials have been reported.

- **Dosage:** It is given as 3–5 mg/kg per daily dose by IV infusion for 3–5 days up to a total dose of 15 mg/kg or 10 mg/kg as a single dose by infusion
- The total dose administered seems to be more important than the number of infusions or duration of therapy
- **Mechanism of action:** It acts by disrupting the cell membrane by forming pores
- **Resistance:** Reported very rarely. It is mediated by mutation in cysteine protease B gene.

Miltefosine

- **Dosage:** It is given as 150 mg/day; orally for 28 days
- **Mechanism of action:** by interacting with lipids, inhibiting cytochrome c oxidase
- **Resistance:** Resistance to miltefosine is rare, mainly reported from India and Nepal. Two cases from Bihar and Jharkhand were detected in AIIMS, New Delhi in 2017. Resistance is mediated by:
  - Deletion in *LdMT/LdRos3* gene, leads to decreased uptake
  - Over expression of ABC transporter (MDR1 gene), leads to increased efflux.

Paromomycin

It is an aminoglycoside antibiotic with anti-leishmanial activity. It is given IM at a dose of 15 mg per kg per day for 21 days.

Immunotherapy

Interferon-γ has been used in antimonial resistant and in selected relapse cases from Kenya, Brazil, and India.

Leishmania Tropica Complex

It includes three species—*L. tropica*, *L. aethiopica* and *L. major*. They cause **old world cutaneous leishmaniasis** (Table 5.6).

- *L. tropica* is reported from Western India (mainly Rajasthan), Middle East and Mediterranean coast. It mainly affects urban area hence known as agent of urban anthroponotic CL
- *L. aethiopica* infects people from Ethiopia, Uganda and Kenya
- *L. major* is reported from Middle East, India, China, Africa, and central and western Asia. It mainly affects rural area hence known as agent of rural zoonotic CL.

Life Cycle

The life cycle of the *L. tropica* complex is same as *L. donovani* except:

- The species of vector sandfly are different:
  - *L. tropica*—vector is *P. sergenti*
  - *L. aethiopica*—vector is *P. longipes*
  - *L. major*—vector is *P. papatasi*.
- Reservoir of infection:
  - *L. tropica*—is man (anthroponotic)
  - *L. aethiopica*—is *Hyraxes* (zoonotic)
  - *L. major*—is rodents (zoonotic).
- In humans, the amastigote forms reside in reticuloendothelial cells of skin (they do not migrate to viscera).

Table 5.5: WHO recommendation for treatment of VL in different regions of the world

Region	Drug regimen(s)

Indian subcontinent (ranked by preference)	• Liposomal amphotericin B
	• Combinations
	  ➢ Liposomal amphotericin B plus miltefosine
	  ➢ Liposomal amphotericin B plus paromomycin
	  ➢ Miltefosine plus paromomycin
	• Amphotericin B deoxycholate
	• Miltefosine
	• Paromomycin
	• Pentavalent antimonials

East Africa and Yemen	Pentavalent antimonial plus paromomycin
Mediterranean Basin, Middle East, Central Asia and in America (due to *L. infantum*)	Liposomal amphotericin B

Abbreviation: WHO, World Health Organization.

Table 5.6: Various agents of cutaneous leishmaniasis

Species	Geographical distribution	Clinical syndrome	Vector (Sandfly)	Reservoir	Transmission
L. L. tropica (Oriental sore)	Western India, North Africa, and Middle East	CL, LR	*Phlebotomus sergenti*	Humans	Anthroponotic
L. L. aethiopica	Ethiopia, Uganda, and Kenya	CL, DCL	*P. longipes*	Hyraxes	Zoonotic
L. L. major	Middle East, India, China, Africa, Central and Western Asia	CL	*P. papatasi*	Rodents	Zoonotic

Abbreviations: CL, cutaneous leishmaniasis; LR, leishmania recidivans; DCL, diffuse cutaneous leishmaniasis.

Clinical Features

Cutaneous leishmaniasis

It is caused by *L. tropica* complex. This condition is also known as **"Oriental sore"**, Delhi evil, Delhi boil, Aleppo Boil and Baghdad Button, etc. (Fig. 5.8A).

- Incubation period ranges from 2–8 weeks
- Oriental sore usually occurs on face and hands
- It begins as painless papule, becomes nodular and finally it ulcerates
- The margins of the ulcers are raised and indurated
- Lesions in *L. tropica* are more swollen, having a thicker crust and less necrotic, less exudative than the lesions of *L. major*. *L. major* lesions are multiple as compared to *L. tropica*; where lesions appear in single or two
- Mostly, it heals spontaneously leaving behind a scar. However, disfiguring facial lesions of *L. tropica* may be psychologically devastating
- There may be satellite lesions, especially in *L. major* and *L. tropica* infections
- Lymphatic spread may be seen in *L. major* producing nodular lesion, clinically resembling to sporotrichosis.

Leishmaniasis recidivans (LR)

LR is a granulomatous response, that occurs years after healing of primary sore due to *L. tropica*.

- It is characterized by new lesions formed on the face, usually scaly, erythematous papules and nodules develop in the center or periphery of a previously healed sore
- It resembles cutaneous tuberculosis; hence LR is also known as lupoid leishmaniasis
- CMI is intact and skin test is positive
- Very few parasites can be demonstrated in the smears from the lesions (Fig. 5.8B).
- LR is primarily seen in Iran and Iraq.

Diffuse cutaneous leishmaniasis (DCL)

DCL is a rare form of leishmaniasis, caused by *L. aethiopica* in Ethiopia and Kenya (old World).

- It is characterized by the lack of a CMI response to the parasite
- Approximately 100 cases have been reported so far, mainly from Kenya and Ethiopia
- Lack of CMI leads to widespread cutaneous disease—symmetric or asymmetric distribution of various lesions like papules, nodules, plaques, and areas of diffuse infiltration, nonulcerative lesions with heavy load of parasites. Lesions may be confused with that of lepromatous leprosy (LL). The difference is DCL lesions are softer compared to indurated lesions of LL
- The DTH response is negative, so skin test, i.e. Montenegro test is negative
- DCL can also be seen in new world, caused by *L. amazonensis* and *L. mexicana* in South and Central America
- It responds poorly to treatment; disease may last long.

Laboratory Diagnosis of CL

Microscopy

Amastigotes can be demonstrated from punch biopsies taken from the edge of the active lesion stained with Giemsa. Amastigotes are better detected in touch preparation (impression smear) than in tissues section.

Culture

Aspiration from the ulcers can be cultured in NNN medium and Schneider's Drosophila medium for the isolation of promastigote forms.

Montenegro test

Positive leishmanin skin test indicates delayed hypersensitivity reaction to the parasite. However, it is negative in diffuse CL (Table 5.7).

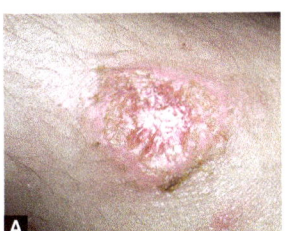
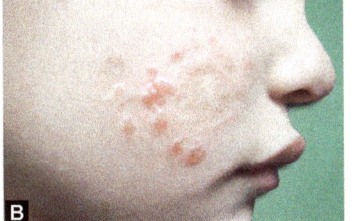

Figs 5.8A and B: Clinical features of: (A) Cutaneous leishmaniasis; (B) Leishmaniasis recidivans

Source: A—World Health Organization, "Manual on visceral leishmaniasis control" (*with permission*); B—Global Skin Atlas/Image Number 2268/Nameer Al-Sudany (*with permission*).

Table 5.7: Differences between various types of leishmaniasis

	MCL, LR	CL	VL, PKDL and DCL
Parasite burden	+	++	+++
Immune response	CMI	CMI	Humoral
Hypergammaglobulinemia	-	-	+++
Delayed hypersensitivity	+++	+	-
Diagnostic tests preferred	PCR, DTH	Culture	Smear Serology

Abbreviations: VL, Visceral leishmaniasis; PKDL, post-kala-azar dermal leishmaniasis; CL, cutaneous leishmaniasis; LR, leishmaniasis recidivans DCL, diffuse cutaneous leishmaniasis; MCL, mucocutaneous leishmaniasis; PCR, polymerase chain reaction; DTH, delayed hypersensitivity; CMI, cell-mediated immune response

Treatment — Cutaneous Leishmaniasis (Old World)

Local therapy is usually recommended. Options available are (i) paromomycin (15%) or methyl benzethonium (12%) ointment for 20 days, (ii) intralesional antimonials, (iii) cryotherapy and (iv) thermotherapy.

Systemic therapy: It is required only for disfiguring or scarring lesions. Various options available are:
- *L. major*— (i) fluconazole for 6 weeks, (ii) pentavalent antimonials with or without pentoxifylline for 10–20 days
- *L. tropica*—Pentavalent antimonials for 10–20 days. In LR cases, it is combined with oral allopurinol
- *L. aethiopica*—Pentavalent antimonials plus paromomycin for 60 days or longer.

Prevention of Leishmaniasis

National vector-borne disease control program

NVBDCP is a national program in India which works for the control of six common vector-borne diseases in India. It has launched the **accelerated plan for kala-azar elimination** in 2017. The target for elimination is to reduce the annual incidence of kala-azar to less than one per 10,000 populations at block PHC level. The blocks in endemic area of India are classified into four categories based on annual incidence of kala-azar; each category has a specific action plan aiming towards kala-azar elimination, as described in Table 5.8.

Vaccine Trials

Currently, no vaccine is available for the prevention of leishmaniasis. However, several trials are going on.
- Both killed and live-attenuated vaccine trials are on going targeting antigens derived from killed promastigotes of several species such as *L. tropica* and *L. amazonensis* and *L. mexicana*
- Trials for recombinant and synthetic vaccines are also on going using gp-63 antigen
- **Vaccine targets for CL include:** *L. major* thiol-specific antioxidant, stress inducible protein-1 and elongation initiation factor

Table 5.8: Categorization of blocks in endemic area* of India based on annual incidence of kala-azar, 2014

Categories	Definition	Measures to be taken
Category I (94 blocks)	Blocks above elimination threshold (high transmission areas) Annual incidence >1 case per 10,000 population	Intensive case detection Vector control activities Case based surveillance
Category II (23 blocks)	Blocks with borderline endemicity Annual incidence 0.8 to <1 per 10,0000 population (low transmission area)	Requires enhanced surveillance
Category III (290 blocks)	Fluctuation blocks with increasing or decreasing trend either year to year or with a gap of few years	Operation factors to be looked in
Category IV (207 blocks)	Silent blocks, i.e. areas reporting nil cases annually for at least two consecutive years	Robust surveillance for validation of nil status Preparedness for detection if cases occur

*Endemic region include Bihar, Jharkhand, Uttar Pradesh and West Bengal

- **Targets for VL include:** Leish-111f + MPL-SE and *Leishmania* methyltransferase
- **Transmission blocking vaccines** are based on salivary gland proteins
- **Leishmanization:** This is an old method, was used for prevention of CL. It involves inoculating into buttock or arm with live promastigotes from culture (Jericho strains of *L. major*); which leads to development of mild skin lesions with subsequent artificial protective immunity thus preventing disfigured lesions on face in future. This is the only method of vaccination available so far with proven efficacy and has been approved for use in Uzbekistan.

Control Measures

Vector control measures should be followed such as:
- Personal prophylaxis by using insect repellents or bed nets
- Control of canine or rodent reservoir
- *Phlebotomus* does not fly high above the ground level and it is nocturnal in habitat. So, sleeping at top floors also can prevent transmission
- Early treatment of all cases (mainly anthroponotic VL and PKDL cases).

NEW WORLD LEISHMANIASIS

New World leishmaniasis is mainly caused by:
- *Leishmania Viannia* (*L.V.*) *braziliensis* complex
- *Leishmania Leishmania* (*L.L.*) *mexicana* complex
- *L.L. chagasi* (new world variant of *L.L. infantum*).

CHAPTER 5 ◆ Flagellates—II (Hemoflagellates)

Table 5.9: *Leishmania Leishmania mexicana* complex and *Leishmania Viannia braziliensis* complex

Leishmania Leishmania mexicana complex			Leishmania Viannia braziliensis complex		
Species	Geographical distribution	Clinical syndrome	Species	Geographical distribution	Clinical syndrome
L. L. mexicana	Central America and northern parts of South America (the Amazon basin)	CL (chiclero ulcer) DCL	L. V. braziliensis	Brazil	CL, MCL (espundia), LR (rare)
L. L. amazonensis		CL, DCL and VL (rare)	L. V. panamensis	Panama, Colombia	CL, MCL
L. L. venezuelensis L. L. garnhami		CL	L.V. guyanensis	Guyana	CL(forest yaws), MCL
L. L. pifanoi		CL, DCL	L. V. peruviana	Peru	CL(Uta), MCL
Reservoir: Forest rodents, marsupial and humans			Reservoir: Dogs, foxes, forest rodents and humans		
Vector: *Lutzomyia* species and Transmission: Zoonotic (for both complexes)					

Abbreviations: CL, cutaneous leishmaniasis; DCL, diffuse cutaneous leishmaniasis; MCL, mucocutaneous leishmaniasis; LR, leishmaniasis recidivans.

The morphology and life cycle of new world *Leishmania* species are identical to that of *L. donovani* except:
- Geographical distribution-restricted to central and south America
- **Vector:** *Lutzomyia* species
- **Reservoir of infection:** Dogs, foxes (zoonotic)
- The amastigote forms in humans reside in reticuloendothelial cells of skin and mucous membrane (do not invade viscera).

Clinical Features of New World Leishmaniasis

Leishmania Mexicana Complex

L. mexicana complex infected people develop CL similar to those seen with old world cutaneous disease (Table 5.9).
- *L. mexicana* causes a specific form of CL called as **chiclero ulcer** (or bay sore) characterized by persistent ulcerations in pinna seen in Central America among workers living in forests harvesting chicle plants to collect chewing gum latex. 30% of people are infected during the first year of exposure
- *L. mexicana* and *L. amazonensis* produce DCL similar to that is described earlier for *L. aethiopica*.

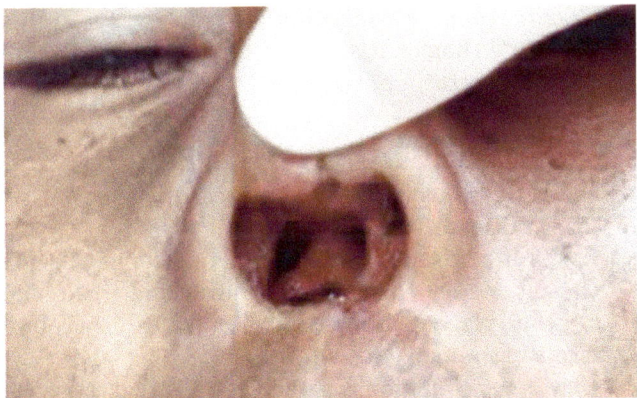

Fig. 5.9: Mucocutaneous leishmaniasis or espundia
Source: Calvopina et al. BMC Infectious Diseases 2006 (*with permission*).

Leishmania Viannia braziliensis Complex

They cause MCL and also CL similar to oriental sore but they are more severe.

Espundia (mucocutaneous leishmaniasis or MCL)

L. braziliensis infects mucous membrane of the nose, oral cavity, pharynx or larynx months to years after the CL.
- It is seen in 1 to 3% of patients infected with *L. braziliensis* after months to years of CL, where the parasite shows metastatic spread to nasal, pharyngeal, and buccal mucosa
- The initial symptoms are often nasal stuffiness, erythema and mucopurulent discharge
- It may eventually involve the upper lip, buccal, pharyngeal, or laryngeal mucosa (Fig. 5.9)
- Ulcerative lesions are formed with erosion of the soft tissue and the cartilages leading to loss of lips, soft part of nose and soft palate. The palatal perforative lesions are called **'Escomel cross'**
- Gradually, the nasal septum may be destroyed, resulting in nasal collapse with hypertrophy of upper lip and nose leading to development of **"tapir nose"**.

Forest yaws and uta: The cutaneous lesions of *L. V. guyanensis* and *L.V. peruviana* are known as forest yaws (pian bois) and uta respectively.

The lesions of *L. guyanensis* and *L. panamensis* are multiple, nodular and have lymphatic spread similar to sporotrichosis.

American CL
The various New World CL which include uta (Peru), dicera de Baurid (Brazil), chiclero ulcer or bay sore (Mexico), and pian bois or forest yaws (Guyana) are collectively called as American cutaneous leishmaniasis (ACL).

Leishmania virus
It is a double stranded RNA virus that persistently infects *L.V. braziliensis* and *L.V. guyanensis*. It has a possible role in alteration of parasitic phenotype and disease pathogenesis. It may be a future target for diagnostic and therapeutic intervention.

Leishmania Leishmania chagasi

L. L. chagasi is the new world variant of *L. L. infantum*. (the agent of Mediterranean VL of Old World).

- Causes American VL (AVL), Atypical CL (ACL) and also PKDL
- AVL occurs in malnourished children <5 years old; whereas ACL occurs in children >5 years and young adults
- Occurs in rural areas of Central and South American region
- It is zoonotic (canine reservoir)
- Vector: *Lutzomyia longipalpis*.

Laboratory Diagnosis of New World Leishmaniasis

Microscopy

Amastigote forms within the macrophages are found abundant in the lesions of DCL followed by VL and CL, when stained with Giemsa or Leishman stain. However in lesions of MCL, fewer parasites are found.

Culture

Skin and mucosal biopsy specimens are first minced to release the organisms and then inoculated onto NNN media and Schneider's *Drosophila* medium.

Montenegro Test

Positive Leishmanin skin test indicates delayed hypersensitivity reaction to the parasites. However, it is negative in diffuse CL and active VL (*L. chagasi*).

Antibody Detection

Antibodies are detected in patients with active VL by various formats described before. However, they show variable sensitivity in CL and poor response in MCL and DCL.

Treatment — New World cutaneous leishmaniasis

In contrast to Old World CL, systemic therapy is recommended for New World CL as the lesions are more chronic, multiple and have tendency for mucosal involvement. **Local therapy** can be given in addition; agents are same as used for Old World CL.
The regimen for **systemic therapy** depends upon the causative agent.
- *L. mexicana*: Ketoconazole or miltefosine for 28 days
- *L. guyanensis* and *L. panamensis*: Pentamidine or pentavalent antimonials or miltefosine for 28 days
- *L. braziliensis*: Pentavalent antimonials for 20 days; or amphotericin B
- *L. amazonensis, L. peruviana* and *L. venezuelensis*: Pentavalent antimonials for 20 days
- Relapse treatment: Amphotericin B or pentavalent antimonials plus topical imiquimod is recommended.

For MCL (all species): (i) pentavalent antimonials with or without oral pentoxifylline for 30 days ; (ii) amphotericin B; (iii) in Bolivia: miltefosine is the agent of choice.

TRYPANOSOMA

Trypanosomes are hemoflagellates that reside in peripheral blood and tissues of their host. Based on their geographical distribution, they can be classified into two types:

African trypanosomes

The African trypanosomes belong to the subgenus *Trypanozoon* and as a group are referred to as the *Trypanosoma brucei* complex. They are transmitted by the vector tsetse fly. They comprise of three subspecies out of which only the first two infect humans.

- ***Trypanosoma brucei rhodesiense:*** It is the causative agent of East African sleeping sickness in man
- ***Trypanosoma brucei gambiense:*** It is the causative agent of West African sleeping sickness in man.
- ***Trypanosoma brucei brucei:*** It causes "nagana", a disease affecting cattle in Africa.

American trypanosomes

Trypanosoma infecting humans in the America belong to two subgenera:

- Subgenus *Schizotrypanum:* It has one species named *T. cruzi*; which is the causative agent of South American trypanosomiasis in man (also called as Chagas' disease) and is transmitted by insect vector reduviid bug
- Subgenus *Tejaraia:* It has one species named *T. rangeli*; which is a non-pathogen, rarely causes asymptomatic infection in man.

Apart from the above, there are few animal trypanosomes which do not infect man

- *T. congolense* and *T. vivax*: They cause disease similar to that of *T. brucei brucei*
- *Trypanosoma evansi*: It causes **"Surra"** in horses and other animals. It is transmitted by flies (tabanidae and stomoxys). Many animal cases have been reported from India
- *Trypanosoma lewisi*: It causes a harmless infection affecting rodents
- *Trypanosoma equiperdum*: It causes **"Stallion's disease"** in horses. It is transmitted by sexual route (not by insect vector).

TRYPANOSOMA CRUZI

It is the causative agent of South American trypanosomiasis or Chagas' disease.

- It was first discovered by Brazilian scientist **Carlos Chagas,** in 1909, isolated from reduviid bug (triatomine bug) and blood of infected monkeys. Later on he found it causing human infection also
- Hence, the condition is named as Chagas' disease. He named the parasite as *T. cruzi* after his guide Oswaldo Cruz.

Habitat

In humans, *T. cruzi* exists in two forms: (1) amastigote and (2) trypomastigote form.

- Amastigotes are intracellular parasite found in reticuloendothelial cells of spleen, liver, lymph node, bone marrow, and myocardium. They are also found in cells of epidermis and striated muscles
- Trypomastigotes are extracellular and found in peripheral blood.

Epidemiology

Chagas' disease is mainly restricted to South and Central American countries like Brazil, Argentina, Venezuela, etc.

- Currently, it is estimated that 16-18 million people are infected with *T. cruzi*. Annual incidence is around 2 Lakhs new cases with 50,000 deaths
- It is a zoonotic disease, having many animal reservoirs like dogs, cats, opossums and rodents.

Morphology

- In vertebrate host, it exists mainly in two forms—(1) trypomastigote form and (2) amastigote form
- In insect vector (reduviid bug), it exists as (1) trypomastigote, (2) epimastigote form.

Trypomastigote Form

It is spindle shaped; measures around 20 μm and appears as C or U shaped

- It is seen in the peripheral blood of the infected patients in two forms—(1) long slender form and (2) short stubby form
- It consists of a central nucleus and large kinetoplast situated posteriorly from which flagellum originates and traverses the whole body as undulating membrane and comes out from the anterior end as free flagellum
- It does not multiply (Figs 5.10A and 5.14).

Amastigote Form

It is found inside the cells of striated muscle (skeletal and cardiac), nervous tissue and reticuloendothelial cells

- When fully developed, a large number of amastigotes may be found in a cyst like cavity
- This is indistinguishable from those found in *Leishmania* infection

- It is round to oval, 2-6 μm in size having a large nucleus, rod shaped kinetoplast and axoneme but no flagella
- It is the multiplying form of the parasite (Fig. 5.10B).

Life Cycle (Fig. 5.11)

Host: *T. cruzi* passes its life cycle in two hosts—(1) humans and (2) vector reduviid bugs or kissing bugs or triatomine bugs (*Triatoma infestans*, *Rhodnius prolixus* and *Panstrongylus megistus*) (Fig. 5.12).

Infective form: Metacyclic trypomastigote form is the infective form, found in feces of reduviid bugs.

Mode of transmission: Reduviid bugs are nocturnal in habitat and humans get infection when abraded skin, mucous membranes, or conjunctivae become

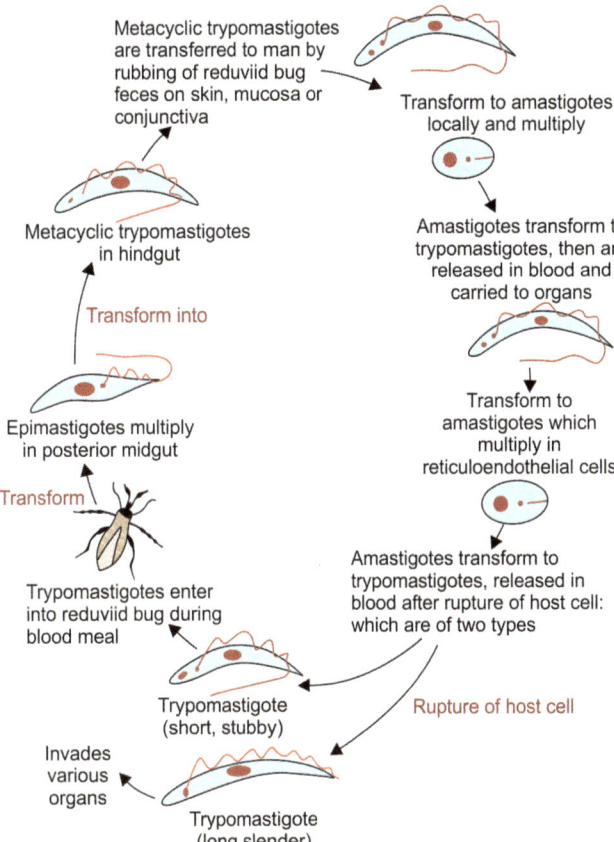

Fig. 5.11: Life cycle of *Trypanosoma cruzi*

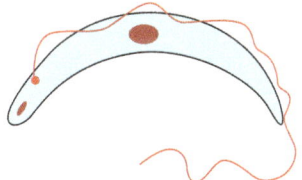 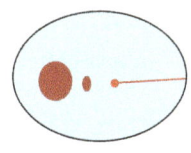

Figs 5.10A and B: *Trypanosoma cruzi* (schematic diagram): (A) Trypomastigote form; (B) Amastigote form

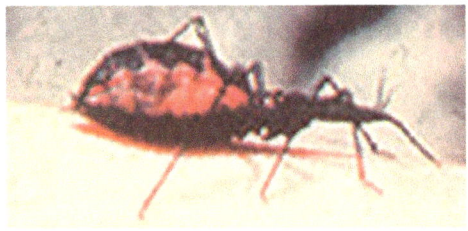

Fig. 5.12: Reduviid bug

Source: DPDx Image Library, Centre for Disease Control and prevention (CDC), Atlanta (*with permission*).

contaminated with reduviid bug's feces containing infective form of the parasite (by rubbing or scratching the feces into the bite wound).

T. cruzi can also be transmitted by the blood transfusion, organ transplantation, from mother to fetus or very rarely by ingestion of contaminated food or drink, and most importantly by laboratory accidents.

Human cycle

On entry into the body, metacyclic trypomastigotes invade local tissues where they lose their flagella and transform to amastigote forms

- ❖ Amastigotes are the replicating form, multiply inside the cells by binary fission and transform to trypomastigotes, which are released in to circulation and carried to various organs where they again transform back to amastigotes
- ❖ The amastigotes multiply preferably in reticuloendothelial cells and other tissues like muscle (cardiac, skeletal and GIT muscles) and nervous tissue. When they intend to invade other sites, they transform to motile C-shaped non-multiplying trypomastigote forms which are released into blood following rupture of the host cells
- ❖ Trypomastigotes in blood occur in two forms; a long slender and a short stubby
    - Long slender forms are the invasive forms, migrate to many organs and continue the life cycle
    - Short stubby forms persist in the blood, to be taken up by the insect vector during a blood meal.

Vector Cycle

During the blood meal, the trypomastigotes are ingested by the reduviid bug.

- ❖ Trypomastigotes transform into epimastigotes, which multiply in the posterior midgut
- ❖ After 8 to 10 days, the epimastigotes transform into metacyclic trypomastigotes in the hindgut and are excreted in the bug's feces
- ❖ The insect cycle takes about 10-15 days (extrinsic incubation period). There is no transovarian transmission seen in the bugs and once infected, they retain the infection throughout the life by the molting cycles.

Pathogenesis and Clinical Feature

Average incubation period is around 1-2 weeks. *T. cruzi* causes American trypanosomiasis (also called as Chagas' disease) which can be divided into four stages.

Early Stage Disease

It is characterized by:

- ❖ **Chagoma:** An erythematous subcutaneous nodule is formed at the site of deposition of bug's feces. It

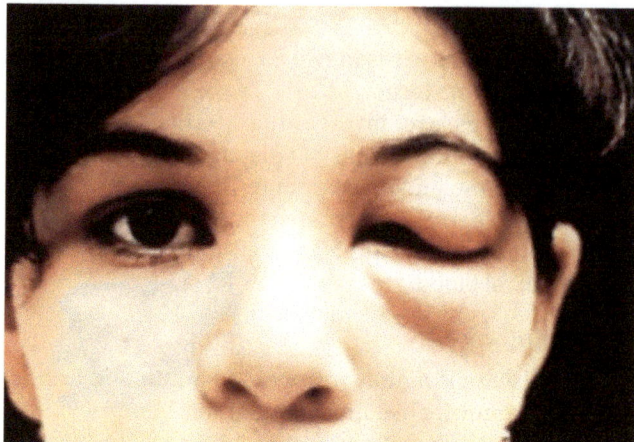

Fig. 5.13: Romana's sign in the eyelid
Source: Centers for Disease Control and Prevention (CDC), Atlanta and WHO/TDR (*with permission*).

is painful, commonly occurs on face and may take 2-3 months to resolve
- ❖ **Romana's sign:** When the parasites enter through conjunctiva, there occurs an unilateral painless edema of the eye lid and conjunctivitis (Fig. 5.13). Though pathognomonic, it is observed only in 48% of cases.

Acute Chagas' Disease

About 1% of patients, commonly the younger children progress to acute stage disease, characterized by:

- ❖ High fever, hepatosplenomegaly
- ❖ Acute myocarditis leading to conduction defects resulting in deaths
- ❖ Meningoencephalitis and generalized lymphadenopathy
- ❖ Usually within 4-8 weeks, patient either succumbs death or recovers spontaneously or develops chronic infection.

Indeterminate Stage

It is the initial asymptomatic phase of the chronic stage.

- ❖ It lasts for years to decades before progressing into symptomatic chronic stage. Some cases, it does not progress further if infected strain is of low virulent
- ❖ **Immune evasion:** The longer persistence of the parasite is related to (i) intracellular location, (ii) invasion to large number of different cell types, (iii) plasticity of the parasites resulting in frequent transformation between extracellular trypomastigotes and intracellular amastigotes.

Chronic Chagas' Disease

About 30% of cases progress to the symptomatic phase of chronic stage, usually years to decade later. Genetic susceptibility of the host may play a role in the progression of the disease. The parasite multiples in the muscles (cardiac and GIT) and nervous tissue; producing various types of manifestation.

- ❖ **Cardiac form:** Occurs in 30% of the patients. Patient develops dilated cardiomyopathy, rhythm disturbances like right bundle-branch block, and thromboembolism
- ❖ **Gastrointestinal form:** Involvement of muscles of GIT leads to megaesophagus (manifested as dysphagia, chest pain, and regurgitation) and megacolon (manifested as abdominal pain and chronic constipation)
- ❖ Megaesophagus may lead to aspiration pneumonia
- ❖ Colon cancers have been associated with chagasic megacolon, though the evidence is conflicting
- ❖ Mixed forms are observed in 10% of the patients.

Autoimmune hypothesis

Though not fully proved, an autoimmune mechanism has been suggested for the pathogenesis of chronic Chagas' disease. T. cruzi antigens cross react with mammalian antigens (molecular mimicry) and many autoantibodies have been detected in infected patients.

- ❖ EVI antibody (an antibody that reacts with endocardium, vascular structures, and interstitium of striated muscle)
- ❖ Antibodies that react with the Schwann sheaths of somatic and autonomic peripheral nerves.

Congenital Trypanosomiasis

Rarely, *T. cruzi* can be transmitted transplacentally both in acute and chronic stage of the disease. It manifests as low birth weight, still birth, rarely myocarditis and neurological alterations.

Association with HIV and HTLV-II

HIV-infected people are at a greater risk of reactivation of underlying *T. cruzi* infection and are more prone to develop meningoencephalitis. Human T-lymphotropic virus 2 (HTLV-II)-infected people have higher association (2.3 times) with *T. cruzi* infection.

Immune Response

Both cell-mediated and humoral immunity are involved against the parasite. IgM antibodies appear early during acute infection. Then the class switch over occurs and IgG and IgA antibodies predominate in the chronic stage of the disease. Antigenic variation which is the characteristic feature of African trypanosomiasis, is rarely observed in *T. cruzi*. CMI, to be particular antibody-dependent cell cytotoxicity (ADCC) is mainly involved in tissue destruction in the chronic stage such as cardiomyopathy and megacolon.

Laboratory Diagnosis *Trypanosoma cruzi*

- ❑ **Peripheral blood microscopy** by wet mount, thick or thin smear—detects trypomastigotes (C' shaped, 20 μm)
- ❑ **Culture**—NNN medium or Yager's liver infusion tryptose medium (epimastigote forms)
- ❑ **Antibody detection** in serum—ELISA, IFA, RIPA, western blot, enzyme strip assay
- ❑ **Antigen detection** from serum, urine—by CLIA and ELISA
- ❑ **Molecular methods**—PCR, using 88 bp TCZ1–TCZ2 primers
- ❑ **Animal inoculation**—mice
- ❑ **Xenodiagnosis**—nymph of reduviid bugs.

Laboratory Diagnosis

Peripheral Blood Microscopy

In acute Chagas' disease, the trypomastigotes (Fig. 5.14A) are frequently found in peripheral blood which can be detected by:

- ❖ **Wet mount** preparation of anticoagulated blood or buffy coat can be done to see the rapid movements of trypomastigotes
- ❖ **Thick and thin smear** (Giemsa staining): Thick smear is more sensitive in detecting the trypomastigotes whereas the thin smear helps in differentiating *T. cruzi* with morphologically similar looking *T. rangeli* (Table 5.10)
- ❖ **Blood concentration techniques** like microhematocrit method and Strout method of buffy coat preparation may be employed if the parasite count is low. Strout method is the most sensitive, involves examination of centrifuged deposit of serum stained with Giemsa stain.

Microscopy from other specimens

- ❖ Amastigotes can be demonstrated in heart tissue obtained at autopsy stained by histopathological stain (Fig. 5.14B)
- ❖ Aspirate from chagoma and enlarged lymph nodes can be examined for amastigotes and trypomastigotes.

Table 5.10: Differences between trypomastigote form of *Trypanosoma cruzi* and *Trypanosoma rangeli*

	Trypanosoma cruzi	*Trypanosoma rangeli*
Pathogenicity	Pathogen, causes Chagas' disease	Nonpathogenic
Size of trypomastigote	Average 20 μm	Average 30 μm
Shape	Often 'C' shaped	Rarely 'C' shaped
Kinetoplast	Large and terminal	Small and subterminal
Posterior end	Short blunt	Long pointed
Location in reduviid bug	Hindgut (feces) Transmitted by rubbing of reduviid bug's feces on abraded skin	Usually found in salivary gland Transmitted by bite of bugs

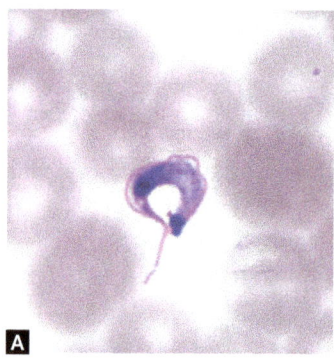 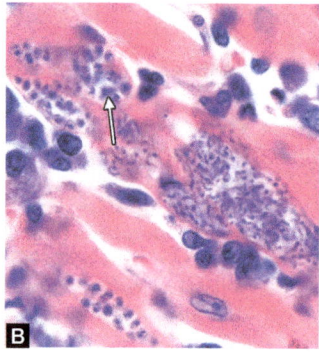 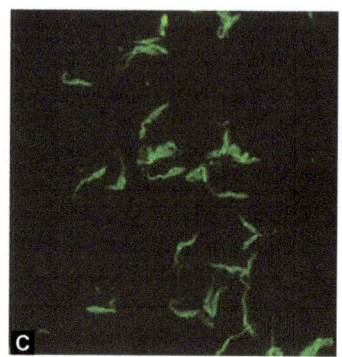 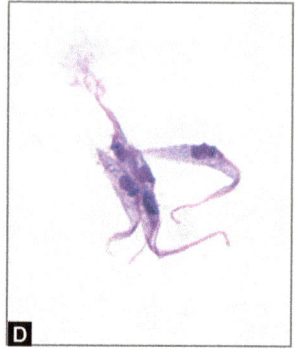

Figs 5.14A to D: *Trypanosoma cruzi*: (A) Trypomastigote form (thin blood smear stained with Giemsa); (B) Amastigote forms in heart tissue stained by hematoxylin and eosin; (C) Indirect fluorescent antibody test showing trypomastigote forms; (D) Epimastigotes from culture
Source: DPDx Image Library, Centers for Disease Control and Prevention (CDC), Atlanta (*with permission*).

Culture

Blood is inoculated onto NNN medium or Yager's liver infusion tryptose medium, incubated at 25°C and observed for the epimastigote forms for up to 30 days before they are considered negative. Culture is more sensitive than smear microscopy (Fig. 5.14D).

Antibody Detection

Chronic Chagas' disease is diagnosed by the detection of specific IgG antibodies against *T. cruzi* antigens. IgM antibodies are diagnostic for congenital infection.
- ❖ Several methods are employed like CFT (Guerreiro Machado test), ELISA and IFA (Fig. 5.14C)
- ❖ Confirmatory serologic assays are:
  - Western blot
  - Chagas' RIPA (Radioimmunoprecipitation assay): It is highly sensitive and specific.
  - Enzyme strip assay (ESA) using recombinant antigen.
- ❖ However, false positive reactions may occur in patients with *T. rangeli* infection, leishmaniasis, syphilis, etc.
- ❖ Detection of IgM and IgA is useful in arriving diagnosis of congenital infection.

Antigen Detection

T. cruzi specific antigens from serum and urine of the infected patients are detected by ELISA which are very useful for diagnosing acute infection and congenital transmission. Recently, a chemiluminescence immunoassay (CLIA) based assay has been developed for blood bank screening and for the monitoring the response to treatment.

Molecular Methods

PCR is available that detects *T. cruzi* specific kinetoplast or nuclear DNA (e.g. 188 bp TCZ1-TCZ2 primer and 330 bp S35-S36 primer) in blood. It is more sensitive than microscopy and serology for the diagnosis of chronic disease. It can detect as low as one trypomastigote per 20 mL of blood. It is also useful in monitoring the response to treatment and for the diagnosis of congenital infection.

Animal Inoculation

Blood or CSF of the patients is inoculated intraperitoneally into mice. Trypomastigotes can be demonstrated from the blood of mice within 10 days of inoculation.

Xenodiagnosis

The infected patients are exposed to 20 numbers of laboratory maintained nymphs of uninfected reduviid bugs daily for 3 days and the feces of the insects are examined by microscopy, monthly for 3 months for the presence of the epimastigote forms. PCR (most sensitive) or antigen detection by using monoclonal antibody can also be done. Xenodiagnosis is more sensitive, useful for detection of light chronic infection.

Treatment — *Trypanosoma cruzi*

Therapy for Chagas' disease is still unsatisfactory.
In acute disease:
- ❑ Benznidazole is considered as the drug of choice in Latin America. The recommended oral dosage is 5 mg/kg per day for adults and 5–10 mg/kg per day for children for 60 days
- ❑ Nifurtimox is given 8–10 mg/kg for adults and 15–20 mg/kg for children in four divided doses for 90–120 days
- ❑ Allopurinol—limited trials showed its efficacy.

In chronic disease: These drugs lack efficacy and may cause many side effects. Supportive treatment such as pacemakers to manage arrhythmias and surgery for correction of megaesophagus and megacolon may be useful.

Prophylaxis

Prevention of the disease in endemic countries depends on control of vector. This includes residual insecticides, health education, measures to reduce insect exposure and housing improvement. No vaccines are available, however several experimental vaccines (such as DNA vaccine or recombinant proteins) are under trial.

TRYPANOSOMA BRUCEI COMPLEX

T. brucei was first demonstrated in human by Sir Forde, near Gambia river in 1901. In 1902, Dutton proposed the name *T. gambiense*. Sir Bruce in 1909, proved that the disease is transmitted by tsetse fly. *T. rhodesiense* was first discovered in the blood of a patient in Rhodesia by Stephans and Fantham in 1910.

T. brucei complex consists of three subspecies:
1. **T. brucei gambiense:** Agent of West African sleeping sickness.
2. **T. brucei rhodesiense:** Agent of East African sleeping sickness.
3. **T. brucei brucei:** Causes "nagana", a disease affecting cattle in Africa. It does not infect humans.

Epidemiology

African trypanosomiasis is endemic in 36 countries of Africa with 60 million people at risk. Approximately 50,000 new cases occur annually.

Life Cycle (Fig. 5.15)

Host: *T. brucei* passes its life cycle in two hosts.
1. The **vertebrate host** is man and other animals.
2. **Invertebrate host** is the **tsetse fly** (genus *Glossina*) (Fig. 16.6.) Both male and female flies bite man and serve as vectors. *Glossina palpalis* group serves as the vector for *T. brucei gambiense;* whereas *Glossina morsitans* group is the vector for *T. brucei rhodesiense*.

Infective form: The metacyclic trypomastigote forms are found in salivary gland of tsetse fly.

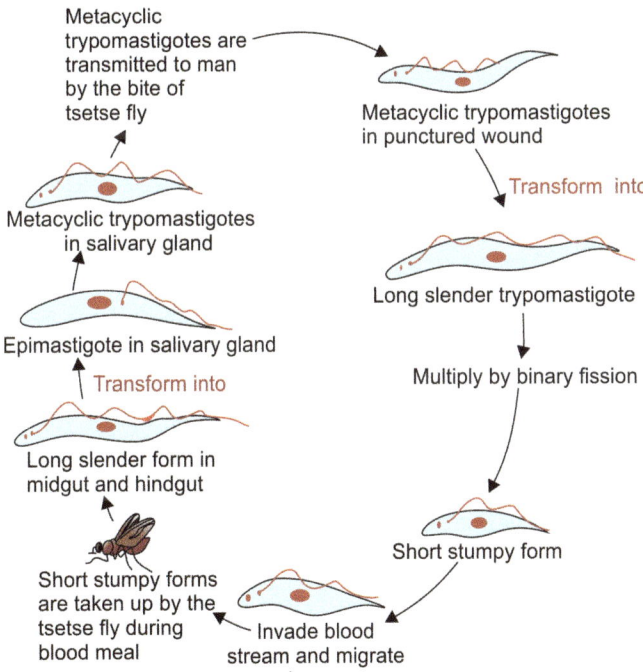

Fig. 5.15: Life cycle of *Trypanosoma brucei*

Mode of transmission: By the bite of tsetse fly, trypomastigote forms are transmitted to the punctured wound from the saliva of the tsetse fly.

Development in Man

At the site of inoculation, they transform into long slender trypomastigote forms of 30 μm long, which multiply by binary fission
- They transform into an intermediate stage and then into nondividing short stumpy form (15 μm long) without free flagellum
- Subsequently, the parasites invade the blood stream resulting in parasitemia and migrate to various organs including CNS
- The short stumpy forms are the infective form to the tsetse fly, hence the transformation of long slender trypomastigotes into short stumpy forms is critical for the transmission of the parasite.

Development in Tsetse Fly

The short stumpy trypomastigote forms are taken up by the tsetse fly along with the blood meal
- They become long slender forms in the midgut and hindgut of the insect where they multiply for two weeks and finally reach the salivary gland
- They attach to the epithelial cells of salivary ducts and transform into broad epimastigote forms
- Finally, the epimastigotes develop into metacyclic trypomastigote forms which are the infective forms to man
- It takes around 3 weeks from the time of blood meal till the fly becomes infective (extrinsic incubation period), then the fly remains infected throughout the life.

Antigenic Variation

Trypomastigotes undergo periodic antigenic variation leading to frequent change of antigenic nature of variable surface glycoprotein (VSG) antigens present on their surface. This serves as the key mechanism of evading host immune (humoral) response.
- Genome of *Trypanosoma brucei* contains thousands of genes that undergo gene switching (like mutations, deletions, additions or recombinations) leading to formation of new **serotype**
- Every 5-7 days, a new wave of genes evolves, that codes for a new batch of serotype. More than 100 serotypes can be present in a single infection. Host immunity is strain specific hence, is not able to eliminate the new waves of parasitemia
- The VSG secreted following antigenic switching are shed into the blood and cause various immune dysregulations such as release of interferon-γ (which stimulates parasite growth), suppression of interleukin-2, and hypergammaglobulinemia.

Table 5.11: Comparison between *Trypanosoma brucei gambiense* and *Trypanosoma brucei rhodesiense*

	Trypanosoma brucei gambiense	*Trypanosoma brucei rhodesiense*
Disease	West African sleeping sickness	East African sleeping sickness
Vectors	Tsetse flies (*Glossina palpalis* group)	Tsetse flies (*Glossina morsitans* group)
Primary reservoir	Humans	Animals (Antelope and cattle)
Human illness	Chronic central nervous system (CNS) disease	Acute (early CNS disease) up to 9 months
Duration of illness	Months to years	<9 months (before that the death occurs)
Lymphadenopathy	Frequent, cervical lymphadenopathy (winter bottom sign)	Minimal (Axially and inguinal)
Parasitemia	Low	High
Virulence	Less	More
Rodent inoculation	Not useful	Diagnostic
Epidemiology	Rural populations	Workers in wild areas, rural populations, and tourists in game parks
Response to drugs	Less resistant	More resistant

Pathogenesis and Clinical Feature

In general, *T. brucei gambiense* develops a chronic course with slow progression; whereas *T. brucei rhodesiense* runs an acute course with rapid progression and early death (Table 5.11).

Trypanosomal Chancre

A self-limited inflammatory lesion may appear a week after the bite of an infected tsetse fly.

Stage I Disease (without CNS involvement)

- **Trypanosomal chancre:** First, a self-limited inflammatory lesion may appear a week after the bite of an infected tsetse fly; called as trypanosomal chancre which lasts for 1–2 weeks
- **Asymptomatic period:** Following this, the parasites enter into the bloodstream causing a symptom free low-grade parasitemia which lasts for few months
- **Systemic febrile illness:** Months to years later, a systemic febrile illness develops; due to dissemination of the parasite through the lymphatics and bloodstream. It is characterized by:
  - Remittent irregular fever with night sweats
  - Lymphadenopathy—the lymph nodes appear as soft, rubbery and nontender. The posterior cervical nodes are commonly involved and called as **Winterbottom's sign**. Lymphadenopathy is a consistent feature of West African trypanosomiasis; which differentiates it from the Eastern variety
  - Pruritus, maculopapular rashes and transient edema are common
  - Delayed sensation to pain is noted (**Kerandel's sign**)
  - **Hematologic manifestations**—include moderate leukocytosis, thrombocytopenia, anemia and production of high levels of polyclonal IgM.

Stage II Disease (CNS invasion)

It involves invasion of the CNS, particularly pons, medulla and frontal; which leads to steady progressive chronic meningoencephalitis. It is characterized by:

- Patients develop characteristic progressive daytime somnolence (hence called as "sleeping sickness"), with restlessness and insomnia at night which may be related to increased prostaglandin D2 level in the body
- Behavioral and personality changes with apathy, confusion, fatigue and loss of coordination may be observed
- Other features include listless gaze, loss of spontaneity, and abnormal speech with few extrapyramidal signs like choreiform movements, tremors and fasciculations
- In the terminal stage, the patient becomes emaciated progressing to coma and death, usually from secondary infection.

Laboratory Diagnosis   *Trypanosoma brucei*

- **Direct microscopy**—detects trypomastigotes
  - Serial blood sample examination
  - CSF examination
  - Lymph node aspirate
- **Antibodies** from serum and CSF—card agglutination test, IFA, ELISA detecting VSG antibodies and TLTF antibodies
- **Antigen** from serum and CSF—ELISA and CIATT
- **Molecular method**—PCR, FISH, LAMP and real-time PCR
- **Culture**—inoculated into KIVI
- **Animal inoculation**—mice.

Laboratory Diagnosis

Direct Microscopy

Specimen

Useful samples are multiple blood samples collected during febrile period (due to periodic release of trypomastigotes in

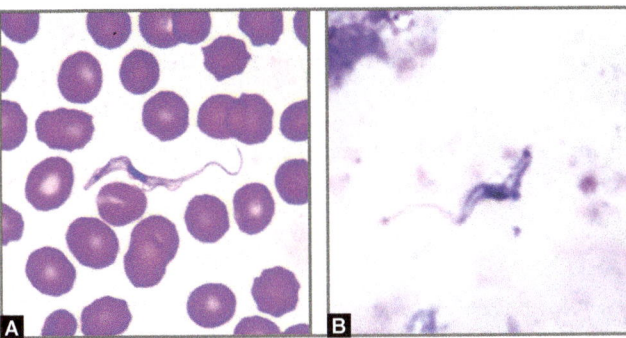

Figs 5.16A and B: Trypomastigote form of *T. brucei* in peripheral blood smear examination (Giemsa stain): (A) Thin smear; (B) Thick smear

Source: A and B—DPDx Image Library, Centers for Disease Control and Prevention (CDC), Atlanta (*with permission*).

blood), chancre fluid, CSF, lymph node aspirate and bone marrow aspirate.

Serial blood sample examination

- **Wet mounting:** It is done to demonstrate highly motile trypomastigotes
- **Thin and thick films:** Smear is fixed and stained with Giemsa stain to visualize the trypomastigote forms
  - Detection limit of thin smear is 1 parasite/200 high power field and that of thick smear is 2000 parasite/mL (or 100/mL following centrifugation) (Fig. 5.16)
  - Trypomastigotes are elongated 14–33 μm long, 1.5–3.5 μm having a flagellum with undulating membrane. Cytoplasm stains pale blue containing dark blue granules with nucleus stained red.
- **Concentration methods:** If the parasitemia is low, then blood concentration methods are followed such as:
  - **Microhematocrit centrifugation:** It uses QBC capillary tube coated with Acridine orange. It claims sensitivity of 55–90% (refer Chapter 6 for procedure)
  - **Mini anion exchange centrifugation:** Involves separation of trypomastigotes from blood using anion exchange chromatography followed by low speed centrifugation. It can detect as low as <100 organisms/mL of blood. Buffy coat examination has a better sensitivity than blood.

CSF examination

CSF examination is done for the following purposes:
- **Staging of the disease:** Stage II disease is confirmed either by detection of trypomastigotes in CSF or by WBC count of >20 cells/μL of CSF with parasite detected in blood or lymph node
- **Mott cells:** Centrifuged deposit of the CSF is examined for the presence of Mott cells (also called as Morula or Mulberry cells). Mott cells are abnormal plasma cells containing large eosinophilic inclusions (called Russell bodies) of IgM; which should be differentiated from leukocytes
- Other CSF findings include increased protein level, lymphocytosis, increased pressure and elevated IgM levels.

Lymph node aspirate

It is useful for *T. brucei gambiense* and shows variable sensitivity of 40–80%.

Antibodies from Serum and CSF

- **Card agglutination test** for trypanosomes (CATT) for *T. brucei gambiense*: It has been developed for field use and mass screening. It detects antibodies to VSG antigen. This is highly sensitive (87–98%) but less specific. It is widely used for mass population screening; titer of ≥1:16 is considered significant
- **Semi-quantitative ELISA** using VSG antigen of *T.b. gambiense* is available to detect various Ig isotypes (IgG1, IgG3 and IgM) in serum and CSF
- **TLTF antibodies:** ELISA format is available detecting anti-trypanosome-derived lymphocyte triggering factor (TLTF) antibodies in serum and CSF
- **Other tests** include indirect fluorescent antibody (IFA) test and latex agglutination test.

Antigens from Serum and CSF

- **ELISA:** Antigen detection by ELISA in serum or CSF is useful for clinical staging of disease to determine CNS infection and for monitoring the response to treatment (antigens are rapidly cleared following improvement)
- **CIATT:** The card indirect latex agglutination trypanosomiasis test (TrypTect CIATT) is simple and rapid test detecting circulating invariant common antigen in serum. It has a good sensitivity of 95.8% for *T.b. gambiense* and 97.7% for *T.b. rhodesiense*; however, the specificity is variable.

Molecular Methods

- PCR assays have been developed which show a detection limit of 5 parasites/mL
- FISH (fluorescence in situ hybridization) using peptide nucleic acid probe appears to be an excellent diagnostic tool with detection limit same as PCR
- Other molecular methods available are branched DNA assay, real-time PCR and LAMP (loop mediated amplification technique).

Culture

Samples can be inoculated into KIVI (kit for *in vitro* isolation) and trypomastigotes are recovered in 7–10 days. However, culture is not routinely performed.

Animal Inoculation in Mice

It is highly sensitive for the isolation of *T.b. rhodesiense* but not useful for *T.b. gambiense*.

Other non-specific Findings

Measurement of levels of the following provides confirmation of CNS involvement.
- Sustained high levels of IgM may be seen; due to antigenic switching in parasite. Absence of elevated IgM levels in serum in an immunocompetent host rules out trypanosomiasis
- Increased prostaglandin D2.

Treatment — *Trypanosoma brucei* complex

The drugs used for treatment of African sleeping sickness are pentamidine and suramin. Alternate drugs are eflornithine, and the organic arsenical melarsoprol. Treatment is based on type of disease (West or East African) and presence or absence of CNS invasion (Table 5.12).

Table 5.12: Treatment of African trypanosomiasis

Causative organism	Stage I (Hemolymphatic stage)	Stage II (neural stage)
Trypanosoma brucei gambiense (West African)	Pentamidine Alternative: Suramin	Eflornithine Alternative: Melarsoprol
Trypanosoma brucei rhodesiense (East African)	Suramin	Melarsoprol

Note: Drugs that can cross blood brain barrier are used in stage II of the disease.

Prophylaxis

Vector control strategies like destruction of the insect's habitats, elimination of reservoir sources, etc. can be done to control African trypanosomiasis. Vaccines are not available as the parasite undergoes frequent antigenic variations.

EXPECTED QUESTIONS

I. Write essay on:
 a. A 31-year-old man from Bihar presented with splenomegaly, anemia, and fever. The bone marrow aspirate collected was subjected to Giemsa staining which revealed amastigotes filled within a macrophage.
  1. Identify the etiological agent and the clinical diagnosis.
  2. Write briefly about the life cycle of the etiological agent.
  3. Describe the pathogenesis and clinical manifestations produced.
  4. What are the various diagnostic modalities?
  5. How will you treat this condition?
 b. Describe the life cycle, clinical feature and laboratory diagnosis of *Trypanosoma cruzi*.

II. Write short notes on:
 a. Post-kala-azar dermal leishmaniasis.
 b. Cutaneous leishmaniasis.
 c. African sleeping sickness.
 d. New world Leishmaniasis.
 e. Chagas' disease.

III. Multiple choice questions (MCQs):
1. Vector for leishmaniasis:
 a. Sandfly
 b. Reduviid bugs
 c. Tsetse fly
 d. *Anopheles* mosquito
2. Old World leishmaniasis is caused by:
 a. *Leishmania donovani*
 b. *Leishmania tropica*
 c. *Leishmania infantum*
 d. All of the above
3. New World leishmaniasis is caused by:
 a. *Leishmania donovani*
 b. *Leishmania braziliensis*
 c. *Leishmania tropica*
 d. *Leishmania major*
4. Amastigote form of *Leishmania donovani* resides in the:
 a. Gastrointestinal tract of insect vector
 b. Salivary gland of mosquito
 c. Cells of reticuloendothelial system
 d. NNN culture media
5. Oriental sore is caused by:
 a. *Leishmania mexicana*
 b. *Leishmania braziliensis*
 c. *Leishmania tropica*
 d. *Leishmania chagasi*
6. *Leishmania donovani* can be cultivated in:
 a. Blood agar
 b. NNN medium
 c. Diamond's medium
 d. RPMI 1640 medium
7. Chiclero's ulcer is caused by:
 a. *Leishmania mexicana*
 b. *Leishmania braziliensis*
 c. *Leishmania peruviana*
 d. *Leishmania chagasi*
8. Espundia is caused by:
 a. *Leishmania mexicana*
 b. *Leishmania braziliensis*
 c. *Leishmania peruviana*
 d. *Leishmania chagasi*
9. Best animal model used for inoculation of *Leishmania donovani*:
 a. Hamster
 b. Guinea pig
 c. Rabbit
 d. Mouse
10. American trypanosomiasis (Chagas' disease) is caused by:
 a. *T. brucei gambiense*
 b. *T. rangeli*
 c. *T. brucei rhodesiense*
 d. *T. cruzi*

Answers
1. a 2. d 3. b 4. c 5. c 6. b 7. a 8. b 9. a 10. d

Apicomplexa—I (Malaria Parasite and Babesia)

CHAPTER OUTLINE

- Classification
- Malaria Parasite
- Babesia

CLASSIFICATION

Phylum Apicomplexa (the sporozoan parasites) distinguished morphologically by the presence of a specialized complex of apical organelles (micronemes, rhoptries, polar ring, conoids and dense granules) which help in invasion into the host cell.

- Phylum Apicomplexa contains one Class Coccidea which in turn has three Orders—(1) Eimeriida, (2) Haemosporida, (3) Piroplasmida
- Order Haemosporida and order Piroplasmida include the blood parasites belonging to the genus *Plasmodium* (the causative agent of malaria) and *Babesia* (rare parasites infecting humans) respectively (Table 6.1).

MALARIA PARASITE

History

Malaria is one of the oldest documented diseases of mankind.

- Cases of malaria were recorded in the ancient Indian, Chinese textbooks and evidences of patients died of malaria were found from Egyptian mummies of more than 3,000 years old
- The name "Malaria" ("Mal" means bad and "aria" means air) was derived from the ancient false belief that "disease is spread by air pollution through stagnant water and marshy lands"
- French army surgeon Alphonse Laveran (1880) was the first to discover the causative agent *Plasmodium*, in the red blood cell (RBC) of a patient in Algeria
- Golgi had described the asexual cycle of the parasite in RBC
- Sir Ronald Ross, in 1897 had described the sexual cycle of the parasite in female *Anopheles* mosquito in Secunderabad, India
- Both Alphonse Laveran in 1902 and Sir Ronald Ross in 1907 won the Nobel Prize for their contributions in malaria
- Ms Tu Youyou, a chemist was awarded Nobel prize in Medicine (2015), for the discovery of artemisinin, which is used for treatment of falciparum malaria.

The Causative Agent of Malaria

More than 125 species of *Plasmodium* exist infecting wide range of birds, reptiles and mammals. However, human infection is mainly caused by five species such as:

1. *P. vivax* causes benign tertian malaria (periodicity of fever is once in 48 hours, i.e. recurs every third day)
2. *P. falciparum* causes malignant tertian malaria (severe malaria, periodicity of fever is once in 48 hours, recurs every third day)
3. *P. malariae* causes benign quartan malaria (periodicity of fever is once in 72 hours, i.e. recurs every fourth day)
4. *P. ovale* causes ovale tertian malaria (periodicity of fever is once in 48 hours, i.e. recurs every third day)
5. *P. knowlesi* causes quotidian or simian malaria (fever periodicity is once in 24 hours, i.e. recurs every day). It is a parasite of monkey but can also infect humans and many cases affecting man were recently reported from Asia.

Other *Plasmodium* species are mainly of animal importance like *P. cynomolgi*, *P. simium*, etc.

Table 6.1: Classification of Phylum Apicomplexa

Higher taxa	Order	Genus
Kingdom: Protozoa Subkingdom: Neozoa Phylum: Apicomplexa Class: Coccidea	Eimeriida	Eimeria Toxoplasma Cryptosporidium Cyclospora Cystoisospora Sarcocystis
	Haemosporida	Plasmodium
	Piroplasmida	Babesia

Life Cycle (Fig. 6.1)

Host: *Plasmodium* completes its life cycle in two hosts:
1. **Definitive host:** Female *Anopheles* (*Anopheline*) mosquito is the definitive host where the sexual cycle (sporogony) takes place
   - Male *Anopheles* does not feed on man and feeds exclusively on fruit juices, i.e. why male *Anopheles* mosquito does not transmit the disease. Whereas female *Anopheles*, needs at least two blood meals before laying eggs
   - Out of 45 species of *Anopheline* mosquitoes in India, only a few are regarded as vectors of primary importance. These are: *Anopheline culicifacies* in rural areas, *A. stephensi* in urban areas and *A. fluviatilis* in hilly areas. Others are *A. minimus*, *A. philippinensis*, *A. sundaicus* and *A. maculatus*.
2. **Intermediate host:** Man acts as intermediate host where the asexual cycle (schizogony) takes place

Human Cycle

Infective form: The sporozoites are the infective form of the parasite. They are present in the salivary gland of female *Anopheles* mosquito.

When *Plasmodium* species is transmitted by blood transfusion or through placenta, trophozoites (or merozoites) act as infective form.

Mode of transmission: Man gets infection by the bite of female *Anopheles* mosquito. Sporozoites from the salivary

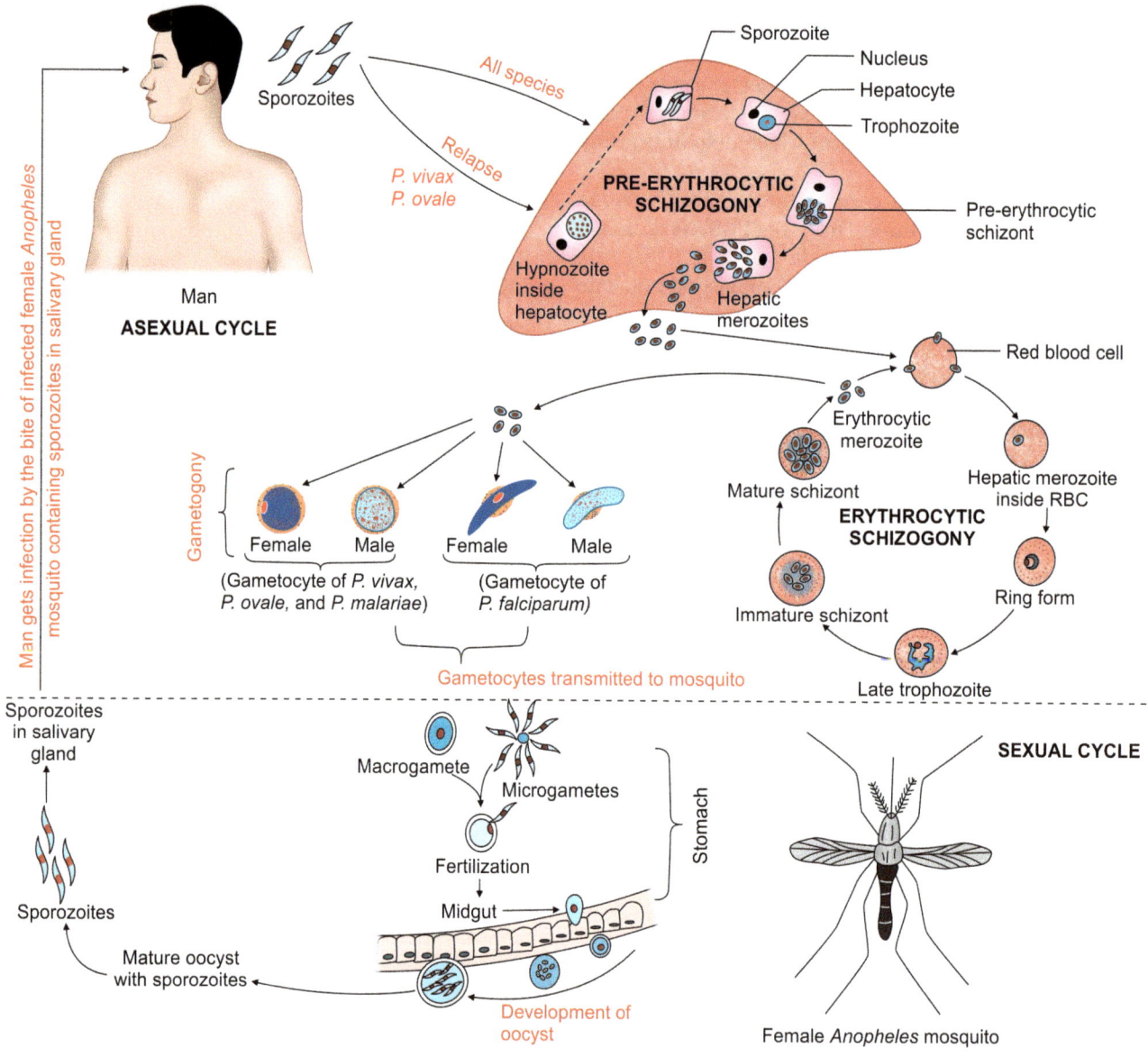

Fig. 6.1: Life cycle of malaria parasite

gland of the mosquito are directly introduced into the blood circulation.

Rarely, it can also be transmitted by:
- Blood transfusion
- Transplacental transmission.

In humans, the asexual cycle takes place through the following stages:
- Pre-erythrocytic schizogony
- Erythrocytic schizogony
- Gametogony.

Pre-erythrocytic schizogony

This stage occurs in liver and it is so named because it occurs before the invasion of RBC.
- It is also called exoerythrocytic stage or intrahepatic or tissue stage
- The motile sporozoites leave the circulation within 30 minutes and enter liver
- **Attachment:** The circumsporozoite protein present on the surface of sporozoites binds noncovalently to the thrombospondin receptors, present on the basolateral surface of hepatocytes facilitating the entry of sporozoites
- After entering into hepatocytes, the spindle shaped sporozoites become rounded and lose their apical complex and transform into trophozoites
- **Trophozoite** is the feeding stage of the parasite which later on undergoes several nuclear divisions (**schizogony**) and transforms into pre-erythrocytic schizont
- **Pre-erythrocytic schizont** contains several merozoites; released outside on rupture of hepatocyte. Merozoites then attack RBCs to perform erythrocytic schizogony
- As only few hepatocytes are infected by *Plasmodium*, so hepatic damage does not occur in malaria
- Duration of pre-erythrocytic schizogony varies from 5 days to 15 days depending on the species (Table 6.2)
- Some sporozoites of *P. vivax* and *P. ovale* do not develop further and may remain in liver as hypnozoites and cause relapse of malaria after many years
- **Relapse** should be differentiated from another phenomena seen in *P. falciparum* and *P. malariae* called as **recrudescence** (Table 6.3).

Erythrocytic schizogony

The hepatic merozoites after released from pre-erythrocytic schizont, attack RBCs.
- Merozoites bind to the **glycophorin receptors** on RBC surface, enter by endocytosis and are contained within a parasitophorous vacuole inside the RBCs. The process of entry into RBC takes about 30 seconds
- **Trophozoite:** Soon the pear-shaped hepatic merozoites round up, lose their internal organelle and transform into trophozoites
- **Ring form:** Early trophozoite form is known as ring form. It is annular or signet ring appearance containing a central vacuole and peripheral thin rim of cytoplasm and a nucleus
- Ring form occupies one-third of RBC except in *P. falciparum*, where it occupies one-sixth of RBC

Table 6.2: Characteristic features of pre-erythrocytic schizogony				
Characteristic feature	**Plasmodium falciparum**	**Plasmodium vivax**	**Plasmodium ovale**	**Plasmodium malariae**
Duration of pre-erythrocytic schizogony	5.5 days	8 days	9 days	15 days
Number of merozoites per infected pre-erythrocytic schizont	30,000	10,000	15,000	15,000
Pre-erythrocytic schizont size	60 μm	45 μm	60 μm	55 μm

Table 6.3: Relapse and recrudescence in malaria	
Relapse	*Recrudescence*
• Seen in *Plasmodium vivax* and *P. ovale* infections	• Although seen in all species, more common in *P. falciparum* followed by *P. malariae*
• Few sporozoites do not develop into pre-erythrocytic schizont, but remain dormant (known as *hypnozoites*) for 3 weeks to one year	• Falciparum malaria—recrudescence is due to persistence of drug resistant parasites, even after completion of treatment
• Reactivation of hypnozoites leads to initiation of erythrocytic cycle and relapse of malaria	• In *P. malariae* infection, long-term recrudescences are seen for as long as 60 years This is due to long-term survival of erythrocytic stages at a low undetectable level in blood
Concept of secondary exo or pre-erythrocytic stage: • Formerly, it was postulated that relapse occurs due to secondary exo or pre-erythrocytic stage where a proportion of hepatic merozoites released from pre-erythrocytic schizont, again attack the liver cells • But now, it is believed that secondary pre-erythrocytic stage does not occur and relapse occurs due to sporozoites undergoing dormancy during the primary pre-erythrocytic stage	

- ❖ **Prepatent period:** Ring forms are the first asexual form that can be demonstrated in the peripheral blood. The time interval between the entry of the parasite into man and demonstration of the parasite in the peripheral blood is called as **prepatent period**. It varies between the species:
  - *P. vivax*—8 days
  - *P. falciparum*—5 days
  - *P. malariae*—13 days
  - *P. ovale*—9 days.
- ❖ **Malarial pigment**
  - *Plasmodium* feeds on hemoglobin. The undigested product of hemoglobin metabolism like hematin, excess protein and iron porphyrin combine to form malarial pigment (hemozoin pigment)
  - The appearance of malarial pigment varies, mostly it is brown black in color and numerous (except in *P. vivax* it is yellowish-brown in color and in *P. falciparum,* it is few in number).
- ❖ **Late trophozoite:** Ring form enlarges and becomes more irregular due to amoeboid movement and transforms into late trophozoite or amoeboid form
- ❖ **Schizogony:** Late trophozoite undergoes multiple nuclear divisions (erythrocytic schizogony or merogony) and produces 6-30 daughter merozoites arranged in the form of rosette. This form is known as **erythrocytic schizont**
- ❖ Number of merozoites per mature schizont varies:
  - *P. vivax*—12-24 number (average 16)
  - *P. falciparum*—18-24 number (average 20)
  - *P. malariae*—6-12 number (average 8)
  - *P. ovale*—8-12 number (average 8).
- ❖ RBCs then rupture to release the daughter merozoites, malarial pigments and toxins into the circulation which result in malarial paroxysm of fever at the end of each erythrocytic cycle
- ❖ Each merozoite is potentially capable of invading a new RBC and repeating the cycle. Intraerythrocytic life cycle takes roughly 48 hours for *P. falciparum, P. vivax* and *P. ovale*, 72 hours for *P. malariae* and 24 hours for *P. knowlesi*
- ❖ **Incubation period:** The time interval between entry of the parasite to the body and appearance of the first clinical feature is known as **incubation period**. It varies between the species:
  - *P. vivax*—14 days (ranges 8-17 days)
  - *P. falciparum*—12 days (ranges 9-14 days)
  - *P. malariae*—28 days (ranges 18-40 days)
  - *P. ovale*—17 days (ranges 16-18 days).
- ❖ In *P. falciparum* infection, the later stages of erythrocytic cycle occur in the capillaries of brain and internal organs. Hence, only the ring forms are found in the peripheral blood by microscopic examination but not late trophozoites and schizonts
- ❖ However, for other species, the entire erythrocytic stage takes place in peripheral blood vessel.

Gametogony

After a series of erythrocytic cycles, some merozoites after entering into RBCs, instead of developing into trophozoites, they transform into sexual forms called as **gametocytes.**

- ❖ The gametocytic development takes place in the blood vessels of internal organs such as spleen and bone marrow and only the mature gametocytes appear in the peripheral blood
- ❖ The gametocytes of all the species are round in shape, except in *P. falciparum* in which they are crescent or banana-shaped
- ❖ They are of two types—(1) male gametocyte (or microgametocyte) and (2) female gametocyte (or macrogametocyte)
- ❖ Microgametocytes in all the species are smaller in size, lesser in number, their cytoplasm stains pale blue, and nucleus is larger, stains red and diffuse
- ❖ In contrast, macrogametocytes are larger, numerous, their cytoplasm stains deep blue, nucleus is small, red and compact
- ❖ The time of appearance of gametocytes in the circulation from the first appearance of asexual forms (i.e. ring forms) in the peripheral blood varies between the species
  - *P. vivax*—4-5 days
  - *P. falciparum*—10-12 days
  - *P. malariae*—11-14 days
  - *P. ovale*—5-6 days.
- ❖ Gametocytes neither cause any clinical illness nor they divide
- ❖ Individuals harboring gametocytes are considered as carriers or reservoirs of infection and play an important role in the transmission of the disease
- ❖ A patient can be a carrier of several *Plasmodium* species at the same time
- ❖ However, gametocytes are effective in transmission of the infection if they are:
  - **Mature;** immature forms are not transmitted
  - **Viable,** i.e. dead gametocytes are ineffective
  - Present in **sufficient density** to infect mosquitoes. The number of gametocytes necessary to infect mosquitoes is **12 per cubic mm** of blood.

Mosquito Cycle

A female *Anopheles* mosquito during the blood meal, takes both the asexual forms and the sexual forms.

- The asexual forms get digested whereas the sexual forms, i.e. the gametocytes undergo further development (hence considered as infective form of the parasite to mosquito)
- **Exflagellation:**
  - Nucleus of the male gametocytes divides into eight flagellated actively motile bodies (15-20 μm length) called as **microgametes**.
  - Microgametes protrude out as thread-like filaments, lash out for some time and then, break free
  - This process is called as **exflagellation**. At 28°C, it is completed in 15 minutes for *P. vivax* and 15-30 minutes for *P. falciparum*
  - Female gametocytes neither divide nor undergo exflagellation but each undergoes maturation to form one **macrogamete or female gamete.**
- **Zygote:** The male microgamete fertilizes with the female macrogamete by fusion of their pronuclei and the zygote is formed. Fertilization occurs in about 30 minutes to 2 hours after the blood meal
- **Ookinete:** Within 24 hours, the nonmotile rounded zygote transforms into vermicular motile elongated form with an apical complex (the ookinete stage). Till this stage, the development takes place in the midgut of the mosquito
- **Oocyst:** The ookinete penetrates into the stomach wall of the mosquito and lies just beneath the basement membrane. It becomes rounded and covered by a thin elastic membrane to form oocyst. This is the stage discovered by Sir Ronald Ross. Several thousands of mature oocysts can be found; each measuring 500 μm
- **Sporozoites:** Oocysts undergo sporogony (meiosis) to produce thousands of spindle-shaped sporozoites measuring 10-15 μm length with apical complex anteriorly
- On rupture of the mature oocyst, the sporozoites are released and migrate to salivary gland
- Mosquito is said to be infective to man only when the sporozoites are present in salivary gland. Once infected, it remains infective throughout the life
- **Extrinsic incubation period:** Time required to complete the life cycle in mosquito is called as extrinsic incubation period and it varies from 1 week to 4 weeks. At 25°C, it is:
  - *P. vivax*—8-10 days
  - *P. falciparum*—9-10 days
  - *P. malariae*—25-28 days
  - *P. ovale*—14-16 days.
- **Mixed infection:** Different species of *Plasmodium* can infect the same mosquito which in turn can transmit mixed infections to man, accounts for 4-8% of total infection. The mixed infection is seldom observed in endemic areas; most common being *P. vivax* and *P. falciparum* mixed infection
- Differences between the four malaria parasites are described in Tables 6.4 and 6.5 and Figure 6.2.

Pathogenesis and Clinical Feature

Benign Malaria

Benign malaria is milder in nature, can be caused by all four species. It is characterized by a triad of febrile paroxysm, anemia and splenomegaly.

Febrile paroxysm

Fever comes intermittently depending on the species. It occurs every fourth day (72 hour cycle for *P. malariae*) and every third day (48 hour cycle for other three species).
- Paroxysm corresponds to the release of the successive broods of merozoites into the bloodstream, at the end of RBC cycle
- Each paroxysm of fever is comprised of three stages—(1) cold stage (2) hot stage and (3) sweating stage
  - **Cold stage:** Lasts for 15 minutes to 1 hour. The patient feels lassitude, headache, nausea, intense cold, chill and rigor

Table 6.4: Differences between the four malaria parasites

Properties	Plasmodium vivax	Plasmodium falciparum	Plasmodium malariae	Plasmodium ovale
Relapse (Hypnozoites)	Seen	Not seen	Not seen	Seen
Recrudescence	Not seen	Seen	Seen (Up to 60 years)	Not seen
Erythrocytic cycle	48 hours	36–48 hours	72 hours	48 hours
Prepatent period	8 days	5 days	13 days	9 days
Incubation period	14 days	12 days	28 days	17 days
R-G interval[a]	4–5 days	10–12 days	11–14 days	5–6 days
Extrinsic IP[b]	8–10 days	9–10 days	25–28 days	14–16 days

Abbreviations: [a]R-G interval, interval between appearance of ring form and gametocyte; [b]IP, incubation period.

Table 6.5: Differences between the four malaria parasites

Parasitic changes	Plasmodium vivax	Plasmodium falciparum	Plasmodium malariae	Plasmodium ovale
Forms seen in peripheral blood smear examination	Trophozoites (early and late), gametocytes and schizonts	Ring forms (early trophozoites) and gametocytes	Similar to that of P. vivax	Similar to that of P. vivax
Ring form (Early trophozoite)	Ring 2.5 μm size, vacuole in the center, peripheral thin rim of blue cytoplasm, surrounding the red nucleus with heavy chromatin dot. Ring occupies 1/3rd of the RBC size. Cytoplasm opposite to the nucleus is thick	Ring 1.5 μm size, smaller than in P. vivax, occupying 1/6th of RBC, with small chromatin dot. *Variants of ring forms*: Multiple rings, Accole (appliqué) forms Double dot/head phone shaped ring forms	Similar to that of P. vivax but thicker, occupy 1/8th of RBC	Similar to that of P. vivax, more compact
Late trophozoite	Large, amoeboid, cytoplasm, prominent vacuole	Small, compact, rounded, slightly amoeboid, vacuole inconspicuous, not seen in smear peripheral smear	Small, compact, band forms seen, vacuole inconspicuous	Small, compact, rounded, coarse pigment, vacuole inconspicuous
Schizont	Large, 9-10 μm, completely fills the enlarged RBC	Small, 4.5–5 μm size, Fills 2/3rd of normal sized RBC	Small, 6.5–7 μm size, almost fills a normal sized RBC	Small, 6.2 μm size, fills 3/4th of enlarged oval RBC
Merozoites/schizont (numbers)	16 (12–24)	18–24 (not seen in peripheral smear)	8 (6–12)	8 (6–12)
Gametocyte	Spherical, almost occupies the RBC	Banana-shaped, larger than RBC size	Similar to that of P. vivax	Similar to that of P. vivax
• Female gametocyte	• Spherical • Larger than male • Cytoplasm stains deep blue • Nucleus stains red compact and eccentric • Pigments- coarse, diffuse	• Crescentic (banana) • Long slender and pointed tips • Larger than RBC • Cytoplasm stains deep blue • Nucleus stains red, compact and central • Pigments- compact	Similar to that of P. vivax	Similar to that of P. vivax
• Male gametocyte	Same as female but • Smaller • Cytoplasm—pale blue • Nucleus—diffuse, chromatin mass surrounded by pale or colorless halo	Same as female but • Broader and shorter • Rounded tips • Cytoplasm stains pale blue • Both nucleus and pigments—diffuse and scattered	Similar to that of P. vivax	Similar to that of P. vivax
Changes in RBCs				
RBCs infected	Young RBCs	RBCs of all age	Old RBCs	Young RBCs
RBC size	Enlarged, round (frequently bizarre form)	Normal in size	Normal in size	Enlarged, oval, fimbriated margin
Schüffner's dots* (eosinophilic stippling)	Present in all stages except in early ring forms	None. Coma like red dots (Maurer's dots) rarely seen	None Ziemann's dots (small red dots) may be present, not considered true stippling	Present in all stages (dots are larger and darker than P. vivax, sometimes called as James dots)
Malarial pigments	Yellowish-brown	Dark brown	Dark brown	Dark yellowish-brown

*****Schüffner's dots:** Pink to red colored eosinophilic dots on the surface of RBCs, are seen when stained properly. They are membrane bound structures in the cytoplasm of RBCs infected with *Plasmodium;* which help in protein transport from the parasite to the erythrocyte surface.

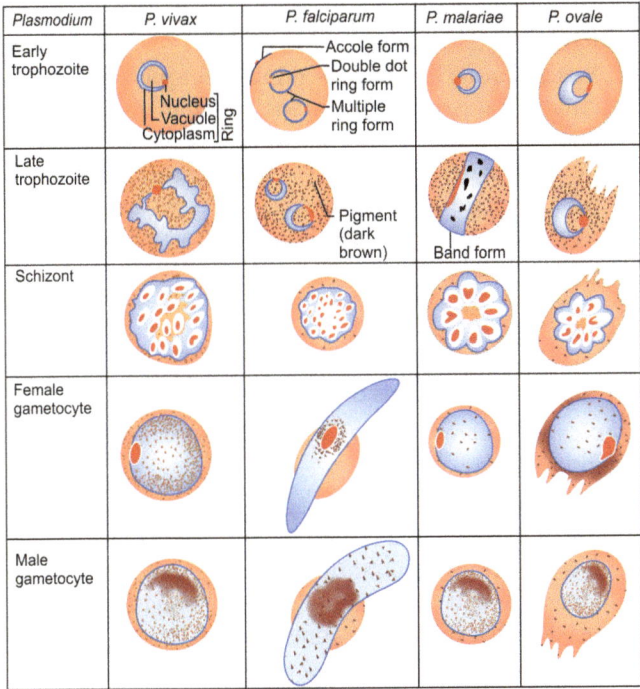

Fig. 6.2: Morphological forms of malaria parasites

- **Hot stage:** Patient develops high grade fever of 39–41°C and dry burning skin. Headache persists but nausea diminishes
- **Sweating stage:** Fever comes down with profuse sweating. Skin becomes cold and moist. Patient feels relieved and often asleep. This stage lasts for 2–4 hours.
- ❖ The classical paroxysm may not be present always due to maturation of generations of parasites at different times
- ❖ In *P. falciparum*, the fever is more irregular or even continuous with marked prostration, headache and nausea.

Anemia

After a few paroxysms of fever, patient develops a normocytic normochromic anemia. Various factors can attribute to the development of anemia such as:
- ❖ Parasite induced RBC destruction—Lysis of RBC due to release of merozoites
- ❖ Splenic removal of both infected RBC and uninfected RBC coated with immune complexes
- ❖ Bone marrow suppression leading to decrease RBC production
- ❖ Increased fragility of RBCs
- ❖ Autoimmune lysis of coated RBCs.

Splenomegaly

After a few weeks of febrile paroxysms, spleen gets enlarged and becomes palpable. Splenomegaly is due to massive proliferation of macrophages that engulf parasitized and nonparasitized coated RBCs.

Falciparum Malaria (Malignant Tertian Malaria)

Pathogenesis of falciparum malaria

Plasmodium falciparum possesses a number of virulence factors and its pathogenesis is different from other species. Hence the disease is more acute and severe in nature with more complications than the benign malaria.

Sequestration of the parasites: An important feature of the pathogenesis of *P. falciparum* is its ability to sequester (holding back) the parasites in the blood vessels of deep visceral organs like brain, kidney, etc. This leads to blockade of vessels, congestion and hypoxia of internal organs. Sequestration is mediated by:
- ❖ **Cytoadherence:** It refers to binding of infected erythrocytes to endothelial cells. It is mediated by a specialized antigen called as *P. falciparum* **erythrocyte membrane protein-1 (PfEMP-1)**
    - Infected RBCs become sticky and develop protuberances in their cell membrane called as **Knobs** that express high level of PfEMP-1 antigen
    - PfEMP-1 binds to specific receptors present on the endothelium leading to adherence of parasitized RBCs to the vascular endothelium of deep organs
    - The endothelial receptors are CD36 molecule (present in most of the organs), ICAM-1 (intracytoplasmic adhesion molecule-1, usually expressed on cerebral vessels) or chondroitin sulfate (on placental endothelium)
- ❖ **Rosetting:** It refers to binding of infected erythrocytes to uninfected erythrocytes. PfEMP-1 also plays an important role in rosetting, as it can adhere to complement receptor 1 (CR1) and blood group A antigen present on the uninfected erythrocytes
- ❖ **Deformability:** Parasitized RBCs become more spherical and rigid, and are less filterable than uninfected cells
- ❖ Since the parasites are sequestrated back in deep vessels, they can avoid frequent spleen passage, hence can escape splenic clearance
- ❖ PfEMP undergoes frequent antigenic variation, thus helps the parasite in evading the host immune response.

High level of parasitemia: *P. falciparum* infection is associated with high level of parasitemia (30–40% of total RBC are infected) compared to other species (<2%).

Other virulence factors like:
- ❖ Knob associated histidine rich protein II (HRP-II)
- ❖ **Glycosyl phosphatidyl inositol (GPI):** Parasitic GPI stimulates the host immune system to release cytokines like IL-1, TNF and IFN-γ.

Complications

Complications of Falciparum Malaria

- **Cerebral malaria:**
  - Occurs due to plugging of brain capillaries by the rosettes of sequestered parasitized RBCs leading to vascular occlusion and cerebral anoxia
  - Cerebral malaria manifests as diffuse symmetric encephalopathy characterized by generalized convulsion in 10% of adults and up to 50% of children
  - Muscle tone and tendon reflexes are reduced
  - Other defects are retinal hemorrhages, neurologic sequelae, repeated seizures, and rarely deep coma
  - Signs of focal neurologic and meningeal irritations are absent
  - High mortality rate—20% among adults and more than 15% among children.
- **Pernicious malaria:** It is characterized by blackwater fever, algid malaria and septicemic malaria
- **Black water fever:**
  - This syndrome is characterized by sudden intravascular hemolysis followed by fever, hemoglobinuria and dark urine
  - It occurs following quinine treatment to subjects previously infected with *P. falciparum*
  - The precise mechanism is not known
  - Autoimmune mechanism has been suggested. Antibodies develop against parasitized and quininized RBCs. With subsequent infection and quinine treatment, there is immunocomplex formation followed by complement mediated massive destruction of both parasitized and nonparasitized RBCs.
- **Algid malaria:** Characterized by cold clammy skin, hypotension, peripheral circulatory failure and profound shock
- **Septicemic malaria:** Characterized by high degree of prostration, high grade fever with dissemination of the parasite to various organs leading to multiorgan failure
- **Pulmonary edema and adult respiratory distress syndrome:** Severe falciparum malaria in adults may lead to noncardiogenic pulmonary edema often aggravated by over hydration. Usually it does not respond to antimalarial therapy; mortality rate is more than 80%
- **Hypoglycemia:** It is associated with a poor prognosis and is particularly problematic in children and pregnant women and following quinine therapy
- **Renal failure:** It occurs due to erythrocyte sequestration in renal microvasculature leading to acute tubular necrosis. It is common among adults than children
- **Bleeding/disseminated intravascular coagulation:** Patient presents with significant bleeding and hemorrhages from the gums, nose and gastrointestinal tract with or without evidence of disseminated intravascular coagulation
- **Severe jaundice:** More common among adults than children; it results from hemolysis, hepatocyte injury and cholestasis
- **Severe normochromic, normocytic anemia:** Characterized by hematocrit of less than 15% or hemoglobin level of less than 5 g/dL with parasitemia level of more than 100,000/μL (>2%)
- **Acidosis:** Results from accumulation of organic acids like lactic acid.

Chronic Complications of Malaria

Tropical splenomegaly syndrome (hyper-active malarial splenomegaly)

- It occurs in people of malaria-endemic areas in tropical Africa and Asia (including India)
- It results from an abnormal immunologic response to repeated malaria infections and is characterized by:
  - Elevated IgM (due to polyclonal B cell activation)
  - Massive splenomegaly
  - Hepatic sinusoidal lymphocytosis
  - Peripheral B cell lymphocytosis (in Africa).
- Patients respond well to antimalarial chemoprophylaxis (proguanil).

Quartan malarial nephropathy

It is a chronic complication seen with *P. malariae* (and possibly with other malarial species). It occurs due to injury to the renal glomeruli by the immune complexes, resulting in nephrotic syndrome. *P. knowlesi* is also known to cause nephrotic syndrome.

Promotes Burkitt's lymphoma

Malaria induced severe immunosuppression in African children provoke Epstein-Barr virus infection to develop Burkitt's lymphoma.

Malaria in Special Situations

Transfusion malaria

Malaria can be transmitted by blood transfusion, needle-stick injury, or organ transplantation. The clinical features and management of these cases are same as for naturally acquired infections (mosquito borne) but differs in many other ways:

- The infective form can be free merozoites, intraerythrocytic forms such as trophozoites or schizont but not gametocytes
- There is no pre-erythrocytic stage of development and no relapse
- The incubation period is often short
- Radical chemotherapy with primaquine is unnecessary as there is no relapse.

Malaria in pregnancy

Malaria during pregnancy increases the risk of fetal distress and can result in premature labor low birth weight and still birth. In areas with high malaria transmission, pregnant women are particularly vulnerable to severe anemia, hypoglycemia and acute pulmonary edema.

Malaria in children

Nearly one million children die of falciparum malaria each year in endemic countries.

Certain complications are relatively common among children like convulsions, coma, hypoglycemia, metabolic acidosis and severe anemia; whereas other complications like jaundice, acute renal failure, and acute pulmonary edema are unusual in children.

Plasmodium knowlesi

It is a malaria parasite of monkeys (long tailed *Macaca fascicularis* and pig tailed *Macaca nemestrina*), but can also rarely affect humans.
- *Anopheles leucosphyrus* is the main vector
- The first human case was documented in 1965, however, recently many cases affecting men have been reported from Asia since 2008
- **World:** Maximum cases have been reported from Malaysia (highest), Thailand, Myanmar followed by few reports from Indonesia, Vietnam, Philippines and Singapore. The largest foci is located at Malaysian Borneo; 3,122 cases have been reported between 2004–2015
- **India:** The only report of *P. knowlesi* infection has documented from Andamans, where 11% of archived samples showed positive for P. knowlesi 18S rRNA gene. However, India has all the potential of getting cases because *A. leucosphyrus* is found in the South-West zone (costal region of Kerala and Maharashtra)
- **Clinical features:** *P. knowlesi* produces an acute illness and relatively high parasitemia
  - Paroxysms of fever occur daily (quotidian malaria) because of short RBC cycle (24 hours)
  - Clinically it resembles *P. vivax*, but severe malaria is seen more frequently (7–10%), compared to 3% of *P. vivax*
  - Common complications seen are respiratory distress (most frequent) and renal failure. No cerebral malaria has been reported so far.
- **Laboratory diagnosis:**
  - On blood smear examination, early trophozoite of *P. knowlesi* is indistinguishable from *P. falciparum*, sometimes shows multiple ring forms, accole forms and double dot ring forms
  - The late trophozoites (with band forms), and round gametocytes of *P. knowlesi*, are morphologically similar to that of *P. malariae*
  - Schizonts contain 16 merozoites without arranged in a rosette.
  - It infects RBCs of all ages. No Schüffner's dots seen. Faint clumpy dots may appear late
  - Currently, no commercially available rapid diagnostic tests (RDTs) are designed to specifically detect *P. knowlesi*
  - *P. knowlesi* specific nested polymerase chain reaction (PCR) assays are available using the primers Pmk8 and Pmkr9 targeting small subunit rRNA.
- **Treatment:** It responds well to chloroquine or primaquine. As the disease rapidly progresses, treatment should be promptly started.

Plasmodium ovale

- In general, *P. ovale* infection is clinically similar to *P. vivax*, except that it is less severe, tends to relapse less frequently, and usually ends with spontaneous recovery
- *P. ovale* has two subspecies (classic type *P. ovale curtisi* and variant type *P. ovale wallikeri*); the latter is associated with a more severe thrombocytopenia.

Immunity Against Malaria

Both innate and acquired immunity contribute to the resistance against malaria.

Innate Immunity

This refers to the inherent and nonimmune mechanisms of host resistance against malaria parasite. This could be due to various factors:
- **Age of RBCs:** *P. falciparum* attacks RBCs of any age, *P. vivax* and *P. ovale* attack the young RBCs and reticulocytes; whereas *P. malariae* attacks older RBCs
- **Nature of hemoglobin:** Sickle cell disease, hemoglobin C and E, fetal hemoglobin and thalassemia hemoglobin are resistant to falciparum malaria
- **Hereditary ovalocytosis:** In this condition, the rigid RBCs are resistant to falciparum malaria
- **RBCs with glucose-6-phosphate dehydrogenase (G6PD) deficiency** are resistant to falciparum malaria
- **Duffy negative red blood cells:** Duffy blood group antigens present on RBC membrane act as receptors for *P. vivax*. So, people with duffy negative RBCs (West Africans) are resistant to vivax malaria
- **HLA-Bw53** and haplotypes bearing DRW13.02 antigen and R111 gene are protected from cerebral malaria
- **Nutritional status:** It has a paradoxical effect. Severe malaria is rare in children suffering from malnutrition.

Acquired Immunity

Both cellular and humoral immunity contribute to the resistance against malaria.
- **Humoral immunity:** Circulating antibodies (IgA, IgM and IgG) against asexual forms give protection by inhibiting the red cell invasion and sequestration, whereas antibodies against sexual forms help in reducing the transmission of malaria
- **Cellular immunity:** It also plays role in providing protection against malaria. Cytokines released from T cells stimulate the macrophages and also stimulate the B cells to produce antibodies
- Immunity against malaria attack is species specific, stage specific and strain specific. Immune defense of the host is sufficient to resist further infection but insufficient to destroy the parasite. Immunity lasts till the original infection remains active and prevents further infection. This is called as **infection immunity** or **premunition** or **concomitant immunity** or **incomplete immunity**.

Epidemiology of Malaria

Malaria is the most lethal parasitic disease of humans, transmitted in 108 countries containing 3 billion people.

- **World:** In 2016, 216 million cases of malaria with 4.45 lakh deaths occurred worldwide
- **WHO region:** Tropical zone is affected the most. According to WHO malaria report 2017, WHO African Region (90%) affected the worst, followed by the South-east Asia Region (7%) and Eastern Mediterranean Region (2%)
- **Incidence rate:** It is about 63 cases per 1000 population at risk, (incidence decreased by 18%, as compared to 2010). The WHO South-East Asia Region recorded the largest decline (48%)
- **Most common species:** In 2016, *P. falciparum* is the most common species worldwide; accounting for 99.7% of malaria cases in sub-Saharan Africa, South east Asia (66%), Eastern Mediterranean regions (58%) and Western Pacific region (77%). *P. vivax* is the predominant parasite only in American region (64%)
- **Age:** Children are more prone to infection and complications. However, newborn are protected from falciparum malaria because of high concentration of fetal hemoglobin in first few months of life
- **Predisposing factors:** The transmission of malaria is directly proportional to:
  - Density of the vector
  - Number of human bites per day per mosquito
  - Time of mosquito bite (more after the dusk)
  - Mosquito longevity (as sporogony lasts for 7–30 days, thus, to transmit malaria, the mosquito must survive for >7 days)
  - Optimum temperature (20–30°C)
  - Optimum humidity (60%)
  - Rainfall (July to November)
  - Altitude below 2,000 meters.

Malaria Situation In India (NVBDCP Report 2016)

India accounts for 6% of total malaria burden in the year 2016. According to National Vector Borne Disease Control Programme (NVBDCP) malaria report 2016:

- In 2016, 1.09 million malaria cases were reported from India with 331 deaths. The mortality rate declined by 70% compared to 2001
- *P. falciparum* was the predominant species; accounted for 65.53% of total cases followed by *P. vivax* (34%)
- Odisha accounted for the maximum malaria cases (41%); followed by Chhattisgarh (13.5%) and Jharkhand (13%). In Odisha, 85% of cases were due to *P. falciparum*; accounted for 23% of total deaths in India
- *P. malariae* infections are <1% and are reported time to time from various places such as Karnataka (Tumkur and Hassan districts, largest foci), Chhattisgarh (Bastar area), Odisha, West Bengal, Madhya Pradesh, Tamil Nadu, Kerala and Assam
- *P. ovale* is mainly confined to tropical Africa. Only few cases are reported from India such as Odisha (Koraput district, 1st case of India), Chhattisgarh (Bastar area), Delhi, Assam, Gujarat and Kolkata.

Malaria Elimination in India

The malaria control in India has been operated through the NVBDCP since 2006.

- WHO has initiated The Global Technical Strategy for Malaria (2016–2030), which aims at elimination of malaria by year 2030. Till date 32 countries have already achieved the elimination status from WHO
- In line with WHO, NVBDCP India has launched **National Framework for Malaria Elimination (NFME)** in 2016 with vision of malaria elimination by 2030. In 2015, all the districts of India are stratified into four categories based on annual parasite incidence (API), (Table 6.6).

The objective set for malaria elimination in India include:

- Eliminate malaria (zero indigenous cases) by 2022 in all existing category 1 and 2 districts (i.e. districts having API <2)
- Category 3 districts (having API ≥2) will be brought into pre-elimination and elimination phase by 2022
- Maintain malaria free-status in category zero districts or in districts where malaria transmission has been interrupted and prevent re-introduction of malaria by strengthening surveillance.

Table 6.6: Stratification of districts based on reported API* for the year 2015, India

Categories	Definition	No. (%) of districts
Category 0 (Prevention of re-establishment phase)	• Districts historically considered to be without local transmission and reporting no case for last 3 years • Vigilance will be maintained to prevent reintroduction of malaria in view of climate change	75 (11)
Category 1 (Pre-elimination phase)	Districts having API <1/1,000 population	448 (66.1)
Category 2 (Elimination phase)	Districts having API ≥1 to ≤2/1,000 population	48 (7.1)
Category 3 (Intensified control phase)	Districts having API >2/1,000 population	107 (15.8)

*Note: API (Annual Parasite Incidence) is defined as = (confirmed cases during 1 year/population under surveillance) x 1000.

Observations

- World Malaria Day: Every year, 25th April is being celebrated as "World malaria day"
- Antimalarial month is celebrated every June.

Laboratory Diagnosis — Malaria parasite

Microscopic tests:
- **Peripheral blood smear**—gold standard
  - **Thick smear**—more sensitive
  - **Thin smear**—speciation can be done based on the following features:
    - *P. vivax*—amoeboid ring form and schizont
    - *P. falciparum*—ring forms (multiple ring form, accole form, headphone shaped ring forms), banana shaped gametocyte
    - *P. malariae*—band forms
    - *P. ovale*—enlarged fimbriated oval RBC with ring forms
- **Fluorescence microscopy** (Kawamoto's technique)
- **Quantitative buffy coat examination**—parasitized RBCs appear as brilliant green dots.

Nonmicroscopic tests:
- **Antigen detection tests** (RDTs) or ICTs—detects pan malarial Ag (LDH, aldolase), falciparum specific Ag (HRP-II)
- **Culture**—RPMI 1640 medium
- **Molecular diagnosis**—PCR using PBRK1 primer.

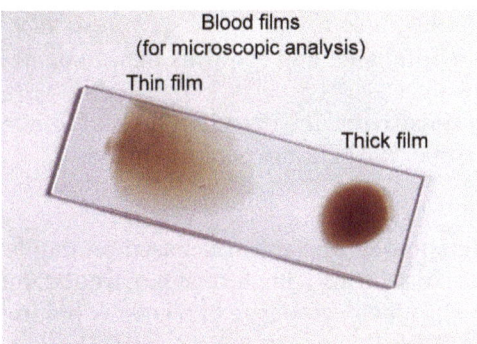

Fig. 6.3: Glass slide showing thin and thick blood smear

Laboratory Diagnosis

The diagnostic tests for malaria can be divided into microscopic and nonmicroscopic tests (see the box above).

Peripheral Blood Smear

Peripheral smear study still remains the simple and gold standard confirmatory test for detection of malarial parasites.

Specimen

Peripheral blood is collected from ear lobe or by finger prick in older children and adults and from the great toe in infants. Blood films should be prepared directly from the capillary blood. In case of ethylenediaminetetraacetic acid (EDTA) anticoagulated blood, smears should be made within an hour of collection of blood. In pregnant women, cord blood and placental impression smears are used. In postmortem cases, smears from cerebral gray matter can be used.

- **Time for taking blood:** Blood should be collected few hours after the height of the paroxysm of fever and before taking antimalarial drugs. Parasite density is maximum during this period
- **Frequency:** Smears should be examined at least twice daily until parasites are detected.

Types of peripheral blood smear

It is of two types—(1) thin and (2) thick smears. Both the smears are made at the same time from capillary blood either on the same or different slides (Fig. 6.3). At least two thick and two thin smears should be made.

- For thick smear, a big drop of blood is spread over 1–2 cm square area on a clean glass slide. The thickness of the film should be such that it allows newsprint to be read. The film is dried and kept in distilled water in a koplin jar for 5–10 minutes for dehemoglobinization
- For thin smear, a small drop of blood is taken on a corner of a slide. It is spread by another spreader slide at an angle of 45° and then is lowered to an angle of 30° and is pushed gently to the left, till the blood is exhausted
- The surface of a good thin film is:
  - Even and uniform
  - Consist of a single layer of RBCs
  - The "feathery tail end" is formed near the center of the slide
  - Margins of the film should not extend to the sides of the slide.
- They are stained with one of the Romanowsky's stains such as Leishman's, Giemsa and Field's, Wright's or JSB (Jaswant Singh and Bhattacharya) stain (for staining procedure, see Chapter 15)
- Thin smear has to be screened first. It is screened near the feathery tail end. At least 200–300 oil immersion fields should be examined before the smears are considered as negative
- Thick smear has to be examined if no parasites are found in thin smear.

Advantages

- Peripheral smear is simple, rapid and cheap
- Thick smear is useful in:
  - **Detecting the parasites:** It is 40 times more sensitive than thin smear, can detect as low as 5–10 parasites per μL of blood
  - Quantification of parasitemia
  - Demonstrating the malaria pigments.
- Thin smear is useful in speciation of malaria parasite. (Speciation is not possible by thick smear as the RBCs are dehemoglobinized).

Disadvantages

- Labor intensive and requires experienced microscopist
- **Low sensitivity:** The detection limit of thin smear is more than 200 parasites per μL of blood.

Speciation

The speciation by thin smear is based on the detection of the asexual forms (ring forms, late trophozoites and schizonts), gametocytes, type of pigments produced and RBC size (Table 6.5 and Figs 6.2, 6.4 and 6.5).

- However, in falciparum malaria, only the gametocytes and ring forms are demonstrated (but not schizonts and late trophozoites) in peripheral blood
- Detection of pigments is considered as peripheral indicator of parasite biomass and the level correlates with severity of disease.

Quantification of parasites

Thick smear is preferred to thin smear for quantification of parasitemia.

- Previously, the "plus system" was used, which is simple but far less accurate for establishing parasite density in thick blood films. Now it is obsolete
- Currently, the quantification is done by calculating the number of parasites counted compared to number of white blood cells (WBCs) in the thick smear or number of RBCs counted in thin smear (Table 6.7)
- Quantification is helpful for:
  - Assessing the severity of infection
  - Monitoring the response to the treatment
  - Detecting drug resistance of *P. falciparum*.

Percentage of parasitemia should be reported to the clinicians as it has direct clinical implication.

- WHO defines severe malaria, if % of parasitemia is >2% with severe anemia (hemoglobin, <5 g/μL)
- Exchange transfusion may be considered if parasitemia ≥10%, as it is associated with highest mortality
- Prognosis is poor if >20% of parasites and/or if >5% of neutrophils contain visible pigment.

Fluorescence Microscopy

- **Kawamoto technique** is a fluorescent staining method for demonstrating malaria parasites. Blood smears are prepared on a slide and are stained with acridine-orange and examined under a fluorescence microscope. Nuclear DNA is stained green
- Nowadays, several other fluorescent dye are used such as benzothiocarboxypurine and 4′,6-diamidine-2-phenylindolo-propidium iodide
- Advantages: Fluorescence staining has several advantages over Giemsa stain—(i) it does not penetrate

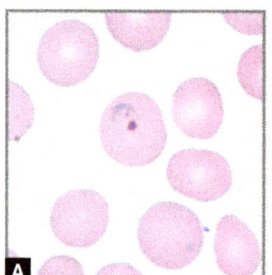 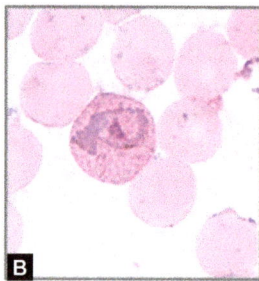 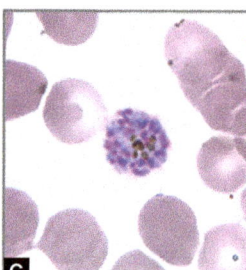 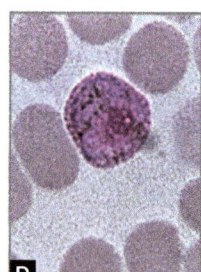 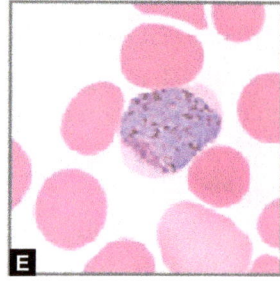

Figs 6.4A to E: Thin blood smear showing different forms of *Plasmodium vivax*; (A) Ring form; (B) Amoeboid form; (C) Schizont; (D) Male gametocyte; (E) Female gametocyte

Source: DPDx Image Library, Centre for Disease Control and prevention (CDC), Atlanta (*with permission*).

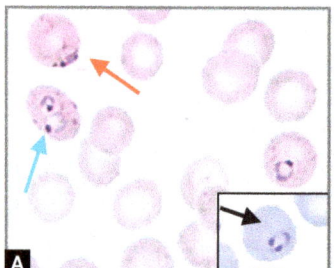 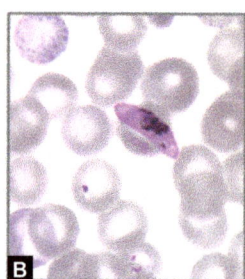 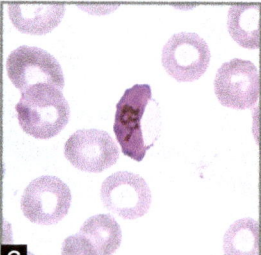 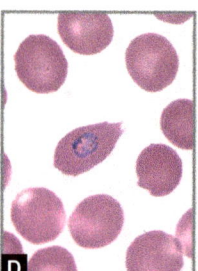 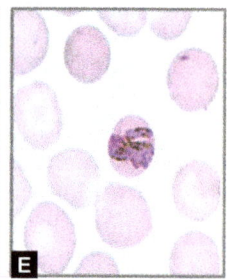

Figs 6.5A to E: Thin blood smear showing: (A) *P. falciparum* ring forms such as multiple rings (blue arrow), accole form (red arrow) and head phone-shaped ring form (black arrow); (B) Female gametocyte of *P. falciparum*; (C) Male gametocyte of *P. falciparum*; (D) Ring form of *P. ovale*; (E) Band form of *P. malariae*

Source: DPDx Image Library, Centers for Disease Control and Prevention (CDC), Atlanta (*with permission*).

CHAPTER 6 ◆ Apicomplexa—I (Malaria Parasite and Babesia)

Table 6.7: Quantification of malaria parasites by thick smear

Plus system (by thick smear)

Parasite count is graded as follows:
+ = 1–10 parasites per 100 OIF
++ = 11–100 parasites per 100 OIF
+++ = 1–10 parasites per single OIF
++++ = > 10 parasites per single OIF

No. of parasites detected per μL of blood

(1) By thick smear

$$= \frac{\text{No. of parasites counted}}{\text{No. of WBCs counted (500 or 200)}} \times \text{Total WBC count (8000)}$$

(2) By thin smear

$$= \frac{\text{No. of parasites counted}}{\text{No. of RBCs counted (5000)}} \times \text{Total RBC count (5,000,000)}$$

Percentage of Parasitemia

$$= \frac{\text{No. of parasites detected per μL of blood}}{50,000}$$

Adapted from World Health Organization.
Abbreviation: OIF, oil immersion field.
Note:
- The number of WBCs counted is up to 500 (if ≤99 parasites are counted) or up to 200 if ≥100 parasites are counted.
- The number of RBCs counted is fixed at 5,000. One should examine 20 fields, with each field containing on an average 250 RBCs/field.
- Only ring forms and schizonts are counted. If gametocytes are seen, do not count them, but report them.
- In mixed infection, count all parasites in RBCs together.
- Always, the actual total WBC count or total RBC count of the patient should be used in formula. If not available, then the average count can be taken as total WBC count (8,000/μL) or total RBC count (5,000,000/μL).

Table 6.8: Procedure of quantitative buffy coat

The commercially available quantitative buffy coat (QBC) capillary tube is precoated internally with acridine orange stain
↓
60 μL of peripheral blood is collected from one end of the tube, which is then closed by a plastic closure (Fig. 6.6A)
↓
A cylindrical float is inserted to the other end of the QBC tube. The tube is centrifuged at 12,000 rpm for 5 minutes
↓
The components of the blood are separated according to their densities, forming discrete bands (Fig. 6.6B)
↓
Because the cylindrical float occupies 90% of the interior lumen of the tube, it forces all the surrounding blood cells into 40 μm space between its outside circumference and inside of the tube
↓
Following centrifugation, the buffy coat region of the QBC tube, i.e. at the RBC/WBC interface is examined under UV light source
↓
The whole 60 μL blood sample can be visualized by rotating the QBC tube under the fluorescent microscope.

into WBCs (unless the smear is fixed) and therefore nucleus of WBCs do not take up the stain, (ii) faster staining and screening of smear, (iii) relatively lesser training is required for interpretation.

Quantitative Buffy Coat Examination

The quantitative buffy coat (QBC) malaria test is an advanced microscopic technique for malaria diagnosis. It consists of three basic steps—(1) concentration of blood by centrifugation, (2) staining with acridine orange stain and (3) examination under ultraviolet (UV) light source (Table 6.8).

Interpretation

Acridine orange has a property of staining the nuclear DNA fluorescent brilliant green. Normal RBCs don't take up the stain (as they are a nucleated). However, parasitized RBCs appear as brilliant green dots. WBCs also take up the stain (Figs 6.6A to D).

Advantages

QBC is faster (the entire tube can be screened within minutes), more sensitive (at least as good as a thick film), uses more blood (60 μL) than thick smear and quantification is possible.

Disadvantages

It is expensive, less specific and speciation is difficult.

Antigen Detection by Rapid Diagnostic Tests

Rapid diagnostic tests (RDTs) have revolutionized the diagnosis of malaria. Several malarial antigens can be detected like:

- **Parasite lactate dehydrogenase (pLDH):** It is produced by trophozoites and gametocytes of all *Plasmodium* species. Currently available test kits can differentiate pan malarial pLDH common to all species and pLDH specific to *P. falciparum*
- **Parasite aldolase:** Produced by all *Plasmodium* species
- ***Plasmodium falciparum* specific histidine rich protein-2 (Pf-HRP-II):** It is produced by trophozoites and young (but not mature) gametocytes of *P. falciparum*
- Most of the kits are designed to detect a combination of two antigens, one is *P. falciparum* specific antigen (i.e. HRP2 or pLDH specific for *P. falciparum*) and other is a pan malarial antigen (like aldolase or pan malarial pLDH)
- Recently, RDT detecting *P. falciparum/P. vivax* is also available. Here, the advantage is, if both the bands appear, indicates mixed infection (*P. falciparum* and *P. vivax*). However, infection due to *P. malariae* or *P. ovale* will be missed by this test
- The principle and procedure of RDTs are described in Table 6.9 and Figures 6.7A and B.

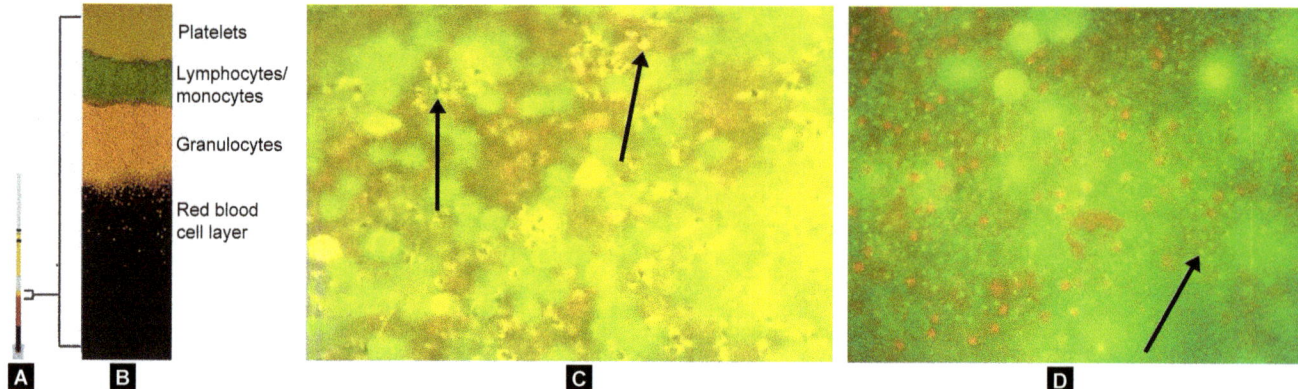

Figs 6.6A to D: (A) QBC capillary tube; (B) Magnified view of QBC capillary tube after centrifugation; (C) Crescent shaped gametocyte of *Plasmodium falciparum*; (D) Ring forms of *Plasmodium falciparum* seen as fluorescent dots

Source: C and D—Department of Microbiology, Sri Siddhartha Medical College, Tumkur, Karnataka.

Table 6.9: Principle and procedure of rapid diagnostic tests

Rapid diagnostic tests (RDTs) are based on lateral flow assay [also called as immunochromatographic test (ICT)]
• Test kits currently available use a nitrocellulose membrane containing a sample pad, an absorbent pad and three detection lines coated with:
  ➢ Test line-1: Coated with capture antibodies specific for *Plasmodium falciparum*
  ➢ Test line-2: Coated with capture antibodies common to all *Plasmodium* spp.
  ➢ Control line: Coated with antibody raised in rabbit sera against polyclonal malarial antibody
• Sample: 5–50 μL of peripheral blood (anticoagulated), serum or plasma is collected according to the manufacturer's instructions
• Blood is mixed with a buffer solution provided by the kit. The buffer solution contains a hemolysing compound that lyses the RBCs to release the malaria antigens
• Buffer solution also contains a polyclonal malarial antibody labeled with colloidal gold (visually detectable marker) which forms antigen antibody complexes with malarial antigen
• Both labeled antigen antibody complexes and unbound polyclonal malarial antibody migrate through the nitrocellulose membrane by capillary action
• *In positive cases:* The labeled antigen antibody complexes will be immobilized at the corresponding pre-deposited lines coated with capture antibody specific for *P. falciparum*, pan malarial capture antibody
• *In both positive and negative cases:* The control band is formed due to binding of the labeled polyclonal malarial antibody to the control antibody. Absence of control band indicates the test is invalid (Figs 6.7A and B).

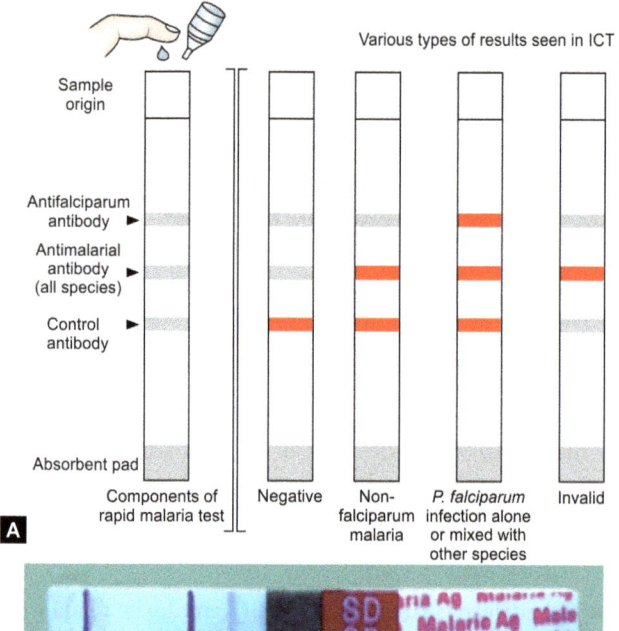

Figs 6.7A and B: (A) Schematic diagram of rapid diagnostic test kit showing negative, non-*falciparum*, pure or mixed infection with *Plasmodium falciparum* and invalid result of malaria; (B) Real image of rapid diagnostic test kit

Source: B—Department of Microbiology, Sri Siddhartha Medical College, Tumkur, Karnataka.

Advantages of rapid diagnostic tests

❖ Rapid diagnostic tests are simple to perform, do not need extra equipment or trained microscopist (Table 6.9)
❖ **Sensitivity:** Rapid diagnostic tests are more than 90% sensitive at >100 parasites/μL. But the sensitivity is markedly reduced at <100 parasites/μL

❖ pLDH is produced by the viable parasites, hence it is used to monitor the response for treatment (microscopy is the best to assess prognosis). However, HRP2 remains positive even after treatment up to 3 weeks
❖ HRP2 is a reliable marker to diagnose malaria in pregnancy

❖ Intensity of the band is directly proportional to the parasitemia and severity of the disease.

Disadvantages of rapid diagnostic tests
Rapid diagnostic test kits are expensive
- Cannot differentiate between the non-falciparum malaria species
- Gametocytes cannot be detected
- False positive bands appear in rheumatoid arthritis factor positive cases
- The lower limit to detect HRP2 is 40 parasites/µL and pLDH is 100 parasites/µL
- RDT has not been developed for *P. knowlesi* yet
- **HRP2/HRP3 gene deletion:** Deletion of HRP2/HRP3 gene has been recently reported from various countries including India; resulting in false negative *P. falciparum* RDT result. A multicentric study conducted in India showed HRP2 and HRP3 gene deletions in 2.4% and 1.8% cases respectively.

RDT under NVBDCP
Governement of India has recently introduced RDT under NVBDCP for areas where microscopy is not available. The following guidelines are recommended.
- RDT based on HRP2 or LDH should be used; aldolase based RDTs are not recommended
- The RDT to be selected should have the following sensitivity and specificity
    - *P. falciparum:* Sensitivity and specificity should be minimum 95% at parasite density level of 200 asexual parasites/uL of blood
    - For *P. vivax:* Sensitivity: ≥75% and specificity: ≥90% at density of 200 parasites/uL.
- RDT should be used only in those villages/areas which satisfy the following criteria
    - *P. falciparum* accounts for >30% of total malaria burden and slide positivity rate is >2%
    - Consistently high annual parasite incidence (API >2) and deaths due to malaria have been reported
    - Inaccessible areas.

Note: Smear microscopy remains the method of choice under NVBDCP in all other remaining areas.

Antibody Detection
ELISA (enzyme-linked immunosorbent assay), IFA (indirect fluorescent antibody test) and rapid diagnostic test formats are available using soluble malarial antigens. Antibodies persist even after the clinical cure. Serology does not detect current infection, but only measures past exposure. Therefore, Government of India has banned the use of antibody detection tests for malaria diagnosis.

Culture
Culture techniques for malaria are mainly used for preparation of malaria antigens. However, they are not used for diagnosis.
- **Trager and Jensen** (1976) discovered a simple method for continuous culture of *P. falciparum*, which has been extended for the cultivation of other species of malaria
- He used **RPMI 1640** medium (Roswell Park Memorial Institute and 1640 denotes the number of passages) in a continuous flow system mixed with a thin layer of RBC and an overlay medium consists of human serum maintained with 7% CO_2 and 1–5% O_2
- All current culture techniques are the modifications of the Trager and Jensen method
- RPMI 1640 medium is the most commonly used and found superior to other media for cultivation of *P. falciparum*
- The other media used are Dulbecco's Modified Eagle Medium (DMEM), RPMI 1630, and Medium 199.

Molecular Methods
Various molecular tests have recently gained attention for malaria diagnosis.
- **Nested multiplex PCR** targeting 18S rDNA has been developed for detection of all five human malaria parasites including *P. knowlesi*. It has a detection limit of 10 to 100 copies/µL. Compared with microscopy, it showed 95.8 to 100% sensitivity and 98.6 to 100% specificity
- PCR can also be used to detect drug resistant genes
- **Real time PCR** is useful for quantification and speciation of parasites. Various gene targets include *P. falciparum Cox-1* gene, 18S rDNA, and mitochondrial DNA sequence
- **LAMP assay:** Recently loop-mediated amplification (LAMP) kit has been developed. Like RDT, it can differentiate *P. falciparum* and non-*P. falciparum* but cannot further speciate. It showed sensitivity of >90%.

Automated Systems
- Automated differential instruments such as Parasite F digital cytometry have been recently developed
- Automated microscopy methods are under development for the semiautomated or automated detection and identification of *Plasmodium* species from digitally stained blood film images
- These methods though sound promising; give false negative results in low parasitemia and therefore requires further validation.

Other Nonspecific Tests

Other nonspecific tests include:
- Normochromic and normocytic hemolytic anemia
- Leukopenia (due to decrease in granulocytes and lymphocytes) and Metabolic acidosis
- Raised erythrocyte sedimentation rate (ESR)
- Raised serum C-reactive protein
- Prolonged prothrombin and partial thromboplastin time in severe infection
- Decreased antithrombin III levels in mild infection
- Hypoglycemia: Lower blood glucose levels are associated with higher mortality
- Severe falciparum malaria is also associated with low plasma concentrations of sodium, calcium, magnesium and albumin; and high levels of lactate, creatinine, muscle and liver enzymes, and conjugated and unconjugated bilirubin
- **Human lysozyme** is a potential biomarker for detection of severity of malaria. It is elevated double than normal value in various samples such as urine, saliva, tear and serum. It is detected by photometric assays, radioimmunoassay and ELISA
- Hypergammaglobulinemia.

Comparison of peripheral smear, quantitative buffy coat and rapid diagnostic tests are described in Table 6.10.

> **Treatment** — **Malaria**
>
> Various antimalarial drugs are depicted in Table 6.11. NVBDCP, India has given guideline for the treatment of vivax malaria and falciparum malaria, as described in Tables 6.12 and 6.13.

Severe malaria (Table 6.14) is an emergency, develops quickly over 1–2 days and may lead to death. Hence, the treatment should be given promptly. The drug of choice include IV artemisinin derivatives or IV quinine (Table 6.15).

Antimalarial Drug Resistance

Antimalarial drug resistance has emerged as one of the greatest challenges facing malaria control today.

Drug Resistance in Falciparum Malaria

Drug resistance in *P. falciparum* is widespread and is described against all the available drugs, however, there are geographical variations (Table 6.16).

Table 6.10: Comparison of peripheral smear, quantitative buffy coat and rapid diagnostic tests

Features	Peripheral smear	Quantitative buffy coat	Rapid diagnostic tests
Method	Cumbersome	Easy	Easy
Time	Longer, 60–120 minutes	Faster, 15–30 minutes	Faster, 15–30 minutes
Sensitivity	Detection limit: • 5 parasites/μL in thick film • 200 parasites/μL in thin film	Claimed to be more sensitive, at least as good as a thick film	• >100 parasites/μL, sensitivity >90% • <100 parasites/μL, sensitivity falls
Specificity	Gold standard	False positives—artifacts may be reported as positive by nontrained technicians	False positive in RA factor (rheumatoid arthritis) positive cases
Speciation	Accurate, gold standard	Difficult	Detect *Plasmodium falciparum* but cannot differentiate non-*falciparum* species
Cost	Inexpensive	Costly equipment and consumables	Kits are costly but no extra equipment required. Good for field study
Experienced Microscopist	Required	Not required, minimal training is sufficient	Not required, minimal training is sufficient

Table 6.11: Antimalarial drugs and their activity

Class	Drugs	Active against parasitic stages
Quinolines and related compounds	Chloroquine Quinine Mefloquine Primaquine	Asexual RBC stages Gametocytes (except *Plasmodium falciparum*) Asexual RBC stages Liver stages and hypnozoites, gametocytes
Artemisinin and its derivatives	Artemisinin, artemether and arte-ether	Asexual RBC stages and gametocytes
Hydroxynaphthoquinones	Atovaquone	Asexual RBC stages,
Biguanide derivative	Proguanil	Liver stages (only for *P. falciparum*)
Diaminopyrimidines	Pyrimethamine	Asexual RBC stages,
Sulfonamides	Sulfadiazine and sulfadoxine	Liver stages (+/-)
Tetracyclines	Tetracycline and doxycycline	Asexual RBC stages (+/-)

Abbreviations: (+/-) indicates doubtful activity; RBC, red blood cell.
Note: **Newer antimalarial drugs:** Arterolane, tetraoxanes, N-tert-Butyl isoquine, cycloguanil-pyrimethamine, azithromycin-chloroquine combination, spiroindolones, albitiazolium and AQ-13 (a next generation 4-aminoquinoline) are some of the newer antimalarial drugs in the pipeline.

Table 6.12: Treatment of Vivax Malaria (NVBDCP guideline, India)

Chloroquine	25 mg/kg, divided over three days, i.e. 10 mg/kg on day 1 and 2 and 5 mg/kg on day 3
Primaquine	0.25 mg/kg body weight; daily for 14 days; should be given under supervision, aiming to kill hypnozoites of *P. vivax* (to prevent relapse) Contraindicated in infants, pregnant women and individuals with G6PD deficiency

* *P. vivax* infection in pregnancy, chloroquine is treatment of choice.
Abbreviation: NVBDCP, National Vector Borne Disease Control Programme.

Table 6.13: Treatment of Falciparum Malaria (NVBDCP guideline, India)

North-Eastern States	**ACT-AL,** i.e. co-formulated tablet of *artemether and lumefantrine*; total dose of 80 mg/480 mg (in adults), given over twice daily for 3 days *plus* Primaquine (0.75 mg/kg) single dose on second day aiming to kill gametocytes of *P. falciparum*. (ACT-AL is contraindicated in 1st trimester pregnancy and children <5 kg weight)
Other states	**ACT-SP,** i.e. artesunate (4 mg/kg) for 3 days *plus* sulfadoxine (25 mg/kg)/ pyrimethamine (1.25 mg/kg), 1 tablet given on first day *plus* Primaquine (0.75 mg/kg) single dose on second day

In uncomplicated *P. falciparum* cases in pregnancy:
First trimester: Quinine salt 10 mg/kg 3 times daily for 7 days
Second/third trimester: Area-specific ACT; as given above

In mixed infection (*P. vivax* plus *P. falciparum*)
ACT-AL and ACT-SP as per geographical area as given above plus Primaquine (0.25 mg/kg) for 14 days

Abbreviations: ACT-AL, artemisinin combination therapy artemether-lumefantrine; ACT-SP, artemisinin combination therapy artesunate-sulfadoxine/pyrimethamine; NVBDCP, National Vector Borne Disease Control Programme
Northeastern states includes Arunachal Pradesh, Assam, Manipur, Meghalaya, Mizoram, Nagaland, and Tripura.

Table 6.14: Severe Malaria

Characterized by ≥1 of the following features:
- Impaired consciousness/coma
- Repeated generalized convulsions
- Renal failure (Serum creatinine >3 mg/dL)
- Jaundice (Serum bilirubin >3 mg/dL)
- Severe anemia (Hb <5 g/dL)
- Pulmonary edema/acute respiratory distress syndrome
- Hypoglycemia (Plasma glucose <40 mg/dL)
- Metabolic acidosis
- Circulatory collapse/shock (Systolic BP <80 mm Hg, <50 mm Hg in children)
- Abnormal bleeding and disseminated intravascular coagulation (DIC)
- Hemoglobinuria
- Hyperpyrexia (Temperature >106°F or >42°C)
- Hyperparasitemia (>5% parasitized RBCs)

Table 6.15: Treatment options available for severe malaria

Drugs	Dosage
Artesunate	2.4 mg/kg IV, given on admission (time = 0), then at 12 and 24 hours, then once a day
Quinine	Loading dose of 20 mg/kg at admission (IV infusion in 5% dextrose over a period of 4 hours) followed by maintenance dose of 10 mg/kg 8 hourly
Artemether	3.2 mg/kg IM, given on admission then 1.6 mg/kg body weight per day
Arteether	150 mg daily IM, for 3 days in adults only (not recommended for children)

Note:
- In pregnancy, quinine is preferred in first trimester.
- In severe *P. vivax* malaria, treatment is same as of *P. falciparum*, except primaquine is given for 14 days.
- For artemisinin derivatives, switch over to oral therapy when the patient becomes stable or after 24 hours of parenteral therapy whichever is later.

Table 6.16: Drug resistance in *Plasmodium falciparum* from World (adapted from World Health Organization, 2018)

	CQ	SP	MQ
South America	++	++	+
Western Africa	++	+	+
Eastern and Southern Africa	++	+	–
Indian subcontinent	++	–	–
South-East Asia* and Oceania	++	++	++
East Asia (South China)	++	++	?

CQ, chloroquine; SP, sulfadoxine-pyrimethamine; MQ, mefloquine
*includes border areas of Thailand, Cambodia, and Myanmar. They show resistance to quinine and halofantrine also.

World's highest burden: Border areas of Thailand, Cambodia, and Myanmar possess the highest risk for resistance to chloroquine and other classes such quinine, sulfadoxine-pyrimethamine, halofantrine and mefloquine.
❖ Many of the strains of *P. falciparum* are multiple-drug-resistant (MDR), which is defined as resistance to at least ≥3 classes of antimalarial drugs
❖ Resistance to artemisinin has not be reported from World; although slow clearance phenotypes have been documented from Mekong river region.

India: Chloroquine resistance in *P. falciparum* has been reported since 1973 (first case from Assam).
❖ Highest chloroquine resistance in India has been reported from northeast states
❖ Currently, 117 districts are considered highly endemic for chloroquine resistance in *P. falciparum* (≥10% treatment failure); which include 67 districts of 7 North-east states and 50 districts from Andhra Pradesh, Chhattisgarh, Jharkhand, Madhya Pradesh and Odisha.

The important factors that contribute to emergence of resistance are:
- Longer half-life of drug
- Mutation of the parasite for resistance (described below)
- Inadequate and irregular usage of drug
- Host immunity.

The development of resistance can be *delayed by combination of drugs,* i.e. combining one drug that rapidly reduces parasite biomass with a partner drug that can remove any residual parasites, e.g. ACT.

Drug Resistance in Vivax malaria

Only sporadic cases of resistance to chloroquine and/or primaquine in some areas have been reported such as India, Burmah, Indonesia, Papua, New Guinea, Brazil, Guyana, Colombia and Solomon Islands.

Mechanism of Drug Resistance

- **Chloroquine resistance in *Plasmodium falciparum*:** Occurs due to mutations in the genes encoding the transporter proteins such as PfCRT (*P. falciparum* chloroquine transporter) and PfMDR1 (*P. falciparum* multidrug resistance gene 1). These proteins help in chloroquine influx into the parasitic food vacuoles. Such mutation results in impaired transport of chloroquine
- More so, mutation in PfMDR1 gene leads to resistance to other antimalarials like amodiaquine, mefloquine and halofantrine
- **Resistance to antifolates** such as sulfadoxine, pyrimethamine and proguanil is due to point mutation in DHFR (dihydrofolate reductase) gene
- **Resistance to artemesinins** has not be reported yet however it is observed in animal experiments and may be linked to *PfKelch13* (K13) mutations. Monotherapy with artemisinins is banned in India as it promotes resistance.

WHO Guideline for Assessing Degree of Resistance

Antimalarial drug resistance is defined as the "ability of a parasite strain to survive and/or to multiply despite administration and absorption of a drug given in doses equal to or higher than those usually recommended but within tolerance of the subject and the drug must be able to gain access to the parasite".

In vivo method (2002): The degree of resistance is divided into four categories:

1. **Early treatment failure (ETF):** Development of danger sign or severe malaria (fever >37.5°C) on day 0–3 and parasitemia on day 3 is 25% higher than day 0 count.
2. **Late clinical failure (LCF):** Development of danger sign or severe malaria (fever >37.5°C) in the presence of parasitemia from day 4 to day 28, without previous meeting of any criteria of ETF.
3. **Late parasitological failure (LPF):** Presence of parasitemia on any day from 7 days to 28 days and fever less than 37.5°C; without previous meeting of any criteria of early and late treatment failure.
4. **Adequate clinical and parasitological response (ACR):** Absence of parasitemia on day 28 irrespective of fever, without previous meeting of any criteria of early and late treatment failure.

In vitro tests: Various in vitro methods are also available for antimalarial drug susceptibility testing such as:
- The WHO *in vitro* micro test using RPMI 1640 medium
- ELISA for measurement of HRP2/or pLDH
- Polymerase chain reaction to detect the *P. falciparum* specific drug resistance genes—available for only a few drugs (chloroquine, pyrimethamine, cycloguanil, sulfadoxine and atovaquone).

Prophylaxis Against Malaria

Prophylaxis against malaria includes chemoprophylaxis, vector control strategies and vaccine prophylaxis.

Chemoprophylaxis

Chemoprophylaxis is recommended for travelers, migrant laborers and military personnel exposed to malaria in highly endemic areas.

- **For short-term chemoprophylaxis (<6 weeks):** Doxycycline is recommended, at a dose of 100 mg daily in adults and 1.5 mg/kg for children. The drug should be started 2 days before travel and continued for 4 weeks after leaving the malaria endemic area. Doxycycline is contraindicated in pregnant and lactating women and children less than 8 years
- **Long-term chemoprophylaxis (>6 weeks):** Mefloquine is recommended at a dose of 5 mg/kg weekly and administered two weeks before, during and four weeks after leaving the area. Mefloquine is contraindicated in cases with history of convulsions, neuropsychiatric problems and cardiac conditions.

Vector Control Strategies

Vector control is still one of the prime weapons to control malaria in endemic areas.

Antiadult measures

- **Residual spraying:** Spraying the houses with residual insecticides such as dichlorodiphenyltrichloroethane (DDT), malathion and fenitrothion is highly effective against adult mosquito

- **Space application** of pesticide in the form of fog or mist by ultra-low volume method of pesticide dispersion
- **Individual protection:** Done by reduction of human-mosquito contact by using insecticide treated bed nets, repellents and protective clothing.

Antilarval measures

- **Larvicide:** Use of mineral oil or Paris green has been extensively used to kill mosquito larvae and pupae
- **Source reduction** (to reduce the mosquito breeding sites): Includes environmental sanitation, water management and improvement of the drainage system
- **Biological larvicide:** *Gambusia affinis* (fish) and *Bacillus thuringiensis* (bacteria) can be used to kill the mosquito larva.

Vaccination for Malaria

Despite of intense research, till date, there is no vaccine licensed for human use. Currently, there are 22 vaccine experiments in various phases of trials are going on globally in Africa, Asia and America (Table 6.17). Most (21 trials) are targeted for *P. falciparum* and one for *P. vivax*. Approaches are made targeting the various stages of malaria cycle (Table 6.17). The main problems in malaria vaccine include:

- The vaccine candidates are poor inducer of cell-mediated immune response
- Antigenic variation in malarial antigens such as PfEMP
- Different immune mechanisms occur in different stages of malaria life cycle.

Only one vaccine trial (RTS, S/AS01) has successfully completed phase III trial; described in the highlight box below.

RTS, S/AS01

This is the most successful malaria trial; started in 2005 in Africa (Kenya and Ghana) by GlaxoSmithKline (GSK).

- **Vaccine candidate:** It consists of PfCSP (circumsporozoite protein of *P. falciparum*), hepatitis B surface antigen (HBsAg), combined with a chemical adjuvant (AS01) to boost the immune system response

Contd...

Table 6.17: Malaria vaccine strategies and trials (Adapted from World Health Organization, 2018)

Stage targeted	Aims at	Host immune response	Target antigen for vaccine candidate	
Pre-erythrocytic vaccine: Prevents infection, disease and transmission.				
Sporozoites	Prevents the entry of the parasite into liver	Humoral immunity mediated by antibodies	RTS,S/AS01 (Phase III)	PfCSP (circumsporozoite protein of *P. falciparum*) fused with hepatitis B surface antigen and a chemical adjuvant (AS01)
			ChAd63-MVA ME TRAP (Phase IIb)	PfCSP engineered with viral vectors such as adenovirus 63 and modified vaccinia virus Ankara (MVA) and Multiple epitope thrombospondin adhesion protein (ME-TRAP).
Liver stage schizont	Prevents intrahepatic schizogony	CMI mediated by CD4 T cell, CD8 T cell, NK cell, IFN-γ	PfSPZ (Phase IIb)	*P. falciparum* sporozoite protein
Blood stage vaccine/ erythrocytic vaccine: These vaccines help in preventing the disease thus, are useful for people living in hyperendemic areas of malaria. Prevention of infection is not required for endemic areas as it is unavoidable and all infected people do not develop the disease.				
Merozoites, erythrocytic schizont antigen on infected RBC surface	Inactivates merozoites before invasion	Both CMI and AMI • Neutralizing antibodies • ADCC • CD4 T cells	GMZ2 (Phase IIb)	Recombinant protein consisting of conserved domains of GLURP (glutamate-rich protein) and MSP3 (merozoite surface protein), of *P. falciparum*
			MSP3 (Phase IIb)	Merozoite surface protein antigen-3
			ChAd63/MVA PvDBP (Phase Ia)	*P. vivax* Duffy binding protein (PvDBP) conjugated with ChAd63/MVA
Transmission blocking/sexual stage vaccine: They do not have direct impact on the individual taking the vaccine, but antibodies are passed to the mosquito during blood meal, block the further transmission of the parasite.				
Gametocyte, ookinetes and mosquito midgut binding sites	Antibodies react with the target sites and block the transmission	AMI in mosquito IgG antibodies taken up during blood meal	Pfs25/EPA (Phase Ib)	25 kDa ookinete specific surface protein, conjugated to a detoxified form of *Pseudomonas aeruginosa* exotoxin A
			Pfs25/VLP (Phase Ia)	Same target as above, but recombinant to virus-like particles (VLPs)

Note: Phase Ia, studies in non-immune subjects; phase Ib, studies in malaria immune subjects; phase IIa, studies in malaria naïve subjects; phase IIb, proof of concept studies in the field; phase III, confirmatory efficacy trial for licensure; phase IV, pilot introduction in selected areas through routine immunization program.
Abbreviations: CMI, cell-mediated immune response; AMI, antibody-mediated immune response; ADCC, antibody-dependent cell-mediated cytotoxicity; IFN, interferon.

Contd...

- Infection is prevented by inducing high antibody titers that block the parasite from infecting the liver
- **Dosage:** 25 μg dose is administered for 3 doses with or without booster
- **Result of Phase III trial:** It was conducted from 2009 to 2014; enrolled 15,000 children of sub-Saharan African countries. It prevented 39% cases of malaria (and 29% cases of severe malaria) among children aged 5–17 months over 4 years with reduction in hospital admissions.
- **Currently in phase IV trial:** The vaccine has been recommended by WHO for pilot introduction in selected areas of three African countries (Ghana, Kenya and Malawi) in 2018; will be given to young children through routine immunization program.

BABESIA

Babesia is an intraerythrocytic protozoa of animals, causes tick born malaria like illness in cattle and sheep. It rarely affects humans causing opportunistic infection.

- *Babesia* is named after a Romanian Scientist, Sir V Babes who described the causative parasite inside the RBC of cattle and sheep in 1888
- Later on, Kilbourne (1893, USA) had demonstrated the parasite to cause Texas cattle fever, a tick-borne hemolytic disease of cattle
- The first human case was reported in 1957 in a farmer in Yugoslavia
- *Babesia* species are grouped into (based on size and genetic basis):
  - Small *Babesia* species (1-2.5 μm): *B. microti, B. gibsoni* and *B. rodhaini*. They are close to a nematode, named *Theileria* species
  - Large *Babesia* species (2.5-5 μm): *B. caballi, B. canis* and *B. bovis. B. divergens* though genetically is related to large group, it appears small in size.
- **Newer species:** There are few newer unnamed species of *Babesia* recently reported to cause human infection in various places; such as WA1 (now called as *B. duncani,* Washington), CA1 (California), and MO1 (Missouri), EU1 species (now called *B. venatorum*, Italy, Austria).

Life Cycle

Host: The nymph stage of the deer tick (hard tick) *Ixodes scapularis* is the primary vector (definitive host) of the parasite. Occasionally, it is transmitted by blood transfusion. Humans act as intermediate host.

Mode of transmission: Man acquires infection by the bite of ticks where the sporozoites enter through the site of bite and are discharged into circulation. Other modes of transmission include blood transfusion and transplacental transmission.

Asexual Cycle in Man

Sporozoites enter into RBCs where they transform into trophozoites and then multiply asexually by budding giving rise to two or four pear-shaped trophozoites (ring forms in tetrad called as **Maltese cross form**); arranged inside RBCs.

- They feed on hemoglobin but pigments are not produced
- Some of the asexual forms transform into gametocytes.

Sexual Cycle in Tick

Following the blood meal, the gametocytes reach the intestine where they multiply sexually and later migrate to salivary gland where they transform into sporozoites.

Pathogenesis and Clinical Features

The incubation period varies from 1 to 6 weeks.
Transmission occurs in warm months (May to September)

- **Mild *Babesia microti* illness:** It is characterized by malaise, fatigue, and weakness and fever. Later on the patient develops chills, sweats, headache, myalgia, anorexia, dry cough, arthralgia and nausea
- **Severe *Babesia microti* illness:**
  - Seen when parasitemia exceeds more than 4%
  - Predisposing factors include age >50 years, males, patients with splenectomy, HIV/AIDS, malignancy, and immunosuppression
  - Patient presents as severe anemia (hemoglobin level < 10 g/dL)
  - Complications may occur like acute respiratory distress syndrome, disseminated intravascular coagulation, congestive heart failure, renal failure and splenic infarcts and rupture.
- **Infections by *Babesia divergens*, *Babesia bovis* and *Babesia duncani*:** Usually seen in splenectomized and immunocompromised patients. Infection is more severe and fulminant with 42% mortality.

Epidemiology

- Babesiosis is highly endemic in the North Eastern United States like Nantucket Island. In Europe almost all cases of babesiosis are due to *B. divergens*
- It is an emerging infectious disease in other countries
- In India, babesiosis is not reported yet.

Laboratory Diagnosis

Peripheral Blood Microscopy

As parasitemia is low in babesiosis, both thick and thin blood smears should be examined.

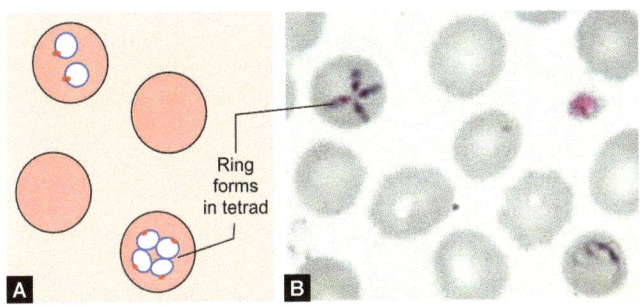

Figs 6.8A and B: Giemsa stained blood smear showing Maltese cross form (A) Schematic diagram; (B) Peripheral blood smear

Source: B—DPDx Image Library, Centers for Disease Control and Prevention (CDC), Atlanta (with permission).

- **Diagnostic feature:** Demonstration of two or four rings of 1–5 μm size inside the RBCs (called as Maltese cross forms) is characteristic feature seen in babesiosis (Figs 6.8A and B)
- It is often confused with the multiple ring forms of *P. falciparum*, but can be differentiated by lack of pigments, lack of crescentic gametocytes, and the presence of pear-shaped rings (Table 6.18).

Serology

Indirect fluorescent antibody (IFA) test for *B. microti* is available. IgG titers of 1:1024 or more signify active or recent infection. Titers typically decline over 6–12 months. Titers of less than 1:64 suggest complete clearance. Titers that remain positive (1:64) suggest persistent low-level parasitemia. IFA may give false-positive result due to cross reactivity to other *Babesia* species and *Plasmodium* species.

ELISA is now available, which detects antibody by using various synthetic peptide antigens such as BMN1-17, MN-10 and circulating BmSA1 antigen.

Molecular Methods

PCR can be done targeting amplification of 18S rRNA gene, has a detection threshold of 20 parasites/μL of blood. It is useful when microscopy fails (low parasitemia). Real-time PCR assay is also available, has a detection limit of 13 parasites in 2 mL blood.

Table 6.18: Differences between *Babesia* and falciparum malaria

Feature	Babesia	Falciparum malaria
Vector	Tick	Female *Anopheles* mosquito
Ring forms	Pear-shaped and in tetrad (maltese cross form); seen both inside and outside RBC	Round and may be single or multiple, seen mainly inside RBCs
Gametocyte	Not seen	Crescentic gametocyte
RBC	Does not contain pigments, no Maurer's stippling seen	Contains pigments, sometime Maurer's stippling seen
Asexual cycle	By budding Schizogony -asynchronous	Binary fission Schizogony—synchronous
Hemolysis	Less severe	More severe
Cerebral features	Not seen	Seen
Parasitemia	Usually low (1–10%)	Usually high
Fever cycle	No periodicity seen	24–36 hours
Endemic area	Temperate area	Tropical and subtropical area
Treatment	Atovaquone plus azithromycin is given	Artemesinin combination therapy

Animal Inoculation

Blood of the patients can be inoculated intraperitoneally into golden hamsters for *B. microti* or gebril for *B. divergens*. After 2–4 weeks, the hamster's blood smear examination is done weekly at least for 6 weeks to demonstrate the parasite. Though cumbersome, it is more sensitive and specific.

Treatment — Babesia

- For mild *Babesia microti* illness: The recommended regimen is oral atovaquone plus azithromycin for 7–10 days
- For severe *Babesia microti* illness: Intravascular (IV) clindamycin plus oral quinine should be given for 7–10 days and blood transfusion to be considered if required
- Other *Babesia* infections by *Babesia divergens* and *Babesia duncani*: Immediate complete RBC exchange transfusion is recommended followed by IV clindamycin plus oral quinine for 7–10 days.

EXPECTED QUESTIONS

I. Write essay on:
a. A 54-year-old male from Chhattisgarh presented with fever, chills and rigor for four days. The patient developed convulsions prior to admission. He was started on ceftriaxone by a private medical practitioner, but did not improve. On physical examination, signs of meningeal irritation, anemia and splenomegaly were present. The blood sample was collected and was subjected to peripheral blood smear examination which showed accole form, multiple ring forms and crescent-shaped gametocytes inside RBCs.
1. What is the etiological agent based on history?
2. Write briefly about the life cycle of the etiological agent.
3. Describe the pathogenesis, clinical manifestations and complications produced.
4. What are the various diagnostic modalities?
5. How will you treat this condition?

b. A 18-year-old female from Udupi, Karnataka, presented with high-grade fever which rises every third day with chills and rigor. Her serum sample was subjected to a rapid diagnostic test which revealed bands near pLDH line and control line, but no band near HRP-II line.
   1. What is the probable etiological agent based on history?
   2. Describe a note on epidemiology of this clinical condition.
   3. What are the various diagnostic modalities?
   4. How will you treat this condition?

II. Write short notes on:
   a. Cerebral malaria.
   b. *Plasmodium knowlesi*.
   c. Prophylaxis of malaria.
   d. Babesiosis.
   e. Vaccine approaches against malaria.
   f. Drug resistance in malaria.

III. Multiple choice questions (MCQs):
   1. Which is the infective form of the malaria parasite to man?
      a. Merozoite
      b. Sporozoite
      c. Trophozoite
      d. Gametocyte
   2. Which is the infective form of the malaria parasite to mosquito?
      a. Merozoite
      b. Sporozoite
      c. Trophozoite
      d. Gametocyte
   3. Which stage of the malaria parasite causes relapse?
      a. Sporozoite
      b. Trophozoite
      c. Merozoite
      d. Hypnozoites
   4. For infection of mosquito, the blood of human carrier must contain atleast:
      a. 12 gametocytes/µL
      b. 10 gametocytes/µL
      c. 16 gametocytes/µL
      d. 18 gametocytes/µL
   5. Which is true about *Plasmodium falciparum*?
      a. High level of parasitemia
      b. It invades erythrocytes of all ages
      c. Its erythrocytic schizogony takes place in the capillaries of internal organs
      d. All of the above
   6. Crescent-shaped or banana-shaped gametocytes are seen in infection with:
      a. *Plasmodium vivax*
      b. *Plasmodium falciparum*
      c. *Plasmodium ovale*
      d. *Plasmodium malariae*
   7. Maurer's dots in red blood cells are seen in infection with:
      a. *Plasmodium vivax*
      b. *Plasmodium falciparum*
      c. *Plasmodium malariae*
      d. *Plasmodium ovale*
   8. Appearance of fever paroxysm every 72 hours (Quartan periodicity of malaria) is seen in infection with:
      a. *Plasmodium vivax*
      b. *Plasmodium falciparum*
      c. *Plasmodium malariae*
      d. *Plasmodium ovale*
   9. Babesiosis is transmitted by bite of:
      a. *Anopheles*
      b. Sandfly
      c. Mite
      d. Tick
   10. Maltese cross form is seen in:
      a. Babesiosis
      b. *Plasmodium ovale*
      c. *Plasmodium malariae*
      d. *Toxoplasma*

Answers
1. b   **2.** d   **3.** d   **4.** a   **5.** d   **6.** b   **7.** b   **8.** c   **9.** d   **10.** a

Apicomplexa—II (Opportunistic Coccidian Parasites)

CHAPTER 7

CHAPTER OUTLINE

- Introduction
- *Toxoplasma gondii*
- *Cryptosporidium* species
- *Cyclospora* species
- *Cystoisospora* species
- *Sarcocystis* species

INTRODUCTION

- Coccidian parasites can be divided into three orders—(1) Eimeriida, (2) Haemosporida and (3) Piroplasmida. The latter two are described in Chapter 6
- **Order Eimeriida contains five genera:** *Toxoplasma, Cryptosporidium, Cyclospora, Cystoisospora* and *Sarcocystis* (refer Chapter 6, Table 6.1)
- *Toxoplasma* is an intracellular parasite that can cause congenital infections and also opportunistic infections (encephalitis) in HIV (human immunodeficiency virus) infected patients
- *Cryptosporidium, Cyclospora* and *Cystoisospora* are acid fast parasites that can cause opportunistic infections (diarrhea) in HIV infected patients
- *Sarcocystis* is a rare parasite infecting man and forms cystic lesions in muscles.

TOXOPLASMA GONDII

Toxoplasma gondii is an obligate intracellular parasite affecting a wide range of mammals and birds including humans.

- Though human infection is very common affecting nearly one-third of world's population; clinical manifestations are relatively rare, mostly restricting to opportunistic infections in immunocompromised persons and congenital infection in fetus
- Charles Nicolle and Louis Manceaux (1908) were the first to discover *T. gondii* in Tunisia from a North African rodent called as *Ctenodactylus gundi*
- The name *Toxoplasma* is derived from a Greek word "*Toxon*" meaning arc or bow referring to the curved shape of the trophozoites (tachyzoites).

Morphology

It exists in three morphological forms—two asexual forms (tachyzoite and tissue cyst) and a sexual form (oocyst).

Tachyzoite

It is an actively multiplying form (trophozoite), usually seen in acute infection.

- **Crescent shaped**, having a pointed anterior end and a rounded posterior end
- It measures approximately 4–8 μm in length and 2–3 μm in breadth; contains several **dense granules** and a round nucleus situated between center and posterior end
- They can infect all mammalian (nucleated) cells; therefore they do not infect RBCs
- At the anterior end, the tachyzoites contain special organelles like rhoptries, and micronemes which are crucial for the adhesion and invasion into the host cell (Fig. 7.1A)
- Inside the host cell, tachyzoites are surrounded by a parasitophorous vacuole within which they divide asexually by a process called as **internal budding** or **endodyogeny** by which daughter trophozoites are formed within the parent cell. They often form **rosettes** surrounding the host nucleus
- Host cell becomes distended by the proliferating tachyzoites and appears as **pseudocyst** (Fig. 7.1B). They are not strongly PAS positive. Later on, the host cell ruptures releasing the tachyzoites that infects other adjoining cells.

Tissue Cyst

It is the resting stage of the parasite, usually seen in chronic infections.

- The parasite multiplies within the host cells and produces a round to oval tissue cyst containing many crescent shaped slowly multiplying trophozoites called as **bradyzoites**, surrounded by a cyst wall
- Tissue cysts vary in size (Fig. 7.1C):
    - Younger ones that measure 2–5 μm in size and contain few bradyzoites
    - Older tissue cysts may reach more than 100 μm size and contain several thousand bradyzoites.
- **Bradyzoites:** They measure 7 μm in length and 1.5 μm in breadth
    - More slender, crescent shaped with a nucleus situated posteriorly
    - Contains several strongly periodic acid-Schiff stain (PAS) positive amylopectin granules
    - Multiply slowly with long generation time
    - They contain cytoplasmic vacuoles
    - Seen in chronic infection
    - More resistant to gastric juice.
- The cyst wall of the tissue cyst is eosinophilic and weakly PAS positive
- Conversion of the tachyzoites to bradyzoites can be triggered by many factors like interferon-γ (IFN-γ), nitric oxide (NO), heat shock proteins, pH, and temperature changes
- Most common site of the tissue cysts—muscles and brain (can be found in any organs)
- They appear spherical in the brain and oval inside the muscle tissue.

Oocyst

Oocyst is the sexual form of the parasite found in cats and other felines.

- It measures 11–14 μm long and 9–11 μm wide; surrounded by a refractile and resistant double layered colorless cyst wall (Fig. 7.1D)
- Unsporulated oocyst excreted in cat's feces is noninfectious (Fig. 7.1E). In the environment, they transform into sporulating oocyst that contains two sporocysts (8 μm × 6 μm) each containing four elongated sporozoites (6–8 μm × 1–2 μm).

Life Cycle (Fig. 7.2)

Host: The life cycle involves two hosts:
1. **Definitive hosts** are cat and other felines; where the sexual cycle takes place.
2. **Intermediate hosts** are man and other mammals (goat, sheep, pig, cattle and certain birds); where the asexual cycle takes place.

Asexual Cycle or Exoenteric Cycle (The Human Cycle)

- **Transmission and infective form:** *T. gondii* is unique among the protozoa as all the three morphological forms can transmit the infection. Transmission to man occurs (in the decreasing order of frequency):
    - Ingestion of tissue cyst containing bradyzoites (infective form) from undercooked meat (most common route)
    - Ingestion of sporulated oocysts (infective form) from contaminated soil, food, or water
    - By blood transfusion, needle stick injuries, organ transplantation, transplacental transmission or laboratory accidents. Tachyzoites are the infective form.
- **Transform into tachyzoites:** In the intestine, sporozoites are released from sporulated oocyst and bradyzoites are released from the tissue cyst. They invade the intestinal epithelium and transform into tachyzoites
- **Transform into tissue cyst:** Tachyzoites multiply actively by endodyogeny and spread locally to the mesenteric lymph node. Subsequently, they also spread to distant extraintestinal organs like brain, skeletal and cardiac muscles, eye, liver, etc. where they transform into bradyzoites which multiply slowly to form tissue cysts, approximately 8–10 days following infection.

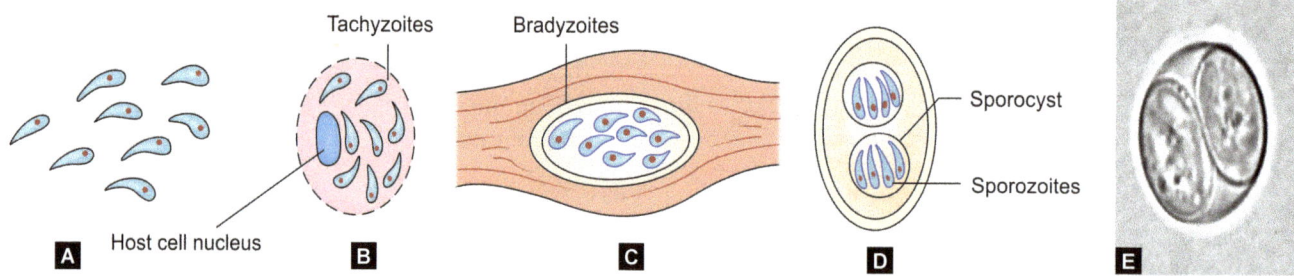

Figs 7.1A to E: *Toxoplasma gondii* (schematic diagram); (A) Tachyzoites; (B) Pseudocyst; (C) Tissue cyst; (D) Sporulated oocyst; (E) Sporulated oocyst in cat's feces (saline mount)

Source: E—DPDx Image Library, Centers for Disease Control and Prevention (CDC), Atlanta (*with permission*).

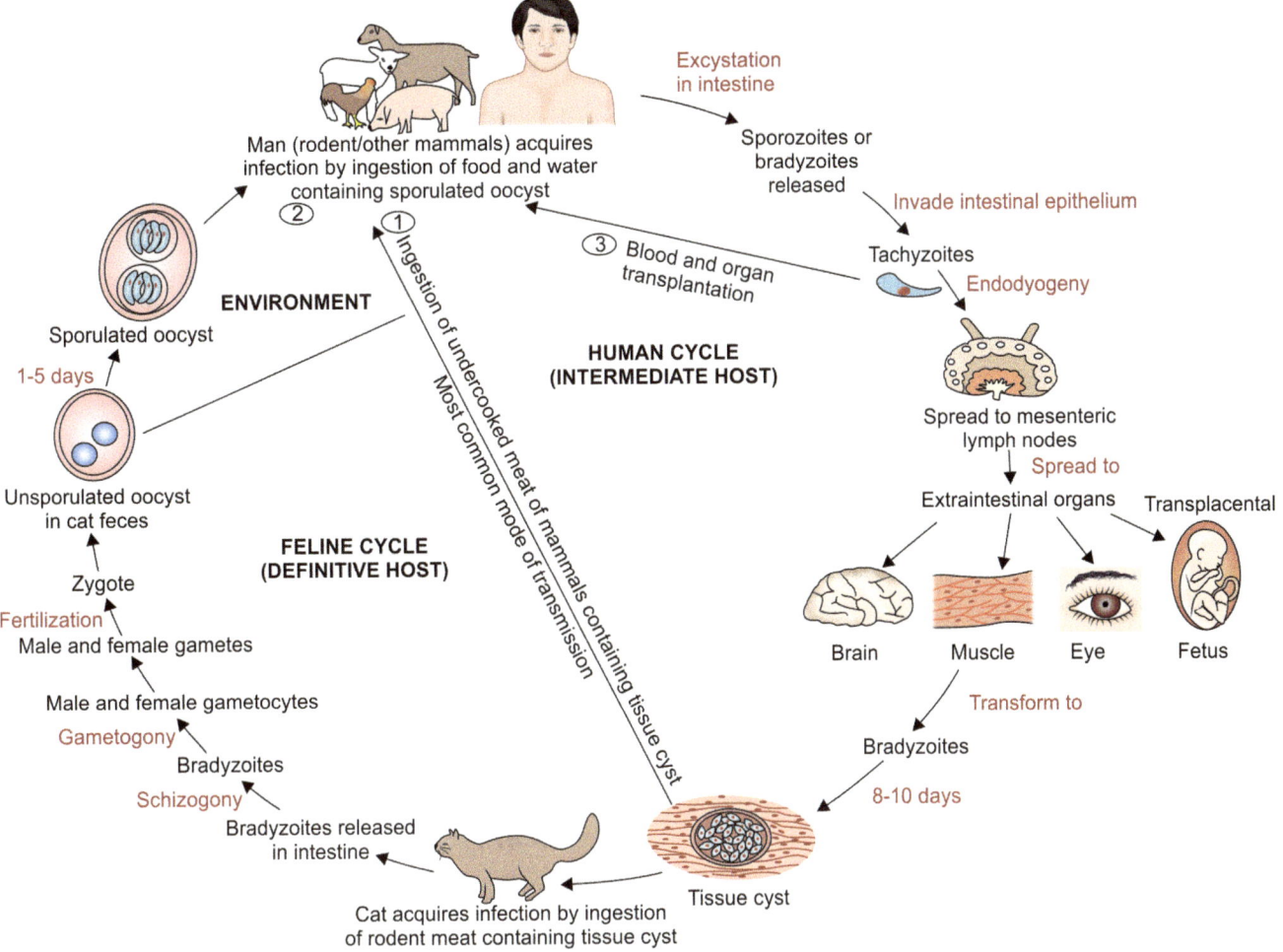

Fig. 7.2: Life cycle of *Toxoplasma gondii*

Sexual Cycle or Enteric Cycle (The Feline Cycle)

Cat and other felines (definitive host) acquire infection by ingestion of tissue cysts in the meat of rodents and other animals. However, tachyzoites and oocysts can also be the infective form to cat.

- Bradyzoites are released from the tissue cysts, which invade the intestinal epithelium, undergo several cycles of asexual generations (schizogony) before the sexual cycle begins
- Sexual cycle (gametogony) begins when the parasite differentiates to form male and female gametocytes which then transform into male and female gametes respectively
- Fertilization of male and female gamete results in formation of zygote which later gets surrounded by a thin, resistant rigid wall to form oocyst
- Oocysts are released in cat's feces after 20 days of consumption of tissue cyst; 4-6 days, if infection to cat is tachyzoites mediated
- Freshly passed oocysts are unsporulated and noninfective. The maturation takes place 1-5 days later, in the humid environment. The mature sporulated oocyst containing two sporocysts is infectious to man for about 1 year (Fig. 7.1 D)
- The feline cycle takes about 3-10 days or 19-48 days following ingestion of tissue cysts and oocysts respectively.

Pathogenicity

Toxoplasmosis is one of the most common parasitic zoonotic infections affecting a wide range of mammals and birds.

Prevalence: Global prevalence is about 25-30%. World is divided into:

- Low seroprevalence (10-30%): Observed in North America, South-east Asia, North Europe, and Sahelian countries of Africa
- Moderate prevalence (30-50%): Found in countries of central and Southern Europe.

❖ **High prevalence (>50%):** Have been found in Latin America and tropical African countries.

Various risk factors for infection are:
❖ The geographical area (cold area, hot arid climatic conditions, high altitudes are associated with a low prevalence)
❖ **Age:** It commonly affects elderly and fetus
❖ Exposure to cat and cat's feces
❖ **Food habits:** Ingestion of uncooked cat and other animal meat (seen in countries like France)—at higher risk
❖ **Immune status:** Patients associated with HIV, malignancies and other immunocompromised conditions are at high risk
❖ Patients undergoing blood transfusion, and organ transplantations are at higher risk
❖ Genetic factor: HLA DQ3 is associated with encephalitis in AIDS patient and hydrocephalus in fetus infected with *Toxoplasma*, whereas HLA DQ1 appears to be protective.

> **Pathogenesis involves the following steps**
> (1) Rhoptries, and micronemes present at the anterior end of sporozoites help in attachment to the host intestinal cells → (2) leads to internalization into the host cell → (3) resides inside parasitophorous vacuoles → (4) prevents phagolysosome fusion → (5) transforms to tachyzoites → (6) spreads to adjacent cells by actin myosin filaments.

Clinical Manifestation

The clinical manifestation of toxoplasmosis can vary depending upon the patient population affected.

Immunocompetent Patients

In the immunocompetent host, both the humoral and the cellular immune responses control the infection. The various mechanisms include activated macrophages, production of parasiticidal antibody, production of IFN-γ, and stimulation of CD8+ cytotoxic T lymphocytes.
❖ Hence, acute toxoplasmosis in the immunocompetent host is usually asymptomatic and self-limited
❖ **Lymphadenopathy:** The most common manifestation of acute toxoplasmosis is cervical lymphadenopathy. Other lymph nodes may also be affected like sub occipital, supraclavicular and inguinal nodes
❖ Other symptoms include headache, malaise, fatigue and fever
❖ Rare complications are maculopapular rash, pneumonia, myocarditis and encephalopathy
❖ Acute infection usually resolves within several weeks, although lymphadenopathy may persist for some months.

Immunocompromised Patients

In contrast, in the immunocompromised host such as patients infected with HIV, heart and bone marrow transplant recipients, malignancies or in fetus, the clinical manifestations are more severe due to the lack of the immune system to control the infection.
❖ The tachyzoites are disseminated to a variety of organs, particularly lymphatic tissue, skeletal muscle, myocardium, retina, placenta and CNS
❖ At these sites, the parasite infects host cells, replicates, leading to cell death and focal necrosis surrounded by an acute inflammatory response.

Toxoplasmosis in Patients with HIV

Toxoplasmosis is one of the common opportunistic parasitic infections in patients with AIDS (15-40%)
❖ Infection occurs either due to reactivation of latent infection (more common) or as a newly acquired infection from an exogenous source such as blood or transplanted organs
❖ It mainly targets CNS leading to *Toxoplasma* encephalitis (TE). Other manifestations include pulmonary infections and chorioretinitis.

Toxoplasma encephalitis

❖ Most common areas involved in TE are the brainstem, basal ganglia, pituitary gland and corticomedullary junction
❖ TE develops when the CD4+ T cell count falls below 100/μL
❖ Pathogenesis is due to the direct invasion by the parasite leading to necrotizing encephalitis and also due to secondary pressure effects on the surrounding area of the CNS
❖ Patients may present with altered mental status, seizures, sensory abnormalities, cerebellar signs and focal neurologic findings including motor deficits, cranial nerve palsies and visual-field loss.

Congenital Toxoplasmosis

Mother acquiring *Toxoplasma* infection in pregnancy is usually asymptomatic. However, she can transmit the infection to the fetus.
❖ **Gestational age:** It is the main factor influencing the fetal outcome. As the gestation proceeds, the chance of transmission increases but the severity of the infection declines
  ▪ If the mother becomes infected during the first trimester, the incidence of transplacental infection is lowest (15%), but the disease in the neonate is most severe

- If maternal infection occurs during the third trimester, the incidence of transplacental infection is maximum (65%), but the infant is usually asymptomatic at birth
- If the mother is infected before pregnancy, then the fetus is mostly uninfected, except when the mother is immunocompromised

❖ Initially though asymptomatic, but the persistence of infection in the newborn child can result in severe disease
❖ The **classical triad** comprises of chorioretinitis, hydrocephalus, and intracranial calcifications
❖ **Other manifestations** include stillbirth, psychomotor disturbance and microcephaly
❖ **Ocular involvement:** Eyes are involved later in life (2nd-3rd decade) when the cysts ruptures
  - Most frequently, it causes bilateral chorioretinitis leading to profound visual impairment. Other ocular manifestations include blurred vision, scotoma, photophobia, strabismus and glaucoma.
  - In contrast, if ocular involvement occurs without history of congenital infection, it is mostly unilateral (Fig. 7.3).
❖ **"TORCH" infection**: *Toxoplasma* is included as one of the component (T) of **"TORCH"** infection, a term used to denote the agents causing congenital infections. Other components are: (R) Rubella, (C) Cytomegalovirus, (H) Herpes simplex virus, (O) Others which include *Treponema pallidum* (syphilis), Varicella, etc.
❖ The incidence of congenital toxoplasmosis is approximately 1 per 1000 live births
❖ It is an important cause of repeated abortion and infertility. Hence, routine antenatal screening for *Toxoplasma* antibodies is advised in many advanced countries.

Laboratory Diagnosis	*Toxoplasma gondii*
❑ **Direct microscopy**—detect tachyzoites in blood and tissue cyst in tissue biopsy: ➤ Giemsa, PAS, silver stains, immunoperoxidase stain ➤ Direct fluorescent antibody test ❑ **Antibody detection** ➤ Detection of IgG in serum (ELISA, IFA)—four-fold rise indicates recent infection ➤ Detection of IgM in serum (ELISA, IFA and IgM-ISAGA)—marker of acute and congenital infection ➤ IgG avidity test (ELISA, ELFA)— low avidity indicates recent infection ➤ Detection of IgA in serum (ELISA or IgA-ISAGA)—useful for acute and congenital infection ➤ Detection of IgE in serum—useful for acute and congenital infection ➤ Sabin-Feldman dye test— specific, but cannot differentiate recent and past infection	

Contd...

Laboratory Diagnosis	*Toxoplasma gondii*
❑ **Detection of *Toxoplasma* antigen**—ELISA ❑ **Molecular diagnosis** (e.g. PCR)— useful for diagnosis (for acute, congenital infection) and for genotyping ❑ **Animal inoculation**—intraperitoneal inoculation into mice ❑ **Tissue culture**—murine alveolar and peripheral macrophage cell line ❑ **Imaging methods**—CT and MRI to detect *Toxoplasma* encephalitis.	

Laboratory Diagnosis

Direct Microscopic Examination

❖ **Specimens:** The specimens frequently examined are peripheral blood, body fluids, lymph node aspirate, bone marrow aspirate, CSF and bronchoalveolar lavage for HIV infected patients, biopsy material from spleen, liver and brain. These specimens are stained with Giemsa, PAS, silver stains, immunoperoxidase stain
❖ **Direct fluorescent antibody test (DFA):** Tachyzoites can be detected by using fluorescein conjugated antibody against *T. gondii* surface antigens
❖ Comma-shaped tachyzoites are detected in the smear made from blood, body fluid and tissue; their presence indicates acute infection (Figs 7.4A and B)
❖ Tissue cyst containing strongly PAS positive bradyzoites can be detected in various tissues like brain or muscle (Fig. 7.4C). This denotes the presence of infection but cannot differentiate acute and chronic infection.

Antibody Detection

Serological tests to detect antibodies remain the most widely used method for diagnosis of toxoplasmosis.

Acute infection with *T. gondii* can be established by simultaneous detection of IgG and IgM antibodies in serum. However, other antibodies such as IgA and IgE also can be detected. Interpretation of IgM and IgG antibody detection tests for diagnosis of toxoplasmosis has been depicted in Table 7.1.

IgG antibody detection

The IgG-ELISA method is now most widely used for the demonstration of IgG antibodies to *T. gondii*.

❖ IgG appears 4 weeks after the infection, peaks at 6–8 weeks and declines slowly to a baseline level that persists for life, hence single rise of IgG cannot differentiate acute with past infection
❖ A fourfold rise in IgG titer is necessary for diagnosis of acute febrile toxoplasmosis. Titre usually exceeds >1:1,000 during late infection or if lymphadenopathy is present

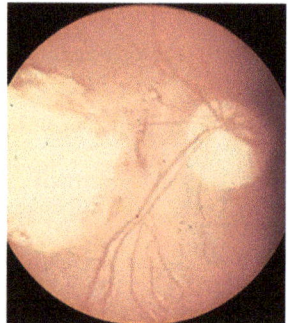
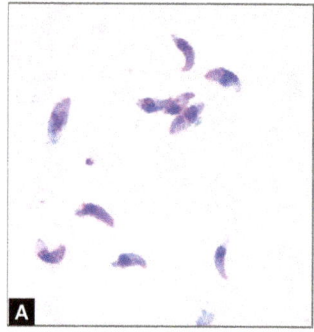
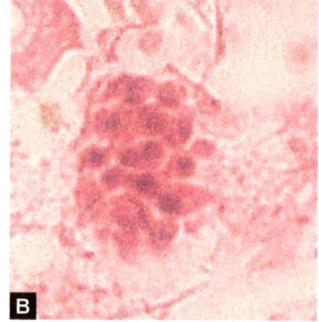
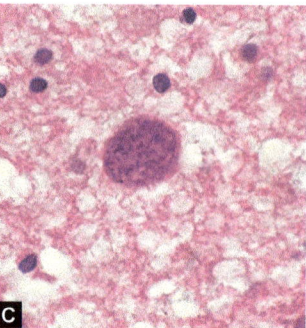

Figs 7.3: Chorioretinitis seen in toxoplasmosis

Figs 7.4A to C: *Toxoplasma gondii* (A) Giemsa stain showing comma-shaped tachyzoites in the blood smear; (B) Histopathology of brain shows pseudocyst containing numerous tachyzoites; (C) Tissue cyst containing bradyzoites (section of brain stained with hematoxylin and eosin)

Source: 7.3 and 7.4A and C—DPDx Image Library; 7.4B—Public Health Image Library, ID# 575/ Dr Edwin P Ewing; Centers for Disease Control and Prevention (CDC), Atlanta (*with permission*).

Table 7.1: Interpretation of IgM/IgG antibody detection test for toxoplasmosis

IgG Result*	IgM Result*	Report/interpretation	Follow up to be done
Negative	Positive	Possible early acute infection (<2–3 weeks) or false-positive IgM result	Retest with a new specimen after 2 weeks and if result shows: • IgG (-) and IgM (+): Indicates false-positive IgM • IgG (-) and IgM (-): Indicates technical error • IgG (+) and IgM (+): Indicates acute infection, but needs further confirmation by IgG avidity testing
Positive	Negative	Infected with *T. gondii* more than 6 months before (remote infection)	Nothing more to be done
Positive	Positive	Infection of *T. gondii* within last 6 months	Perform IgG avidity test If low avidity: Indicates recent infection (within 12 weeks)** If high avidity: Indicates remote infection (>12 weeks old)

* If IgM or IgG result becomes equivocal: then repeat the test with fresh specimen collected 2 weeks later.
** If IgG avidity is low, draw a second sample 3 weeks after the first sample; send both specimens to *Toxoplasma* reference laboratory for confirmation of IgG, IgM, and IgG avidity results and possibly differential agglutination and IgA and IgE testing.

- IgG cannot be used to diagnose congenital infection (as IgG crosses placenta)
- **Differential absorption test:** When a mixture of IgG and IgM is present, 6-mercaptopurine can be used that absorbs IgM from the mixture so that the remaining antibody after the absorption is IgG.

IgM antibody detection

Specific IgM normally develops early, within 1–2 weeks after primary infection.
- Though it is a marker of acute infection, but it is not a reliable indicator and has a low predictive value for diagnosis of acute/recent toxoplasmosis. This is because of the variable persistence of detectable IgM levels up to 6 months by ELISA and may be up to 6 years when capture ELISA is used
- The detection of IgM antibodies, which do not cross the placental barrier, provides a much more accurate diagnosis of congenital infection

- **Other methods** to detect IgM includes IgM-capture ELISA, IgM-IFA (indirect immunofluorescence antibody) and IgM immunosorbent agglutination assay (IgM-ISAGA)
- **False positive IgM** may be seen with samples containing rheumatoid factor or antinuclear antibodies.

IgG avidity test

IgG avidity test is a much reliable indicator of recent infection compared to IgG and IgM detection.
- *Principle:* The avidity of IgG antibody with its antigen increases with time and this property can be useful in differentiating recent with past infection
- Low IgG avidity indicates recent infection (<12 weeks); whereas a strong avidity indicates past infection (i.e. infection must have occurred at least 12 weeks earlier)
- Pregnancy: IgG avidity test is of much use in first four months of pregnancy during which a high avidity ratio excludes the possibility of recent *T. gondii* infection.

Hence, it allows the avoidance of unnecessary treatment and follow-up in pregnant women
- Both ELISA and ELFA (enzyme-linked immunofluorescence assay, e.g. VIDAS, bioMérieux) based methods are available.

IgA antibody detection

IgA Antibodies can be detected by ELISA or ISAGA methods.
- IgA antibodies may be detected in sera of acutely infected adults. However, a negative result does not exclude, nor does a positive result confirm, a recent primary infection
- IgA detection is useful for diagnosis of congenital toxoplasmosis.

IgE antibody detection

IgE antibodies are detectable by ELISA, useful for the following purposes:
- *Toxoplasma* encephalitis in HIV infected patients
- Congenital infection (though IgE is less sensitive than IgM and IgA)
- Congenital toxoplasmic chorioretinitis
- *Acutely infected adults:* The duration of IgE seropositivity is less than with IgM or IgA antibodies and hence appears useful as an adjunctive method for identifying recently acquired infections.

Sabin-Feldman dye test

This is the gold standard antibody detection method, usually done in the reference laboratories. Other serological tests are evaluated taking this test as standard.
- It is a complement mediated neutralization test that requires live tachyzoites
- Because of its technical difficulty and inability to differentiate between recent and past infection; this test is seldom used nowadays in routine diagnostics. Refer author's first edition for detail procedure.

Detection of Toxoplasma Antigens

Antigen detection is less commonly used as it lacks sensitivity. It may have a role in situations where antibodies are low—(i) immunocompromised, (ii) early acute stage and (iii) monoclonal gammapathies.

Molecular Diagnosis

Polymerase chain reaction (PCR) can be employed to detect *Toxoplasma* specific DNA from various clinical samples like blood, CSF, bronchoalveolar lavage or amniotic fluid. PCR is highly sensitive, specific; can be used to diagnose TE or congenital infections in resource—poor settings.

Toxoplasma genotypes

Toxoplasma strains fall into three clonal lineages as types I to III. They vary in their geographical distribution and disease they produce. For example,
- Type II is seen in North America and Europe and has been associated with congenital infections and AIDS
- Type III stains are seen in China
- In South America, all three lineages are prevalent.

Animal Inoculation

T. gondii can be isolated from mice by intraperitoneal inoculation of the clinical samples into the healthy (*T. gondii* free) laboratory maintained mice. Mice die in 7-10 days and peritoneal fluid and spleen aspirate smears show tachyzoites. If death does not occur, then the mice are observed for 6 weeks and tail blood is screened for *Toxoplasma* antibodies.

Tissue Culture

T. gondii can be isolated by inoculating into cell lines such as human foreskin fibroblast, continuous cell lines (HeLa, LLC, and Vero).

Imaging Methods

CT or MRI scan of brain can be done to demonstrate multiple ring enhancing lesions in basal ganglia or corticomedullary junction to diagnose TE in HIV patients.

CSF Examination

Evaluation of CSF of patients with TE reveals an elevation of intracranial pressure, lymphocytosis, and a slight increase in protein concentration, occasional increase in the gamma globulin level and a normal glucose level.

Diagnosis of Congenital Toxoplasmosis

Antenatal diagnosis

If acute infection is documented in a pregnant women, then the following diagnostic algorithm should be followed.
- **Ultrasonography** of fetus should be done at 20-24 weeks of gestation and repeated every 2-4 weeks for detecting the lesions of congenital infection
- **PCR and/or isolation:** Amniotic fluid sample is collected, centrifuged and the pellet is subjected to PCR and/or isolation in mouse or tissue culture
    - If either or both found positive, then antenatal diagnosis is confirmed
    - If both negative: Perhaps the neonate may be affected; warrants evaluation of the neonate.

Postnatal diagnosis
- **Isolation of the parasite** at delivery must be attempted from amniotic fluid, placenta and cord leukocyte

- **IgM and IgG:** Newborn and maternal sera are subjected to detection IgG (dye test, IFA or ELISA) and IgM (ELISA or IFA)
  - IgG titer of ≥1,000 in neonate: Indicates possible diagnosis which should be followed by IgM testing
  - IgM titer of neonate ≥1:4 after 2 weeks of age indicates probable diagnosis and guides the clinicians to initiate treatment to the neonate.
- **Other tests include**
  - IgA detection (neonatal and maternal blood): IgA appears to be more sensitive than IgM for the diagnosis of congenital toxoplasmosis. IgA antibodies usually disappear within 10 days of birth, hence persistence of IgA beyond 10 days confirms the diagnosis
  - IgE detection (neonatal and maternal blood)
  - PCR in neonatal and maternal blood detecting specific genes of *T. gondii*
  - Fundus examination should be performed to rule out chorioretinitis.

Diagnosis in Special Situations

Immunocompromised patients

Antibodies are produced at a very low level and irregularly in immunocompromised patients; hence, antibody detection methods are not reliable. All other diagnostic modalities can be employed in immunocompromised patients.

Ocular toxoplasmosis

The serum antibody titer may not correlate with the presence of active lesions in the fundus, particularly in cases of congenital toxoplasmosis.
- In general, a positive IgG titer in serum along with typical lesions establishes the diagnosis
- Antibody production in ocular fluid can also be used for diagnosis
- Antigen detection or PCR can be done for the diagnosis of ocular toxoplasmosis.

Treatment	Toxoplasmosis
Immunocompetent patients	
Immunocompetent patients with only lymphadenopathy do not require specific therapy unless they have persistent, severe symptoms. Patients with ocular toxoplasmosis are usually treated for 1 month with pyrimethamine plus either sulfadiazine or clindamycin and sometimes with prednisolone.	
Congenital toxoplasmosis	
Neonates with congenital toxoplasmosis are treated with daily oral pyrimethamine (1 mg/kg) and sulfadiazine (100 mg/kg) with folinic acid for 1 year.	
Immunocompromised patients	
Toxoplasmosis is rapidly fatal in immunocompromised patients. If not treated, it may progress to encephalitis. So treatment is essential.	

Contd...

Treatment	Toxoplasmosis
i. Primary prophylaxis:	
AIDS patients with *Toxoplasma* infection, having CD4+ T lymphocyte count of less than 100/μL should receive prophylaxis against TE.	
▫ Trimethoprim-sulfamethoxazole (cotrimoxazole) is the drug of choice	
▫ Dapsone-pyrimethamine, atovaquone with or without pyrimethamine can be given as alternate	
▫ Prophylaxis can be discontinued in patients who have responded to antiretroviral therapy (ART) and whose CD4+ T lymphocyte count has been more than 200/μL for 3 months.	
ii. Secondary prophylaxis (Long-term maintenance therapy):	
Required for HIV positive patients who are previously treated for toxoplasmosis.	
▫ Should be started if the CD4+ T lymphocyte count decreases to less than 200/μL	
▫ However, it can be discontinued if the patient is asymptomatic, and have a CD4+ T lymphocyte count of more than 200/μL for at least 6 months.	

Prevention

The various methods recommended to prevent toxoplasmosis include:
- Consumption of thoroughly cooked meat
- Proper hygiene maintenance and hand cleaning of people handling cats and other felines
- Regular prenatal and antenatal screening to detect *Toxoplasma* infection in women of child bearing age
- Avoiding cat's feces (oocyst) contaminated materials (like a cat's litter box)
- Screening of blood banks or organ donors for antibody to *T. gondii*
- No vaccine trials are going on currently.

CRYPTOSPORIDIUM SPECIES

Cryptosporidium is an intestinal coccidian parasite affecting various animals and men.
- It causes self-limiting acute diarrhea in immunocompetent healthy individuals; whereas it is an opportunistic pathogen in immunocompromised patients (including HIV infected patients), causing chronic persistent life-threatening diarrhea
- Tyzzer (1907) was the first to describe it in gastric crypts of laboratory mice. Subsequently it was found to affect many animals like rats, guinea pigs, pigs, horses, etc. The first human case was reported in 1976
- It belongs to the family *Cryptosporidiidae*. It is different from other coccidian parasites in such a way that it does not go deep into the host cells, but is confined to an **intracellular extracytoplasmic location**. All the sexual and asexual stages of development take place within a **parasitophorous vacuole** that lies just below the cell

membrane of the brush border epithelium of the small intestine
- *Cryptosporidium* species infecting man is now classified as two separate species, *C. parvum* (mammals, including humans) and *C. hominis* (primarily humans)
- Other species infect wide range of mammals (*C. felis, C. canis* and *C. muris*), fishes (*C. nasorum*), birds (*C. meleagridis, C. baileyi*) and reptiles (*C. crotali*). They do not cause infection in human although humans may serve as host.

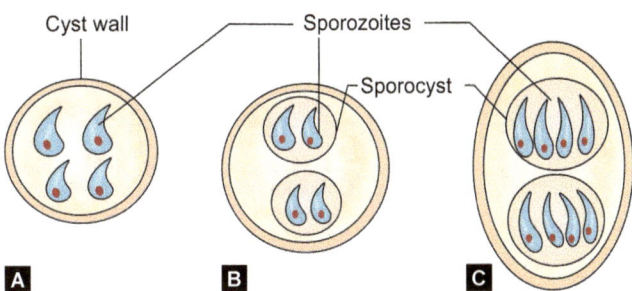

Figs 7.5A to C: Sporulated oocysts (schematic diagram) of (A) *Cryptosporidium*; (B) *Cyclospora*; (C) *Cystoisospora*

Morphology

Oocyst

It is the infective form to man as well as the diagnostic form excreted in the feces.
- It is round, small, 4–6 μm in size, surrounded by a cyst wall and bears four sporozoites (Figs 7.5A to C)
- Each sporozoite is crescentic-shaped with pointed anterior end, blunt posterior end and a nucleus located posteriorly
- Two types of oocysts are demonstrated—(1) thick walled and (2) thin walled
  - **Thick wall oocyst** contains two electrodense cyst wall—outer uniformly thick, moderately coarse layer and an inner fine granular layer with a suture point at one pole. In between the two walls, lies an electroluscent middle zone containing two oocyst membranes
  - **Thin-walled oocysts** are surrounded by a single layered membrane
- The oocysts are acid fast in nature but do not stain by iodine
- They are extremely resistant to routine chlorination, heat and other disinfectants.

Life Cycle (Fig. 7.6)

Cryptosporidium completes its life cycle (both sexual and asexual stages) in single host (man or other animals).

Infective stage: Sporulated oocyst is the infective form of the parasite. Thick walled oocyst is infectious to other persons, where as the thin walled oocysts can cause autoinfection (through contaminated fingers).

Mode of Transmission: Man acquires infection by:
- **Ingestion** of food and water contaminated with feces containing thick-walled oocysts
- **By autoinfection:** Thin-walled oocyst can infect the same host.

Development in Man

- **Excystation:** In the small intestine, the suture present in the inner wall of the oocyst gets dissolved and four slender crescent shaped sporozoites are released from each oocyst. Various factors like pancreatic enzymes and bile salts help in excystation
- **Invasion:** Sporozoites invade the brush border epithelium of the small intestine and lie inside a parasitophorous vacuole near the microvilli surface, within which all the stages of development take place
- **Schizogony:**
  - The sporozoites subsequently differentiate into trophozoites which then undergo asexual multiplication (schizogony) to produce type I meronts
  - Each type I meront undergoes schizogony to release eight merozoites, which then again invade the adjacent enterocytes and undergo repeated schizogony to produce type II meronts
  - Four merozoites are released by the schizogony of each type II meront.
- **Gametogony:**
  - The merozoites undergo gametogony and transform into sexual forms (microgamont and macrogamont)
  - Each microgamont releases 16 microgametes while only one macrogamete is produced from each macrogamont.
- **Sporogony:**
  - Fertilization takes place between microgamete and macrogamete to produce the zygote
  - Subsequently, about 80% of zygote transform into highly resistant double layered thick walled oocyst and remaining 20% transform into single layered thin walled oocyst
  - Within the host cell, the oocysts undergo sporogony to produce four sporozoites
  - Sporulated oocysts are excreted in the feces. Thick walled oocysts infect the new hosts where as the thin walled oocysts infect the same host (autoinfection).
- **Prepatent period:** It is the period from the time of ingestion of oocyst to completion of the life cycle and release of newly developed oocyst in human feces (approximately 4–22 days).

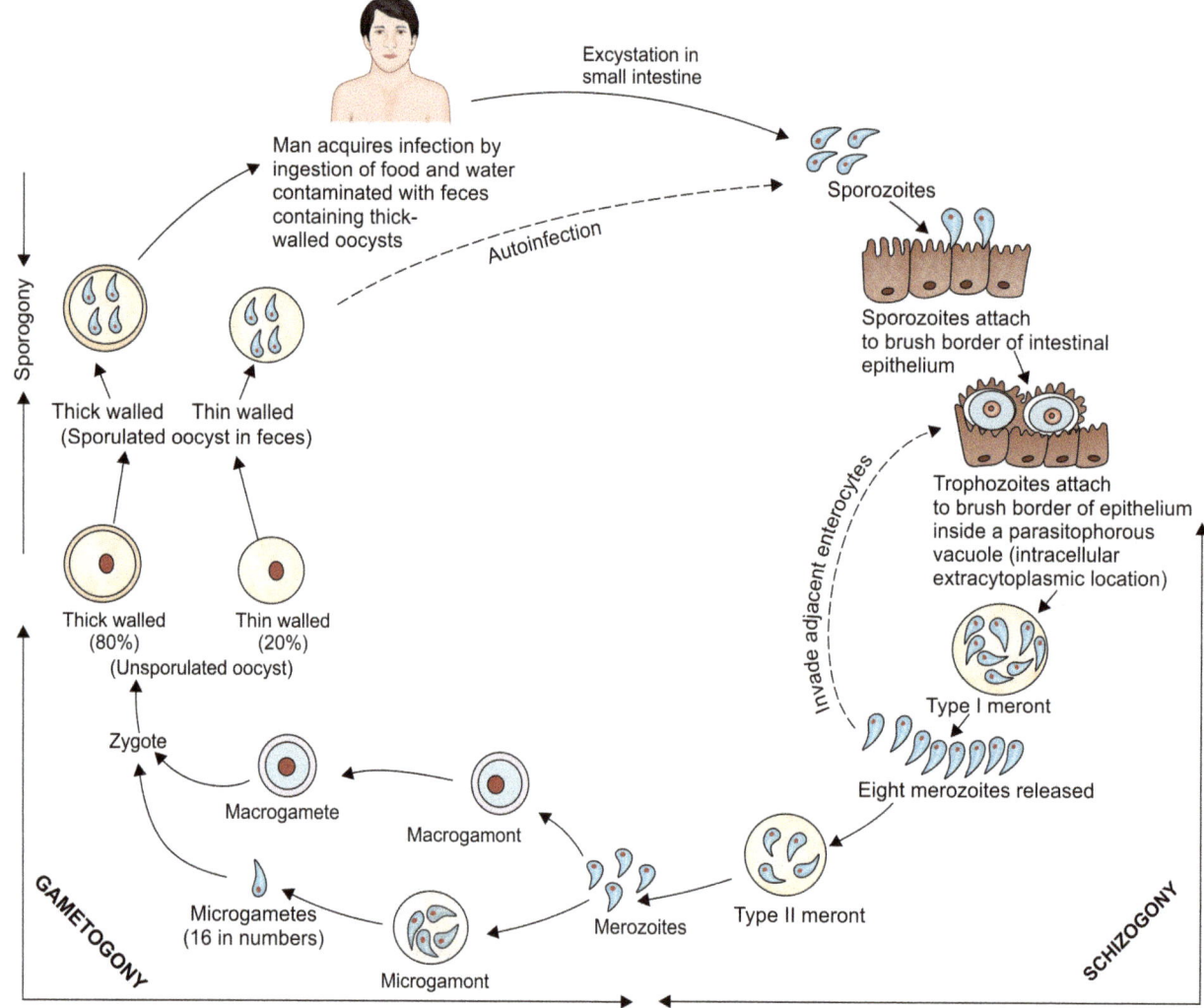

Fig. 7.6: Life cycle of *Cryptosporidium*

Epidemiology

Cryptosporidiosis is a zoonotic disease.
- *C. parvum* is common in rural area; transmission is associated with contact with animals and exposure to surface water. Subtype IIc commonly infects man
- *C. hominis* is mainly a human parasite, more commonly seen in urban setting with high population density and children
- **Seasonality:** *C. parvum* infection is common in spring whereas *C. hominis* in autumn
- **Source of infection** includes rain water lodges and swimming pool recreational water
- A massive outbreak occurred in Milwaukee, USA in 1993 affecting >4 lakh people; transmitted through contaminated public water supply
- **Prevalence:** Cryptosporidiosis is found in most region of the world except Antarctica. The prevalence depends upon the immunity of the host
- In immunocompetent people, the prevalence in developing countries like India varies from 2.4 to 15%; where as in the western countries it is 1.4–6%
- In immunocompromised hosts (HIV positive patients), the prevalence is 12–46% in developing countries (46% in Haiti) and 7–21% in developed countries.

Factors that contribute to the disease include
- Low infective dose of *Cryptosporidium* (10–100 oocysts can initiate the infection)
- Large multiplication capacity ($>10^{10}$) in single host
- Small size of the oocyst (4–6 μm)
- **Oocysts viability:** Oocysts remain viable up to six months if kept moist; however the viability is lost if dessicated or with freezing
- Resistant to the available drugs and disinfectants including chlorination

- Large animal and human reservoir
- Lack of appropriate immune response
- Poor sanitary conditions
- Travel to underdeveloped countries
- Zoonotic contact
- Peak age of infection: Infants and children.

Pathogenesis

The pathogenesis involves the following steps.
- **Excystation:** Following infection, the oocysts undergo excystation in small intestine releasing four sporozoites. This is mediated by proteases and aminopeptidases released by oocysts
- **Attachment:** Sporozoites attach to the brush border epithelium of the small intestine (ileum) with the help of a unique protein called as **CP47** (47 kDa *Cryptosporidium* protein)
- **Penetration:**
  - Discharges from the apicomplex (rhoptries, micronemes and dense granules) present in the anterior end of the sporozoites help in invasion
  - Following penetration, the parasite forms a parasitophorous vacuole near the microvilli surface of the host cells (intracellular extracytoplasmic location).
- Then, the parasite activates the host cell kinase signaling pathway that liberates proinflammatory cytokines like tumor necrosis factor (TNF)-α, IL-8, prostaglandins, etc.
- Cytokines released from the inflammatory site can activate the phagocytes; attract fresh leukocytes which in turn liberate soluble factors
- These factors increase intestinal secretion of chloride and water and decrease the sodium absorption coupled to glucose transport. But sodium-glutamine transport is not affected. So, glutamine based ORS (oral rehydration solution) are more affective in treatment.

Clinical Features

Immunocompetent Hosts
- Usually the infection is asymptomatic
- Sometimes, patient develops self-limiting watery nonbloody frothy diarrhea 5-6 times a day
- Other features like abdominal pain, nausea, anorexia, fever, and/or weight loss may be present
- Symptoms develop after an incubation period of 1 week and subside within 1-2 weeks
- *Cryptosporidium* accounts for 2-6% of cases of traveler's diarrhea
- Respiratory cryptosporidiosis may occur occasionally.

Immunocompromised Hosts
Host immune status is not a primary factor for initiating the infection, but play an important role in determining the length and severity of the illness once the infection is established.
- Disease is more severe in immunocompromised hosts especially in patients with AIDS having CD4+ T cell counts less than 100/μL
- It produces a chronic, persistent remarkably profuse diarrhea (1-25 L/day), leading to significant fluid and electrolyte loss (resembling cholera and diarrhea)
- Severe weight loss, wasting and abdominal pain may be seen
- Autoinfection by thin-walled oocyst is a key factor for the chronic diarrhea which maintains the infection
- **In HIV infected patients,** extraintestinal manifestations are common such as biliary tract infection (sclerosing cholangitis), respiratory tract infection, and pancreatitis
- Other immunocompromised conditions where cryptosporidiosis is common include severe combined immunodeficiency syndrome, hematological malignancies and solid organ transplant recipient.

Laboratory Diagnosis — *Cryptosporidium*

- **Direct microscopy** (Stool examination)— shows round 4–6 μm size oocyst containing four sporozoites
  - Direct wet mount
  - Wet mount after concentration—Sheather's sugar floatation technique is preferred
  - Acid fast staining and calcofluor white staining
  - Direct fluorescent antibody staining.
- **Antigen detection** from stool—ELISA, ICT (Triage parasite panel detecting protein disulfide isomerase Ag)
- **Antibody detection** from serum—ELISA
- **Molecular diagnosis**—PCR detecting 18S rRNA and β-tubulin gene
- **Histopathology** of intestinal biopsy specimen—appears as blue beads.

Laboratory Diagnosis

Direct Microscopy (Stool Examination)
- **Sample collection:** Three stool samples should be collected. Rarely (in the HIV positive patients), sputum, bronchial wash, duodenal or jejunal aspirate can be collected
- **Direct wet mount:** Direct wet mounting from the mucus plug of the stool sample is done to demonstrate highly refractile, round, double walled 4-6 μm size oocyst
- **Concentration technique:** If the oocyst load is less, then various techniques are used to concentrate the stool sample. They are two types of stool concentration techniques:
  1. Floatation technique like Sheather's sugar floatation technique (widely used for coccidian parasites), zinc sulfate floatation technique or saturated salt floatation technique

2. Sedimentation technique like formalin ether or formalin ethyl acetate sedimentation technique.
- ❖ **Staining procedures:**
  - **Acid fast staining:** The oocysts of *Cryptosporidium* are acid fast to 1% sulfuric acid or acid alcohol and appear as round, 4-6 μm red color oocyst against blue back ground. The sensitivity of acid fast staining is low and it requires a minimum concentration of more than 50,000 and 500,000 oocysts/mL of liquid stool and formed stool respectively (Fig. 7.7A)
  - Commonly used modified acid fast staining methods are:
    - Kinyoun's method (cold acid fast staining)
    - Rapid safranin methylene blue method
    - Carbol fuchsin negative staining method.
  - **Direct fluorescent antibody staining** is done to detect *Cryptosporidium* oocyst by using fluorescent labeled monoclonal antibody directed against cyst wall antigens. This is more sensitive (10 times) and specific than acid fast staining. It is also useful to detect oocyst from water and other environmental samples. Currently, this method is considered as the gold standard test for cryptosporidiosis (Fig. 7.7B)
  - **Optical fluorescent brighteners** such as Uvitex 2B, Calcofluor white can also be used to improve detection
  - **Combined acid-fast trichrome staining** has been developed for simultaneous detection of *Microsporidia* and *Cryptosporidium*; this coinfection is found up to 30% of cases in AIDS patients with CD4 T cell count <100/μL.

Antigen Detection from Stool

- ❖ **ELISA** has been developed to detect *C. parvum* specific coproantigen (oocyst antigen) from stool; shows a sensitivity ranging from 66% to 100% with excellent specificity
- ❖ **Immunochromatographic test (ICT)** is also available (e.g. Triage parasite panel) for simultaneous detection of antigens of *Cryptosporidium* (detecting protein disulfide isomerase antigen), *Giardia* and *E. histolytica*. It shows sensitivity (83–96%) and specificity (99–100%).

Antibody Detection

- ❖ **ELISA** is used to detect *Cryptosporidium* specific antibodies (IgM and IgG) in patient's serum for seroepidemiological purpose
- ❖ **Indirect fluorescent antibody** test is also available detecting antibodies against oocyst antigens.

Molecular Diagnosis

- ❖ **PCR** is available to detect specific *Cryptosporidium* genes from both clinical and environmental samples targeting genes such as 18S rRNA and β-tubulin gene
- ❖ PCR is more sensitive, takes less time and can differentiate the *Cryptosporidium* genotypes which plays an important role in outbreak situations
- ❖ Other methods available are BioFire FilmArray (a commercial automated multiplex PCR), and real time PCR.

Histopathology

Various developmental stages of the parasite can be demonstrated from the intestinal biopsy specimens (jejunum). When stained by H&E stain, *Cryptosporidium* appears as 1–3 μm basophilic round bodies within the cell membrane of enterocytes called as **"blue beads"** (Fig. 7.7C).

Culture Isolation

Cryptosporidium can grow in cell lines such as primary human intestinal epithelial cell lines, human colonic tumor

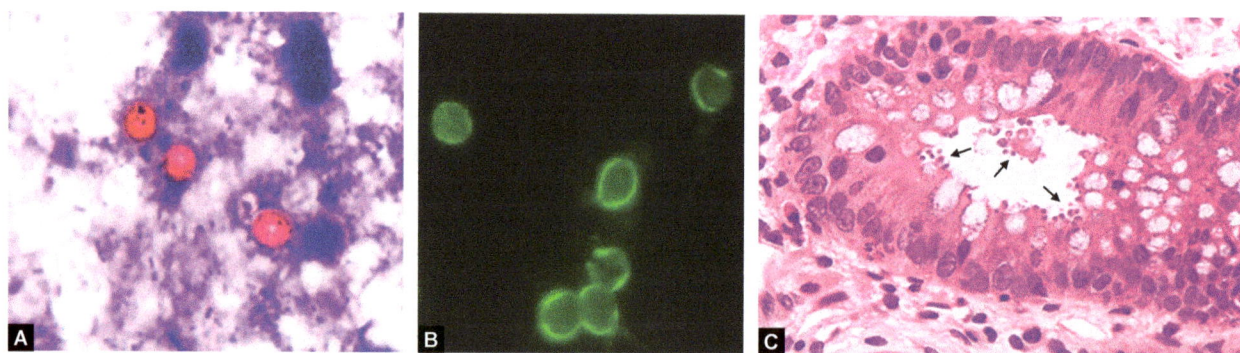

Figs 7.7A to C: *Cryptosporidium* species (A) Acid fast stain shows red color oocyst against blue back ground; (B) Direct fluorescent antibody staining shows brilliant green fluorescent oocysts; (C) Hematoxylin and eosin stain of intestinal biopsy shows numerous oocysts at the luminal surface of the intestinal crypt (marked by arrows)

Source: A to C—Swierczynski G, Milanesi B. Atlas of human intestinal protozoa Microscopic diagnosis (*with permission*).

CHAPTER 7 ❖ Apicomplexa—II (Opportunistic Coccidian Parasites)

cells (HCT-8, CCL-224), Madin Darby canine kidney cells (MDCK, CCL-34). However, culture is limited for research purpose; not used for routine diagnosis.

Flow Cytometry

It is useful for the quantitation of *Cryptosporidium* oocysts in stool. It is 10 times more sensitive than conventional immunofluorescence assays.

Other Methods

- Low CD4-T lymphocyte count (especially in HIV positive patient)
- Fecal leukocyte marker—lactoferrin is increased in 75% of cases indicating increase pus cells in feces.

Water and environmental testing

When an outbreak is suspected, drinking water and other environmental water samples can be subjected to the following tests to detect *Cryptosporidium* oocysts.
- Immunofluorescence method: 100L of water passed through a polypropylene yard cartridge filter or membrane filter and the filtrate is then subjected immunofluorescent staining
- Fluorescence in situ hybridization technique
- PCR detecting oocyst specific gene
- Immunomagnetic separation coupled with immuno-fluorescence microscopy
- Oocyst viability can be assessed by (i) cell culture and (ii) Beta tubulin mRNA which is as a marker of oocyst viability.

Treatment — Cryptosporidiosis

- Mild cases are self-limited, requires fluid replacement like ORS, with lactose-free glutamine supplemented diet
- Severe cases: Nitazoxanide is given to adults (500 mg twice daily for 3 days). It is not effective in HIV infected patient. Paromomycin can be given as an alternate. Macrolide antibiotics including spiramycin, azithromycin and clarithromycin and diclazuril have some activity against *Cryptosporidium* species.

Prevention

- Requires minimizing exposure to infectious oocysts in human or animal feces
- Proper hand washing, use of submicron water filters, use of appropriate disinfectants/sterilants to kill the oocysts (such as hydrogen peroxide, steam sterilization), improved personal hygiene are some of the efforts to prevent transmission.

CYCLOSPORA CAYETANENSIS

History

Cyclospora cayetanensis is the most recently described coccidian parasite as human intestinal pathogen. It is named by Schneider in 1881 and human infection was described by Ashford in 1979.

Life Cycle

Humans are the only known host. Man gets infection by ingestion of food and water contaminated with sporulated oocyst in soil.

Life cycle is not fully understood, but believed to be similar to that of *Cryptosporidium* except (Table 7.2):
- The oocysts released in the human feces are unsporulated
- The sporulation of oocyst takes place in the soil (environment) whereas in *Cryptosporidium*, the sporulation of oocyst takes place in the human intestine
- **Morphology of sporulated oocyst:** Mature oocyst is round, 8–10 μm size, contains two sporocysts, each containing two sporozoites (see Fig. 7.5B).

Clinical Features

Incubation period ranges from 2–11 days.
- It causes self-limiting diarrhea resembling *Cryptosporidium* infection

Property	Cryptosporidium	Cyclospora	Cystoisospora
Infective form	Sporulated oocyst	Sporulated oocyst	Sporulated oocyst
Diagnostic form	Sporulated oocyst	Unsporulated oocyst	Unsporulated oocyst
Outbreaks	Frequent, large	Common, large	Occasional, small
Zoonotic potential	Yes	Uncertain	No
Oocyst size	4–6 μm	8–10 μm	23–36 μm
Oocyst shape	Round	Round	Oval
Sporulated oocyst contain	Four sporozoites	Two sporocysts, each having two sporozoites	Two sporocysts, each having four sporozoites
Acid fastness	Uniformly acid fast	Variable acid fast	Uniformly acid fast
Autofluorescence	No, but can be stained with fluorescent dye	Autofluorescence ++	Autofluorescence +/-
Sporulation of the oocyst	Occurs inside the host cells (enterocytes)	Occurs in soil (environment)	Occurs in soil (environment)
Treatment	Nitazoxanide	Cotrimoxazole	Cotrimoxazole

Table 7.2: Differences between *Cryptosporidium*, *Cyclospora* and *Cystoisospora*

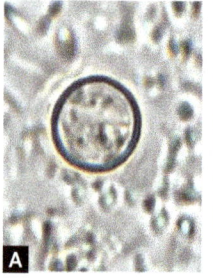 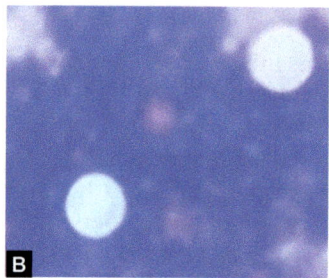 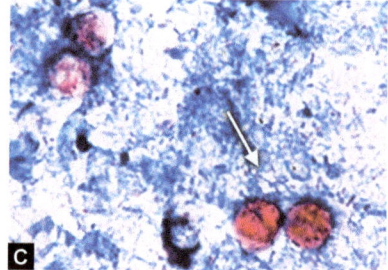 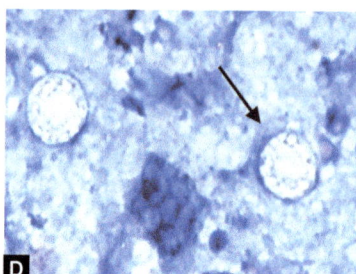

Figs 7.8A and B: *Cyclospora* species (A) Saline mount preparation showing unsporulated oocyst; (B) Epifluorescence microscopy showing autoflourescent oocysts; (C) Acid fast oocysts; (D) Non-acid fast oocysts (variable acid-fastness)
Source: A—Dr Anand Janagond, Associate Professor of Microbiology, S Nijalingappa Medical college, Bagalkot, Karnataka; B to D—Swierczynski G, Milanesi B. Atlas of human intestinal protozoa microscopic diagnosis (*with permission*).

- Disease is more severe with biliary tract involvement in immunocompromised (HIV positive patients).

Epidemiology

- Disease is prevalent in Central and South America (Haiti, Guatemala, Peru and Venezuela) and South Asia (India and Nepal)
- More cases have been reported from Haiti (11% of AIDS related diarrhea), children of Nepal (32%) and travelers coming to India, Pakistan and Morocco
- Food-borne outbreaks of cyclosporiasis have been linked to various types of imported foods including raspberries, basil and mesclun lettuce.

Laboratory Diagnosis

Stool Examination

Stool examination is done similar to that for cryptosporidiosis. Multiple stool specimens are examined by direct microscopy (Figs 7.8A) or stained by acid fast stains or fluorescent stains.
- *Cyclospora* oocysts are approximately twice the size of *Cryptosporidia* oocysts. It is round, 8–10 μm size and **variably acid fast** (i.e. 50% of oocyst are acid fast, rest are nonacid fast) (Figs 7.8C and D)
- **Autofluorescence** of the oocysts under ultraviolet epifluorescence microscopy is both rapid and sensitive, although not specific (Fig. 7.8B)
- Additional stains includes auramine, safranin and lactophenol cotton blue.

Molecular Diagnosis

- Conventional PCR and nested PCR assays are available targeting small subunit rRNA and 70-kDa heat shock protein (HSP70) of *Cyclospora*. Its showed a sensitivity of 62%
- *Cyclospora* may be misidentified as *Eimeria* species by PCR; which should be further differentiated by performing PCR-RFLP.

- BioFire Film Array Gastrointestinal Panel is also available commercially.

Flow cytometry has been proposed as an alternate method of diagnosis.

Serology

Antibodies to *Cyclospora* can be detected, however serological tests are not commercially available.

Histopathology

Biopsy specimens from the intestine show villous atrophy, acute and chronic inflammatory changes in the lamina propria. Inside the enterocytes, *Cyclospora* is supranuclear in location, whereas *Cryptosporidium* is located on the surface of the enterocytes.

Treatment	Cyclosporiasis
❑ Cyclosporiasis is treated with cotrimoxazole (trimethoprim 160 mg/sulfamethoxazole 800 mg twice daily for 7 days). HIV-infected patients may experience relapses and may require long-term suppressive maintenance therapy ❑ Patients who cannot tolerate cotrimoxazole may be treated with ciprofloxacin or nitazoxanide.	

CYSTOISOSPORA (ISOSPORA) BELLI

Introduction

Isospora belli has been recently renamed as *Cystoisospora belli*.
- Though more than 200 *Cystoisospora* species are identified, but *C. belli* is the only species that infects man. No other animal reservoir is known
- It belongs to the family Sarcocystidae
- It was first described by Virchow in 1860 and was named by Wenyon (1923)
- A second species called *C. natalensis* have been reported from South Africa, but further studies are required for validation.

Morphology

Oocyst

The sporulated oocyst is oval/elliptical, 20-33 µm × 10-19 µm in size, contains two sporocysts, each with four sporozoites. The oocyst is surrounded by a thin, smooth, two layered cyst wall (Fig. 7.5C).

Life Cycle

Man gets infection by ingestion of food and water contaminated with sporulated oocyst in soil.

- In the proximal small intestine, eight sporozoites are released from each oocyst. They invade the duodenal and jejunal epithelium and transform into trophozoites
- Trophozoites multiply and transform into schizont that undergoes asexual multiplication (schizogony) to produce merozoites
- Merozoites again attack fresh enterocytes to repeat the asexual cycle. Some of the merozoites transform into microgametocyte and macrogametocyte **(gametogony)**
- Eventually, they form macrogametes and microgametes which fuse to form the zygote **(fertilization)**
- Zygotes secrete the cyst wall and develop into immature oocysts, excreted in the feces
- In the soil, the sporulation occurs within 3-4 days and immature oocyst transform into sporulated oocyst which bears two sporocysts each containing four sporozoites.

Epidemiology

C. belli is found worldwide but predominantly in tropical and subtropical climates, especially in South America, Africa, and Southeast Asia including India. Humans are the only host; there is no other animal reservoir.

It is frequently associated in AIDS patients, prevalence ranging from 3% (USA) to 37% (Zambia). However, it is rare in HIV infected children (different from cryptosporidiosis).

Clinical Feature

Acute infections can begin abruptly with fever, abdominal pain, and watery nonbloody diarrhea and can last for weeks or months.

- Disease is less severe and outbreaks are less common compared to cryptosporidiosis
- In immunocompromised or HIV positive patients, disease is more severe resembling cryptosporidiosis; with chronic, profuse watery diarrhea and extraintestinal infections such as involvement of biliary tract.

Laboratory Diagnosis

Laboratory methods are similar to that for cryptosporidiosis.

- Stool examination—diagnosis can be established by demonstration of characteristic oval oocyst in patient's stool by:
    - Saline wet mount of stool (Fig. 7.9A)
    - **Acid fast stained smears:** The oocyst is uniformly acid fast, oval/elliptical, 20-33 µm × 10-19 µm in size, surrounded by a thin, smooth, two layered cyst wall (Fig. 7.9B)
    - Other stains like lactophenol cotton blue and safranin can be used
    - **Fluorescent stained smears:** By auramine rhodamine stain (Fig. 7.9D)
    - **Autofluorescence** can be seen under 330-380 nm ultraviolet filter. However, this property is not consistent like in *Cyclospora*
    - Phase contrast microscopy is also useful (Fig. 7.9C)
- If the oocyst load is less, then stool samples are concentrated by Sheather's sugar floatation technique
- Examination of small bowel specimens (e.g. duodenal aspirates) may be helpful if stool examination is negative
- **Other tests:**
    - Peripheral blood eosinophilia

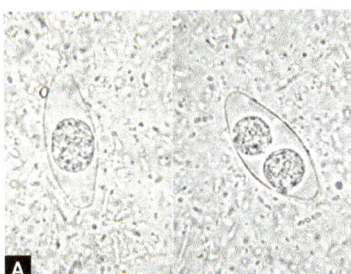 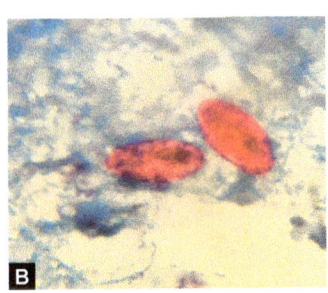 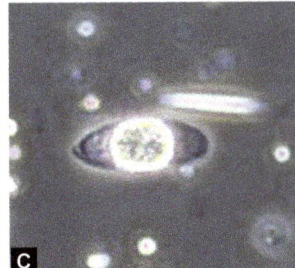 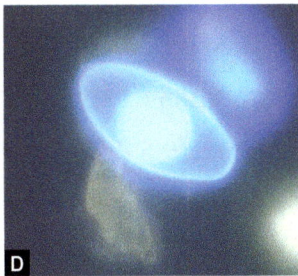

Figs 7.9A to D: *Cystoisospora belli* (A) Saline mount preparation shows left—unsporulated oocyst and right—sporulated oocyst; (B) Modified acid fast stain showing unsporulated oocyst; (C) Phase contrast microscopy showing unsporulated oocyst; (D) Fluorescent stained smears showing unsporulated oocyst

Source: B—Dr Anand Janagond, Associate Professor of Microbiology, S Nijalingappa Medical college, Bagalkot, Karnataka (*with permission*); A, C and D—Swierczynski G, Milanesi B. Atlas of human intestinal protozoa Microscopic diagnosis (*with permission*).

- Charcot-Leyden crystals in stool
- Low CD4- T cell count (in HIV infected patients).
- **Molecular methods:** PCR and real-time PCR using *C. belli* specific primers (based on small-subunit rRNA) is highly sensitive and specific but its use for routine diagnosis requires further study
- **Histopathologic examination:** Tissue sections from the small bowel of infected patients reveal villous atrophy, crypt hyperplasia and inflammatory cells (eosinophils) infiltration of lamina propria. Asexual and sexual stages of the parasite can be identified within the parasitophorous vacuoles of the enterocytes.

Treatment	*Cystoisospora belli*
□ Cotrimoxazole (160 mg trimethoprim/800 mg sulfamethoxazole) is the treatment of choice. It is administered four times daily for 10 days □ Patients with HIV infection usually require longer courses but have more chance of relapse □ Alternatives treatment: Pyrimethamine (75 mg/day) together with folinic acid (10–25 mg/day), or ciprofloxacin (500 mg twice daily for 7 days followed by suppressive therapy three times weekly) □ Nitazoxanide has also been used successfully.	

SARCOCYSTIS SPECIES

Sarcocystis is a zoonotic parasite. Though more than 120 species of *Sarcocystis* have been reported infecting a wide range of domestic and wild animals but the frequency of human infection is relatively low.
- It was first described in the skeletal muscle of a house mouse in 1843 in Switzerland
- Two well-described species are *S. hominis* (infects cattle) and *S. suihominis* (infects pigs). They produce two types of human infection: (1) intestinal sarcocystosis and (2) muscular sarcocystosis
- The muscular disease causing species were grouped under the term *Sarcocystis "lindemanni"* previously. However, this name is no longer used.

Morphology

It exists in three morphological forms.

Oocyst

Oocysts are found usually in the intestine of the definitive host. They sporulate within the lamina propria of the intestinal epithelium.
- The sporulated oocyst is elongated and spherical, colorless thin walled (<1 μm), measures 15–20 μm
- It contains two elongated sporocysts and each sporocyst contains four elongated sporozoites.

Sporocyst

From the sporulated oocyst, sporocysts are released and are excreted in the feces of definitive host. It is the infective form to the intermediate host. It is oval 9–16 μm size and contains four elongated sporozoites.

Sarcocyst

Sarcocysts (muscular cysts) are found in the cardiac and skeletal muscles (of diaphragm, esophagus) of the intermediate host.
- It is elongated, measures 100–325 μm in size; found longitudinally along the muscle fiber
- It has a thick cyst wall and is always surrounded by a parasitophorous vacuole within the cytoplasm of the muscle cells
- The cyst is divided into many compartments that contain numerous banana-shaped **bradyzoites** or metrocytes (7–16 μm long) containing prominent PAS (periodic acid-Schiff stain) positive amylopectin granules.

Life Cycle (Fig. 7.10)

Host: Unlike other coccidian parasites, *Sarcocystis* has an obligatory two hosts life cycle.
- *Definitive host:* Carnivorous animals such as dogs, cats and others (including man) act as a definitive host
- *Intermediate host:* Cattles and pigs serve as intermediate hosts. Man can also accidentally acts as intermediate host.

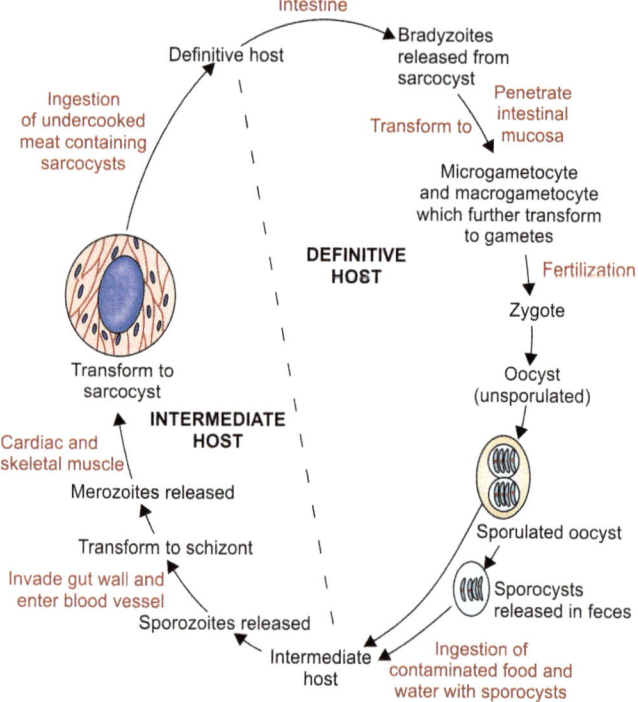

Fig. 7.10: Life cycle of *Sarcocystis* species

CHAPTER 7 ◆ Apicomplexa—II (Opportunistic Coccidian Parasites)

Transmission and infective form:
- Definitive hosts acquire the infection through ingestion of raw or undercooked beef (*S. hominis*) or pork (*S. suihominis*) infected with sarcocysts
- Intermediate host becomes infected by ingestion of food or water contaminated with sporocysts or oocysts excreted in the feces of carnivorous animals.

Cycle in Definitive Host

Following ingestion of sacrocysts infected meat; bradyzoites are released from sacrocysts and penetrate the intestinal mucosa, multiply and transform into microgametocyte (male) and macrogametocyte (female).
- The gametocytes transform to gametes which then undergo fertilization and zygote is formed which later on undergo meiosis to transform into an oocyst
- Oocysts are initially unsporulated; undergo maturation to form sporulated oocysts in the lamina propria, which bear two sporocysts each containing four sporozoites
- The sporocysts released from oocysts or the oocysts per se are passed in the human feces and are infective to the intermediate host.

Cycle in Intermediate Host

Sporocysts or oocysts ingested by the intermediate host rupture, releasing sporozoites. Sporozoites enter endothelial cells of blood vessels and undergo schizogony, resulting in first-generation schizonts.
- Merozoites derived from the first-generation schizont invade small capillaries and blood vessels, becoming second-generation schizonts
- The merozoites released from second generation schizont invade muscle cells and develop into sarcocysts containing bradyzoites, which are the infective stage for the definitive host.

Cycle in Humans

In man, the cycle of definitive host is usually seen resulting in intestinal sarcocystosis. However, accidental ingestion of food or water contaminated with sporocysts or oocysts excreted in the feces of carnivorous animals such as dogs and cats can result in muscular sarcocystosis.

Clinical Features

Intestinal Sarcocystosis

It is usually asymptomatic but patient may develop nausea, vomiting, abdominal pain and diarrhea.
- Symptoms appear early after ingestion of beef (3-6 hours) than pork (24 hours)
- Various studies have shown a natural prevalence of 2-10% throughout the world, including India (14 cases due *S. suihominis* were reported from Indian children).

Muscular Sarcocystosis

It is also usually asymptomatic; symptoms depend on the size of the muscle cysts that varies from 50 µm to 5 cm
- Larger cysts can cause muscle pain, weakness in muscle or rarely focal myositis and eosinophilic myositis
- Myocarditis and pericarditis are rare findings
- It has been associated with malignancies, primarily involving the tongue and nasopharynx
- Nearly 200 cases of human muscular sarcocystosis have been reported from the world (which includes an outbreak of nearly 100 cases in Malaysia in 2011-12). In India, 11 cases have been reported.

Laboratory Diagnosis

Intestinal Sarcocystosis

It is diagnosed by stool examination demonstrating the sporocysts or sporulating oocysts of *Sarcocystis* (Figs 7.7.11A and B).
- Speciation is not possible as the oocysts of all the species are morphologically similar
- The sporocysts are excreted in the feces of the infected patient as long as 14-18 days and 11-13 days after ingestion of uncooked beef and pork respectively
- Stool concentration is done if the parasite count is low. Zinc sulfate flotation is preferred over sedimentation

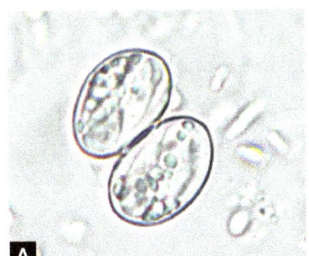 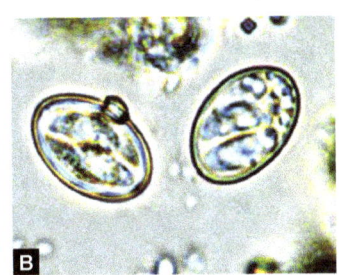 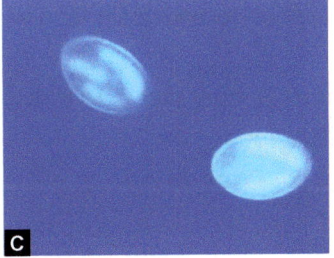 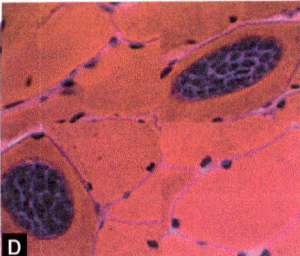

Figs 7.11A to D: *Sarcocystis* (A) Oocyst containing two sporocysts in saline mount; (B) Sporocysts containing sporozoites in saline mount; (C) Sporocysts autofluoresce under UV light-sporozoites are clearly seen; (D) Sarcocysts in skeletal muscle biopsy

Source: A and D—DPDx Image Library, Centers for Disease Control and Prevention (CDC), Atlanta (*with permission*); B and C—Swierczynski G, Milanesi B. Atlas of human intestinal protozoa Microscopic diagnosis (*with permission*).

❖ *Sarcocystis* sporocysts exhibit autofluorescence under UV light (Fig. 7.11C).

Muscular Sarcocystosis

Histological examination

Histological examination of muscle biopsy can be done to demonstrate the sarcocysts in cardiac and skeletal muscle (Fig. 7.11D).

- ❖ They measure 100–325 µm in size, contain numerous PAS positive bright red bradyzoites measuring 7–16 µm
- ❖ An active infection is characterized by immature sarcocysts associated with an inflammatory response, whereas mature sarcocysts without any inflammation indicates past infection

❖ Myositis and myonecrosis, tissue eosinophilia, and inflammatory changes may be seen in cases of eosinophilic myositis.

Serology

Detecting antibodies using Western blot suggests past exposure, but is not diagnostic of acute disease.

Treatment	Sarcocystosis
☐ No specific treatment for *Sarcocystis* infection is known. Infection, if symptomatic, is generally self-limited ☐ Cotrimoxazole, furazolidone and albendazole are used, but their efficacy is doubtful ☐ Corticosteroids may provide symptomatic relief in cases of eosinophilic myositis.	

EXPECTED QUESTIONS

I. **Write essay on:**
  a. A 61-year-old person reactive for HIV, presented with altered mental status, seizures, sensory abnormalities. The bone marrow aspirate collected was sent for Giemsa stain which revealed crescent shaped tachyzoites (6 × 2 µm in size).
    1. Identify the etiological agent and diagnose the clinical condition.
    2. Write briefly about the life cycle of the etiological agent.
    3. What are the various diagnostic modalities?
    4. How will you treat this condition?
  b. A 46-year-old female patient infected with HIV presented to the casualty with severe profuse diarrhea, with a frequency of 15 times a day for past 10 days. She also complained of weight loss and abdominal pain. The stool specimen was subjected for modified acid-fast staining, which revealed round sporulated oocysts (4–6 µm in size), containing four sporozoites.
    1. Identify the etiological agent.
    2. Write briefly about the life cycle of the etiological agent.
    3. What are the various diagnostic modalities?
    4. How will you treat this clinical condition?

II. **Write short notes on:**
  a. Cyclosporiasis.
  b. Muscular sarcocystosis.
  c. Congenital toxoplasmosis.

III. **Multiple choice questions (MCQs):**
  1. Oocysts of *Toxoplasma gondii* are excreted in the feces of:
     a. Cat   b. Sheep
     c. Cattle   d. Humans
  2. Congenital toxoplasmosis is more severe in which trimester of pregnancy?
     a. First   b. Second
     c. Third   d. During delivery

  3. Most common manifestation of *Toxoplasma gondii* in immunocompetent adult:
     a. Lymphadenopathy   b. Chorioretinitis
     c. Myocarditis   d. Encephalitis
  4. Most common manifestation of *Toxoplasma gondii* in immunocompromised adult:
     a. Lymphadenopathy   b. Chorioretinitis
     c. Myocarditis   d. Encephalitis
  5. Most common manifestation of congenital toxoplasmosis:
     a. Lymphadenopathy   b. Chorioretinitis
     c. Myocarditis   d. Encephalitis
  6. Sporulated oocyst of *Cystoisospora belli* contains:
     a. One sporocyst and two sporozoites
     b. One sporocyst and four sporozoites
     c. Two sporocysts and four sporozoites
     d. Two sporocysts and eight sporozoites
  7. Sporulated oocyst of *Cyclospora cayetanensis* totally contains:
     a. One sporocyst and two sporozoites
     b. One sposrocyst and four sporozoites
     c. Two sporocysts and four sporozoites
     d. Two sporocysts and eight sporozoites
  8. Which statement is false about *Cryptosporidium* species?
     a. Developmental stages of the parasite occur inside a parasitophorous vacuole
     b. High infective dose
     c. Large number of animal reservoir
     d. It causes diarrhea in AIDS patients
  9. Intermediate host for *Sarcocystis suihominis* is:
     a. Pig   b. Dog
     c. Man   d. Cattle
  10. For muscular sarcocystosis, man acts:
     a. Intermediate host   b. Definitive host
     c. Only host   d. Paratenic host

Answer
1. a   2. a   3. a   4. d   5. b   6. d   7. c   8. b   9. a   10. a

Miscellaneous Protozoa

CHAPTER 8

CHAPTER OUTLINE
- Microsporidia
- *Balantidium coli*
- *Blastocystis* species

MICROSPORIDIA

Classification

Microsporidia are lower eukaryotic, spore forming obligate intracellular parasites, infecting a broad range of vertebrates and invertebrates.
- In humans, they are opportunistic pathogens affecting HIV positive patients
- Microsporidia have a unique character of entering into the host cell via a polar tube within a spore.

Taxonomical classification: Microsporidia were once classified under parasite; are now considered to be evolved from the fungi, being most closely related to the zygomycetes.
- They resemble fungi in having chitin and trehalose, similarities in cell cycles, and certain gene organizations
- They belong to Kingdom Fungi, Phylum Microspora, Class Microsporea and order Microsporida
- Though Microsporidia are in a transition stage from parasite to fungi; at this point, it is discussed under parasitology in this text book.

Classification based on their habitat: Microsporidia include over 170 genera comprising 1400 species. However, only nine genera comprising fifteen species are found to infect man (Table 8.1).

Morphology of Spores

Spore is highly resistant extracellular form (survives in the environment) and also is the infective stage.
- It is oval, variable in size ranging from 1–1.5 μm length and 0.5 μm width in human tissue (Fig. 8.1)
- It has a double layered cyst wall. Outer layer (exospore) is proteinaceous and electron dense. Inner layer (endospore) is chitinous and electron-lucent
- Inner side of the cyst wall is lined by plasma membrane
- Cytoplasm contains various organelles like coiled polar tube (six coils), polar sac, polaroplast, nucleus and a posterior vacuole
- Coiled polar tube has a spring like tubular extrusion mechanism by which the infective material, **sporoplasm** is injected into the host cell
- The polar tube ends anteriorly into a **polar sac** (Fig. 8.1)
- Near the anterior pole, **polaroplast** is situated on both the side of the polar tube, which is a component of the extrusion apparatus.

Life Cycle (Fig. 8.2)

Mode of transmission: Humans acquire infection by ingestion (or rarely inhalation or ocular contact) of spores of microsporidia.

Extrusion of Sporoplasm

The infective material of the spore (sporoplasm) is injected into the host cell (**enterocyte**). The polar tube comes out of the spore as a long flexible cylindrical structure and injects the sporoplasm by the extrusion mechanism (helped by the polar sac, polaroplast, raised pH and calcium ion) into the host cell in two ways:
1. By punching a hole in the host cell plasma membrane, e.g. *Enterocytozoon*.
2. Or by the expansion of the host cell plasma membrane to cover the emerging sporoplasm, e.g. *Encephalitozoon*.

Asexual Cycle

Inside the host cell, the sporoplasm multiplies to generate a number of meronts.
- Multiplication occurs either by merogony (binary fission) or schizogony (multiple fission) or plasmotomy (division of cytoplasm without their relation to nuclei to produce multinucleated offspring)

Table 8.1: Classification and clinical manifestations of microsporidia

Genus	Species	Habitat and infections
Enterocytozoon	E. bieneusi	Most common species infecting man Small intestine: Enteric infection (diarrhea, acalculous cholecystitis) Rarely cause nasal polyp, infections of bile duct, liver and respiratory system It has zoonotic potential. More than 90 genotypes are described; only 17 infect humans, most common being group 1
Encephalitozoon	E. intestinalis	Second most common species infecting man Small intestine: Enteric infection
	E. cuniculi	Extraintestinal infections such as: • Disseminated systemic infection • Eye: Keratoconjunctivitis, • Sinuses: Chronic sinusitis • CNS: Brain abscess • Heart: Myocarditis and endocarditis • Respiratory and genitourinary tract infections
	E. hellem	Disseminated infection involving eyes (keratoconjunctivitis), urinary tract and respiratory tract Transmission is from birds
Pleistophora	P. ronneafiei	Skeletal muscle (myositis)
Trachipleistophora	T. hominis	Myositis, sinusitis and conjunctivitis
	T. anthropophthera	Brain, heart and kidney
Brachiola	B. vesicularum	Skeletal muscle and eye (corneal stroma)
Anncaliia	A. connori	Eye: Corneal stroma Smooth and cardiac muscle
	A. algerae	Eyes, muscle and possible disseminated infection Mosquito-borne transmission documented
Nosema	N. ocularum	Eye: Corneal stroma
Vittaforma	V. corneae	Eye: Corneal stroma and rarely urinary tract (UTI) Water-borne transmission documented
Tubulinosema	T. acridophagus	Systemic disseminated infection Grasshoppers are the non-human host
Microsporidium	M. ceylonensis	Eye: Corneal stroma (corneal ulcer)
	M. africanum	Eye: Corneal stroma (corneal ulcer)

Note: Most of the species are zoonotic having various animal reservoir.

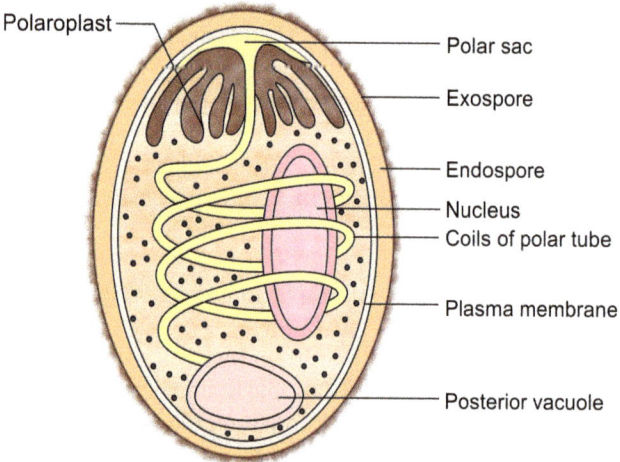

Fig. 8.1: Morphology of Microsporidia spore (schematic diagram)

❖ Meronts are round to elongated. They remain free in the host cell cytoplasm (in most species) or lie inside a parasitophorous vacuole (e.g. *Encephalitozoon*).

Sexual Cycle (Sporogony)

Finally, the meronts develop into sporonts; which then eventually get surrounded by a double layered cyst wall and directly transform into sporoblasts or may become multinucleated to form sporogonial plasmodia that later transform into sporoblasts.

❖ Sporoblasts undergo sporogony and develop into spores
❖ Spores are present either free in the host cytoplasm or enclosed by a sporophorous vesicle (e.g. *Pleistophora* and *Trachipleistophora*)
❖ Most of the species, the spores are liberated by lysis of the host cell except in *Encephalitozoon hellem*, where the spores germinate without host cell lysis.

CHAPTER 8 ◆ Miscellaneous Protozoa

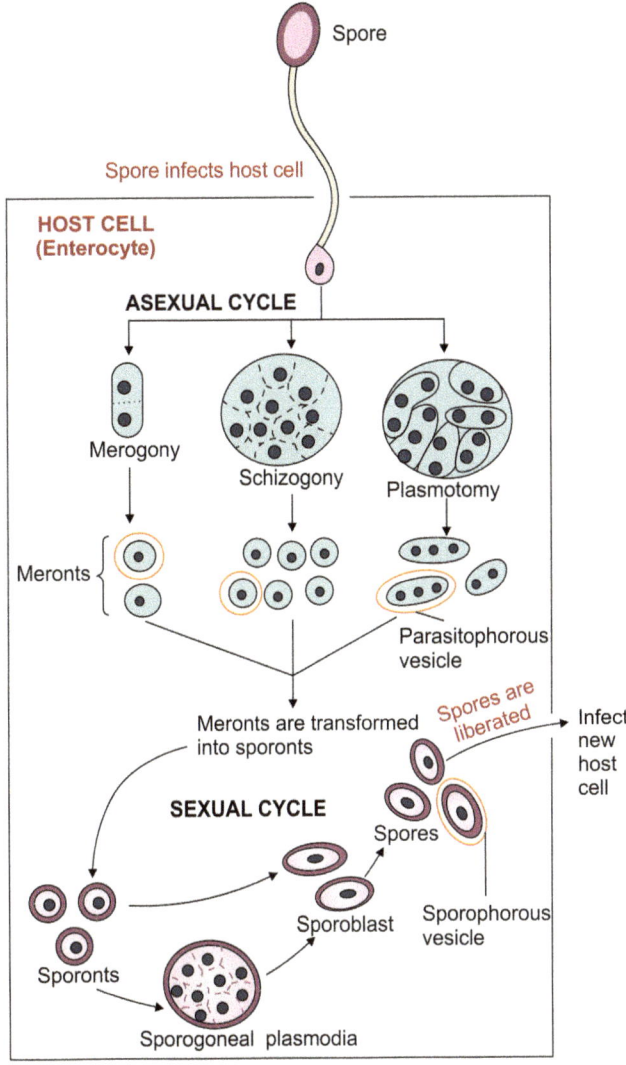

Fig. 8.2: Life cycle of Microsporidia

Pathogenesis and Clinical Feature

Microsporidia mainly cause opportunistic infections in HIV-infected patients, when their CD4 T cell count falls below 100 μL or in any other patients with immunosuppression like recipients of organ transplant. Depending up on the species causing infection, clinical presentation of microsporidiosis may be of various types: (i) enteric infection, (ii) ocular infection, (iii) musculoskeletal infections and (iv) disseminated infections (see Table 8.1).

Epidemiology

Though, the first human case of microsporidian infection was reported in 1959, but it is being increasingly recognized as opportunistic infectious agent worldwide since the advent of HIV AIDS.

- The largest number of cases have been reported in AIDS patients from North America, Western Europe and Australia where the prevalence ranges from 2% to 50% or higher
- In addition, it has also been reported in patients receiving organ transplants, elderly debilitated persons
- In India, few clusters of cases have been reported so far. The first case of enteric microsporidiosis was reported in 2001 (Sehgal et al.) and ocular microsporidiosis was reported in 2003 (S Sharma et al.)
- In a study done at PGI, Chandigarh (Saigal K et al., 2012), Microsporidia were the most common parasites detected (15%) in the stool samples of HIV infected patients, *E. intestinalis* being the most common species.

Laboratory Diagnosis — Microsporidiosis

- **Light microscopy** for the spore detection—by modified trichrome stain, modified acid fast stain, Gram stain (Brown-Brenn modification), Giemsa, PAS stain
- **Fluorescence microscope**—detects spores
- **Electron microscopy**—detects spores
- **Cell culture**—in Vero, RK13 and MRC-5 cell lines
- **Antibody assays**—IFA, ELISA, Western blot (Ab to C1 Hsp70 protein)
- **Antigen assays**—DAF (detects Ag on the spores surface)
- **Molecular methods**—PCR (detecting small and large subunit rRNA)
- In-situ hybridization.

Laboratory Diagnosis

Light Microscopy for the Spore Detection

- **Samples:** Various samples can be collected like stool, small intestinal contents (collected by Entero-test) corneal smear or small intestinal biopsies, sputum, urine, etc.
- **Modified trichrome stain (MTS):** It is the recommended stain for Microsporidia (Fig. 8.3A)
  - Microsporidia appear as red oval refractile spores against a blue background
  - Various modification of MTS are Weber green MTS, Ryan blue MTS and Kokoskin hot method of MTS
  - It differs from routine trichrome stain, as it contains higher concentration of chromotrope 2R (10 times) component.
- **Modified acid fast stain (using 1% acid alcohol):** Microsporidia spores are acid fast and appear red, 1–1.5 μm size, with darker cell wall and polar tubule as diagonal belt like stripe within the cell. (Fig. 8.3B)
- **Gram stain** (Brown-Brenn and Brown-Hopps modification): Microsporidia spores stain gram positive
- **Other stains:** Giemsa stain (Figs 8.3D and 8.4A), periodic acid Schiff stain (PAS) and Gram chromotrope stain can be used (Fig. 8.3C).

Fluorescence Microscope

Fluorochrome stain like Calcofluor white (Fig. 8.4B), Fungi-Fluor, and Uvitex 2B stain can be used. These reagents are sensitive but nonspecific.

Electron Microscopy

Transmission electron microscopy is considered as the **gold standard** method for the definitive diagnosis of microsporidiosis (Fig. 8.4C).

- ❖ It is highly specific, but lacks sensitivity, time consuming, labor-intensive and expensive
- ❖ Microsporidia can be identified to the genus and species level based on ultrafine structure of the spores (number of coils in polar tubes), method of division and nature of the host cell parasite interface (whether grow directly or inside a parasitophorous vacuole).

Cell Culture

Microsporidia have been successfully cultivated in a number of mammalian cell lines including monkey and rabbit kidney cells (Vero and RK13), human fetal lung fibroblasts (MRC-5) and MDCK cell line.

- ❖ Its use in routine clinical diagnosis is limited as it is time consuming and laborious
- ❖ However, it is useful for antigen preparation and drug susceptibility test.

Serology

Antibody assays

Various methods like indirect immunofluorescence, immunoperoxidase, ELISA and Western blot [detecting antibody (75-kDa band) against C1 Hsp70 protein of *E. cuniculi* and *E. intestinalis* spores] are used to detect antibodies. They are not very useful as they lack specificity and give false positive results in unrelated infections.

Antigen assays

Direct antibody fluorescent test (DAF) is available for detecting the antigens on Microsporidia spores by using fluorescent tagged monoclonal antibodies (Fig. 8.4D) Spores have a darker cell wall with coiled polar tubule appear as diagonal lines or cross lines within the cell.

Molecular Methods

Several polymerase chain reaction (PCR)-based methods have been developed, targeting different genes like small subunit and large subunit gene of rRNA and intergenic spacer region (ISR) gene for diagnosis and speciation of Microsporidia infecting humans.

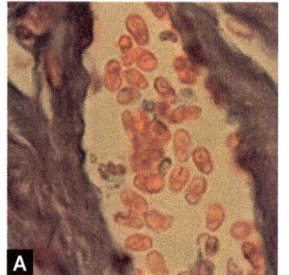 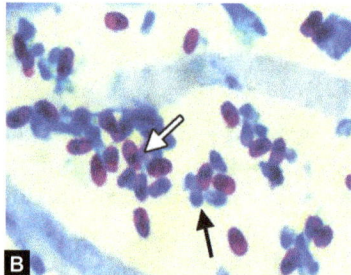 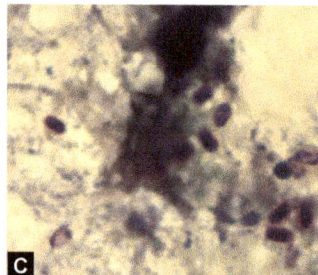 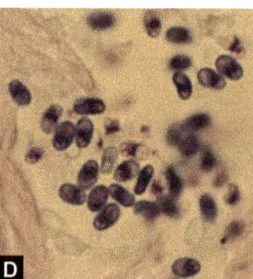

Figs 8.3A to D: Microsporidia spores in corneal section stained with (A) Modified trichrome stain; (B) Acid fast stain (showing red stained mature spores and blue stained (non acid-fast) immature or degenerating spores); (C) Gram Chromotrope; (D) Giemsa stain

Source: A, C, D—DPDx Image Library, Centers for Disease Control and Prevention (CDC), Atlanta (*with permission*); B—Savitri Sharma, LV Prasad Eye Institute, Hyderabad.

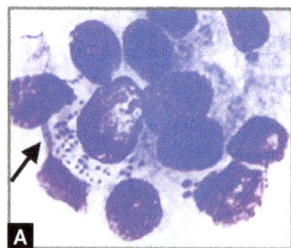 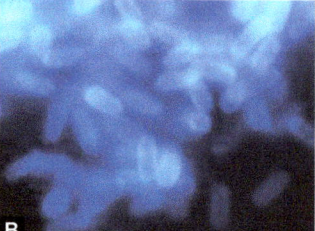 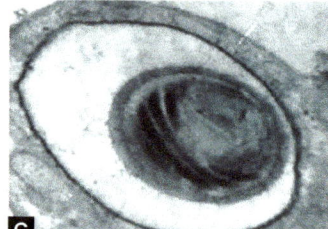 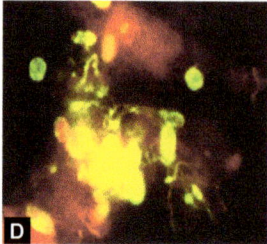

Figs 8.4A to D: Microsporidia spores: (A) Duodenal biopsy (Giemsa stain) shows numerous spores inside the enterocyte (marked by arrow); (B) Calcofluor white stain; (C) Electron microscopic picture; (D) Direct antibody fluorescent test showing fluorescing spores

Source: A—Giovanni Swierczynski, Bruno Milanesi. "Atlas of human intestinal protozoa Microscopic diagnosis" (*with permission*); B, C, D—Savitri Sharma, LV Prasad Eye Institute, Hyderabad.

Random amplified polymorphic DNA amplification has also been available.

In situ Hybridization

In situ hybridization has been established for the detection of *E. bieneusi* in humans by using probes directed against the small subunit rRNA of *E. bieneusi*, present directly in the biopsy specimens.

It is time-consuming, not been described for other species and its sensitivity and specificity have not been evaluated.

Treatment	Microsporidiosis
❑ Albendazole is effective for the treatment of enteric, muscular and ocular microsporidiosis. It is given 400 mg twice daily for 2–4 weeks. Relapse may be seen in some cases ❑ Other alternate drugs which are tried include Octreotide, nitazoxanide, fumagillin and itraconazole ❑ Nutritional therapy: To reduce malabsorption in case of enteric microsporidiosis ❑ Topical agents can be applied for the corneal lesions like topical itraconazole, metronidazole and topical propamidine ❑ Control of AIDS by antiretroviral therapy (ART) is important to reconstitute the immune system and to prevent remissions.	

BALANTIDIUM COLI

Balantidium coli, is the largest protozoan and the only ciliated parasite of humans.

Though it was observed by AV Leeuwenhoek earlier while examining a dysentery stool but the proper description was given later by Malmsten (Sweden) in man, in 1857.

Taxonomy: It belongs to the Phylum Ciliophora, Class Litostomatea, Order Vestibuliferida and Family Balantidiidae. There is a recent change in nomenclature to *Neobalantidium coli*.

Habitat: It resides in the large intestine of man, pig (main reservoir) and other animals.

Morphology

It exists in two forms—(1) trophozoite (found in dysenteric stool) (2) cyst (found in carriers and chronic cases). Both the forms are binucleated having a large macronucleus and a small micronucleus.

Trophozoite

It is found in the active stage of the disease and considered as the invasive form (Fig. 8.5A).
- It is oval shaped, 50–100 μm in length and 40–70 μm in breadth
- The whole body is covered with a row of tiny delicate **cilia** (organ of locomotion); causing a rotary and boring motility

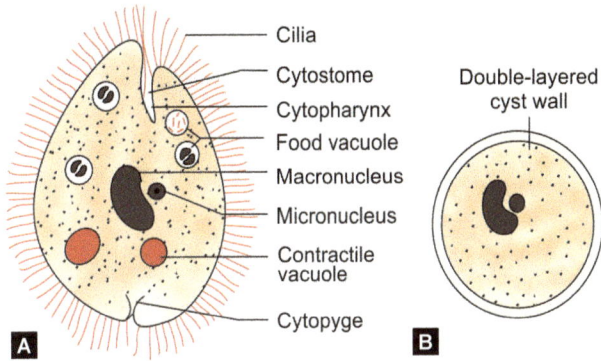

Figs 8.5A and B: Morphology of *Balantidium coli* (schematic diagram): (A) Trophozoite; (B) cyst

- **Cilia** present near to the mouth part appear to be longer and called as **"adoral cilia"**
- Anterior end is narrow and the posterior end is broad
- Anterior end bears a groove (**peristome**) that leads to a mouth (**cytostome**) followed by a short funnel-shaped gullet (**cytopharynx**) extending up to one-third of the body
- Posterior end is broad, round and bears an excretory opening called a **cytopyge**
- The cytoplasm is divided into outer clear ectoplasm and inner granular endoplasm
- The endoplasm contains:
  - Two nuclei: Large kidney-shaped macronucleus in the center and a small micronucleus lies in the concavity of the macronucleus
  - Two contractile vacuoles
  - Numerous food vacuoles.

Cyst

It is round, measures 50–70 μm in size, surrounded by a thick and transparent cyst wall. It also contains two nuclei (macronucleus and micronucleus) and vacuoles (Fig. 8.5B).

Life Cycle (Fig. 8.6)

Host: Life cycle is completed in a **single host**.
- Pig is the **natural host**
- Man is the **accidental host**.

Infective form: Cysts are the infective form

Mode of transmission: Man gets infection by ingestion of food and water contaminated with cysts.

Development in Large Intestine

- **Excystation:** Probably occurs in the small intestine but multiplication takes place in the large intestine
- A single trophozoite is formed from each cyst

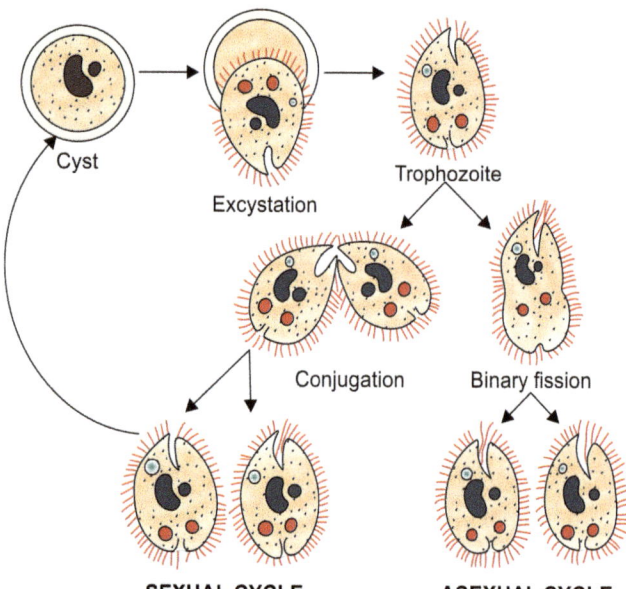

Fig. 8.6: Life cycle of *Balantidium coli*

- Trophozoites are the feeding stage of the parasite; they multiply either in the gut lumen or enter the submucosa of the large intestine
- Trophozoites divide by both sexual and asexual methods:
  - **Asexual reproduction:** Trophozoites divide by binary fission. Micronucleus divides first followed by the macronucleus and finally a transverse septum is formed that separates the cytoplasm into two halves (see Fig. 8.6)
  - **Sexual reproduction:** Trophozoites also replicate sexually (**syngamy**) by conjugation (Fig. 8.6)
    - Two trophozoites come in contact with each other at their anterior ends and exchange the nuclear material for few moments after which they detach
    - There is no increase in numbers of trophozoites
- Both trophozoites and cysts are excreted in the feces
- Trophozoites disintegrate but the cysts are resistant and are infective to man and pig.

Clinical Feature

Asymptomatic Carriers

Majority of infections lead to asymptomatic carriers; they harbor the cysts and spread the infection.

Acute Disease

This stage is similar to acute amoebic dysentery except that it is less severe, invasion is limited to muscularis mucosa and extraintestinal involvement occurs very rarely.

- Trophozoites invade the gut submucosa and form multiple tiny superficial ulcers (due to hyaluronidase secreted by the parasite) with necrotic base and undermined edge
- Microscopically, cluster of trophozoites are found in submucosa along with inflammatory cells (predominantly lymphocytic)
- Patients have frequent profuse diarrhea resembling cholera and dysentery with mucous and blood, weeks to months later. Other features include fever, nausea, vomiting and abdominal pain.

Chronic Disease

These patients have periods of increased bowel movements (mucous or rarely bloody) with alternate periods of constipations. Organism load is less and requires repeated stool examination.

Complications

Complications are seen in immunocompromised and malnourished people.
- These include perforation of the large intestine, involvement of appendix, peritonitis, severe dehydration leading to renal failure
- Extraintestinal manifestations may be rarely seen like liver abscess, pleuritis and pneumonia, etc.

Epidemiology

B. coli is worldwide in distribution particularly in tropical and subtropical countries where pig to human contact is more.
- Highest prevalence (20%) has been reported from the mountain districts of West Irian (Indonesia)
- So far only one outbreak of **balantidiasis** in humans is reported from Pacific Island of Truk in 1973
- In India, balantidiasis is quite rare.

Laboratory Diagnosis

Stool Examination

Repeated stool examination should be done as the parasite is excreted intermittently.
- Trophozoites are detected in acute disease (dysenteric stool) (Fig. 8.7C)
- Saline mount: Trophozoites are easy to identify by its rotatory motility, large size kidney shaped macronucleus and presence of cilia (Fig. 8.7A)
- Cysts are seen in chronic cases or carriers (Fig. 8.7D).
- Cyst is round, measures 50–70 μm in size, surrounded by a cyst wall and has two nuclei.

In pulmonary infection, trophozoites may be demonstrated in bronchopulmonary lavage. It should be differentiated from ciliated epithelial cells; which are smaller in size (<30 μm) with fewer cilia.

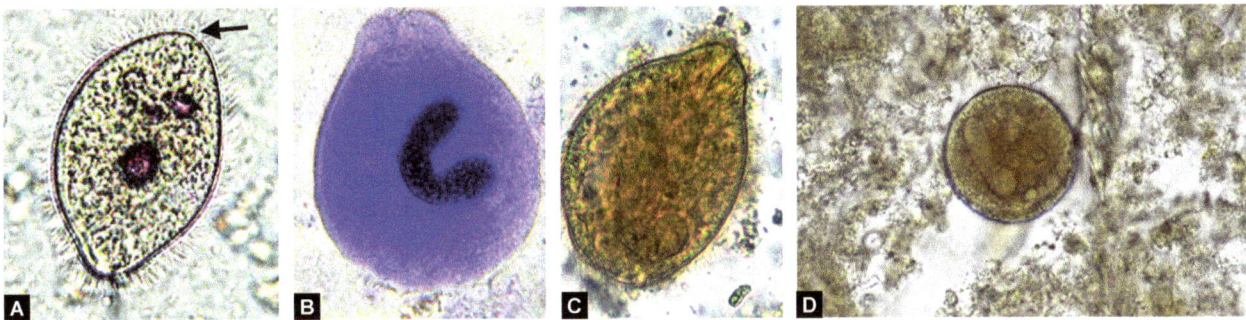

Figs. 8.7A to D: *Balantidium coli* (A) saline wet mount preparation shows trophozoite with cilia; (B) Mayer's hematoxylin stain shows trophozoite with prominent macronucleus; (C) Iodine stain showing trophozoite; (D) Iron hematoxylin stain shows cyst with prominent macronucleus

Source: Giovanni Swierczynski, Bruno Milanesi. "Atlas of human intestinal protozoa Microscopic diagnosis" (*with permission*).

Histopathology

Histopathological staining of the biopsy tissue or scrapping of the ulcers taken by sigmoidoscopy reveals cluster of trophozoites, cysts and lymphocytic infiltration in submucosa (Figs 8.7B).

Culture

The culture media like Boeck and Drbohlav egg serum media and Balamuth's media that support the growth of *Entamoeba histolytica* can be used for cultivation of *B. coli*. Culture is rarely necessary as the parasite is easily detected by stool microscopy or histopathology.

Treatment	*Balantidium coli*

- Tetracycline is the drug of choice. It is given 500 mg four times a day for 10 days
- Alternatively, metronidazole can be given. It is given 750 mg three times a day for 5–7 days
- No relapse or drug resistance is reported so far
- Treatment of carriers is also recommended to prevent the spread of the disease.

Prevention

Balantidiasis can be prevented by:
- Treatment of carriers shedding the cysts
- Hygienic rearing of pigs and prevention of pig to human contact
- Prevention of contamination of food or water with pig and human feces.

BLASTOCYSTIS SPECIES

Habitat

Blastocystis species (earlier called as *B. hominis*) is single-celled anaerobic protozoan parasite resides in the intestine of many animals including humans

It was considered as the most common commensal protozoa of intestine; however, recently its pathogenic role is described.

Taxonomic Status

Taxonomic status of *Blastocystis* was uncertain for longtime:
- Over the years, *Blastocystis* has been classified under various groups such as under yeasts, sporozoa and amoeba
- Recently, according to Cavalier and Smith's six kingdom classification, *Blastocystis* was placed under kingdom Chromista, subkingdom Chromobiota, infrakingdom Hetrokonta (stramenopiles), phylum Bigyra and class Blastocystea
- **Subtypes or Species:** Based on small subunit rDNA analysis, *Blastocystis* is classified into at least 17 lineages or species or subtypes (ST)
    - ST1 to ST4 account for >90% of human carriage
    - ST3 is the commonest subtype in world, as well as from India
    - ST9 is found in nonhuman hosts also.

Life Cycle

Blastocystis species shows great morphological variations; occur in six forms—vacuolar, avacuolar, multi-vacuolar, amoeboid, granular and cyst forms.
- **Transmission:** Humans acquire infection by consumption of food or water contaminated with feces containing cysts (infective form)
- **Excystation** occurs in the large intestine to release the vacuolar form
- **Multiplication:** The vacuolar form multiplies by binary fission (or by other modes of reproduction such as plasmotomy and budding) and also can transform into other forms and vice versa
- **Encystation:** The vacuolar form undergoes encystation in the lumen of the large intestine to produce the cysts, which are shed in the feces
- **Infective form:** Cysts are of two types; thick walled and thin walled. Thick-walled cysts are the infective form. Thin-walled cysts die soon; may cause autoinfection but the data is inconclusive.

Pathogenesis and Clinical Feature

Blastocystis species is considered as a gut commensal when it is found in stool of asymptomatic individuals or symptomatic individuals co-infected with other enteric pathogens. In the absence of any other gut pathogen; *Blastocysts* may present clinically as below:

- Asymptomatic infection with passage of vacuolar form in stool
- **Intestinal infection:** Presents with symptoms of irritable bowel syndrome (such as abdominal pain, bloating and flatulence) and diarrhea. Hydrolytic enzymes and proteases secreted by *Blastocystis* induce release of interleukin-8 by activating the gut mucosa; which in turn is responsible for the intestinal symptoms. Traveling to developing tropical country appears to be a risk factor
- **Extraintestinal infection** such as urticaria, angioedema, iron deficiency anemia and arthritis may be associated with *Blastocystis* infection.

Laboratory Diagnosis

Stool Microscopy

Stool microscopy by permanent stained smear (trichrome stain) is the procedure of choice; which demonstrates various forms of Blastocystis (Figs 8.8A to E).

- **Vacuolar forms** are the most common form seen in stool microscopy. They measure 5–15 μm in size with 1–4 nuclei. They contain a large central body (or vacuole) comprised of carbohydrate and lipid, occupying 70–90% of the cell with a thin peripheral cytoplasm
- **Granular forms** are the next common form to be seen in stool microscopy. They contain granules within the central vacuole
- **Amoeboid forms** (10 μm) are often confused with pus cells and macrophages; hence are easily missed in stool microscopy. They may possess pseudopods, but are nonmotile. They are usually seen in symptomatic individuals
- **Cysts** may also be seen in stool microscopy, but often get missed due to their small size (3–6 μm)
- **Avacuolar and multi-vacuolar forms** (both measure 5–8 μm): Though they are the predominant form in vivo, are often missed in stool microscopy. Multi-vacuolar forms have multiple interconnected small vacuoles of different sizes. Avacuolar forms do not contain the central body
- **Ruling out other enteric parasites:** A minimum of three stool microscopy (including the permanent stained smear) and/or some of the immunoassays should be performed to ensure that no other protozoa are found before attributing symptoms to *Blastocystis*
- **Quantitation:** As the parasite load may correlate with clinical symptoms; *Blastocystis* should be quantitated as follows: few (≤2), moderate (3–9) and many (≥10) per 10 oil immersion field in permanent stained smear.

Antibody Detection

ELISA and IFA (Immunofluorescent assay) have been available for antibody detection in serum. Strong antibody response indicates the ability of the organism to cause symptoms.

Molecular Methods

PCR: Two methods are currently in use for screening of fecal samples by PCR.
- Subtype-specific primers targeting small subunit rDNA
- Genus-specific primers with subsequent sequencing for ST identification.

Real-time PCR: Quantitative real time PCR (TaqMan) has been developed for the detection of *Blastocystis* and is found to be more sensitive.

Treatment	*Blastocystis hominis*
☐ Metronidazole is found to be effective used alone or in combination with paromomycin or nitazoxanide. ☐ If failed with metronidazole treatment, then cotrimoxazole and nitazoxanide can be tried.	

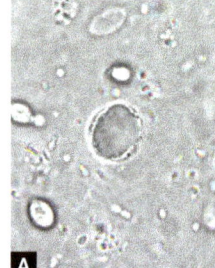 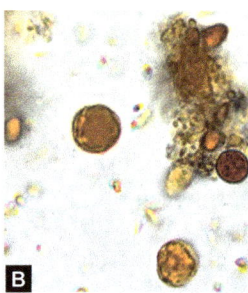 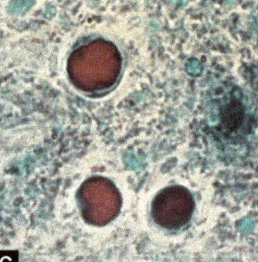 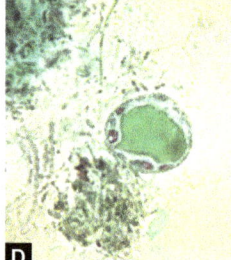 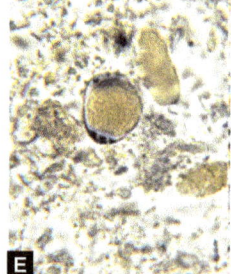

Figs 8.8A to E: *Blastocystis* species showing vacuolar forms: (A) Saline wet mount; (B) Iodine mount; (C and D) Trichome stain; (E) Iron hematoxylin stain

Source: A to C—DPDx Image Library, Centers for Disease Control and Prevention (CDC), Atlanta (*with permission*); D and E—Giovanni Swierczynski, Bruno Milanesi." Atlas of human intestinal protozoa Microscopic diagnosis" (*with permission*).

CHAPTER 8 ◆ Miscellaneous Protozoa

EXPECTED QUESTIONS

I. **Write short notes on:**
   a. Life cycle of Microsporidia.
   b. Infection caused by Microsporidia.
   c. Laboratory diagnosis of Microsporidia.
   d. Balantidiasis.
   e. *Blastocystis hominis.*

II. **Multiple choice questions (MCQs):**
   1. **Microsporidia spores are better stained by which of the following stain?**
      a. Albert stain
      b. H and E stain
      c. Modified trichrome stain (MTS)
      d. Iodine stain
   2. **Gold standard method for the diagnosis of Microsporidiosis:**
      a. Electron microscopy
      b. Modified trichrome stain (MTS)
      c. Direct antibody fluorescent test (DAF)
      d. ELISA
   3. **The main reservoir of *Balantidium coli*:**
      a. Cattle
      b. Man
      c. Sheep
      d. Pig
   4. **The largest protozoa parasitizing human intestine:**
      a. *Trichomonas hominis*
      b. *Balantidium coli*
      c. *Entamoeba coli*
      d. *Isospora*
   5. **Which of the following bears two nuclei named as macronucleus and micronucleus?**
      a. *Balantidium coli*
      b. *Dientamoeba fragilis*
      c. *Isospora*
      d. *Entamoeba coli*

Answer
1. c   2. a   3. d   4. b   5. a

SECTION 3

HELMINTHOLOGY

Section Outline

9. Introduction to Helminths *123*
10. Cestodes *125*
11. Trematodes or Flukes *152*
12. Nematodes—I (Intestinal Nematodes) *174*
13. Nematodes—II (Nematodes of Lower Animals that Rarely Infect Man) *198*
14. Nematodes—III (Somatic Nematodes) *209*

Introduction to Helminths

CHAPTER 9

CHAPTER OUTLINE
- General characteristics
- Morphology
- Life cycle

GENERAL CHARACTERISTICS

Helminths are elongated flat or round worm-like parasites measuring few milimeters to meters.
- They are eukaryotic multicellular and bilaterally symmetrical
- They belongs to two phyla (Table 9.1)
  - Phylum Platyhelminths (flat worms)—it includes three classes:
    1. Class: Cestoidea (tapeworms).
    2. Class: Trematodea (flukes or digeneans).
    3. Class: Monogenea (ectoparasite of fishes, do not infect man).
  - Phylum: Nemathelminths.

The classification of all the medically important helminths according to their habitat in man is depicted in Table 9.2.

MORPHOLOGY

In general, helminths exist in three morphological forms—(1) adult form (or the worm), (2) larval form and (3) eggs.

Adult Form

Phylum Platyhelminths
- Shape is tape like (in cestodes) or leaf like (in trematodes)
- They have a definite head end called as **suckers**
- They lack body cavity
- Alimentary canal is absent in cestodes but incomplete (rudimentary) in trematodes
- They are monoecious or hermaphrodite (i.e. both the sexes are present in the same worm), except in *Schistosoma* (diecious).

Table 9.1: Differences between cestodes, trematodes and nematodes

Properties	Cestodes	Trematodes	Nematodes
Shape	Tape-like and segmented	Leaf-like and unsegmented	Elongated, cylindrical and unsegmented
Head end	Suckers present, some have attached hooklets	Suckers present No hooklets	No sucker, no hooklets. Some have well developed buccal capsule
Alimentary canal	Absent	Present but incomplete	Complete from mouth to anus
Body cavity	Absent	Absent	Present
Sexes	Monoecious	Monoecious (except schistosomes)	Diecious
Life cycle	Requires two hosts (except *Hymenolepis* and *Diphyllobothrium*)	Requires three hosts (except *Schistosoma*)	Requires one host (except filarial worms and *Dracunculus*)
Larva forms	Cysticercus, hydatid cyst, coenurus, cysticercoid, coracidium, plerocercoid and procercoid	Cercaria, metacercaria, redia, miracidium and sporocyst	Rhabditiform larva, filariform larva and microfilaria

Table 9.2: Classification of helminths based on habitat

Cestodes	Trematodes	Nematodes
Intestinal cestodes • Diphyllobothrium species • Taenia solium and Taenia saginata causing intestinal taeniasis • Hymenolepis species • Dipylidium species	**Blood trematodes** • Schistosoma **Hepatic trematodes** • Fasciola hepatica • Clonorchis species • Opisthorchis species	**Intestinal nematodes** **Large intestine** • Trichuris trichiura • Enterobius vermicularis **Small intestine** • Ascaris lumbricoides • Ancylostoma duodenale • Necator americanus
Somatic/tissue cestodes • Taenia solium causing cysticercosis • Taenia multiceps • Echinococcus species • Spirometra species	**Intestinal trematodes** • Fasciolopsis buski • Heterophyes species • Metagonimus species • Watsonius species • Gastrodiscoides species **Lung trematodes** • Paragonimus westermani	**Tissue nematodes** • Filarial worm ➢ Wuchereria bancrofti ➢ Brugia malayi ➢ Loa loa ➢ Onchocerca species ➢ Mansonella species ➢ Trichinella spiralis ➢ Dracunculus medinensis

Phylum Nematoda

- They are evolutionary more developed than Platyhelminths
- They possess a definite body cavity (space between body wall and alimentary canal)
- Alimentary canal is complete, starting from mouth leading to esophagus, intestine and ending at anus
- They are diecious, i.e. male and female worms are separate
- The nervous system and excretory system are rudimentary and there is no circulatory system.

Larval Form

There are various larval forms of helminths found in man and other hosts (see Table 9.1).
- **In cestodes:** Cysticercus, hydatid cyst, coenurus, cysticercoid, coracidium, procercoid and plerocercoid forms
- **In trematodes:** Cercaria, metacercaria, redia, miracidium and sporocyst
- **In nematodes:** Rhabditiform larva, filariform larva and microfilaria.

Eggs

Based on their reproduction, helminths can be classified into the following:

- **Oviparous:** Most of the helminths (cestodes, trematodes and many nematodes) are oviparous, i.e. after fertilization, the adult worm lay eggs (e.g. all cestodes, trematodes and intestinal nematodes except *Strongyloides*)
- **Viviparous:** Some higher helminths do not have egg stage. After fertilization, they directly discharge larvae (e.g. tissue nematodes such as filarial worms, *Dracunculus* and *Trichinella*)
- **Ovoviviparous:** They lay egg containing larva, that immediately hatches out (e.g. *Strongyloides*).

- Various helminths have distinct morphology of eggs which can be used to differentiate the helminths **(Details have been discussed in the respective chapters).**

LIFE CYCLE

Life cycle of helminths gets completed in one or more hosts.
- Cestodes complete their life cycle in two hosts (definitive host and intermediate host) except **Hymenolepis** (requires only one host—man) and **Diphyllobothrium** requires three hosts (one definitive host— man, and two intermediate hosts—First, cyclops and second, fish)
- Most of the trematodes require three hosts (one definitive host—man, and two intermediate hosts—first snail and second aquatic plant or fish) except schistosomes (need two hosts, definitive host—man and intermediate host—snail)
- Nematodes complete their life cycle in one host (man) except filarial worms (need two hosts, definitive host—man and intermediate host—mosquito) and **Dracunculus** (need two hosts, definitive—host man and intermediate host—cyclops).

Pathogenesis, clinical manifestations, epidemiology, laboratory diagnosis and treatment of various helminths have been discussed in detail in the respective chapters.

EXPECTED QUESTIONS

I. **Write short notes on:**
   a. Various larval forms of helminths found in man.
   b. List out general properties of nematodes.

II. **Differentiate between:**
   a. Cestodes and trematodes.
   b. Trematodes and nematodes.

Cestodes

CHAPTER 10

CHAPTER OUTLINE

- Classification of cestodes
- Morphology of cestodes
- Pseudophyllidean cestodes
  - *Diphyllobothrium* species
- *Spirometra* species
- Cyclophyllidean cestodes
  - *Taenia* species
  - *Echinococcus* species
- *Hymenolepis nana*
- *Dipylidium caninum*

CLASSIFICATION OF CESTODES

Systemic Classification

Cestodes belong to Phylum Platyhelminths, Class Cestoidea, Subclass Eucestoda and two orders—Pseudophyllidea and Cyclophyllidea; each comprises of several genera (Table 10.1).

Classification Based on the Habitat

Based on habitat, cestodes are classified into:

1. **Intestinal cestodes:** Here, the adult worms inhabit in human Intestine. Examples include:
   - *Diphyllobothrium* species
   - *Taenia solium* and *Taenia saginata* causing intestinal taeniasis
   - *Hymenolepis* species
   - *Dipylidium* species.
2. **Somatic/tissue cestodes:** Here, the larvae forms are found in human muscles or organs. Examples include:
   - *Taenia solium* causing cysticercosis
   - *Taenia multiceps*
   - *Echinococcus* species—the agent of hydatid disease affecting liver
   - *Spirometra* species.

Table 10.1: Classification of medically important cestodes

Order	Family	Genus
Pseudophyllidea	Diphyllobothriidae	*Diphyllobothrium* *Spirometra*
Cyclophyllidea	Taeniidae	*Taenia* *Echinococcus*
	Hymenolepididae	*Hymenolepis*
	Dipylidiidae	*Dipylidium*

MORPHOLOGY OF CESTODES

In their life cycle, cestodes exist in three morphological forms: (1) adult worm, (2) egg, (3) larva.

Adult Worm

Adult worm is usually found in the intestine of men and animals (Fig. 10.1).

Shape

Cestodes are long, segmented, flattened dorsoventrally, tape like worms hence also called as tapeworms.

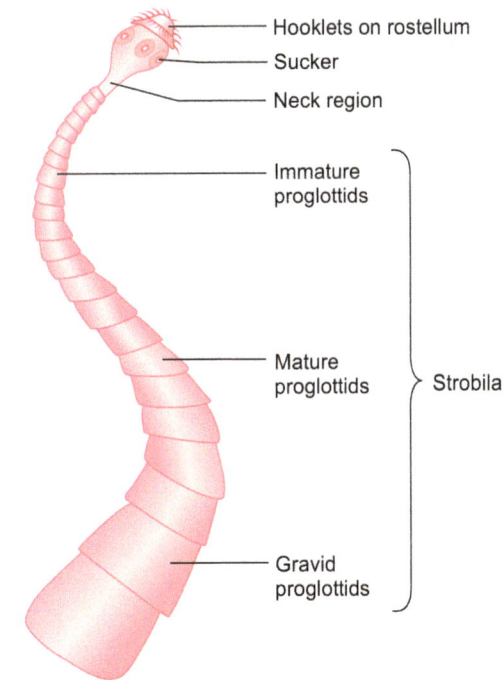

Fig. 10.1: Adult worm of cestode (schematic diagram).

Size

Cestodes vary from few milimeters to several meters. *Hymenolepis nana* is the smallest tapeworm (1–4 cm) where as *Diphyllobothrium* is the longest cestode measuring 10 meters or more.

Body Structure

Adult worm consists of three parts: (1) head or scolex, (2) neck, (3) strobila (body or trunk).

Head or scolex

Scolex is the organ of attachment.

- In cyclophyllidean cestodes, the scolex bear four cup like muscular suckers (or *acetabula*). In some species like *T. solium* and *H. nana*, scolex has a beak like apical protrusion called as **rostellum**, which may be armed with hooklets. (These species are called as **armed tapeworms**)
- In pseudophyllidean cestodes, the scolex does not possess suckers but it bears a pair of longitudinal groove called as **bothria** by which it attaches to small intestine.

Neck

Next to head, the portion is called as **neck** from which the segments (proglottids) arise.

Strobila

This is the body or trunk of the cestodes, which is surrounded by a body wall called as **tegument**.

- It consists of a number of segments (or proglottids). The length of the tapeworm varies based on the number of segments
- Proglottids bear the reproductive organs (both male and female); there are three types of proglottids—(1) immature, (2) mature and (3) gravid segments
  - **Immature segments:** Male and female reproductive organs are not differentiated
  - **Mature segments:** Contain male and female organs in the same segment, male organ appear first (Fig. 10.2)
  - **Gravid segments or fertilized segments:** Following fertilization, the uterus gets filled with eggs. Other organs are atrophied.

Female Reproductive Organs

They are present on the ventral side and consist of:

- **A bilobed ovary:** Present in the middle and posteriorly
- **Oviduct:** Arises from ovary, joins with spermatic duct and opens into the ootype
- **Ootype:** It is the chamber where fertilization takes place. There may be self-fertilization or cross fertilization between the segments
- **Vagina:** A tube that connects genital pore to the ootype through which the sperm enters. At its inner end, it contains seminal receptacle (for storage of sperm) and spermatic duct
- **Uterus:** Straight tube arises from the ootype where the eggs are stored after fertilization in the gravid segment. Its end may be opened (in pseudophyllideans) or closed as blind sac (in cyclophyllideans)
- **Vitelline gland (vitellaria)** and **Mehlis' gland** are present near the ootype. They occur as single mass (in cyclophyllideans) or scattered mass (in

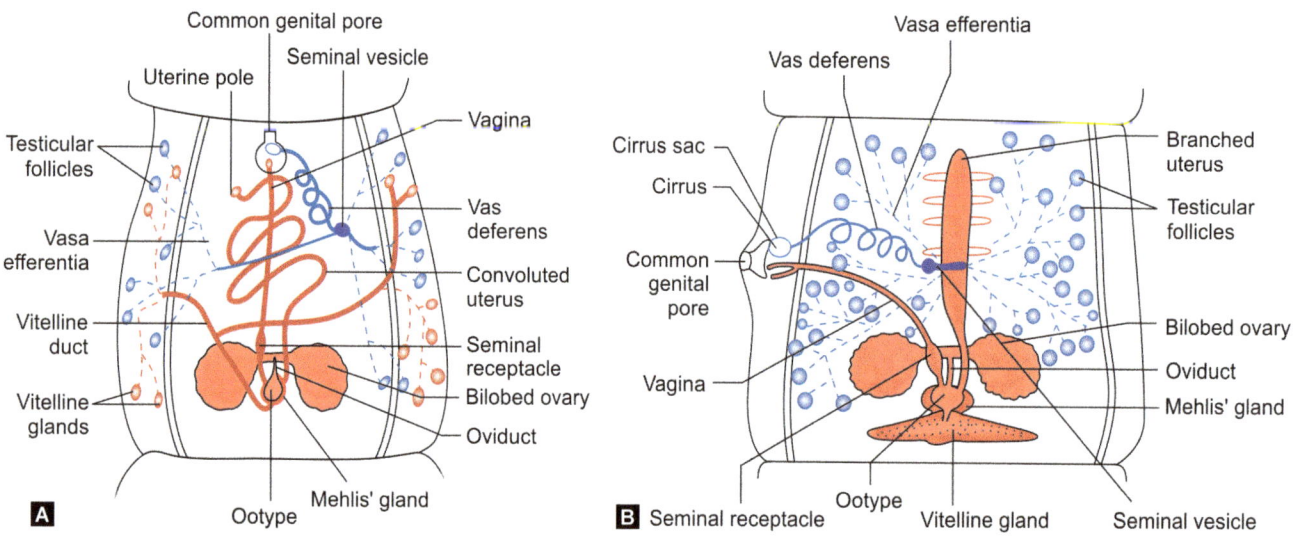

Figs 10.2A and B: Mature proglottids (schematic diagram) of: (A) Pseudophyllidean cestodes; (B) Cyclophyllidean cestodes

pseudophyllideans). They release their secretion through their ducts into the ootype.

Male Genital Organs

They are present on the dorsal side and consist of:
- **Testes:** They exist as multiple follicles (except in *Hymenolepis* which are three in number). Sperms are released to vasa efferentia which join together to form vas deferens
- **Vas deferens:** It is a convoluted tube, opens in the common genital pore. It bears a seminal vesicle and ends in the common genital pore as a swollen muscular and protrusible organ called as **cirrus** (equivalent of penis) surrounded by a **cirrus sac.**

Nervous System

It is rudimentary, consists of brain-like structure (central ganglion, lateral and rostellar ganglia connected by central nerve ring) present in the scolex from which the longitudinal nerve trucks arise and pass through all the segments and joined by transverse nerves in each segment.

Excretory System

It is also rudimentary and present in each segment. It consists of two lateral canals (dorsal and ventral) connected by transverse canals in each segment. The excretory canals are built up of **flame cells** (terminal cells) and **canal cells.**

Circulatory System

There is no circulatory system and no body cavity.

Body Wall (or Tegument)

It is made up of three layers—outer microvillus like structure called as **microthrix**, middle **basal plasma membrane** and inner **muscular layer** (outer circular and inner longitudinal muscle coats).

Eggs

Eggs are released into the uterus following fertilization and fill the gravid proglottids (Fig. 10.3).

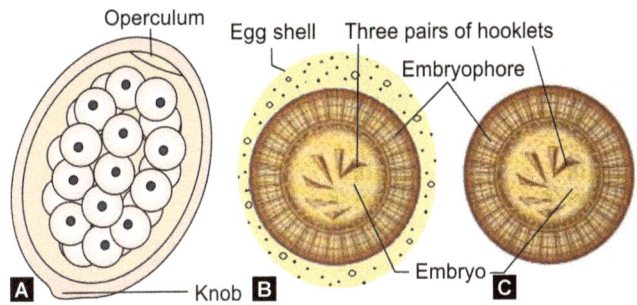

Figs 10.3A to C: Schematic diagram of eggs of cestodes: (A) Pseudophyllidean cestodes; (B) Cyclophyllidean cestodes; (C) Cyclophyllidean cestodes after the loss of egg shell

- **In pseudophyllidean cestodes:** Eggs are ovoid, operculated, surrounded by a single layer called as **egg shell** (or capsule), inside which the embryo is present containing hooklets (three pairs). Membrane lining the embryo is **ciliated**. The eggs when laid first in the feces, are not embryonated. Maturation takes place later in water (Fig. 10.3A)
- **In cyclophyllidean cestodes:** Eggs are round to oval, covered by two layers—an outer egg shell (or capsule) filled with yolk material (thin, so might be lost) and an inner thick radially striated embryophore surrounding the embryo. Eggs are embryonated from the beginning, contains six hooklets but the lining membrane is not ciliated (Figs 10.3B and C).

Larva

Embryonated eggs undergo further development to form larvae (Fig. 10.4).
- **Pseudophyllidean cestodes:** Larva is solid without any sac. They are:
  - **Coracidium:** First stage larva of *Diphyllobothrium*
  - **Procercoid:** Second stage larva of *Diphyllobothrium*
  - **Plerocercoid:** Third stage larva of *Diphyllobothrium*
  - **Sparganum:** Larval stage of *Spirometra*.
- **Cyclophyllidean cestodes:** Larvae contain bladder like sacs. They are:
  - **Cysticercus:** Larval stage of *Taenia*

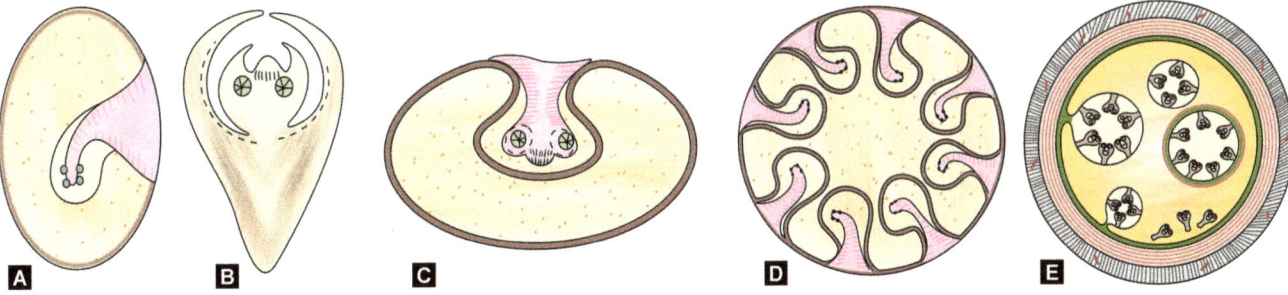

Figs 10.4A to E: Larvae of cyclophyllidean cestodes: (A) Cysticercus bovis; (B) Cysticercoid; (C) Cysticercus cellulosae; (D) Coenurus; (E) Hydatid cyst

Table 10.2: Differences between Pseudophyllidean cestodes and Cyclophyllidean cestodes

	Pseudophyllidean cestodes	Cyclophyllidean cestodes
Scolex	Bears two grooves (bothria)	Bears four suckers (Some species bear rostellum with hooklets)
Uterus	Convoluted (rosette-shaped), unbranched, opens at the uterine pole	Branched and closed as a blind sac, No uterine pole
Genital pore	Situated ventrally in the midline	Situated laterally
Vitelline gland	Scattered throughout the segment	Single mass behind ovary
Eggs	• Covered by one layer—egg shell • Freshly passed eggs in feces are unembryonated • Eggs are operculated and the embryo is ciliated	• Covered by two layer—egg shell and embryophore • Embryonated from the beginning • Eggs are not operculated and the embryo is not ciliated.
Larval form	Solid	Contains bladder like sac

- **Hydatid cyst:** Larval stage of *Echinococcus*
- **Coenurus:** Larval stage of *Multiceps*
- **Cysticercoid:** Larval stage of *Hymenolepis*.

LIFE CYCLE OF CESTODES

Cestodes complete their life cycle in two hosts (definitive host and intermediate host) except:
- *Hymenolepis* (requires only one host—man)
- *Diphyllobothrium* requires three hosts (one definitive host—man and two intermediate hosts—cyclops and fish).

Pathogenesis, clinical features, laboratory diagnosis and treatment of cestodes are discussed in detail later individually.

Differences between pseudophyllidean cestodes and cyclophyllidean cestodes have been discussed in the Table 10.2.

PSEUDOPHYLLIDEAN CESTODES

DIPHYLLOBOTHRIUM SPECIES

Diphyllobothrium latum, is the largest known parasite found in human intestine.
- It is also known as **fish tapeworm** or **human broad tapeworm** (proglottids are broader than longer, latum means broader)
- Its life cycle was described by Rosen in 1917
- Currently, there are 14 species of *Diphyllobothrium*. Human infection is caused by *D. latum* (most common); followed by *D. dendriticum, D. pacificum, D. nihonkaiense* and *D. ursi*.

Classification

D. latum belongs to the Order Pseudophyllidea and Family Diphyllobothriidae (Table 10.1).

Epidemiology

- Though *D. latum* infection occurs worldwide; high incidence has been reported from Northern Europe (Scandinavia countries such as Russia and Finland), North America (Canada and Alaska) and recently from South America (Chile)
- Other species: Infection with *D. dendriticum* is seen in Arctic, Australia and New Guinea; *D. pacificum* in Peru and Southern Pacific; *D. nihonkaiense* in Japan, Northern Pacific and emerging in Europe and *D. ursi* in Alaska and Canada
- **India:** *D. latum* is very rare in India. Three cases of diphyllobothriasis have been reported so far from Southern India (Vellore 1998 and Pondicherry 2007, Karimnagar 2011).

Habitat

The adult worm of *D. latum* resides in the small intestine [jejunum (mostly) and duodenum].

Morphology

Adult Worm

D. latum is the **longest tapeworm** infecting man, measuring up to 15 meters or more with over 3,000 proglottids. It consists of head, neck and body (strobila). The normal life span can be up to 25 years (Fig. 10.5).

Head or scolex

It is spoon-shaped, 3 × 1 mm, bears two longitudinal grooves called as **bothria** (one on ventral and other on dorsal surface) by which it attaches to the small intestine. There are no suckers and rostellum (Figs 10.6 A and B).

Neck

It is situated next to scolex and represents the growing end, from which the proglottids arise. It is unsegmented and longer than the head.

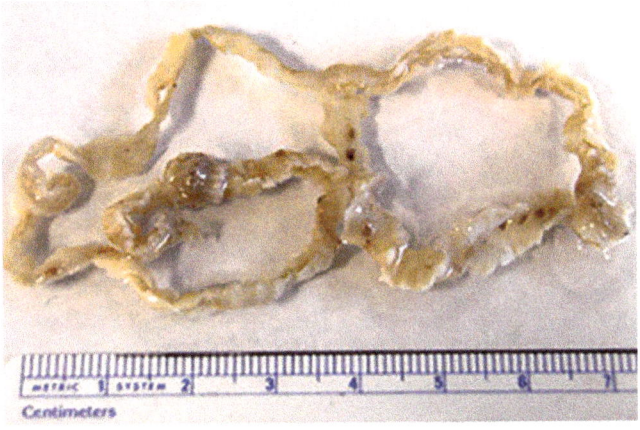

Fig. 10.5: Section of an adult *Diphyllobothrium latum* containing many proglottids (scale is in centimeters)
Source: DPDx Image Library, Centers for Disease Control and Prevention (CDC) Atlanta (*with permission*).

Strobila

- There are more than 3,000 segments divided into immature, mature and gravid segments (in that order starting from neck) (Fig. 10.6C)
- The mature segment is broader (10–20 mm) than longer (2–4 mm) and contains the male and the female reproductive organs. Female organs consist of bilobed ovary, coiled and rosette-shaped uterus, vitelline gland scattered throughout the segment and a vagina. Genital pore is situated midventrally. Male organs consist of testes (follicles), vas deferens and cirrus (Fig. 10.2A)
- **Gravid segment:** Uterus is filled with eggs which are discharged periodically through the uterine pole
- Some terminal gravid segments become shrunken and empty due to constant discharge of eggs and break off from the body and passed in the feces. (This is known as **pseudoapolysis**).

Eggs

- Fertilized eggs are oval, measuring 58–75 μm length and 40–50 μm width (Figs 10.3A and 10.8A and B)
- Eggs are operculated at one end and bear a knob at the other end
- When freshly passed in the feces, they are unembryonated, surrounded by egg shell
- Embryonated egg contains a hexacanth **oncosphere** lined by a ciliated membrane.

Larva

There are three larval stages:
1. First stage larva (coracidium).
2. Second stage larva (procercoid).
3. Third stage larva (plerocercoid).

Life Cycle (Fig. 10.7)

Host: Humans are the definitive host. Dogs, cats and foxes are the other rare definitive hosts. There are two intermediate hosts:
1. **First intermediate hosts:** Fresh or marine water copepods mainly of the genera *Cyclops* and *Diaptomus*.
2. **Second intermediate hosts:** Fresh or marine water fishes (pike, salmon, perch and trout).

Infective form: Third stage plerocercoid larvae
Mode of transmission: Humans get infection by ingestion of undercooked fresh water fish or marine fish containing third stage plerocercoid larva.

Development in Definitive Host (Intestine)

The plerocercoid larvae undergo further development to form adult worms which attach to the small intestine by the help of bothria. Adult worms become sexually mature in 4 weeks, fertilization takes place and they begin to lay eggs. Million of eggs are released every day (Fig. 10.7).

Development in Water

- **Embryonation and formation of L1 larva (coracidium):** Eggs are unembryonated when freshly passed in the feces, but become embryonated after 8–12 days in fresh or marine water at 16–20°C. This ciliated embryo is released through the operculum of the egg into water, which is known as the first stage larva (**coracidium**)
- **Development in first intermediate host (L_1 to L_2 transformation):** The coracidium swims in water and survives only for 12 hours within which it has to be ingested by small copepods (*Cyclops* and *Diaptomus*).

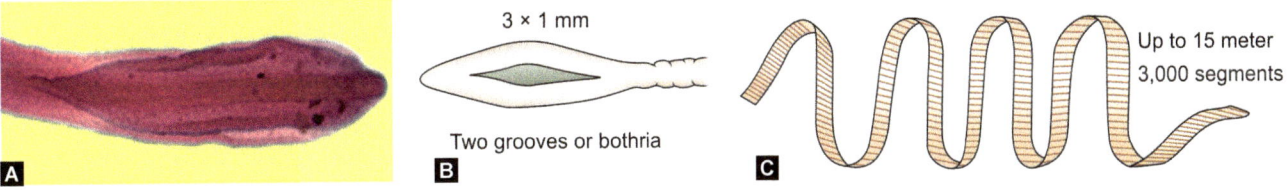

Figs 10.6 A to C: Adult worm of *Diphyllobothrium latum* (A) Scolex, carmine-stained; (B) Scolex (schematic); and (C) Strobila (schematic)
Source: A—DPDx Image Library, Centers for Disease Control and Prevention (CDC) Atlanta (*with permission*).

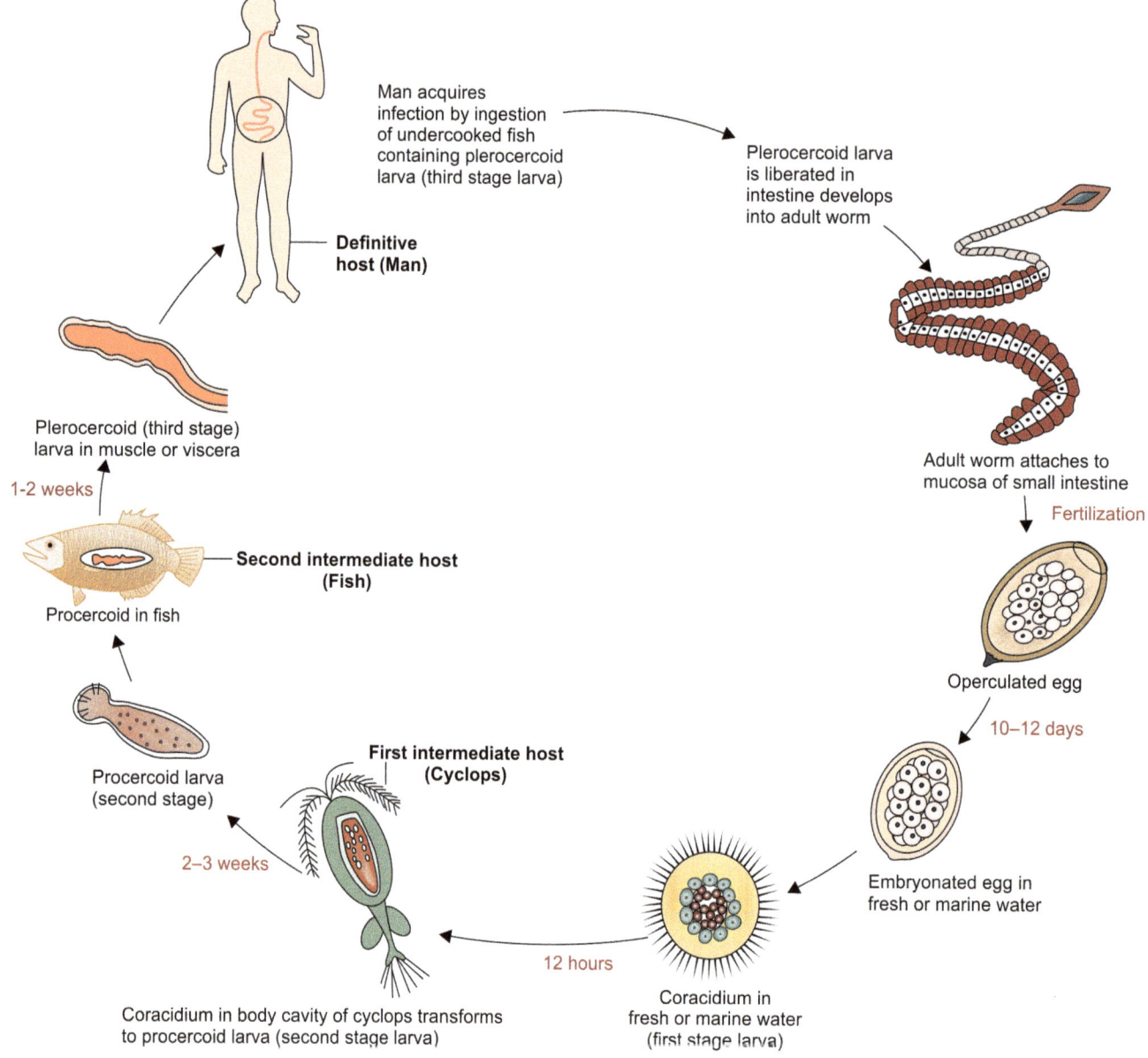

Fig. 10.7: Life cycle of *Diphyllobothrium latum*

It loses cilia and penetrates the intestine; enters the body cavity of copepods where it transforms within 2-3 weeks into 0.5 mm long, second stage **procercoid larva** (infective stage to the fresh or marine water fish)

❖ **Development in second intermediate host (L_2 to L_3 transformation):** The fresh or marine water fishes are infected by ingestion of copepods containing procercoid larva. The procercoid penetrates the intestine of fish; migrates to muscle, liver and fat of the fish where it transforms within 1-2 weeks into an elongated 10-20 mm × 2-3 mm size, L_3 stage **(plerocercoid larva)**. This stage is infective to man and the cycle is repeated

❖ **Paratenic host:** If small fishes are eaten by a big suitable fish, then the plerocercoid penetrates the intestine of the bigger fish and survives without further development. This type of host is called as **paratenic host** (A host in which the parasite survives without any development and is not essential for its life cycle).

Pathogenesis and Clinical Features

❖ Most of *D. latum* infections are asymptomatic
❖ Minor manifestations may include abdominal discomfort, diarrhea, vomiting, weakness and weight loss or rarely acute abdominal pain and intestinal

obstruction, **cholangitis** or **cholecystitis** (may be produced by migrating proglottids)

- **Vitamin B_{12} deficiency:** The adult worm causes dissociation of the vitamin B_{12}-intrinsic factor complex within the gut lumen, which leads to a decrease in absorption of B_{12} at ileum
  - Vitamin B_{12} deficiency leads to development of **megaloblastic anemia** and some people may exhibit neurologic sequelae like paresthesia
  - This effect has been noted only in Scandinavia (exclusively in Finland), where up to 2% of infected patients, especially the elderly, have megaloblastic anemia. This may be attributed to genetic predisposition of the individuals.

Laboratory Diagnosis

Stool Examination

The diagnosis is made readily by the detection of:
- Characteristic eggs in the stool—surrounded by egg shell and an operculum at one end and a knob at the other end (Figs 10.8A and B)
  - Eggs are bile-stained; do not float in saturated salt solution
  - Operculated eggs of *D. latum* should be differentiated from eggs of *Nanophyetus salmincola*, a trematode found in Pacific northwest region of US and in eastern Siberia (Fig. 10.8C) and from eggs of *Paragonimus westermanni* (see Fig. 11.16A) (Table 10.3)
- Proglottids may be discharged in the stool in some cases. The proglottids of *D. latum* has two characteristic features which help in identification (Fig. 10.8D):
  - They are are released in chain of segments of few cm to 0.5 meter long; not in single
  - They are wider than long (3 × 11 mm)
  - Possess rosette shaped uterus.
- Species identification is reliably done by PCR with sequencing.

Blood Examination

- Eosinophilia mild to moderate
- Evidence of megaloblastic anemia such as:
  - Increased mean corpuscular volume (MCV > 95 fl)
  - Increased mean corpuscular hemoglobin (MCH)
  - Normal mean corpuscular hemoglobin concentration (MCHC = 32–36 g/dL)
  - Macrocytes (enlarged RBCs) are present.

Treatment	*Diphyllobothrium latum*
❏ Praziquantel (5–10 mg/kg once) is highly effective (drug of choice) ❏ Niclosamide is given alternatively ❏ Parenteral vitamin B_{12} should be given if B_{12} deficiency is manifested.	

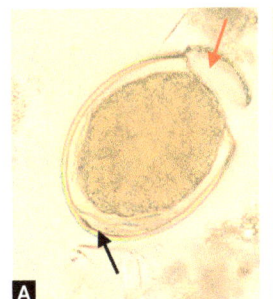 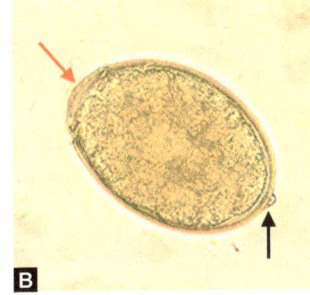 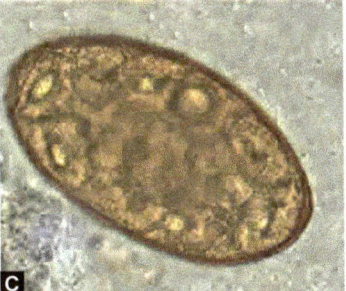 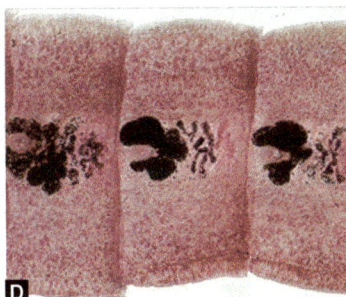

Figs 10.8A to D: (A and B) Egg of *Diphyllobothrium latum*—note the operculum (red arrow) and posterior knob (black arrow); (C) Egg of *Nanophyetus salmincola*; (D) Carmine-stained gravid proglottids of *Diphyllobothrium latum* (broader than longer, rosette-shaped ovaries)
Source: A to D—DPDx Image Library, Centers for Disease Control and Prevention (CDC), Atlanta (with permission).

Table: 10.3: Difference between eggs of *Diphyllobothrium latum, Nanophyetus salmincola* and *Paragonimus westermani*

	Diphyllobothrium latum	*Nanophyetus salmincola*	*Paragonimus westermani*
Shape	Oval and operculated	Broadly oval, operculated	Broadly oval, operculated
Size	58–75 × 40–50 μm	64–97 × 34–55 μm	80–120 × 45–65 μm
Opercular end	Opercular shoulder absent	Opercular shoulder absent	Opercular shoulder present
Abopercular end	Knob	No knob Thickened and darkened area	No knob Thickened and darkened area

Prevention

Preventive measures include thorough cooking of fish or freezing. *D. latum* infection has been called the **Jewish housewives' disease**, since they acquire infection by tasting the uncooked fish while preparing.
- Proper cooking of fish (5 minutes at 55°C)
- Deep freezing (–20°C for 7 days, or –35°C for 15 hours) of fish should be followed for people who eat raw fish.

SPIROMETRA SPECIES

Spirometra and *Diphyllobothrium* species other than *D. latum* and few other species (that are not normal human parasites) can accidentally infect man and cause a disease called as **sparganosis.**
- Disease is so named because; it is caused by the plerocercoid larva (L_3 stage) of these parasites which is called as **sparganum**
- Genus *Spirometra* belongs to Diphyllobothriidae family. Medically important members are *S. mansoni, S. mansonoides, S. erinacei, S. ranarum* and *S. proliferum.*

Life Cycle and Pathogenesis

Host: Its life cycle is similar to *D. latum*. Only hosts are different:
- **Definitive hosts:** Dogs and cats
- **First intermediate host:** Cyclops
- **Second intermediate host:** Frogs, snakes and birds.

Infective form: Plerocercoid larva (L_3 stage) called as sparganum.

Mode of transmission: Man acts as an accidental host and gets infected by:
- Ingestion of undercooked reptiles and birds containing plerocercoid larva L_3 (sparganum). Here, man acts as definitive host
- Or ingestion of cyclops containing procercoid larva (L_2) which gets transformed into sparganum in human intestine. Here, man acts as second intermediate host
- Or by local application of raw infected flesh of any 2nd intermediate host as poultice containing sparganum. Here, man acts as definitive host.

Sparganosis

Disease caused by sparganum larva is called as **sparganosis**.
- The sparganum (L_3 larva) penetrates the intestinal wall and migrates to subcutaneous tissues, muscles, eyes and visceral organs like brain (frontal and parietal lobes) and lymphatics
- Here, the sparganum gets encysted to form painful fibrous nodules measuring 2 cm associated with pruritus and urticaria
- Ocular sparganosis is a serious manifestation and presented as painful edematous swelling of the eyelids (usually upper lids) with lacrimation and pruritus
- Lymphatic involvement can lead to elephantiasis
- **Aberrant sparganosis:** Caused by *Spirometra proliferum*. It is a rare tapeworm larva that grows by budding and continuous branching. The spargana are recovered from subcutaneous tissue, muscle, intestinal wall, etc. The normal tissue organization is lost. The adult form of this parasite is not known. It is reported from Japan, USA and Venezuela. It is fatal in all reported cases.

Epidemiology

Human sparganosis is rare. Cases have been reported from Ethiopia, South Sudan, China, Japan and Southeast Asia like Thailand and less often from America and Australia. *S. mansoni* is the predominant species in Asia whereas *S. mansonoides* is common in USA.

In India, sparganosis is extremely rare. A case of cerebral sparganosis was reported from Hyderabad in 2003 and a case of sparganosis of kidney was reported from UP in 2011.

Laboratory Diagnosis

Diagnosis of sparganosis is made by surgical removal of the nodules and demonstration of the elongated worm like sparganum larva.
- The sparganum is motile, elongated, white and opaque measuring 20–30 cm long × 3 cm width, resembles narrow tapeworm proglottids (Fig. 10.9)
- It can be distinguished from other bladder like larval forms of tissue cestodes by absence of suckers and hooklets.

Treatment	*Spirometra*
▢ Definite treatment is the surgical removal of the nodule ▢ Drugs are not effective, however, praziquantel or triclabendazole is recommended.	

Prevention

Human sparganosis can be prevented by filtering and boiling of drinking water, and eating the properly cooked fish.

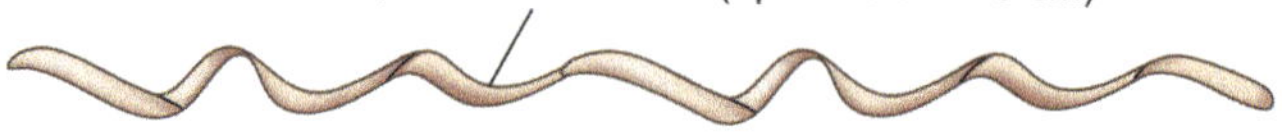

White ribbon-like, motile structures (up to 30 cm × 3 cm)

Fig. 10.9: Morphology of sparganum larva

CYCLOPHYLLIDEAN CESTODES

TAENIA SPECIES

Taenia species cause two types of manifestations in humans—**intestinal taeniasis** and **cysticercosis**.

Classification

Taenia belongs to the order Cyclophyllidea, family Taeniidae (see Table 10.1). Several species are known to infect man (Table 10.4). Two important members are:
* *T. saginata* (also called as **beef tapeworm**): It causes **intestinal taeniasis** in man
* *T. solium* (also called as **pork tapeworm**): It causes both **intestinal taeniasis** and **cysticercosis** in man.

History

Cysticercosis is an ancient disease, has also been described in ancient Indian medical book, the Charaka Samhita.
* It was first described in pigs by Aristophanes and Aristotle in third century BC, latter it was noticed in humans by Parunoli in 1550
* Neurocysticercosis was first reported in a coolie from Madras, died due to seizure (Armstrong 1888)
* In 1912, Krishnaswamy was the first to report the cases of muscle pains and subcutaneous nodules with abundant cysticerci in muscles, heart and brain through autopsy.

Habitat

The adult worms of *T. saginata* and *T. solium* reside in the small intestine (jejunum and ileum) of humans, where as the larva of *T. solium* (cysticercus cellulosae) reside and form cystic lesions in the muscle, brain and eyes.

Table 10.4: Taenia species infecting humans

Taenia species	Definitive host	Intermediate host	Organ affected	Disease
T. saginata	Man	Cattle	Intestine	Intestinal taeniasis
T. solium	Man	Pig	Intestine	Intestinal taeniasis
T. solium	Man	Man	Muscle, CNS and eye	Cysticercosis
T. asiatica	Man	Pig	Liver	Intestinal taeniasis
T. multiceps	Dog	Sheep and rarely man	CNS	Coenurosis

Abbreviation: CNS, central nervous system.

Morphology

It exists in three forms—(1) adult worm, (2) egg and (3) larva.

Adult Worm

The adult worm consists of head (scolex), neck and strobila (body) (Figs 10.1 and 10.10C).
* The description of the adult worm is similar to any cyclophyllidean cestodes (given in detail earlier)
* The important features of *T. saginata* and *T. solium* are slightly different to each other and are given in Table 10.5 and Figures 10.10 and 10.11.

Head or scolex

The scolex bears four cup like muscular suckers (or acetabula) which helps in attachment (Figs 10.10 A and B).

In *T. solium*, the scolex has a beak like apical protrusion called as **rostellum**. The rostellum is armed with two rows of hooklets (hence called as **armed tapeworm**).

Neck

Situated next to the head. It is the narrow growing region from which the proglottids arise. Neck is longer in *T. saginata*.

Strobila

Strobila is the trunk or body, consists of many segments (or proglottids). Segments are of three types—(1) immature, (2) mature and (3) gravid.
* Immature segments are wider than longer, mature segments appear square and gravid segments are longer than wider
* The mature segment contains the male and the female reproductive organs (Fig. 10.11)
    * Female organs consist of ovary, branched and closed uterus, ootype, single mass of vitelline gland and laterally situated genital pore
    * Male organs consist of testes (follicles), vas deferens and cirrus (Fig. 10.2B).

Eggs

Following fertilization eggs are released into the uterus and fill the gravid proglottids.
* *Taenia* eggs are round, 31–43 μm size, covered by two layers (Figs 10.12A and B)
* An outer egg shell (or capsule) filled with yolk material (thin, so might be lost) and an inner embryophore (brown, thick walled and radially striated) surrounding the embryo
* The embryo or oncosphere contains three pair of hooklets

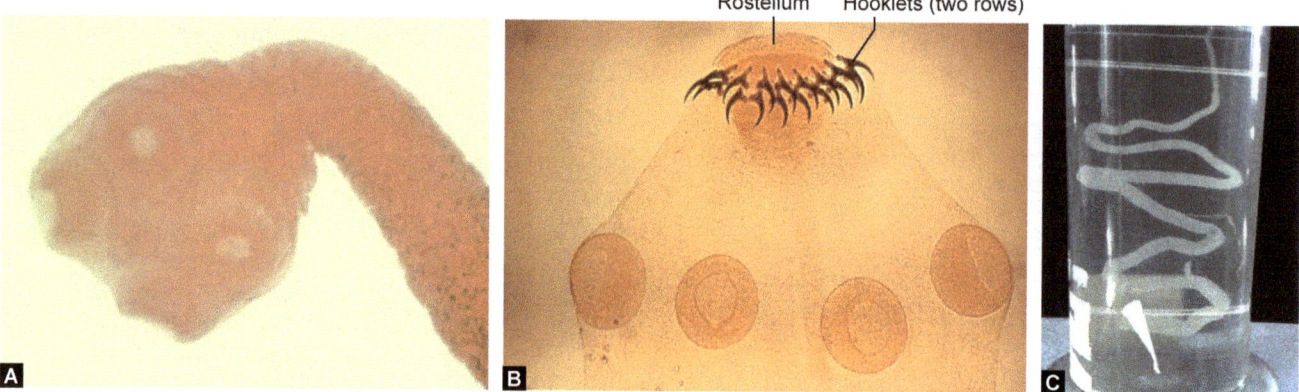

Figs 10.10A to C: (A) Carmine-stained scolex of *T. saginata*; (B) Carmine-stained scolex of *T. solium*; (C) Adult worm of *Taenia* species

Source: A—DPDx Image Library, Centers for Disease Control and Prevention (CDC), Atlanta (*with permission*); B—Public Health Image Library, ID#: 5262, Centers for Disease Control and Prevention (CDC), Atlanta (*with permission*); C—Head of Department, Microbiology, Meenakshi Medical College, Chennai (*with permission*).

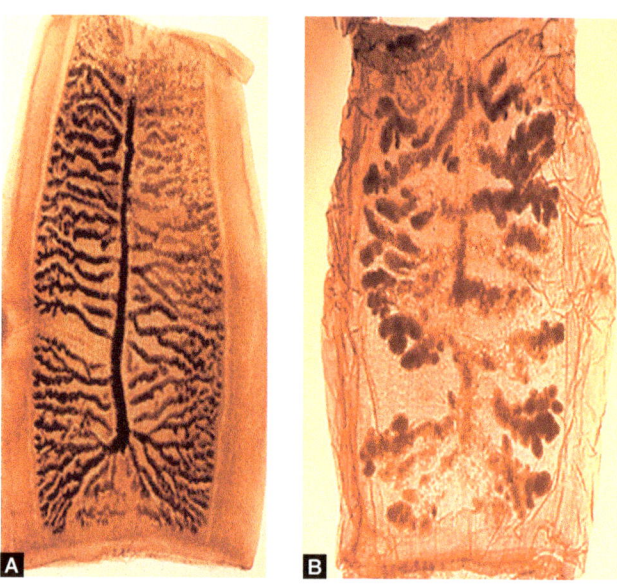

Figs 10.11A and B: Carmine-stained mature proglottids of (A) *T. saginata*; (B) *T. solium*

Source: A—ID#: 5259; B—ID#: 5261: Public Health Image Library, Centers for Disease Control and Prevention (CDC), Atlanta (*with permission*).

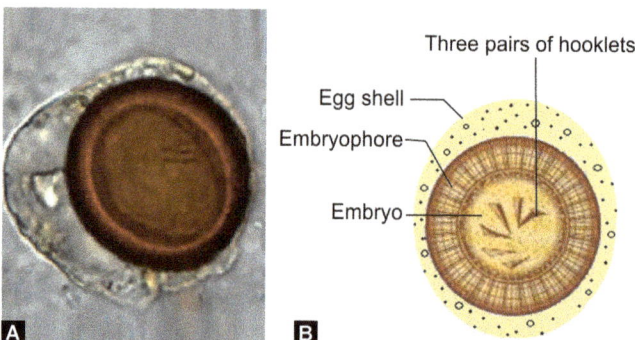

Figs 10.12A and B: Egg of *Taenia* species: (A) In saline mount; (B) Schematic diagram

Source: A—DPDx Image Library, Centers for Disease Control and Prevention (CDC), Atlanta (*with permission*).

- Eggs of *T. saginata* and *T. solium* are indistinguishable from each other (except, *T. saginata* eggs are acid fast), and are infective to cattle and pigs respectively
- Eggs of *T. solium* are also infective to man (to cause cysticercosis).

Larva

Cysticercus is the larval stage of *Taenia*. It contains a muscular organ with bladder like sac. It is called as:
- Cysticercus cellulosae in *T. solium*
- Cysticercus bovis in *T. saginata*.

Larval stage of *T. saginata* and *T. solium* is infective to man (to cause intestinal taeniasis).

Life Cycle of Taenia saginata (Fig. 10.13)

Host: Man acts as the **definitive** and cattle serve as the **intermediate host.**

Infective stage: Cysticercus bovis (larval stage) is the infective stage to man, while eggs are infective to cattle.

The Human Cycle

Mode of transmission: Man acquires the infection by ingestion of undercooked beef containing encysted larval stage (cysticercus bovis).

Larva transforms to adult: The larva hatch out in small intestine, the scolices exvaginate and anchor to the intestinal wall by suckers and gradually develop into the adult worms.

- Adult worms become sexually mature in 10–14 weeks, fertilization occurs (self or cross fertilization within the segments) and eggs are formed and later released in the feces. Eggs are infective to cattle

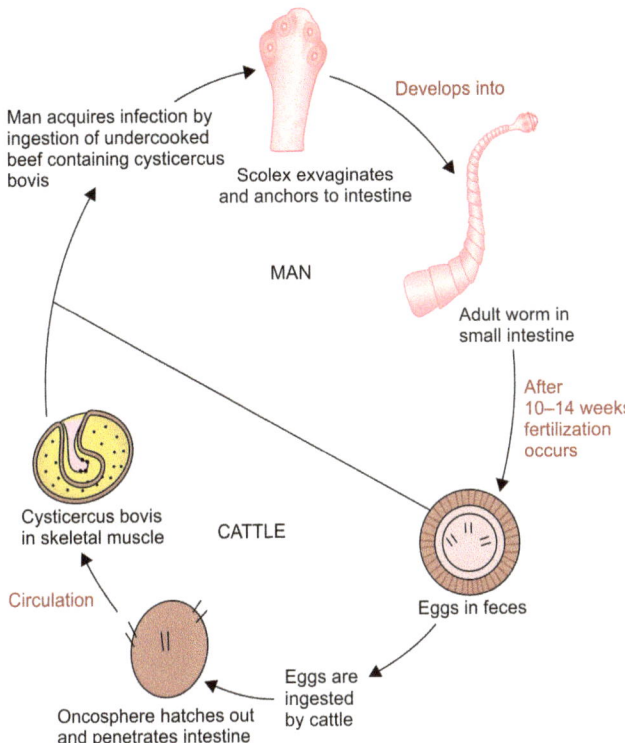

Fig. 10.13: Life cycle of *Taenia saginata*

❖ Sometime, the older gravid segments break off and are released in the feces. They are quite mobile and migrate in the feces.

The Cattle Cycle

Mode of transmission: Eggs are ingested by cows and buffaloes while grazing the field.

Eggs transform to larvae: In the duodenum, the embryophore surrounding the egg ruptures, releasing the oncosphere. With the help of hooklets, the oncospheres penetrate the intestine, and reach the skeletal muscle via blood where they transform into bladder like larvae (cysticercus bovis) which get encysted and deposited as cysts. This takes around 70 days of time.

Cysticercus bovis: Small 7.5–10 mm wide and 4–6 mm long, round, grayish white bladder like worm containing opaque invaginated scolex without hooklets (Fig. 10.4A).

Life Cycle of Taenia solium (Fig. 10.14)

Life cycle of *T. solium* depends on the disease it causes.

When it causes intestinal taeniasis, the life cycle is exactly similar to that of *T. saginata* except:
❖ The intermediate host is pig (hence called as pork tapeworm)
❖ Men harboring the adult worm excrete the eggs in feces which can infect the same individual by autoinfection

❖ In pigs, the development time is shorter (7–9 weeks). But when it causes cysticercosis, the life cycle is different and given as below:
❖ **Host:** Man acts as both **definitive** and **intermediate host**
❖ **Infective stage:** Eggs of *T. solium*
❖ **Mode of transmission:** Firstly man acquires the infection by—(1) ingestion of contaminated food or water containing eggs of *T. solium* and (2) autoinfection (described below)

> **Autoinfection:** Eggs excreted in the feces reinfect the same individual. Autoinfection can be of two types:
> 1. **External autoinfection:** Due to unhygienic personal habit, e.g. contaminated finger
> 2. **Internal autoinfection:** Due to reverse peristaltic movements by which the gravid segments throw the eggs back into the stomach (equivalent to swallowing of the eggs).

❖ **Further life cycle in man is similar to that in pigs:** Oncosphere is released from the eggs, penetrates the intestine and enters into the portal circulation or mesenteric lymphatics and reaches to various organs like subcutaneous tissue, muscle, eye and brain where it is transformed to the larval stage; cysticercus cellulosae in 7–9 weeks and deposited as cyst. Full development to mature cysts takes 2–3 months of time.

Cysticercus Cellulosae

A mature cysticercus cellulosae measures 5 mm long and 8–10 mm wide, spherical (or slightly oval), yellowish-white, separated from the host tissue by a thin collagenous capsule (Fig. 10.15).

❖ **It contains two chambers:** Outer one is a bladder like sac filled with 0.5 mL of vesicular fluid (may go up to 60 mL in brain) and the inner chamber contains the growing scolex with hooklets and a spiral canal (Fig. 10.4C).
❖ **Racemose cysticerci:** In some cases, when the parasites are lodged in spacious area, they grow and transform into larger lobulated cysticerci (>20 cm), containing 60 mL of vesicular fluid
  - They do not contain scolices within the bladder, resemble metastatic tumor
  - Mainly found in brain (fourth ventricle and subarachnoid space), and cervical spinal cord
  - It is associated more frequently with HIV infected patient
  - Patients present with increased intracranial pressure and frequently require surgery
  - The prognosis of racemose cysticerci is poor.

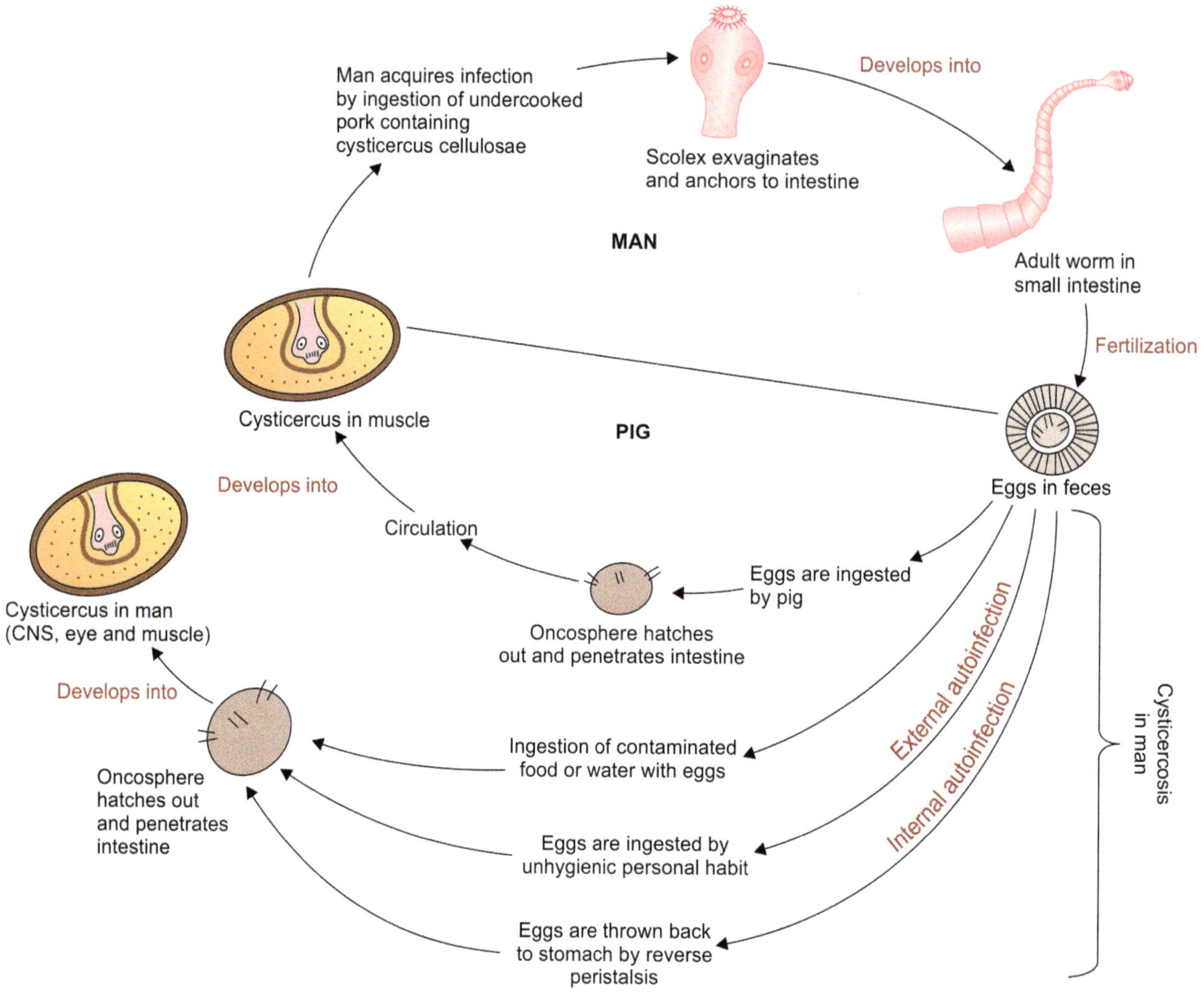

Fig. 10.14: Life cycle of *Taenia solium*

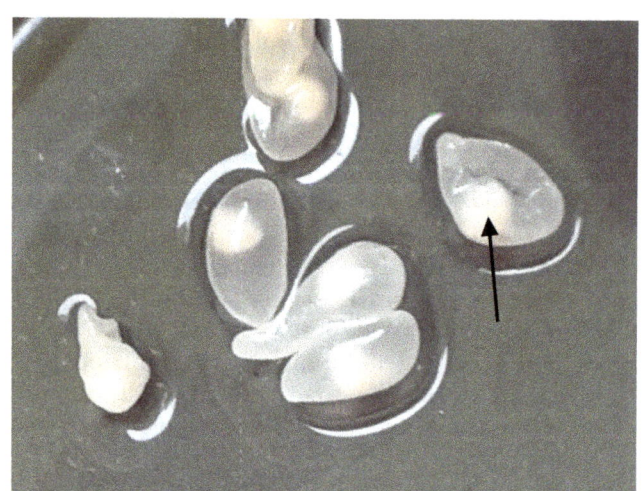

Fig. 10.15: Cysticercus cellulosae (surgically removed)
Source: Head of department, Microbiology, Meenakshi Medical College, Chennai (*with permission*).

Pathogenesis and Clinical Features

Intestinal Taeniasis

Both *T. saginata* and *T. solium* can cause intestinal taeniasis.
* Often, it is asymptomatic; patients become aware of the infection most commonly by noting the passage of proglottids in their feces
* The proglottids are often motile, and patients may experience perianal discomfort (or pruritus) when proglottids are discharged
* Mild abdominal pain or discomfort, nausea, loss of appetite, weakness, weight loss, headache and change in bowel habit (constipation or diarrhea) can occur
* Occasionally obstruction by the migrating proglottids can result in appendicitis or cholangitis.

Cysticercosis

Clinical spectra of the disease depend upon the localization of the cyst. Though it is discovered from any site of the body but the common sites are central nervous system (CNS), subcutaneous tissue, skeletal muscle and eyes.

- **Subcutaneous cysticercosis:** It is frequently asymptomatic but may manifest as palpable nodules
- **Muscular cysticercosis:** Manifest as muscular pain, weakness or pseudohypertrophy
- **Ocular cysticercosis:** Can involve eyelids, conjunctiva and sclera. Common symptoms like proptosis, diplopia, loss of vision and slow growing nodule with focal inflammation
- Neurocysticercosis (see the highlight box below).

Neurocysticercosis

Neurocysticercosis (NCC) is the most common form and accounts for 60–90% cases of cysticercosis

- NCC is considered as the most common parasitic CNS infection of man and the most common cause of adult onset epilepsy throughout the world
- Age: Adults of 30–50 years age are affected commonly
- Based on the site of involvement, NCC is of two types:
  1. **Parenchymal:** Involves brain parenchyma; considered as the most common site of NCC
  2. **Extraparenchymal** sites are meninges, ventricles, spinal cord and subarachnoid space.
- **Asymptomatic neurocysticerosis (NCC):** Sometimes NCC remains in the brain without causing any apparent symptoms
- **Manifestations:** Seizure is the most common manifestation (70% of cases). NCC accounts for 50% cases of late onset epilepsy
- **Other features include:**
  - Hydrocephalus: It is the most common extra parenchymal feature. Its presence carries bad prognosis.
  - Increased intracranial pressure and hypertension- presented as headache, vomiting and vertigo
  - Chronic meningitis
  - Focal neurological deficits
  - Psychological disorders and dementia
  - Cerebral arteritis (associated with subarachnoid cysticercosis)
  - Basal and vetricular involvement: Carries poor prognosis.
- **NCC exists in four morphological stages:** It starts as vesicular form, gradually develops into necrotic, followed by nodular and finally into calcified stage
- The clinical presentation is variable and depends on number, location and size of the cyst, the morphological stage of the cyst and the host immune response.
- **NCC and HIV:** NCC coinfection is likely to be increasingly recognized in patients with HIV and should be included in the differential diagnosis of CNS infections in these patients.

Epidemiology

Taenia saginata Infection

The *T. saginata* infection is common in cattle breeding areas of the world. The areas with the highest prevalence (up to 27%) include Central Asia, Central and East Africa.

Taenia solium Infection

World

Cysticercosis is a major public health problem, especially in the developing world.

- *T. solium* infection is endemic includes Mexico, Central America, South America, Africa, Southeast Asia, India, Philippines, and Southern Europe
- NCC is the most frequent preventable cause of epilepsy worldwide. According to WHO, 30% of all epilepsy cases in endemic countries and 3% epileptic cases globally may be due to NCC
- However, it is reported less from the Muslim countries (as pork eating is not allowed).

India

- NCC is largely underreported in India, accounting for 2–3% of epileptic cases. Reports of NCC has come from places such as NIMHANS, Bengaluru (2%) and Delhi (2.5%). The underreporting is because of lack of systematic population-based studies and unavailability of imaging techniques
- Cysticercosis is highly prevalent in the northern states such as Bihar, Odisha, Uttar Pradesh and Punjab.

Laboratory Diagnosis

Intestinal taeniasis

Stool examination

Wet mount examination of stool is carried out to demonstrate the characteristic eggs and less often proglottids of *Taenia* species.

- Multiple stool examination and concentration techniques (formol-ether sedimentation) can be followed to increase the detection rate
- Anal swabs (cellophane swabs used for *Enterobius*) can be used to collect fecal matter and is superior for detection of eggs than stool
- **Eggs** of *T. saginata* and *T. solium* are morphologically similar except that eggs of *T. saginata* are acid fast
  - Egg is round 31–43 μm size and consists of an oncosphere with six hooklets surrounded by an embryophore
  - Eggs are bile-stained; do not float in saturated salt solution.
- **Proglottids** of *T. saginata* and *T. solium* can be differentiated by lateral branches in uterus, accessory lobe in ovary, vaginal sphincter and expulsion of segments (singly or in chain) (Table 10.5). This can be detected by India ink injection gently into the lateral genital pore of proglottids
- **Scolex** can be detected in feces very rarely. *T. solium* scolex is armed with rostellum and hooklets.

Table 10.5: Differences between *Taenia saginata* and *Taenia solium*

Features	Taenia saginata	Taenia solium
Adult worm		
Length	4–6 meters or more	2–4 meters
Head/scolex	• Large and quadrangular • Four suckers present which may be pigmented • No rostellum, No hooklets	• Small and globular • Four suckers present—not pigmented • Bears rostellum with two rows of 25–30 hooklets • Hence called as armed tapeworm
Neck	Longer	Shorter
Proglottids (Fig. 10.11)		
No. of proglottids	1,000–2,000	800–1,000
Uterus	Bears in 15–20 lateral branches*	Bears in 7–13 lateral branches*
Lobes of ovary	Two, no accessory lobe	Three–two lobes with an accessory lobe
Testes	300–400 follicles	150–200 follicles
Vaginal sphincter	Present	Absent
Measurement	Gravid segment—20 mm × 5 mm	Gravid segment—12 mm × 6 mm
Expulsion of segments	Expelled singly in the feces	Expelled in chain of 5–6 segments
Eggs per segment	80,000 eggs per gravid segment	40,000 eggs per gravid segment
Larva	Cysticercus bovis present in cattle's muscle, but not in man	Cysticercus cellulosae present in pig's muscle and also in man (muscle, eye and brain)
Egg	Acid fast, 31–43 μm size	Non-acid fast, 31–43 μm size
Life cycle		
Disease	Causes intestinal taeniasis	Causes intestinal taeniasis and cysticercosis
Host	Definitive host: Man Intermediate host: Cattle	• For intestinal taeniasis—definitive host is man and intermediate host is pig • For cysticercosis—man acts as both definitive and intermediate hosts
Infective form	Larva (cysticercus bovis)	• For intestinal taeniasis—larva (cysticercus cellulosae) • For cysticercosis—egg
Diagnostic form	Egg	• For intestinal taeniasis—egg • For cysticercosis—larva (cysticercus cellulosae deposited in tissue)
Mode of transmission	Ingestion of contaminated beef	• For intestinal taeniasis—ingestion of contaminated pork • For cysticercosis—(i) contaminated food and water and (ii) auto-infection

Contd...

*Note: The lateral branches at the point of origin from one side of the uterus should be counted (Fig.10.11).

Taenia specific antigen detection in stool

ELISA has been developed to detect *Taenia* specific antigen (coproantigen) in stool by using polyclonal *Taenia* antibodies.

❖ **Advantages:** This test has many utilities:
  ▪ Claims more sensitive than stool examination
  ▪ Can detect *Taenia* carriers; is useful for the control of this zoonotic infection
  ▪ Prognosis: It can be used for treatment follow up; becomes negative after 30 days of effective treatment.
❖ **Disadvantage:** It cannot differentiate between *T. saginata* and *T. solium*.

Molecular methods

PCR targeting mitochondrial DNA followed by sequencing is available; which can distinguish between four distinct *Taenia* species: *T. saginata, T. asiatica*, and two genotypes of *T. solium* (one found in Asia and other in Africa and Latin America).

Laboratory Diagnosis — Cysticercosis

- **Radiodiagnosis**—CT scan and MRI (useful for detecting number, location, size of the cysticerci and the stage of the disease)
- **Antibody detection** in serum or CSF—
  ➢ ELISA (using crude extract of cysticerci)
  ➢ Western blot (using 13 kDa LLGP Ag)
- **Antigen detection** in serum or CSF—ELISA
- Lymphocyte transformation test
- **Histopathology** of muscles, eyes, subcutaneous tissues or brain biopsies—can detect cysticerci
- **FNAC** of the cyst and then staining with Giemsa
- **Fundoscopy** of eye—detects larvae
- Modified Del Brutto diagnostic criteria.

Cysticercosis

Radiodiagnosis (imaging methods)

CT scan and MRI are the two important imaging methods used to detect cysticerci in brain.

❖ Because of the vesicular structure, live cysticerci appear hypodense (low signal intensity) area and the scolex is present eccentric inside the vesicle and gives a hyperdense (high signal intensity) area

- ❖ Imaging methods are useful to identify:
  - The number of cyst (single or multiple cysticerci)
  - Location of the cyst (parenchymal or extraparenchymal)
  - Size of the cyst (small—cysticercus cellulosae and big cyst—cysticercus racemosus)
  - The stage of the disease (vesicular, necrotic, nodular and calcified)
  - Extent of the lesion
  - Active or dormant lesion: Associated inflammation and edema gives a ring like enhancement surrounding the cysts, indicates acute infection.
- ❖ CT scan is useful to detect calcified cysts (appears as hyperdense dots) (Fig. 10.16)
- ❖ MRI has a higher contrast resolution, which makes lesion clearer. It is superior than CT scan to detect the:
  - Extraparenchymal cysts in ventricle and cisterns
  - Inflammatory changes
  - Vesicular and necrotic lesions
  - Noncystic lesions.

Immunodiagnosis

It has the advantage of lower cost than CT and MRI and confirms the etiology.

1. Antibody detection

ELISA: ELISA detects antibodies in serum and CSF by using crude extract of cysticerci or vesicular fluid.
- ❖ It is highly sensitive (75–90%) in serum. CSF ELISA also gives better results

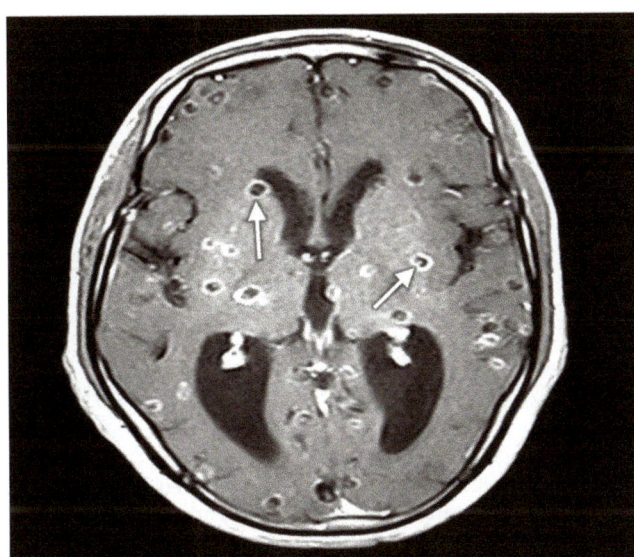

Fig. 10.16: CT scan of brain showing multiple ring enhancing lesions with eccentric scolex (neurocysticercosis)
Source: Dr A Subathra, Department of Radiodiagnosis, JIPMER, Puducherry (*with permission*).

- ❖ Moreover, recent ELISA method using purified glycoprotein antigens has shown better sensitivity but its specificity is low as it gives false positive results in cross reacting helminthic infections such as echinococcosis
- ❖ **QuickELISA:** It is a quantitative ELISA, available commercially. It detects antibodies in serum against T24H recombinant antigen. Results are comparable to western blot, has a sensitivity of 96% and specificity 99%.

Western blot: Western blot assay [also called as enzyme immune transfer blot (EITB)] uses highly specific 50-13 kDa lentil lectin-purified seven glycoprotein (LLGP) antigenic fractions; hence its specificity approaches 100%.
- ❖ Presence of one to seven Gp bands confirms the diagnosis
- ❖ It can be performed on serum, blood, dried blood spot or CSF
- ❖ The sensitivity and specificity are 98% and 100% respectively in persons with multiple viable cyst
- ❖ The sensitivity is directly proportional to the number of live cysticerci.

However, antibody detection methods have disadvantages—(1) Cannot differentiate active and past infection, (2) Antibodies persist even after recovery of the patient.

2. Antigen detection

Antigen detection in CSF or serum by ELISA has been developed using monoclonal *T. solium* antibodies. Antigen disappears following treatment hence, can be used for monitoring.

Lymphocyte transformation test

It is based on the transformation of the lymphocytes when subjected to *T. solium* cyst fluid antigens and showed sensitivity of 93.7% and specificity of 96.2%.

Histopathology

Cysticerci can be detected in muscles, eyes, subcutaneous tissues (or brain during postmortem) by biopsy following surgical removal or fine needle aspiration of the cyst followed by microscopic demonstration of the parasite (Fig. 10.17).

Fine-needle aspiration cytology (FNAC)

Fine-needle aspiration of the cyst can be done followed by staining with Giemsa, or Ryan's modification of trichrome stain.
- ❖ Microscopically, it can differentiate between viable, necrotic and calcified cysticerci through their morphological pattern

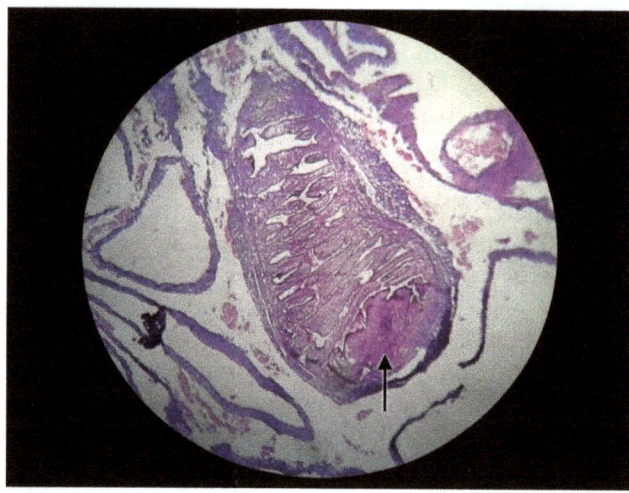

Fig. 10.17: Cysticercus cellulosae in biopsy from the brain (hematoxylin and eosin stain)—An entire cysticercus seen within the bladder walls, [Parenchymatous portion of the cysticercus can be better observed. The extensive folding of the spiral canal and one sucker of the scolex (Arrow)]

Source: Head of Department, Pathology, Meenakshi Medical College, Chennai (with permission).

- Cholesterol crystals are frequently seen which may be attributed to the high lipid content of the lesions. Charcot-Leyden crystals are characteristically absent.

Fundoscopy

Ocular cysticercosis can usually be diagnosed by fundoscopy for the visual identification of the movements and morphology of the larval worm.

Revised DelBrutto's diagnostic criteria

DelBrutto's criteria has been widely used for the diagnosis of NCC in endemic countries since 2001. It has been revised in 2016. It is based on clinical, imaging, immunological and epidemiological data (Table 10.6).

Treatment — Intestinal taeniasis

- **Praziquantel (drug of choice):** Single dose of (10 mg/kg) is highly effective
- Niclosamide (2 g) is also effective but is not widely available.

Treatment — Cysticercosis

Antiparasitic agents:
- For brain parenchymal lesions:
  - Albendazole (15 mg/kg per day for 8–28 days) or
  - Praziquantel (50–100 mg/kg daily in three divided doses for 15–30 days)
- Longer courses are often needed in patients with multiple subarachnoid cysticerci

Symptomatic treatment of:
- Seizures by antiepileptic drugs

Contd...

Table 10.6: Revised DelBrutto's diagnostic criteria and degrees of diagnostic certainty for neurocysticercosis, 2016

Absolute criteria (AC)		1. Histological demonstration of the parasite from biopsy of a brain or spinal cord lesion 2. Fundoscopy—visualization of subretinal cysticercus 3. Neuroimaging—confirmatory presence of scolex within a cystic lesion
Neuroimaging criteria (NIC)	Major (M-NIC)	1. Cystic lesions without a discernible scolex 2. Enhancing lesions 3. Multilobulated cystic lesions in the subarachnoid space 4. Typical parenchymal brain calcifications
	Confirmatory (C-NIC)	1. Resolution of cystic lesions after cysticidal drug therapy 2. Spontaneous resolution of single small enhancing lesions 3. Migration of ventricular cysts documented on sequential neuroimaging studies
	Minor (m-NIC)	Obstructive hydrocephalus or abnormal enhancement of basal leptomeninges
Clinical/ exposure criteria (CEC)	Major (M-CEC)	1. Detection of specific anti-cysticercal antibodies or antigens 2. Cysticercosis outside CNS 3. Evidence of a household contact with *T. solium* infection
	Minor (m-CEC)	1. Clinical manifestations suggestive of neurocysticercosis 2. Individuals coming from or living in an area where cysticercosis is endemic
Degrees of diagnostic certainty	Definitive diagnosis (any one)	• 1 AC • 2M-NIC + any 1CEC • 1M-NIC + 1C-NIC + any 1CEC • 1M-NIC +1M-CEC + any 1 CEC with the exclusion of other similar pathologies
	Probable diagnosis	• 1M-NIC + any 2 CEC or • 1 m-NIC + at least 1M-CEC

Abbreviation: CNS, central nervous system

Contd...

Treatment — Cysticercosis

- High-dose glucocorticoids should be used to reduce the inflammatory reactions caused by dead cysticerci
- Hydrocephalus: Attempts should be made to reduce intracranial pressure. In the case of obstructive hydrocephalus, cysticerci can be removed by endoscopic surgery or ventriculoperitoneal shunting.

Surgery:
- Open craniotomy to remove cysticerci is rarely required nowadays
- Surgery is indicated for ocular, spinal and ventricular lesions because antiparasitic drugs can provoke irreversible inflammatory damage.

Prevention

Intestinal taeniasis can be prevented by:
- Adequate cooking of beef or pork viscera:
  - Thorough cooking at 65°C for 5 minutes
  - Refrigeration at 4°C for >30 days
  - Salting and pickling are not effective.
- **Effective fecal disposal** to prevent infection to cattle and pigs.

The prevention of cysticercosis involves:
- **Good personal hygiene** to prevent autoinfection with eggs
- **Effective fecal disposal** to prevent contamination of food and water with eggs
- Treatment and prevention of human intestinal infections
- **Vaccines to prevent porcine cysticercosis:** Various antigens like *T. solium* oncosphere antigen, *T. crassiceps* and *T. ovis* recombinant antigens are attempted for vaccination of pigs. They are under development.

OTHER TAENIA SPECIES

Taenia saginata asiatica (Asian Tapeworm)

Some authors still regard it as a separate species where as others consider it as a subspecies of *T. saginata* due to similarities of the DNA sequences.
- It is morphologically similar to *T. saginata* except:
  - Intermediate host is pig (not in cow)
  - Cysticerci are located primarily in liver (not in muscle), and man acquires infection through ingestion of pig liver containing infected cysticerci
  - Scolex in cysticerci bears hooklets (may be lost in mature worms)
  - Both the cysticerci and the adult worm are smaller (with 300–1,000 proglottids).
- Human infection has been reported from Taiwan and other Asian countries like Korea, China, Indonesia, Japan, Philippines, Vietnam, Thailand but not reported from India, yet
- Clinical features, diagnosis and treatment are similar to that of *T. saginata*
- It causes intestinal taeniasis; not cysticercosis
- It is differentiated from *T. saginata* by PCR targeting mitochondrial DNA followed by sequencing.

Taenia multiceps (Multiceps multiceps)

It is a rare parasite infecting man.

Morphology

- **Larva (coenurus):** It is characterized by unilocular cyst with multiple scolices. Hence, it is named as multiceps (Figs 10.4D and 10.18)

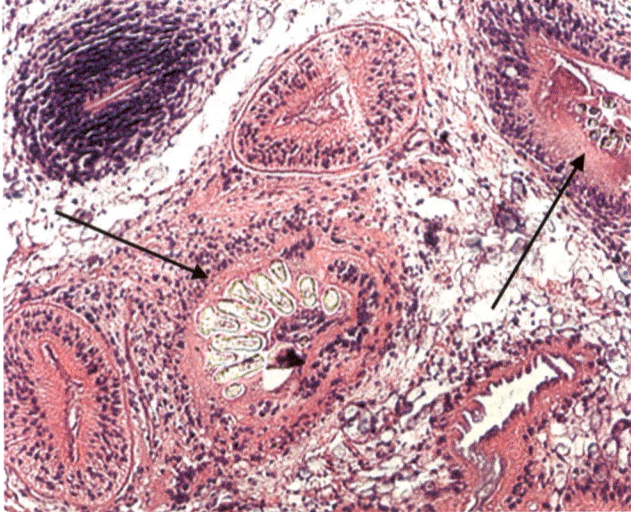

Fig. 10.18: Coenurus removed from a subcutaneous nodule in the shoulder area of a patient, stained with hematoxylin and eosin (H and E). The black arrows point to hooklets in the protoscoleces

Source: DPDx Image Library, Centers for Disease Control and Prevention (CDC), Atlanta (*with permission*).

- Adult worm is 40–60 cm in length. Scolex is pear-shaped with four suckers and armed rostellum with two rows of hooklets
- Eggs are about 30 μm in size, similar to that of other *Taenia* eggs.

Life Cycle

- **Host:** It passes its life cycle through two hosts:
  1. **Definitive host:** Dog, fox and wolf
  2. **Intermediate host:** Herbivorous animals like sheep. Humans act as accidental intermediate host.
- This disease occurs mainly in sheep and other herbivores affecting CNS, where it is called as **gid** (means unstable gait and giddiness)
- Men get infection by ingestion of food and water contaminated with dog's feces containing eggs
- Oncospheres hatch out from the eggs, penetrate the intestine and migrate to various organs, usually CNS where they transform into the larval stage called as **coenurus**.

Manifestations

Symptoms occur as a result of space occupying lesions in CNS which includes headache, vomiting, paralysis, seizure, etc.

Epidemiology

Nearly 175 cases have been reported in humans so far; mainly from developing countries where the dog population is not controlled such as African countries (like

Uganda, Kenya, Ghana and South Africa), Brazil, Mexico, Canada and the United States. Animal cases have been found in many other countries as well.

In India, few cases have been reported so far. Two cases of cerebral coenurosis have been reported from NIMHANS, Bengaluru in 2011.

Diagnosis

Diagnosis is based on gross and histological examination of coenurus following surgical removal.

Treatment	*Taenia multiceps*
Surgical removal is recommended. Praziquantel is also effective.	

ECHINOCOCCUS SPECIES

Echinococcus causes hydatid disease in man. There are four species of *Echinococcus* known to infect humans:
1. **E. granulosus:** Causes cystic hydatid disease or cystic echinococcosis (CE)
2. **E. multilocularis:** Causes alveolar hydatid disease or alveolar echinococcosis
3. **E. vogeli:** Causes polycystic hydatid disease.
4. **E. oligarthrus:** Causes unicystic hydatid disease.

Echinococcus granulosus
History
It is also called as **dog tapeworm.**
- Hydatid cysts were recognized from the time of Hippocrates and Galen
- Hartmann (1695) had demonstrated the adult form in dogs while Goeze (1782) had described the larval form (hydatid cyst).

Genotypes
Recently, it was known from molecular typing that *E. granulosus* complex comprises of 10 genotypes.
- The genotypes differ from each other in their intermediate host, geographic distribution, morphology of adult and larval stage, and protoscolex production
- Genotype G1-G3 cause 88% of human cases. In India, G1 (sheep strain) is more common, followed by G5 (cattle strain).

Habitat
The larval form (hydatid cyst) is found in liver and other viscera of man and other herbivores. The adult worms reside in dog's intestine.

Morphology
Adult Worm

Adult worm of *Echinococcus* is much smaller than other cestodes.

- It measures 3-6 mm long, consists of head, neck and strobila (Fig. 10.20C).
- **Head/scolex:** It is pyriform shaped (300 μm diameter), bears four suckers and a rostellum armed with two rows of hooklets
- **Neck:** Neck is short and thick
- **Strobila:** It is made up of only three proglottids/segments: one immature, one mature and one gravid segment. The gravid segment is broader than others and is filled with 100-1,500 eggs. The structure of the proglottids is similar to other cyclophyllidean cestodes as described earlier
- Life span of adult worm is up to 20 years.

Eggs

E. granulosus eggs are morphologically similar to *Taenia* eggs, consists of an oncosphere with six hooklets surrounded by an embryophore (See Fig. 10.3 C).

Larva

The larval form of *E. granulosus* is called as **hydatid cyst**. (Described later under pathogenicity).

Life Cycle (Fig. 10.19)

Host: *E. granulosus* life cycle passes through two hosts:
1. **Definitive host:** Dogs and other canine animals
2. **Intermediate hosts:** Sheep and other herbivores are the usual intermediate host. Man acts as an **accidental intermediate host** (dead end).

Infective form: Eggs are the infective form.

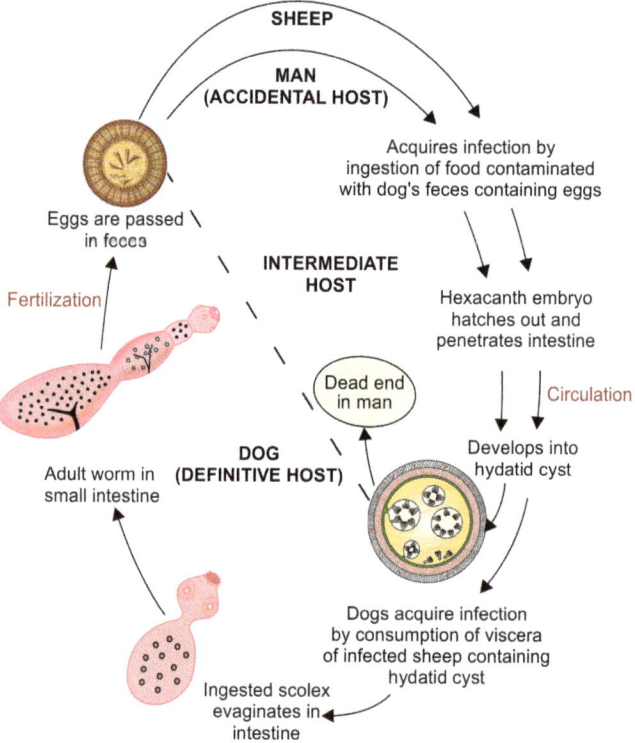

Fig. 10.19: Life cycle of *Echinococcus granulosus*

CHAPTER 10 ◆ Cestodes

Mode of transmission: Man (and other intermediate hosts) acquires the infection by ingestion of food contaminated with dog's feces containing *E. granulosus* eggs. Rarely flies serve as a *mechanical vector* of the eggs.

Development in man

Eggs transform to larva (hydatid cyst): In duodenum, the oncosphere is released by the rupture of embryophore. It penetrates into the intestinal wall, enters the portal circulation and carries to the liver (60–70% of cases) or lungs or rarely to other organs.

- Host-immune response tries to remove the parasite. Hence an inflammatory response takes place surrounding the sites where the oncospheres are settled
- Host-immune response may destroy many oncospheres, but few may escape destruction and develop into hydatid cyst
- The oncospheres are encysted by the fibrous tissue (produced by fibroblasts) and transform into fluid-filled bladder-like cyst called as **hydatid cysts**
- The hydatid cyst undergoes maturation increases in size at a rate of 1 cm/month. Full development takes 10–18 months in sheep (Figs 10.20A and B)
- This stage is infective to dog and other definitive hosts
- Man is a dead end (as dogs do not feed on human viscera).

Development in dog

Dog and other canine animals acquire infection by consumption of the contaminated viscera of intermediate hosts (sheep) containing mature hydatid cysts.

The hydatid cyst (larva) transforms into adult worm in dog's intestine. The adult worm becomes sexually mature, self-fertilizes to produce eggs which are passed in feces and are infective to man.

Pathogenicity

Pathogenicity is related to the deposition of the hydatid cysts (larval form of the parasite) in various organs.

Hydatid cyst

Fully developed hydatid cyst of *E. granulosus* is unilocular, subspherical in shape and size varies from few milimeters to more than 30 cm (usual size 5–8 cm) (Figs 10.20A and B).

- It appears as fluid-filled bladder-like cyst
- Cyst wall consists of three layers (Figs 10.21A to C):
  1. **Pericyst (outer layer, host derived):** Consists of fibrous tissue and blood vessels produced by the host cellular reaction.
  2. **Ectocyst (middle layer, parasite derived):** It is a tough elastic, glycan rich acellular hyaline layer of variable thickness (1 mm). It resembles the white of a hard-boiled egg.
  3. **Endocyst (inner layer, parasite derived):** It is the germinal layer, 22–25 µm thickness. It consists of number of nuclei embedded in protoplasmic mass. Its function is to form the ectocyst outside and on the inner side it forms brood capsule and secretes the hydatid fluid (Fig. 10.21C).
- **Hydatid fluid:** It is clear, colorless to pale yellow
  - It has a pH of 6.7 and specific gravity of 1.005 to 1.010
  - Chemical composition: It contains sodium chloride, sodium sulfate, sodium phosphate and succinates
  - It is antigenic, toxic and anaphylactic
- Brood capsules arise from the inner side of the endocyst and contains number of protoscolices (future head)

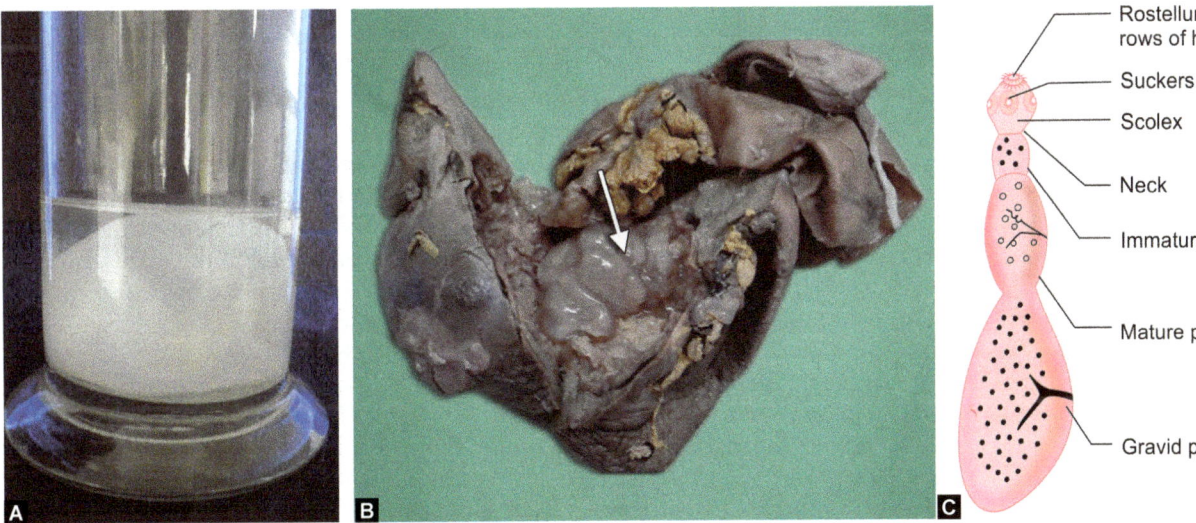

Figs 10.20A to C: *Echinococcus granulosus*: (A) Hydatid cyst, macroscopic picture; (B) Surgically resected hydatid cyst from liver; (C) Adult worm (schematic)

Source: A—Head, Department of Microbiology, Sri Siddhartha Medical College, Tumkur, Karnataka;
B—Head of Department, Pathology, Meenakshi Medical College, Chennai (*with permission*).

- **Hydatid sand:** Some of the brood capsules and protoscolices break off and gets deposited at the bottom as granular deposit to form the hydatid sand
- **Variety of hydatid cyst:**
  - Primary cyst: Formed directly from the oncosphere released from the eggs ingested
  - Secondary cysts: Formed due to the breakage of the primary cyst by trauma. The secondary cysts are carried in the circulations to various organs
  - Acephalocyst: Cysts without brood capsules and protoscolices
  - Endogenous daughter cysts: Formed by the breakage of the brood capsule into the hydatid fluid; surrounded by ectocyst and endocyst.
- **Fate of the hydatid cyst:**
  - Spontaneous resolution may happen to few cysts
  - Rupture of the cyst, which may lead to either:
    - Formation of secondary cysts or
    - Anaphylactic reaction to the hydatid fluid antigens.

Clinical Features

Infection usually occurs in childhood but gets manifested in adult life.
- **Site:** Most common site of location of the cyst is liver (60–70%, right lobe) or lung (20%), kidney (4%), muscle (4%), spleen (3%), soft tissue (3%), brain (3%), bone (2%) and others (1%)
- **Age:** Lung, brain, spinal, and orbital hydatid cysts are more common in younger patients. Multiorgan involvement is increasingly reported in children
- The cysts grow up to 5–10 cm in size within the first year and can survive for years or even decades
- **Asymptomatic:** Many cases are asymptomatic and infection is detected only incidentally by imaging studies
- **Symptoms occur due to:**
  - **Pressure effect of the enlarging cyst:** Leads to palpable abdominal mass, hepatomegaly, abdominal tenderness, portal hypertension and ascites
  - **Obstruction:** Daughter cyst may erode into the biliary tree or a bronchus and enter into the lumen to cause cholestasis, cholangitis, and dyspnea
  - **Secondary bacterial infection** can cause pyogenic abscess formation in the hydatid cysts
  - **Anaphylactic reactions:** Cyst leakage or rupture may be associated with a severe allergic reaction to hydatid fluid antigens; leading to hypotension, syncope and fever.
- **Outcome of the disease:** It depends on the cyst size and location
- Younger children are more associated with extra-hepatic cysts in lungs, brain and orbital sites
- In 20–40% of cases, multiple cysts or multiple organ involvement have been reported
- **Atopic allergy:** Patient sometimes develops hypersensitivity (atopy and anaphylaxis); which is attributed to release of various allergens from the cyst such as 12-kDa AgB (protease inhibitor), Ag5 serine protease, etc.

Epidemiology

E. granulosus is worldwide in distribution.
- **World:** Higher incidence has been reported from Central Asia (>10 per 1 Lakh population); which may be up to 27 per 1 lakh population in Tajikistan.
- **India:** Hydatid disease is reported from various places in India like Andhra Pradesh and Tamil Nadu, Chandigarh, Kashmir, Maharashtra and West Bengal.

Laboratory Diagnosis	Echinococcus granulosus
□ **Hydatid fluid microscopy** (direct mount or staining with acid fast stain)—detects brood capsules and protoscolices	
□ **Histological examination** (H & E)—demonstrates cyst wall and attached brood capsules	
□ **Antibody detection**—ELISA (using B2t antigen), DIGFA (dot immunogold filtration assay) and western blot	
□ **Imaging methods**—X-ray, USG (demon-strates Water lily sign), CT scan, MRI	
□ **Molecular methods**—PCR, PCR-RFLP and molecular typing (10 genotypes, most common in India is type 1)	
□ **Skin test** (Casoni test)—demonstrates type I hypersensitivity reaction.	

Laboratory Diagnosis

Hydatid fluid microscopy

After surgical removal of the cyst, the hydatid fluid is aspirated and examined by direct microscopy or staining with acid fast stain for presence of hydatid sand.
- Diagnostic aspiration is not usually recommended because of the risk of fluid leakage which may lead to anaphylaxis or dissemination of infection
- Drop of centrifuged fluid is placed between two slides and the slides are rubbed over the fluid
- Hydatid sand is felt as grating of the sand grains in between the slides. The hydatid sand comprises of protoscolices and brood capsules
- Purulent material can be examined after treating with hydrochloric acid.

Histological examination

Surgically removed cysts can be subjected to histopathological stains like Giemsa, hematoxylin and eosin (H & E) and periodic acid-Schiff (PAS) stain to

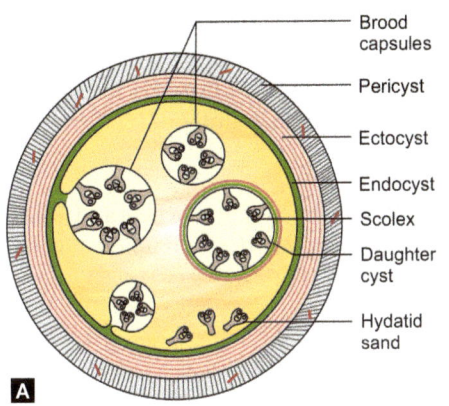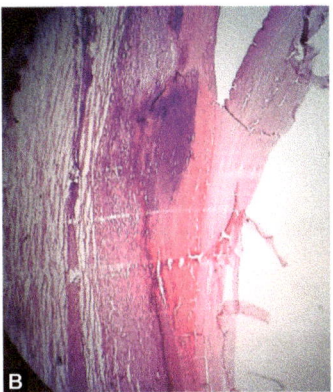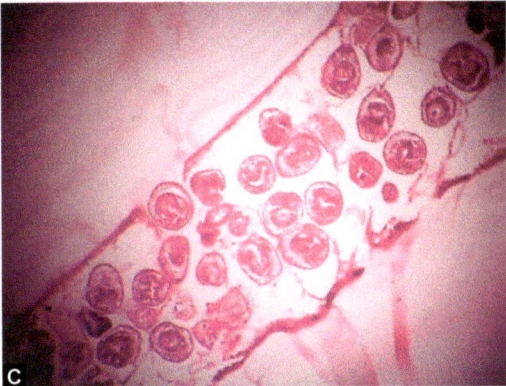

Figs 10.21A to C: Microscopy of hydatid cyst: (A) Schematic; (B and C) Histopathological section (hematoxylin and eosin stain) showing (B) all three layers of cyst wall—pericyst, ectocyst and endocyst; (C) endocyst with attached brood capsules

Source: B and C—Head, Department of Pathology, Meenakshi Medical College, Chennai (*with permission*).

demonstrate the three layers of the cyst wall and attached brood capsules (Figs 10.21B and C).

Antibody detection

Serodiagnosis of hydatid disease follows a two-step approach; first, a more sensitive test (for screening) such as ELISA, DIGFA (dot immunogold filtration assay), IHA (indirect hemagglutination assay) or IFA (indirect fluorescent antibody test) is carried out. If found positive, should be confirmed with more specific test such as immunoblot.

- **ELISA:** ELISA using crude *E. granulosus* cyst fluid antigen is available, but is less commonly used because of its variable sensitivity of 50–98%
    - Currently, ELISA using recombinant B2t antigen (C-terminal truncated recombinant antigen B2) or 2B2t antigen (containing two molecules of B2t) are commercially available; increasingly used
    - 2B2t-ELISA has shown better result with sensitivity 91% and specificity 93% and is also used as an indicator of cure in surgically treated patients.
- **DIGFA:** Dot immunogold filtration assay (DIGFA) has been developed in China for simultaneous detection of serum antibodies against four native antigens; cyst fluid (EgCF), AgB and protoscolex extract (EgP) of *E. granulosus* and Em2 (metacestode antigen) of *E. multilocularis*. Overall sensitivity is 80% and 93% for cystic and alveolar echinococcosis respectively with specificity >90%
- **Immunoblot (Western blot):** Immunoblot is the most specific serological method; used as a confirmatory test when ELISA result is inconclusive
    - **h-HCF-IB** (human hydatid cyst fluid-immunoblot): It is a commercial assay which uses human hydatid cyst fluid antigen. It has a sensitivity of 83%, and a specificity of 98%
    - Immunoblot detecting antibody against antigen B fragment (produces 8–12kDa band) has been in use. This test is 92% sensitive and 100% specific.

Antibody methods are useful for seroepidemiological study but cannot differentiate recent and past infection. Antigen B is the antigen of choice used for seroepidemiological study for detection of antibody.

Patients with liver cysts show better results than extrahepatic cysts. Pulmonary cysts do not produce detectable antibodies. Alveolar echinococcosis shows better results than cystic echinococcosis.

Imaging methods

Imaging methods play an important role as they are noninvasive methods, which can detect the cysts incidentally in asymptomatic individuals and in seronegative cases.

- **X-rays:** It is simple, inexpensive, yet useful technique to detect hepatomegaly and calcified cysts and cysts in lungs
- **Ultrasound (USG):** It is the imaging method of choice because of its low cost and high diagnostic accuracy of 90%
    - It detects both single and multiple cystic lesions
    - **WHO classification of USG imaging:** WHO has classified the USG images of cysts into six types according to its activity (CL and CE1 to CE5) (Table 10.7). This is useful in determining whether the cyst is active or not
    - USG is used to monitor the response to treatment
    - It is also used for epidemiological studies to detect the prevalence of hydatid cyst in population.
- **Computed tomography (CT scan):** It can detect 90–100% of cases (Fig. 10.22)
    - It detects more accurately the number, location of the cyst and the complications

Table 10.7: WHO international classification of ultrasound images of hydatid cyst		
Types	Activity	USG finding
CL	Active	Cystic lesion and no visible cyst wall
CE1	Active	Visible cyst wall and internal echoes (**snowflake sign**)
CE2	Active	Visible cyst wall and internal septation (**honeycomb appearance**)
CE3	Transitional	Have detached laminar membranes or may be partially collapsed, and floating within the cyst cavity (known as **Water lily sign**).
CE4	Inactive	Non-homogeneous mass
CE5	Inactive	Cyst with a thick calcified wall

Abbreviations: WHO: World Health Organization; CE- cystic echinococcosis.
Note: This classification is also applicable for CT scan and MRI images.

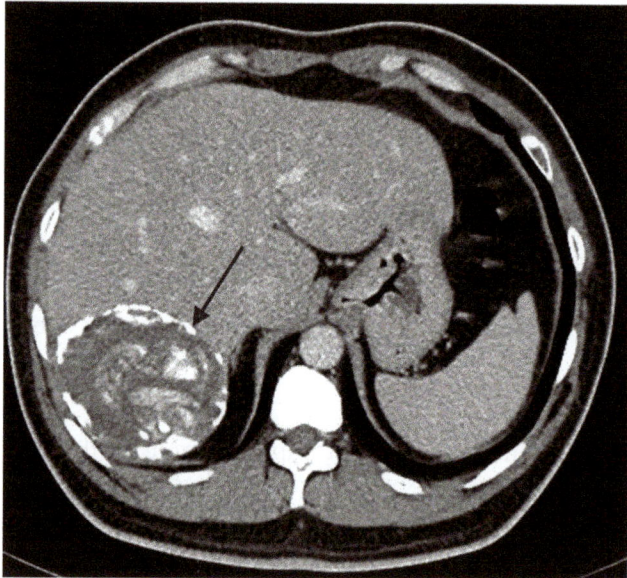

Fig. 10.22: CT scan showing calcifying hydatid cyst in the liver.
Source: Dr A Subathra, Department of Radiodiagnosis, JIPMER, Puducherry (*with permission*).

- It is superior to detect the calcified lesions. Calcification occurs in 10% of cysts and usually requires 5–10 years to develop
- It is superior to USG to detect smaller cysts, extra-hepatic cysts and to differentiate hydatid cyst from other cystic lesions
- CT scan can also be used as a prognostic marker.
❖ **Magnetic resonance imaging (MRI):** It has a higher contrast resolution, which makes cysts clearer. It can be used as an alternate to CT scan. However, it poorly detects the calcified cysts.

Molecular methods
❖ PCR targeting mitochondrial DNA has been developed
❖ PCR-RFLP can be used to detect genotypes of *E. granulosus*
❖ 10 genotypes have been identified from G1 to G10; G1 is the most common genotype in India.

Skin test (Casoni test)
It is an immediate hypersensitivity reaction (wheal and flare), which develops following injection of hydatid fluid antigens. It was developed by Casoni in 1911. Now it is obsolete.

Other tests
❖ Eosinophilia is present in 20–25% cases
❖ Hypergammaglobulinemia.

Assessment of parasite viability
Viability of the parasite can be assessed by:
❖ Ultrasonography differentiating the cyst into active or inactive
❖ Histopathology—evaluating the intact parasite-derived cyst wall including germinal layer
❖ Vital stain (e.g. eosin stain)—evaluate the protoscolices for flame cell activity and morphological integrity
❖ Metabolic viability assessment using high-field MRS (magnetic resonance spectroscopy) of cyst content
❖ Real-time PCR targeting several constitutively expressed genes of *E. granulosus* that determine viability.

Treatment — *Echinococcus granulosus*

Therapy for cystic echinococcosis is based on viability, size and location of the cyst; guided by USG and overall health of the patient.
PAIR (puncture, aspiration, injection and re-aspiration)
It is an alternate method recommended instead of surgery. It involves four basic steps:
1. Percutaneous puncture of the cyst
2. Aspiration of 10–15 mL of cyst fluid
3. Infusion of scolicidal agents like hypertonic saline, cetrimide, or ethanol
4. Re-aspiration of the fluid after 5 minutes

PAIR claims higher cure rate, less recurrence rate, less complications and hospitalization compared to surgery
PAIR is recommended for single hepatic cyst (CE1 lesion and uncomplicated CE3 lesion)
PAIR is contraindicated for:
- Superficially located cysts (because of the risk of rupture)
- CE2: Cyst with multiple thick internal septal division (honeycomb appearance).
- Inaccessible cyst or extrahepatic cysts
- Cysts communicating to biliary tree
- CE4 and CE5 lesions: These are inactive lesions; should be managed with observation only.

Surgery
- Though surgery is the definitive method of treatment, it should be reserved for:
  - Cases where PAIR is contraindicated or refractory
  - Secondary bacterial infection
  - Advanced disease

Contd...

Contd...

Treatment	*Echinococcus granulosus*

- Disadvantages of surgery are high recurrence rate (2–25%) and postoperative complications (10–25%)
- Preoperative use of albendazole is effective in reducing size and to prevent recurrence.

Antiparasitic agents
Albendazole is the drug of choice, given to prevent recurrence and to reduce the size of the cyst before surgery or PAIR and is given at 15 mg/kg daily in two divided doses; 1 week before to 4 weeks after the procedure.
- Complicated and multivesicular cysts may require longer duration.

Pulmonary cyst, preoperative albendazole should be avoided; praziquantel is given alternatively.

Percutaneous thermal ablation
It is a noninvasive method, involves percutaneous radiofrequency ablation of the germinal layer of the cysts.

Prevention

Echinococcosis can be prevented by:
- Administering praziquantel to infected dogs
- To improve personal hygiene to reduce contamination of food and water with dog's feces
- Vaccinating the sheep
- Limitation of stray dogs population.

Echinococcus multilocularis

Morphology

E. multilocularis is morphologicaly similar to *E. granulosus* except it is smaller in size (1.2 –3.7 mm length).

Life Cycle

Life cycle is similar to that of *E. granulosus*. Only the hosts are different.

Host: There are two types of hosts:
1. Definitive host: Foxes and wolves (and also dogs and cats)
2. Intermediate hosts: Small wild rodents like squirrels, voles, mice, etc.
   Man is an accidental intermediate host.

Clinical Features

E. multilocularis is the causative agent of alveolar (or multilocular) hydatid disease.
- So named because the cysts have multiple locules or cavities with no fluid or no free brood capsule/scolices; often with central necrosis and cavitation of the lesion. Man being not a natural host, cysts are usually sterile, do not produce brood capsule and protoscolices
- Liver is the most common organ affected (98% of cases)
- **Symptoms** developed are similar to that of *E. granulosus* such as hepatomegaly and portal hypertension
- Cyst appears as solid, firm mass with irregular outer layer and has an ability to migrate rapidly to other organs so that it mimics a malignant tumor. However, there is no malignant potential. The rapid invasion is due to a **surface protein 14-3-3** found on germinal layer
- Cysts spread by direct extension or via blood or lymphatics. Some cases (2%), piece of the endocyst may migrate to brain and lungs. It is associated with high mortality
- **Disease phases**: The disease can be classified into five phases; initial, progressive, advanced, stable and abortive
- **Geographical distribution:** This disease is found more frequently in Russia, Kazakhstan, China, South-Central Europe and North America.

Laboratory Diagnosis

Imaging methods

Imaging methods like USG, CT Scan and MRI can detect the number and size of the cyst, extension of the lesion and calcification if any.

Antibody detection tests

Different ELISA formats are available using cyst fluid antigen, cyst wall derived glycan (Em2) antigen, recombinant Em-10 and Em-18 antigens. These tests are sensitive but gives false positive results in cross reacting *E. granulosus* infection.

Histopathological diagnosis

Staining with periodic acid-Schiff (PAS) following FNAC (fine needle aspiration cytology) or biopsy can be done to detect the multiloculated sterile cyst and associated necrosis.

Molecular method

Specimen obtained through FNAC can be subjected to PCR; which can differentiate various *Echinococcus* species.

Treatment	*Echinococcus multilocularis*

Surgical resection remains the treatment of choice. Albendazole should be continued for at least 2 years post-surgery and monitored for 10 years for recurrence.

Echinococcus oligarthrus and Echinococcus vogeli

They rarely infect humans and cause polycystic (*E. vogeli*) and unicystic (*E. oligarthrus*) hydatid disease respectively; both together called as neotropical echinococcosis.

- **Host:** There are two types of host:
  1. Definitive host: Wild felids like wild cats, jaguars and pumas (*E. oligarthrus*) or bush dogs (*E. vogeli*).
  2. Intermediate host: Rodents like paca, spiny rats and opossum.
- **Clinical Features:** *E. vogeli* infects most commonly liver (80%) followed by lungs and other viscera. Symptoms are similar to that of cystic echinococcosis
- **Epidemiology**
  - To date, over 200 cases of polycystic hydatid disease have been reported. Most of the cases are seen in humid tropical forest area of South America like Brazil, Colombia, Ecuador, Panama and Venezuela. It has also been reported now from North America
  - Only three cases of *E. oligarthrus* are reported so far, two involving orbit and one in heart.
- **Laboratory Diagnosis:** Depends on imaging methods, histopathology, serology or molecular methods like PCR
- **Treatment** is similar to that of *E. granulosus*.

HYMENOLEPIS NANA

It is the smallest cestode infecting man, hence called as dwarf tapeworm.
- Name *Hymenolepis* refers to a thin membrane covering the eggs (Hymen- membrane, lepis- covering, and nana- small size)
- It was first detected by Bilharz in 1857 in small intestine.
- **Renaming:** There is consideration to rename *H. nana* as *Rodentolepis nana*.

Epidemiology

H. nana is considered as the most common tapeworm infection throughout the world infecting 50-75 million of people. The overall prevalence ranges from 0-4% with higher prevalence in children (16%).

Morphology

Adult Worm

The adult worm is small, 2.5-4 cm in length and consists of head, neck and strobila. It resides in the small intestine (upper two-thirds of ileum).
- **Head/scolex:** It is globular with four suckers and a rostellum bearing single row of 20-30 hooklets
- **Neck:** It is long and gives rise to proglottids
- **Strobila:** Consists of 200 segments (proglottids). Mature proglottids contain both male and female reproductive organs. Genital pore opens laterally on the same side. Uterus has lobulated wall and there are only three testicular follicles (Rest description is similar to any other cyclophyllidean cestodes described earlier).

Egg

Eggs are the infective form as well as the diagnostic form of the parasite.
- Egg is round to slightly oval in shape, 30–47 μm size
- It has two membranes (outer egg shell and an inner embryophore) and an oncosphere with six hooklets. Space between the two membranes is filled with yolk granules
- **Polar filaments:** Both the poles of embryophore are thickened from which four to eight polar filaments emerge
- **Non bile stained (colorless in saline mount):** It is the only cestode egg that is not stained by bile when passed through intestine.

Larva

The larval form is called **cysticercoid** (Fig. 10.4B). It is solid, except the proximal part which is vesicular and contains the scolex.

Life Cycle (Fig. 10.23)

Two life cycles are noted, i.e. direct and indirect cycle.

Direct Cycle

Host: Man is the only host. There is no intermediate host. Rodents (rat and mice) are the other hosts.

Infective form: Eggs are the infective form.

Mode of transmission: Man acquires the infection by:
- Ingestion of food and water contaminated with eggs
- Autoinfection with the eggs released in their small intestine.

In the small intestine, eggs hatch out, penetrate the intestinal wall and develops into cysticercoid larvae in 4-5 days.
- Thereafter, the intestinal villi rupture and cysticercoids larvae become free in the gut lumen and transform into the adult worms in 10-12 weeks
- Adult worm, when fully mature undergoes fertilization to produce eggs
- Eggs are passed in the feces which are infective to man
- Though the adult worm lives only about 4-10 weeks, the infection persists due to autoinfection.

Indirect Cycle

- **Host:** Man is the **definitive host**. Insects act as **intermediate host** such as rat fleas like *Pulex irritans* and *Xenopsylla cheopis*
- **Mode of transmission:** Men acquire the infection rarely, by accidental ingestion of insects containing the cysticercoid larva

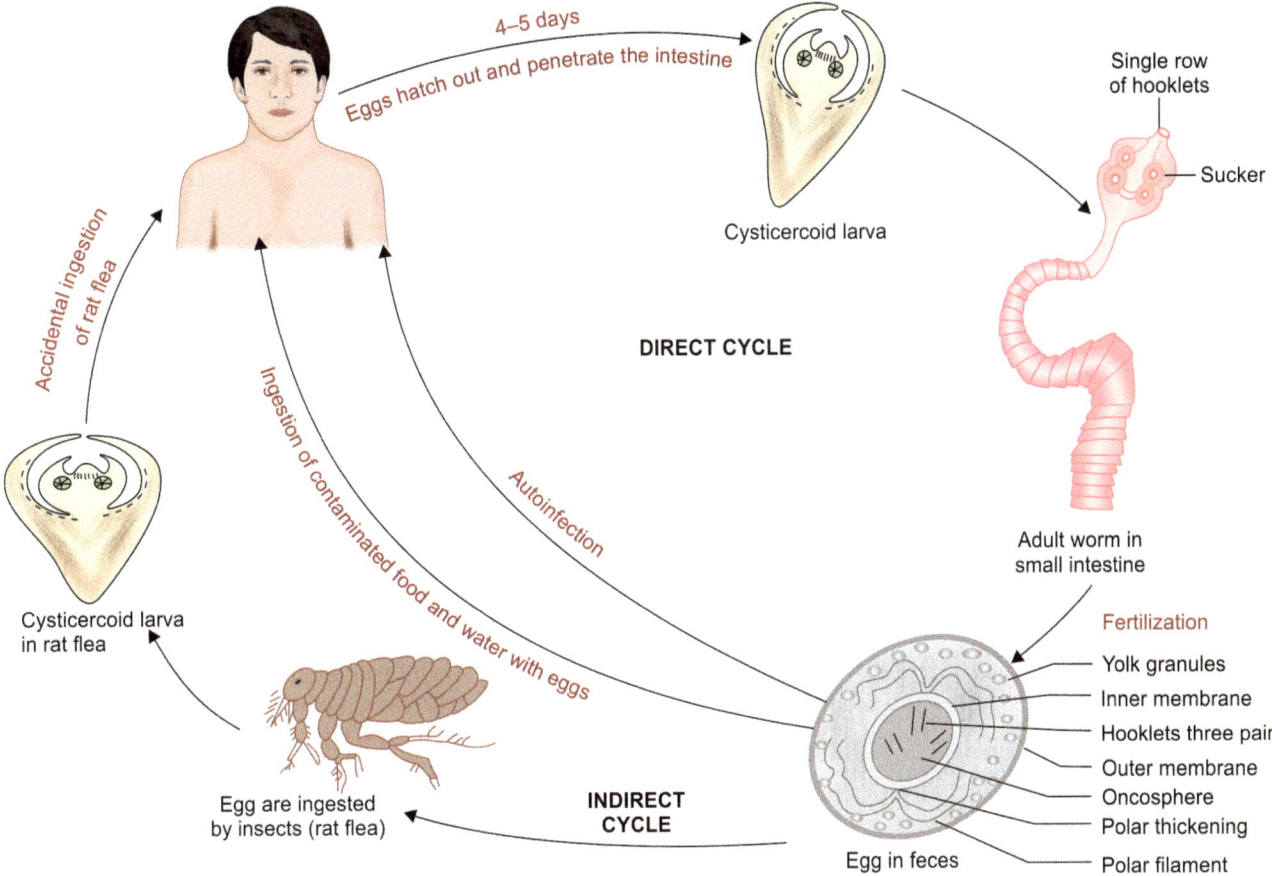

Fig. 10.23: Life cycle of *Hymenolepis nana*

- **In human intestine:** The larva develops into adult worm in human small intestine (upper part of ileum) which then produces eggs that are passed in the feces
- **In rat fleas:** Eggs are ingested by the insects, embryo hatches out, penetrate the intestine and develop into the larval stage-cysticercoid larva in the insect's body cavity. This stage is infective to man.

Treatment	*Hymenolepis nana*
□ Praziquantel (25 mg/kg once) is the treatment of choice, since it acts against both the adult worms and the cysticercoid larvae in the intestinal villi □ Nitazoxanide (500 mg bid for 3 days) may be used as an alternative □ Niclosamide can also be given.	

Clinical Features

H. nana infection is usually asymptomatic. When infection is intense and the worm burden exceeds 1000–2000 worms, patients develop symptoms like anorexia, abdominal pain, headache, dizziness and diarrhea with mucus.

Laboratory Diagnosis

Infection is diagnosed by detection of the characteristic non bile stained eggs with polar filaments between the shell membranes in the stool (as described earlier) (Figs 10.24A and B). Stool concentration can be done if the egg load is less. PVA (polyvinyl-alcohol) should not used for preservation as it distorts the morphology. Some patients have eosinophilia of 5% or more.

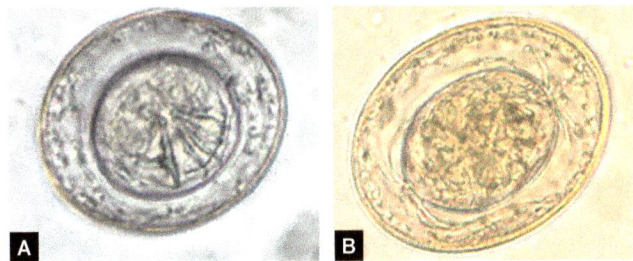

Figs 10.24A and B: Non bile stained egg of *Hymenolepis nana* in (A) saline mount—three pairs of hooklets are seen clearly; (B) iodine mount— polar filaments are seen clearly

Source: DPDx Image Library, Centers for Disease Control and Prevention (CDC), Atlanta (*with permission*).

Prevention

Good personal hygiene and improved sanitation can eradicate the disease. Epidemics have been controlled by mass chemotherapy coupled with improved hygiene.

Hymenolepis Diminuta

Hymenolepis diminuta is also called as rat tape worm.
- It is similar to *H. nana* with some differences as shown in the Table 10.8
- Always, it requires an intermediate host as insects like lepidopterans, myriapods, beetles, etc.
- It undergoes indirect life cycle only, there is no direct life cycle
- Human infection is rare. Only less than 500 cases are reported so far, mainly from India or other places like Japan, Italy, etc.

DIPYLIDIUM CANINUM

D. caninum, also called as double pored tapeworm is a common tapeworm of dogs and cats.
- **Morphology:** Adult worm is 10–70 cm long, scolex contains four oval suckers. It is armed with rostellum and 1–7 rows of hooklets (Fig. 10.25A)
- **Life Cycle:** It resembles with the indirect cycle of *H. nana*
  - Host: There are two types of hosts. Definitive host are dogs and cats (rarely men). Intermediate host are insects (fleas)
  - Man acquires infection by ingestion of flea containing cysticercoid larva (Fig. 10.25B).
- **Clinical Features:** Most infections are asymptomatic, but rarely symptoms like indigestion, loss of appetite, diarrhea, pruritus ani, abdominal pain may be reported. Children are affected commonly
- **Laboratory Diagnosis:** Stool examination is performed to demonstrate proglottids or eggs in feces
  - Eggs: Eggs are of 25–40 μm size, present in groups of 15 (**egg packets**) (Fig. 10.25D)
  - Proglottids: They are typically **barrel-shaped** (3.2 mm wide), looks like cucumber seed when fresh and rice grain when dry. It contains two sets of reproductive organs with two genital pores on both the lateral side, hence named as double pored tapeworm (Fig. 10.25C).
- **Epidemiology:** Human cases are rare and have been reported from Austria, Japan and the USA
- **Treatment:** Praziquantel is the drug of choice
- **Prevention:** It requires flea control.

Table 10.8: Differences between *Hymenolepis* nana and *Hymenolepis diminuta*

	Hymenolepis nana	Hymenolepis diminuta
Common name	Dwarf tapeworm	Rat tape-worm
Host	Man is the only host, occasionally insects act as intermediate host	Rodents (or man) definitive host and Insects are intermediate host
Life cycle	Both direct and indirect cycle	Only indirect cycle occurs, i.e. always needs insects
Person to person spread	Yes	No
Autoinfection	Yes	No
Adult worm		
Length	Small <4 cm, spherical	Large, (20–60 cm), oval
Scolex	Bears four suckers with rostellum and hooklets	Bears four suckers, with rostellum but no hooklets
Proglottids	<200	800–1,000
Egg	Smaller, 30–47 μm, polar filaments present Non-bile stained	Larger 70–85 × 60–80 μm polar filaments absent and bile stained
Human infection	Common	Rare

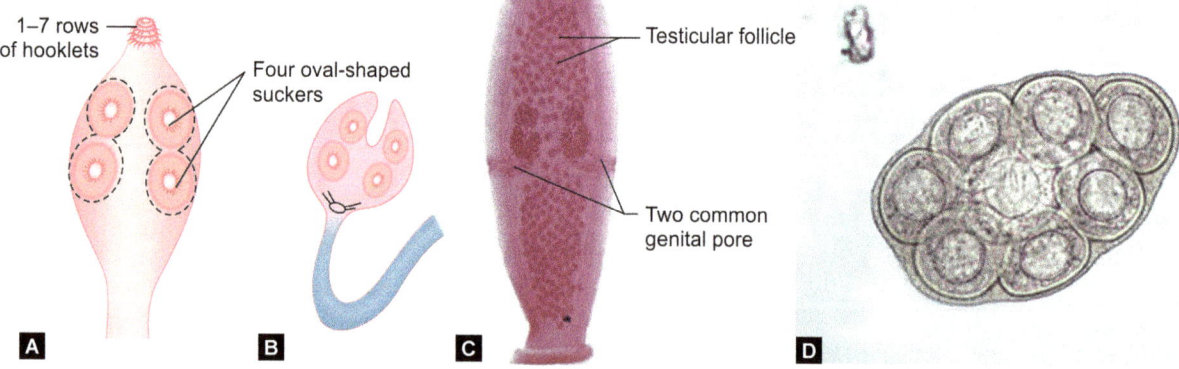

Figs 10.25A to D: *Dipylidium caninum*: (A) Scolex (schematic diagram); (B) Cysticercoid larva (schematic diagram); (C) Proglottids with two genital pores carmine stained; (D) Egg packets (in saline mount of stool)

Source: C and D—DPDx Image Library, Centers for Disease Control and Prevention (CDC), Atlanta (*with permission*).

CHAPTER 10 ◆ Cestodes

EXPECTED QUESTIONS

I. Write essay on:
  a. A 9-year-old child came to the pediatric OPD with history of passing segments of a worm. The stool examination revealed—(i) helminth eggs, described as round to oval, containing an embryo with three pairs of hooklets, surrounded by an embryophore and (ii) proglottids with 15–20 lateral branches from uterus.
    1. Identify the disease and the causative agent.
    2. Name the different species which can infect man and how to differentiate them.
    3. Write briefly about the life cycle of the etiological agent.
    4. What are the various diagnostic modalities?
  b. A 21-year-old vegetarian female presented with recurrent episodes of seizure, headache vomiting and vertigo. MRI scan of brain showed cystic lesion in brain parenchyma, following which surgery was performed. The cysts were surgically removed which appeared yellowish white in color, measuring 0.5–1.5 cm size, slightly oval in shape, containing a bladder like sac with a white spot.
    1. What is the etiological diagnosis?
    2. Write briefly about the life cycle of the etiological agent.
    3. What are the various diagnostic modalities?
    4. How will you treat this condition?
  c. A 24-year-old woman presented with complaints of pain in the right hypochondrium. Ultrasonography revealed a single space occupying cystic lesion in the right lobe of the liver. The cyst was removed surgically and subjected to histopathological examination, which revealed three layered of cyst wall with attached brood capsules.
    1. Identify the disease and the causative agent.
    2. Write briefly about the life cycle of the etiological agent.
    3. What are the various diagnostic modalities?
    4. How will you treat this condition?

II. Short notes on:
  a. Sparganosis.
  b. Diphyllobothriasis.
  c. Double pored tapeworm.
  d. Hydatid cyst.
  e. Laboratory diagnosis of Neurocysticercosis.
  f. Polycystic hydatid disease.
  g. Alveolar hydatid disease.
  h. Coenurosis.

III. Multiple choice questions (MCQs):
  1. Which of the following cestode does not have a rostellum and hooks?
     a. *Echinococcus granulosus*   b. *Taenia solium*
     c. *Taenia saginata*   d. *Hymenolepis nana*
  2. Which of the following cestode eggs are NOT bile stained?
     a. *Hymenolepis nana*   b. *Diphyllobothrium latum*
     c. *Echinococcus granulosus*   d. *Taenia solium*
  3. The larval form of *Hymenolepis nana* is called:
     a. Hydatid cyst   b. Coenurus
     c. Cysticercus   d. Cysticercoid
  4. Humans acquire cysticercus cellulosae infection by all, *except*:
     a. Ingestion of contaminated vegetables
     b. Autoinfection
     c. Reverse peristalsis
     d. Ingestion of contaminated pig's meat
  5. Which of the following cestode does not need an intermediate host to complete the life cycle?
     a. *Hymenolepis nana*   b. *Taenia saginata*
     c. *Diphyllobothrium latum*   d. *Echinococcus granulosus*

Answer
1. c   2. a   3. d   4. d   5. a

Trematodes or Flukes

CHAPTER 11

CHAPTER OUTLINE

- Classification of trematodes
- General characteristics of trematodes
- Blood flukes
  - *Schistosoma* species
- Liver flukes
  - *Fasciola* species
  - *Clonorchis* species
  - *Opisthorchis* species
- Intestinal flukes
- *Fasciolopsis* species
- Other less common intestinal trematodes
- Lung fluke
  - *Paragonimus* species

Trematodes (also called as **flukes**) include the helminths that are unsegmented, flat (flat worms) and leaf-like.

CLASSIFICATION OF TREMATODES

Systemic Classification

Systemic classification of medically important trematodes is proposed by Gibson and Bray (1994) and is outlined in Table 11.1. Trematodes belong to Phylum Platyhelminthes and Class Trematoda or Digenea.

Classification Based on the Habitat

Based on the habitat, trematodes are classified as follows.
- ❖ **Blood trematodes (flukes):** Examples include:
  - *Schistosoma haematobium*: It resides in vesical venous plexus
  - *Schistosoma mansoni* and *S. japonicum*: They reside in rectal venous plexus and portal venous plexus.
- ❖ **Hepatic trematodes (flukes):** Examples include:
  - *Fasciola hepatica* and *Fasciola gigantica*: Both reside in liver
  - *Clonorchis* species and *Opisthorchis* species: Both reside in the bile duct.
- ❖ **Intestinal trematodes (flukes):** Examples include:
  - Small intestine: *Fasciolopsis buski*, *Heterophyes* species, *Metagonimus* species, *Watsonius* species
  - Large intestine: *Gastrodiscoides* species
- ❖ **Lung trematodes (flukes):** *Paragonimus westermani*.

GENERAL CHARACTERISTICS OF TREMATODES

Morphology

Trematodes exist in three morphological forms—adult worm, egg and larva.

Adult Worm

The adult worms are unsegmented and flattened dorsoventrally but some have thick fleshy bodies (schistosomes).
- ❖ **Size:** They range from less than 1 mm to ~60 mm
- ❖ **Suckers:** They attach to host with two suckers—(1) oral sucker (anterior) which surrounds the mouth and (2) ventral sucker (acetabulum) on the ventral surface
- ❖ **Digestive system:** It is incomplete, consists of anterior mouth, muscular pumping pharynx which continues

Table 11.1: Classification of trematodes

Order	Superfamily	Family	Genus and Species
Strigeida	Schistosomatoidea	Schistosomatidae	*Schistosoma haematobium, S. mansoni, S. japonicum S. mekongi, S. intercalatum*
Echinostomida	Paramphistomatoidea	Zygocotylidae	*Gastrodiscoides hominis, Watsonius watsoni*
	Echinostomatoidea	Fasciolidae	*Fasciola hepatica, F. gigantica, Fasciolopsis buski*
Plagiorchiida	Opisthorchioidea	Opisthorchiidae	*Opisthorchis felineus, O. viverrini, Clonorchis sinensis*
		Heterophyidae	*Heterophyes heterophyes, Metagonimus yokogawai*
	Plagiorchioidea	Troglotrematidae	*Paragonimus westermani, Nanophyetus salmincola*

as esophagus. Esophagus bifurcates in front of ventral sucker into a pair of blind intestinal pouches called caeca. The anus is absent
- Most trematodes are hermaphrodites (monoecious) except the schistosomes, which are diecious (sexes are separate)
- **Male reproductive organs:** Consist of number of testes present near the cecal end, vas efferens arise from each testes join to form a common vas deferens which runs via a small seminal vesicle and opens at genital pore situated near the ventral sucker
- **Female reproductive organs:** Consist of an ovary (present near the ventral sucker), vitelline glands surrounding ovary, oviduct, ootype and a uterus containing eggs that opens behind the ventral sucker
- The **excretory system** is bilaterally symmetrical. It consists of flame cells and collecting tubules which lead to a median bladder opening at the posterior end of the body, usually on the dorsal aspect
- The **nervous system** consists of paired ganglia at the anterior end. From this, nerves extend anteriorly and posteriorly.

Eggs

- Trematodes are oviparous, i.e. they lay eggs; which develop into larvae later in the environment
- The eggs of all the trematodes are characteristically operculated except that of schistosomes
- Schistosomes are eggs are non-operculated. Instead, they possess a spine.

Larvae

- Trematodes have five larval forms such as miracidium, sporocyst, redia (first and second generation), cercaria, and metacercaria
- Schistosomes differ from other trematodes as they do not have redia and metacercaria larvae. Instead, they possess two generations of sporocyst larvae.

Life Cycle

Host: Trematodes complete their life cycle in three different hosts, one definitive host (man) and two intermediate hosts. **The first intermediate** host is **fresh water snail** or **mollusc** and the **second intermediate host** is either aquatic **plant** or **fish** or **crab**. However, schistosomes do not need a second intermediate host.

Mode of transmission: Man acquires infection by eating aquatic plants, fishes or crabs harboring infective form (metacercariae larva) or by the penetration of free living cercariae larva (infective form, in schistosomiasis).

Development in Definitive Host (Man)

The young trematodes migrate to their habitat where they grow into adults, sexually mature and begin to lay eggs, which are excreted in feces, urine or sputum (depending on the species) and gain access to water.

Depending on embryonation, eggs show three different types of development:
1. The eggs which are embryonated when laid, hatch to release miracidia, which infect the intermediate host, i.e. snail (e.g. schistosomes).
2. The eggs which are not embryonated when laid, first mature in water and then hatch to release miracidia, which infect suitable intermediate host (e.g. *Paragonimus, Fasciola,* and *Fasciolopsis*).
3. The eggs which are embryonated when laid, but hatch only on ingestion by suitable snail host (e.g. *Clonorchis, Opisthorchis,* and *Metagonimus*).

Developments in First Intermediate Host (Snail)

The miracidium is a free swimming ciliated larva which penetrates suitable intermediate host like snails.
- Miracidium contains apical gland which releases proteolytic enzymes which aids the process of penetration
- In liver or lymph spaces of intermediate host, miracidium transforms into sporocyst
- Asexual multiplication of sporocysts does not occur at this stage except in schistosomes where asexual multiplication gives rise to second generation sporocysts
- The sporocysts develop to become rediae. The rediae multiply to produce second generation rediae; which then transform into cercariae. There is no redia stage in schistosomes
- A single miracidium can give rise to large number of cercariae. Trematodes vary from each other in the morphology of their cercariae larvas; for examples, fork tailed cercariae in schistosomes (Fig. 11.1C).

Developments in Second Intermediate Host (Fish or Crab)

After ingestion by a fish or a crab, the cercarial larvae develop into metacercariae which are the infective forms to the definitive host (man).

The life cycle of schistosomes differs from other trematodes in various ways; which is depicted in the highlight boxes below and Table 11.2.

Treatment	Trematodes
Praziquantel is the drug of choice for all trematodes infection except for *Fasciola*, where triclabendazole is recommended.	

Table 11.2: Differences between schistosomes and other trematodes

Properties	Other trematodes	Schistosomes
Host	Definitive: Man Intermediate: • 1st: Snail • 2nd: Plant or fish*	Definitive: Man Intermediate: Snail There is no 2nd intermediate host
Infective form	Metacercaria lava (present inside 2nd intermediate host)	Cercaria lava (present free in water)
Mode of transmission	Ingestion of 2nd intermediate host	Skin penetration
Eggs	Operculated, no spine	Non-operculated, spine present
Larvae	Five stages: Miracidium, sporocyst, redia, cercaria, and metacercaria	Same except: • No metacercaria • No redia • Sporocyst are present in two generations
Adults	Hermaphrodite (male and female organs present in same worm)	Diecious (sexes are separate), female worm lies in the gynecophoric canal of male worm
Fertilization	Self-fertilization	Cross fertilization

*2nd intermediate host is aquatic plant for *Fasciola* and *Fasciolopsis*; crayfish or crab for *Opisthorchis*, *Clonorchis* and *Paragonimus*

Life cycle of Trematodes except schistosomes

Metacercaria larvae (infective form) present in second intermediate host (aquatic plant or fish) → Transmitted to man by ingestion → Larvae migrate to their habitat (intestine, liver, bile duct or lungs) → Develop into adult worms → Adult worms undergo self-fertilization → Eggs produced, which are passed in feces or sputum → Eggs develop in water into miracidium larvae* → Ingested by snail (1st intermediate host) → Transform to sporocyst → Rediae (1st and 2nd generations) → Cercaria larvae → Infective to second intermediate hosts such as plant or fish (ingestion) → Develop to metacercaria (infective form to man) → Life cycle continues

*Note: In *Clonorchis* and *Opisthorchis*, the eggs hatch to release miracidium only after ingestion by suitable snail host.

Life cycle of schistosomes

Cercaria larvae (infective form) present freely in water → Transmitted to man by skin penetration → Larvae penetrate to venous circulation and migrate to their habitat (intestine or kidney) → Develop into adult worms → Adult worms undergo cross-fertilization → Eggs produced, which are passed in feces or urine → Eggs develop in water into miracidium larvae → Ingested by snail (1st intermediate host) → Transform to sporocyst (1st and 2nd generations) → Transform to cercaria larva → Cercaria larva released in water (infective form to man) → Life cycle continues.

The detail of epidemiology, clinical manifestations, laboratory diagnosis and treatment have been discussed under the individual trematodes in the subsequent text of this Chapter.

BLOOD FLUKES

SCHISTOSOMA SPECIES

The schistosomes are known as **blood flukes** as they live in vascular system of humans and other vertebrate hosts. They cause **schistosomiasis** which is the second most devastating tropical parasitic disease (after malaria), affecting more than 200 million people residing in rural and agricultural areas. *Schistosoma* species belong to:
❖ **Order:** Strigeida
❖ **Superfamily:** Schistosomatoidea
❖ **Family:** Schistosomatidae.

The schistosomes that parasitize humans are categorized into African and Asian species (Table 11.3). The important species are *S. haematobium* and *S. mansoni* (found in Africa) and *S. japonicum* (found in Asia).

Morphology

The general morphology of schistosomes is similar to any trematodes described earlier; exist in three forms: adult worm, larva and egg. However, they differ from other trematodes in many ways which is discussed below and in Table 11.2.

Adult Worm

Adult worms live in the venous plexuses of definitive hosts (hence called as **blood flukes**).
❖ The body is cylindrical, covered by a thick (4 μm), tuberculated and syncytial tegument (except in *S. japonicum* which possesses a smooth tegument)
❖ There is no muscular pharynx and the intestinal caeca reunite behind the ventral sucker to form a single canal
❖ Suckers are armed with delicate spines
❖ Schistosomes are diecious and can live for 20–30 years
❖ **Size:** The male worm is 12-15 mm in length and 0.5-1 mm in breadth. Female worm is slightly longer and slender; 16-22 mm in length and 0.25 mm in breadth
❖ Male worm possesses a sex canal (**gynecophoric canal**) on ventral side in which the female worm reposes (Fig. 11.1A). The female worm matures sexually only in presence of male worm; which may be attributed to selective gene expression in the reproductive tract of the female worm when it comes in contact with male worm
❖ The number of testes in male worms varies from four to nine
❖ The Laurer's canal is absent in female worms.

Table 11.3: Schistosomes that parasitize humans

Schistosomes	Definitive host	Intermediate host (various genera of snail)	Distribution
African schistosomes			
Schistosoma haematobium	Man, monkey, chimpanzee	Bulinus	Africa and Middle East
Schistosoma mansoni	Man, monkey, chimpanzee and dog	Biomphalaria	Africa and South America and Caribbean
Schistosoma intercalatum	Man	Bulinus	West and Central Africa
Asian schistosomes			
Schistosoma japonicum	Man, dog, cat and rodent	Oncomelania	China and Philippines
Schistosoma malayensis	Man and rodent	Robertsiella	Malaysia
Schistsoma mekongi	Man and dog	Neotricula	Laos and Thailand

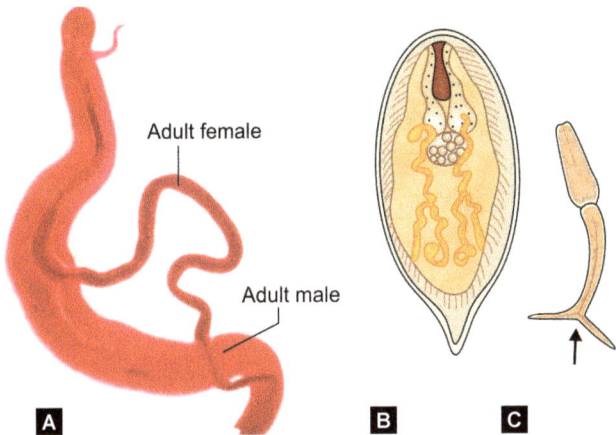

Fig. 11.1A to C: (A) Adult worms of schistosomes (The thin female worm resides in the gynecophoric canal of the thicker male worm); (B) Terminal spined egg of *S. hematobium*; (C) Fork tailed cercaria

Source: A—DPDx Image Library, Centers for Disease Control and Prevention (CDC), Atlanta (with permission).

Eggs

Schistosomes lay non-operculated eggs with a spine like projection. The size of the eggs varies depending up on the species; ranging from 70–180 µm length × 40–73 µm breadth. The location of spine differs between the species; which helps in their identification, for example:
- *S. haematobium*: possesses terminal spine (Fig. 11.1B)
- *S. mansoni*: possesses lateral spine
- *S. japonicum*: possesses lateral rudimentary inconspicuous spine.

Larva

Various larval forms are miracidium, sporocysts (first and second generations), and cercaria.
- There are no rediae and metacercariae stages
- The cercaria larvae are the infective form. They are elongated and oval with 400 × 60 µm size; have a characteristic forked (bifurcated) tail (Fig. 11.1C). They have a life span of 24–72 hours.

Hosts

Humans are the definitive host and snails are the intermediate host. Unlike other trematodes, there is no second intermediate host.

SCHISTOSOMA HAEMATOBIUM

History

Schistosoma haematobium is the causative agent of **urinary schistosomiasis or bilharziasis**. Theodor Bilharz in 1851 detected the adult worm and the terminal spined eggs in the mesenteric veins of a young man at autopsy.

Habitat

Adult male worm holds the female worm and resides in the venous plexus of urinary bladder and ureter.

Epidemiology

Approximately, 200–300 million individuals are infected with schistosomes globally across 74 countries. Large majority (85%) live in sub-Saharan Africa, where >2 Lakh deaths per year occur due to schistosomiasis.

S. haematobium infection is endemic in 53 countries in the Middle East, the African continent (across Nile river valley) and the Indian Ocean islands (Madagascar, Zanzibar and Pemba).

India: Schistosomiasis is extremely rare in India. A confirmed endemic focus of urinary schistosomiasis was demonstrated in Gimvi village of Ratnagiri district, Maharashtra; transmitted by snail of genus *Ferrissia*.

Morphology

Adult worms, eggs and larvae are the three forms. They are morphologically similar to other schistosomes as described earlier, with some minor differences (Table 11.4).

Life Cycle (Fig. 11.2)

Host: There are two types of hosts:
1. **Definitive host:** Man is the definitive host.

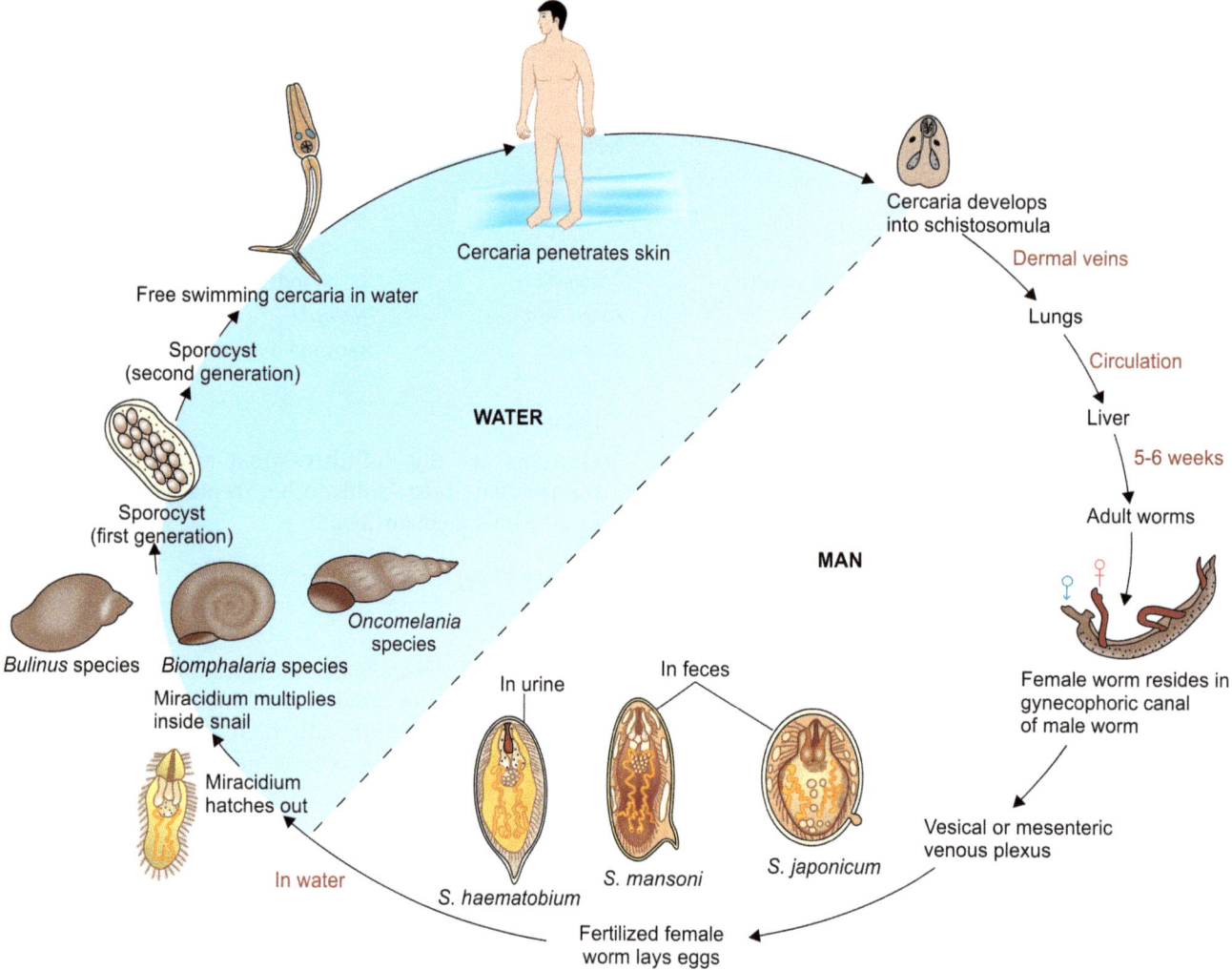

Fig. 11.2: Life cycle of *Schistosoma* species

2. **Intermediate host:** Freshwater snails of genus *Bulinus*.

Mode of transmission: Man acquires infection by penetration of skin by the infective form (cercariae) present in contaminated water.

Development in Man

The free swimming infective cercaria penetrates the intact epidermis with the help of oral and ventral suckers. It loses its tail and outer coating to become the next stage larva, **schistosomula**.

- The schistosomula travels via dermal veins to reach lungs and from there via the systemic circulation, it enters the portal system
- Within liver sinusoids, it feeds and grows for a period of 5–6 weeks to develop into adult worm
- Adult worms become sexually mature, pairing of worms take place, female worms reside in the gynecophoric canal of male worms. They migrate from the portal system, move against the blood flow and reach vesical and ureteric venous plexus
- The young flukes become coated with host red cell antigens and histocompatibility antigens, so that they are not recognized as foreign and escape from the host immune response
- Fertilized female worm lays eggs in these venous plexus. Fertilized female worm contains 20–200 eggs at one time. The eggs penetrate the venules and urinary mucosa with the help of terminal spine and the lytic substances secreted by them. Eggs along with blood are excreted in urine
- **Pre-patent period:** It is the time taken between the penetration of cercariae and the first production of eggs, which is usually within 3 months.

Development in Water

The fully embryonated eggs are passed in urine. When these eggs gain access into the water they hatch after 8–10 days to release free-swimming miracidium.

Development in snail

Miracidium lives in water for 8-12 hours and infect snails of *Bulinus* species.

- ❖ In snail, the miracidium multiplies asexually giving rise to first and second generation sporocysts which on further development, transforms to fork tailed cercaria. Redial stage is absent
- ❖ A single miracidium can give rise to ~10^5 cercariae. The cercariae escape from the snail into water and cause human infection. The cycle is repeated.

Pathogenesis and Clinical Features

Acute Schistosomiasis

The invasion of cercariae in the skin causes dermatitis at penetration site followed by allergic pruritic papular lesion. Migration of schistosomula in lungs causes cough with mild fever.

Chronic Schistosomiasis

Urogenital disease

Light infection may be asymptomatic. Symptoms develop usually after 3–6 months.

- ❖ The adult worms are rarely pathogenic. The main pathogenic mechanism in schistosomiasis is due to the eggs deposited in various tissues
- ❖ The eggs passing into urinary bladder cause the mucosal damage that leads to dysuria and hematuria (seen upto 80% of children infected)
- ❖ The soluble antigens released from the eggs provoke delayed type of hypersensitivity reaction around them. This leads to the formation of egg granuloma composed of egg at the center surrounded by macrophages, lymphocytes, fibroblasts, and multinucleated giant cells
- ❖ The granuloma varies in size. Many granulomas are joined together, to form larger nodules. The urinary mucosa covering the nodules shows glandular metaplasia (**cystitis glandularis**)
- ❖ Later on, in chronic stage fibrotic changes occur, visible as sandy patches on cystoscopy
- ❖ In heavy infection, male genital organs are frequently affected. Deposition of the eggs in scrotal lymphatics may cause elephantiasis in scrotum and penis
- ❖ *S. haematobium* infection may be an important risk factor for potential activation and transmission of HIV.

Obstructive uropathies

Fibrosis may cause obstruction of the lower end of the ureters that result in hydroureter and hydronephrosis, which may be seen in 25–50% of infected children.

Bladder carcinoma

The metaplastic changes in urinary mucosa may lead to carcinoma of bladder.

- ❖ **Predisposing factors**
  - Diet containing nitroso compounds intake, commonly found in Egyptian food (cheese, fava beans, raw salted fish)
  - Secondary bacterial infections, causing cystitis
  - Genetic factors: Such as activation of *H-ras*, inactivation of p53 and retinoblastoma genes.
- ❖ **Type:** Squamous cell carcinoma is the most common type. It is seen with high to moderate worm burden; whereas transitional cell carcinoma may occur in areas with lighter worm load.

Involvement of other sites

Eggs may be carried by venous blood to various parts of the body like spinal cord, liver, lungs or intestine and produce similar granulomas.

> **Laboratory Diagnosis**   *Schistosoma haematobium*
>
> - ❑ **Urine microscopy**—detects terminal spined eggs
> - ❑ **Histopathology** of bladder mucosal biopsy—detects terminal spined eggs
> - ❑ **Antibody detection** (serum)—HAMA-FAST-ELISA, HAMA-EITB, IFA, IHA and cercarial Huller reaction
> - ❑ **Antigen detection** (serum and urine)—CCA and CAA detection by ELISA or dip stick assay.

Laboratory Diagnosis

Urine Microscopy

Diagnosis of *S. haematobium* is made by detection of non-operculated terminal spined eggs in the urine or rarely in feces (Figs 11.1B and 11.3A).

The terminal hematuria portion of urine is collected between 12 pm and 3 pm, concentrated by centrifugation or by membrane filtration and observed under microscope for the presence of non operculated terminal spined eggs.

> **Cross-over infection**
>
> Though eggs of *S. haematobium* and *S. mansoni* are usually found in urine and stool respectively; in heavy infection, *S. haematobium* eggs can be found in stool and *S. mansoni* eggs may be passed in urine. This is due to adult worms may be found in the vessels that are not their normal habitat. This finding is known as "crossover" infection.

Histopathology

S. haematobium eggs can be demonstrated in bladder mucosal biopsy or wet cervical biopsy specimens (in

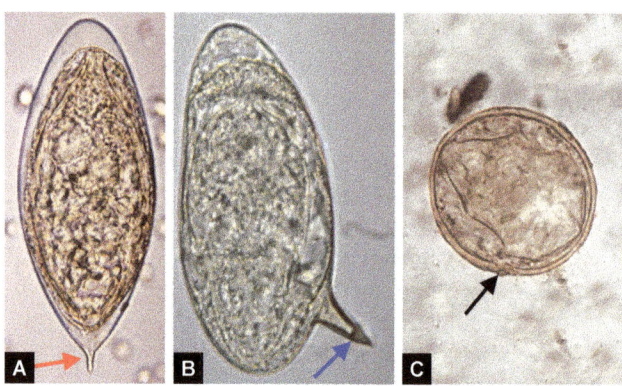

Figs 11.3A to C: *Schistosoma* eggs (A) *S. haematobium*; (B) *S. mansoni*; (C) *S. japonicum*
Source: A—ID# 4843, B—ID# 4841, C—ID#4842. Public Health Image Library, Centers for Disease Control and Prevention (CDC), Atlanta (*with permission*).

females). The number of eggs present in crushed tissue correlates significantly with the size of the genital lesions.

Antibody Detection

The tests for detection of antibody are useful for sero-epidemiology.
- Two assays are available to detect serum antibodies against *S. haematobium* adult worm microsomal antigen (HAMA)
  - **HAMA-FAST-ELISA** [Falcon assay screening test ELISA] is a new test with high sensitivity (95%) and specificity (99%)
  - **HAMA-EITB** (enzyme-linked immunotransfer blot).
- Other antibody detection methods are—cercarial Huller reaction, and indirect fluorescent antibody test (IFA) and indirect hemagglutination (IHA) test
- IgE and IgG4 are elevated in schistosomiasis like any other helminthic infections.

Antigen Detection

Detection of circulating antigen indicates recent infection and can be used for monitoring the treatment response. They are also useful when urine microscopy fails to detect eggs (chronic and ectopic cases).
- Circulating cathodic antigen (CCA) and circulating anodic antigen (CAA) can be detected in serum and urine by ELISA or dip stick assays. CCA levels are much higher in urine than CAA
- ELISA-based assay using specific monoclonal antibodies against soluble egg antigen (M Ab-SEA) shows sensitivity of 90% (serum) and 94% (urine)
- Other ELISA assays are based on antigens such as 290-2E6-A and 128C3/3/21.

| Treatment | *Schistosoma haematobium* |

Praziquantel is the drug of choice; given 20 mg/kg/dose, two doses in single day.
Metrifonate can be give alternatively. It inhibits acetylcholine receptors on tegument surface of adult male worm. It is administered in multiple oral doses over weeks; hence not preferred in control programs.

Prevention

Preventive measures include:
- Proper disposal of human excreta and urine
- Eradication of snails by using molluscicides such as metal salts (iron or aluminum sulfate), metaldehyde, methiocarb and acetylcholine esterase inhibitors
- Treatment of infected persons.

Elimination of Schistosomiasis

The WHO is currently moving towards elimination of schistosomiasis as a public health problem in Africa by 2020 and globally by 2025. This may be achieved through treatment of cases using praziquantel to prevent morbidity in later life and also through mass drug administration in some places (Egypt and China).

SCHISTOSOMA MANSONI

S. mansoni produces intestinal schistosomiasis in humans. Sir Patrick Manson first noted the lateral spined eggs of this parasite in West Indies and Sambon proposed the name *S. mansoni*.

Habitat

Adult male and female worms reside in mesenteric veins draining sigmoidorectal region.

Epidemiology

S. mansoni infection is common in 54 countries; from African countries including Madagascar, South America (Brazil and Argentina), Caribbean Islands (West Indies) and Arabian Peninsula. No cases have been reported from India so far.

Morphology

- Adult worms are similar to other schistosomes with some minor differences (Table 11.4)
- Nonoperculated eggs have characteristic lateral spine. They measure 114–180 μm × 45–73 μm (see Fig. 11.3B)
- Fork tailed cercaria is the infective form.

Life Cycle

Life cycle of *S. mansoni* is similar to *S. haematobium* except:

Table 11.4: Comparison of species of *Schistosoma*.			
Features	Schistosoma haematobium	Schistosoma mansoni	Schistosoma japonicum
Habitat of adult worm	Vesical and pelvic venous plexuses	Mesenteric veins draining sigmoidorectal region	Mesenteric veins draining ileocecal region
Tegument	Small tubercles	Large papillae with spines	Smooth
Size (male)	15 × 0.9 mm	12 × 0.8–1 mm	15 × 0.5 mm
Size (female)	20 × 0.25 mm	16 × 0.25 mm	22 × 0.3 mm
Number of testes	4–5 in cluster	6–9 in cluster	7 in linear
Uterus	With 20–100 eggs at one time	Short; one egg at one time	Long; contain 50 eggs at one time
Egg	Elliptical with sharp terminal spine; 112–170 × 40–70 µm in size. Egg shell is not acid-fast, miracidium larva inside egg is acid-fast	Elliptical with sharp lateral spine; 114–180 µm × 45–73 µm in size. Eggs shell is acid-fast	Oval to almost spherical; rudimentary lateral knob; 70–100 µm × 50–65 µm in size. Egg shell is acid-fast
Egg discharged in	Urine	Feces	Feces

- Humans are the definitive host; sometimes other vertebrate hosts like monkeys, chimpanzees and dogs may act as reservoir and definitive host
- Fresh water snails of *Biomphalaria* species are intermediate hosts
- Prepatent period is about 4–7 weeks
- The adult worm lives in mesenteric veins draining sigmoidorectal region.

Pathogenesis and Clinical Feature

In general, the pathogenesis of mansonian schistosomiasis occurs in three stages.

Cercarial Dermatitis

After 2 or 3 days of cercarial invasion, an itchy maculopapular rash develops on the affected areas of the skin called as cercarial dermatitis **(swimmer's itch)**. This is also observed in *S. japonicum* infection.

Cercarial dermatitis is particularly severe when humans are exposed to avian schistosomes (*Trichobilharzia* species and *Orientobilharizia* species) and mammalian schistosomes (*Gigantobilharzia* species and *Microbilharzia* species). Man being an aberrant host, these parasites don't undergo further development. This condition occurs when a person from non-endemic area visit to an area endemic for these schistosomes. Cercariae die in the skin and evoke severe allergic responses.

Acute Schistosomiasis (Katayama Syndrome)

The acute phase of disease occurs within 4–8 weeks of infection, especially when the schistosomes start producing eggs. It is less common in endemic area.
- The antigens (released from eggs) and the adult worms stimulate the host humoral response, leading to the formation of immune complexes and serum sickness like illness called **Katayama fever**
- It is characterized by fever, generalized lymphadenopathy, and hepatosplenomegaly. Parasite-specific antibodies may be detected. There is a high peripheral blood eosinophilia.

Chronic Schistosomiasis

After eggs are produced, they are trapped in the small venules and are carried into the intestine (or less commonly to bladder) and are excreted in feces. Some are carried through portal circulation into liver and other parts of the body.

Intestinal disease

The eggs are deposited in the intestinal wall. Soluble antigens liberated from eggs induce inflammatory reactions that lead to granuloma formation around the eggs in the intestine.
- Fibrosis and thickening occurs in the intestinal wall along the entire length of colon and rectum
- Patient may present with diarrhea or dysentery.

Hepatosplenic disease

Granuloma formation and fibrosis in liver (called as **Symmers pipestem fibrosis**) seriously impedes the portal blood flow leading to portal hypertension, hepatomegaly (seen in 15-20%), splenomegaly and gastric varices.
- In schistosomiasis, the spleen is enlarged and hard, which should be differentiated from soft spleen of leishmaniasis
- *S. mansoni* is increasingly associated with hepatitis C virus; particularly in Egypt (up to 50% prevalence) and accelerates the occurrence of chronic hepatitis and cirrhosis in these patients.

Other body sites

Eggs are carried in circulation to distant sites such as lungs, brain, spinal cord, causing egg sequestration and granuloma formation.
- **Pulmonary involvement** leads to pulmonary hypertension and right sided heart failure

- **Neuroschistosomiasis** involving brain and spinal cord: Myelopathy of the lumbosacral region is the most common neurological manifestation of *S. mansoni* or *S. haematobium* infection; whereas acute encephalitis is typical of *S. japonicum* infection
- **Kidney:** Nephrosclerosis and kidney failure may occur due to circulating immune complexes deposited in glomerular membrane, (not due to egg deposition)
- Secondary bacterial infection can occur, especially with *Salmonella* species and *Staphylococcus aureus*
- **Liver abscess:** *S. aureus* colonizes the granuloma formed by *S. mansoni* in liver, that leads to liver abscess.

Laboratory Diagnosis

Stool Microscopy

In acute cases, eggs with lateral spine can be demonstrated in stool or rarely in urine (see Fig. 11.3B).

In chronic cases or in patients with low worm burden, the number of eggs excreted in stool is less and intermittent. Hence, the following ways can be employed to increase the sensitivity
- Multiple stool specimens should be examined
- Stool concentration techniques by centrifugal sedimentation should be followed
- **Hatching test:** This involves hatching of motile miracidia when the eggs are diluted in water in a side armed flask and perpendicular beam of light is passed through the water at the top; and inspecting the lighted area with a hand lens, every 30 minutes for four hours. Hatching of miracidium (observed as minute white organisms swimming rapidly in a straight line) confirms the viability of the parasite
- The quantitation of eggs in stool specimens can be done by Kato thick smear technique or by Ritchie's method.

Rectal Biopsy Specimen

- Histopathological demonstration of lateral spined eggs in biopsy material from rectal mucosa confirms the diagnosis of schistosomiasis (Fig. 11.4)
- Alternatively, the biopsy tissue can be crushed between two glass slides and stained without sectioning. This technique is more effective than histologic examination as it allows to determine the viability of the eggs by closely observing the flame cell activity within the miracidium larva, inside the egg
- Egg shell of **S. mansoni** is acid-fast and can be stained by modified Ziehl-Neelsen stain.

Antibody Detection

Antibody detection tests are less useful as they cross-react with other helminth infections, become positive slowly and remain positive even after successful treatment.

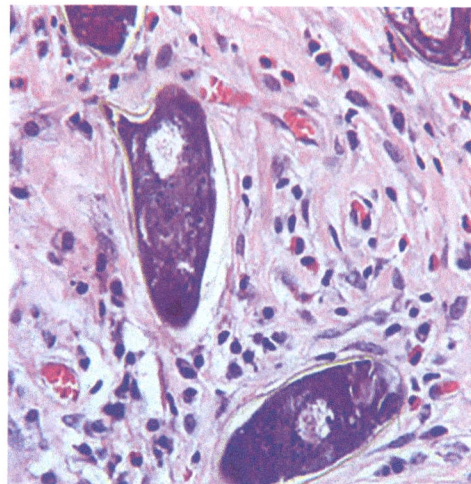

Fig. 11.4: Eggs of *S. mansoni* in liver tissue (stained with H&E)
Source: Dr Munaf Desai, Al Qassimi Hospital, Sharjah, United Arab Emirates; DPDx Image Library, Centers for Disease Control and Prevention (CDC), Atlanta (*with permission*).

- Various tests available are circumoval precipitin test, cercaria-Huller reaction, IFA, IHA, ELISA and EITB
- They detect antibodies by employing antigens such as soluble adult worm or egg antigens.

Antigen Detection

Antigen detection is useful for assessing the severity of disease and to monitor the efficacy of treatment.
- ELISA is available to detect circulating schistosome antigens (CCA and CAA) in the serum and urine
- Dipstick test is available for detecting CCA in urine; showed sensitivity of 92%.

Treatment	*Schistosoma mansoni*
Praziquantel is the drug of choice; given 20 mg/kg/dose, two doses in single day. Oxamniquine is also very effective. **Drug resistance** ☐ Resistance to praziquantel has not been detected yet. However, low-level tolerance has been reported for *S. mansoni*. Resistance to oxamniquine is reported from South America ☐ Artemisinin derivatives used for malaria are active against immature worm (schistosomula) and may be used in future for praziquantel insensitive strains of *S. mansoni*.	

Prevention

Prevention of *S. mansoni* infection is same as that for *S. haematobium*.

SCHISTOSOMA JAPONICUM

It is the most pathogenic species among the schistosomes. It is the only schistosome species that shows zoonotic transmission.

Habitat

Adult worms reside in the mesenteric veins draining the ileocecal region.

Epidemiology

S. japonicum infection occurs most commonly in China, Indonesia and Philippines. It is eradicated from Japan since 1960. Children of 5–10 years of age are commonly affected. No cases have been reported from India so far.

Morphology

Adult worms are similar to other schistosomes (Table 11.4) with the following differences:
- **Tegument:** The body surface is smooth
- The eggs are relatively smaller (70–100 μm length × 50–65 μm width) and more spherical than those of other schistosomes and have rudimentary lateral spine (may be absent in some strains) (*see* Fig. 11.3C).

Life Cycle

Life cycle of **S. japonicum** is similar to that of *S. mansoni* with few exceptions:
- Definitive host is mainly man and sometimes domestic animals like cat, dog and cattle
- Intermediate host—snails of *Oncomelania* species
- The prepatent period is around 5 weeks
- **Higher egg output:** The female worm lays more than 3,000 eggs/day.

Pathogenesis and Clinical Features

Pathogenesis is almost similar to that caused by *S. mansoni*. However, the disease is more severe because of the higher egg production and smaller size of the eggs (easy dissemination). The manifestations seen are as follows.
- **Cercarial dermatitis** (described under *S. mansoni*)
- **Katayama fever:** It is seen after 40 days of infection. It is more severe and sometimes leads to death
- **Intestinal disease:** Deposition of egg granulomas in the intestinal wall (large intestine) leads to mucosal hyperplasia, ulcers, micro abscess formation and sometimes, pseudopolyposis with blood loss
- **Hepatosplenic disease:** Seen due to granulomatous response surrounding the eggs. Left lobe of liver is the most common site involved
- **Cerebral schistosomiasis:** It occurs in 2–4% of cases, due to migration of eggs. Parietal lobe is the most common site
    - Symptoms include Jacksonian convulsions and grand mal seizures
    - The higher incidence of CNS involvement of *S. japonicum* compared to other schistomes is attributed to their small size eggs; which are released in higher numbers from the worm, and can be carried easily to CNS.
- **Carcinoma:** Both colorectal carcinoma and liver carcinoma (and cirrhosis) have been reported from people of China and Japan infected with *S. japonicum*
- Chronic secondary infection with *Salmonella* species and hepatitis B virus have been associated with *S. japonicum*.

Laboratory Diagnosis

The diagnostic methods of *S. japonicum* is similar to that of *S. mansoni*. The additional information is described here.
- **Pyrosequencing:** Egg of *S. japonicum* is difficult to differentiate from that of *S. mekongi*. A **pyrosequencing** assay has been designed to detect DNA specific to *S. japonicum* and *S. mekongi* in fecal samples and in infected snails
- **Magnetic fractionation method:** Here, the magnetic microspheres are used which bind to the eggs in stool specimen and form egg—microsphere conjugate. *S. japonicum* eggs have higher affinity to bind microspheres than *S. mansoni* eggs due to higher localization of iron in its egg shell. This test is useful for screening of large volume of samples with a good diagnostic sensitivity

Treatment	*Schistosoma japonicum*
Praziquantel is given 20 mg/kg/dose, three doses in single day.	

Vaccine

No vaccine is licensed for schistosomiasis yet. However, several trials are going on using various vaccine candidates such as:
- Bilhvax trial: 28-kDa glutathione S-transferase of *S. haematobium* (Sh28GST), tested in human volunteers
- *S. mansoni* surface protein tetraspanin (Sm-TSP-2), tested in mice
- Sm-p80 (large subunit of calpain) of *S. mansoni*; has shown cross protection against *S. haematobium*, tested in baboons
- *S. japonicum* recombinant paramyosin muscle protein antigen.

SCHISTOSOMA INTERCALATUM

S. intercalatum remains endemic in 10 countries in Central and West Africa.
- **Clinical features:** Similar to *S. mansoni* like intestinal, hepatosplenic manifestations and secondary *Salmonella* infections
- **Laboratory diagnosis:** Eggs resemble with that of *S. haematobium* (with a terminal spine), but of large size (140–240 μm × 50–85 μm) and acid-fast positive

❖ **Treatment:** Praziquantel is the drug of choice; given 20 mg/kg/dose, two doses in single day.

Schistosomiasis in India
- Human schistosomiasis is extremely rare in India. This may be due to many reasons such as—absence of appropriate intermediate host (snails), environmental conditions and host immune mechanisms
- A confirmed endemic focus of urinary schistosomiasis was demonstrated in Gimvi village of Ratnagiri district, Maharashtra in 1952. It was found to be transmitted by snail of genus *Ferrissia*. More than 600 cases were reported mainly affecting people of 10–20 years of age. However, with the help of World Health Organization (WHO), it was eliminated from that place
- **Cercarial dermatitis** has been reported in high proportion in rural/tribal population of Assam, Chhattisgarh and Madhya Pradesh in people who use water from ponds and water tanks
- Even cases of **hepatic schistosomiasis** caused by *S. incognitum* were reported by Chandler in 1926
- **Paddy field dermatitis:** Cercarial larvae of many of the avian species can cause dermatitis in the rice filed workers and is called as paddy field dermatitis (farmer's dermatitis). Rice field dermatitis is an occupational health problem in Assam (*S. spindalis*), also seen in other countries like Japan, Malaysia and Thailand.

SCHISTOSOMA MEKONGI

S. mekongi infection occurs in the Mekong river basin of Laos, Thailand and Cambodia.
- Man and dogs are the **definitive hosts**. Snails of the Genus *Neotricula aperta* serve as **intermediate hosts**
- **Clinical features:** It is similar to that caused by *S. japonicum*, with intestinal, hepatosplenic and brain involvement
- **Laboratory diagnosis:** Eggs are spherical, similar to that of *S. japonicum* except that they are smaller (30–55 μm × 50–65 μm). Antibody and antigen detection methods are also available similar to that of other schistosomes
- **Treatment:** Praziquantel is the drug of choice; given 20 mg/kg/dose, three doses in single day.

LIVER FLUKES

FASCIOLA HEPATICA

Fasciola hepatica, also known as the **common liver fluke or sheep liver fluke**. The disease is called **fascioliasis**. In addition to humans, it also infects sheep and other domestic animals. *F. hepatica* was the first trematode to be described and the first for which the entire life cycle was defined (Leuckart and Thomas in 1883).

Habitat
The parasite lives in the liver and bile duct.

Epidemiology
Fascioliasis is a cosmopolitan zoonotic disease. It is particularly endemic in sheep-raising countries.
- **World:** Fascioliasis is an important health problem in Peru, Bolivia, and Chile; although cases have been reported worldwide, affecting over 2.4 million people.
- **India:** Human fascioliasis in India is extremely uncommon. Only few cases are reported so far, mainly from North and Northeastern India including Assam, Uttar Pradesh and Bihar. Recently, few cases are reported from Mumbai and Vellore. Various animal studies indicate that *F. gigantica* is more prevalent in India than *F. hepatica*.

Morphology

Adult Worm
The adult worm is large in size (3 cm length by 1.2 cm breadth), flat, leaf-shaped, brown colored (Figs 11.5 and 11.6A).
- **Suckers:** The anterior end has a conical projection (shoulder) containing oral sucker while the posterior end is rounded. The ventral sucker is situated away from the oral sucker
- Intestine is bifurcated and incomplete and bears lateral branches
- It is hermaphrodite with both male and female reproductive organs.

Egg
Eggs are oval, bile stained, unembryonated and operculated (Fig. 11.6B).

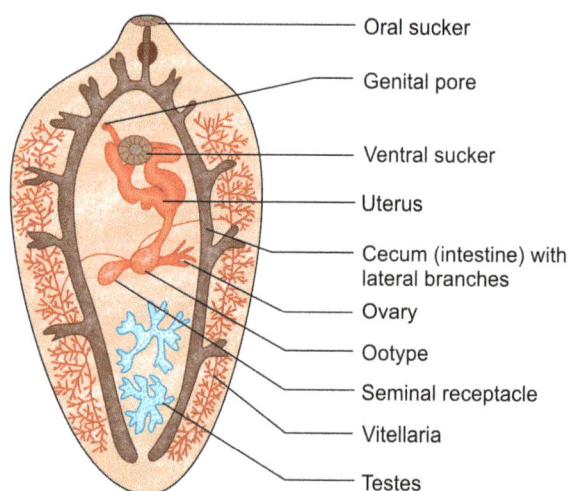

Fig. 11.5: Adult worm of *Fasciola hepatica* (schematic diagram)

CHAPTER 11 ◆ Trematodes or Flukes

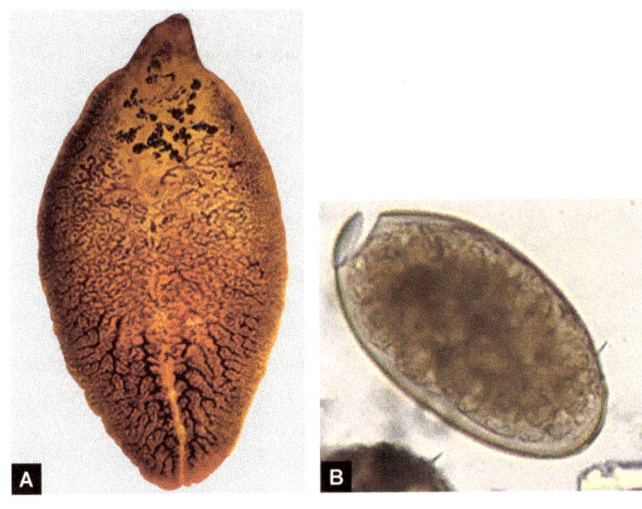

Figs 11.6A and B: *Fasciola hepatica* (A) Adult worm (carmine-stained); (B) Egg (saline mount)
Source: A and B—DPDx Image Library, Centers for Disease Control and Prevention (CDC), Atlanta (*with permission*).

- **Large size:** Measures about 130–150 μm by 63–90 μm size
- The eggs of *F. hepatica* are similar to that of *Fasciolopsis buski* and cannot be differentiated.

Larva

Metacercaria larva is the infective form for man and other definitive hosts. Other larval forms are miracidia, rediae and sporocysts.

Life Cycle (Fig. 11.7)

Host: Sheep is the principal definitive host. Goats cattle and humans are other definitive hosts. The amphibian snails (Genus: *Lymnaea*) are the first intermediate hosts and water plants serve as the second intermediate hosts.

Mode of transmission: The sheep and other definitive hosts including man get infection by eating water plants and water cress containing metacercariae.

Development in Man or Sheep

In duodenum, the metacercariae excyst and penetrate through intestinal wall to reach peritoneal cavity.
- The larvae invade liver tissue and migrate through the liver parenchyma into the hepatic ducts where they mature into adult worms in about 9 weeks of infection
- Inside the hepatic duct the fluke starts laying unembryonated eggs which come back to the intestine and are excreted in the feces.

Development in Water

The eggs further develop in water in 1–2 weeks to release miracidium at 22–26°C.

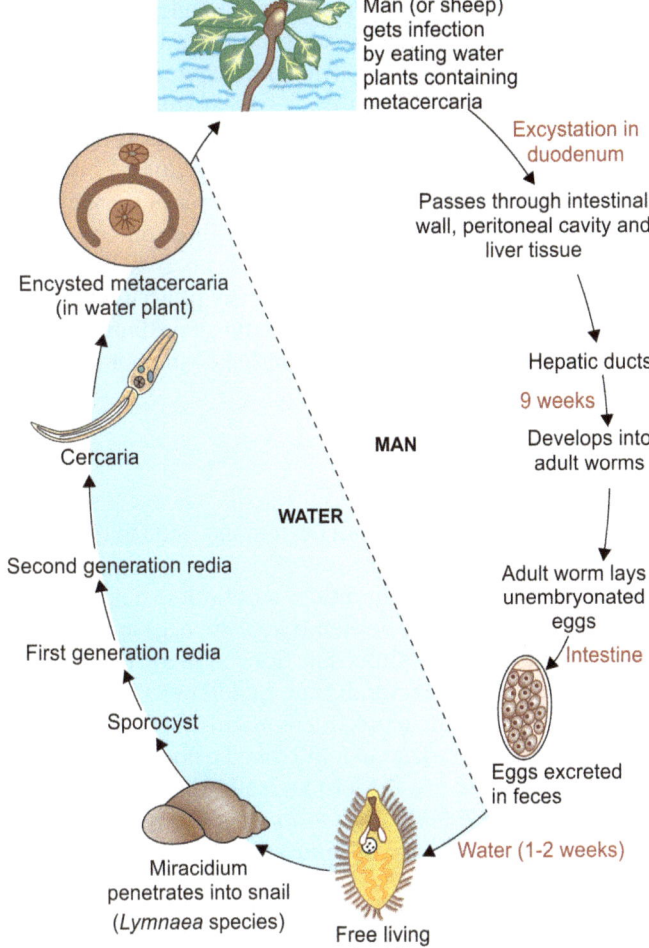

Fig. 11.7: Life cycle of *Fasciola hepatica*

Development in snails

The miracidium penetrates the suitable snail host. Inside the snail host, the miracidium multiplies and transforms into sporocysts, which further develop into two generations of rediae. Finally, the rediae give rise to cercariae.

Development in aquatic plants

The cercariae escape from the snails and infect the water plants where they encyst to form metacercariae. Metacercariae when ingested by the definitive host, cause infection and the cycle is repeated.

Pathogenesis

Incubation period varies from days to few months. *F. hepatica* produces both acute and chronic infections.
- **Acute disease** develops during metacercarial migration (1–2 weeks after infection) and includes fever, right-upper-quadrant pain, hepatomegaly and eosinophilia. CT scan of the liver may show migratory tracks. The adult worm can cause obstruction of the bile duct and

dilatation of the biliary tract. Liver and bile duct damage is possibly as a result of toxins produced by the larvae
- In **chronic phase**, the liver parenchyma is inflamed with formation of multiple subcapsular abscesses (called as **liver rot**). Bile duct obstruction by adult worm and biliary cirrhosis are also reported but less commonly. However, liver malignancy is not associated
- **Halzoun or Marrara syndrome:** In endemic areas where uncooked goat and sheep livers may be eaten, the adult worms may attach to the pharyngeal wall; causing severe pharyngitis and laryngeal edema. This is described as Halzoun syndrome in Lebanon or Marrara in Sudan.

Laboratory Diagnosis

Stool Microscopy

Typical operculated eggs can be demonstrated in the stool specimen (see Fig. 11.6B).
- However in acute condition, stool microscopy is not useful as the worm burden is less and eggs appear late during the course of infection. Concentration techniques (sedimentation methods) can be followed to increase the sensitivity. Floatation methods are not useful
- It should also be kept in mind that the operculated eggs of *F. hepatica* are morphologically similar to that of *F. gigantica*, *F. buski*, *Echinostoma* and *Gastrodiscoides*
- **Spurious infection (pseudofascioliasis):** Sometimes, eggs may be detected in the stool of people who have eaten *F. hepatica* infected liver. This can be differentiated from true infection by stool examination of the patient, 3 days after a liver free diet.

Antibody Detection

Detection of serum antibodies against excretion secretion antigen helps in early diagnosis before the eggs are detected in stool.
- Various serological tests available are ELISA, counterimmune electrophoresis and Western blot techniques
- They are useful for seroepidemiological study and to monitor the response to treatment.

Molecular Methods

Various PCR-based methods are available to detect *F. hepatica* specific genes in stool specimens. PCR is highly sensitive and specific compared to stool examination and serology even in light infection; may serve as a future tool for diagnosis.

Other Methods

- Imaging methods—like ultrasound, CT scan or MRI can be employed to detect the lesions in the liver

- Peripheral blood eosinophilia
- Elevated serum IgE and IgG4 antibodies.

Treatment	*Fasciola hepatica*
☐ Triclabendazole (10 mg/kg once) is the drug of choice for fascioliasis	
☐ Bithionol and praziquantel are the other alternative drugs.	

Prevention

Fascioliasis can be prevented by avoidance of consumption of alfalfa juice, raw water plants and cleaning them before use. Other measures include control of snails, health education and treatment of infected person.

FASCIOLA GIGANTICA

F. gigantica is closely related to *F. hepatica*.
- It is seen in tropics and aquatic environment and is the predominant species in Africa, Southern Europe, and some Pacific Islands
- It is a common parasite of herbivores like cattle and camels. Human infection is also reported but rare
- In India, less than 10 cases have been reported, mainly from Assam, Arunachal Pradesh and West Bengal
- **Life cycle:** Similar to that of *F. hepatica*. Only difference is first intermediate host is aquatic snail (in contrast to amphibian snail for *F. hepatica*)
- **Clinical feature:** Similar to that of *F. hepatica*, characterized by hepatomegaly and abdominal pain
- **Laboratory diagnosis:** Eggs are morphologically similar to that of *F. hepatica* and *F. buski*, but larger in size (160–190 µm × 70–90 µm)
- **Treatment:** Same as that of *F. hepatica*.

CLONORCHIS SINENSIS

Clonorchis sinensis is also called **Chinese or oriental liver fluke**. McConnell was the first to describe the adult worm and the pathologic changes in a Chinese patient who died in a medical college, Kolkata, India in 1875.

Habitat

Adult worm lives in the bile duct, pancreatic duct and common bile duct of man and other domestic animals.

Epidemiology

C. sinensis is found primarily in Eastern Asia like China, Korea, Japan and Malaysia; infects over 35 million people globally. However, infections from India are not reported so far though the first case was detected from Kolkata.

Morphology

Adult worm

Adult worms are dorsoventrally flattened, elongated, lancet-shaped, measure 10–20 mm in length and 3–5 mm in width. The characteristic distinguishing feature is the presence of two deeply lobulated and branched testes one behind another. The uterus is situated anteriorly. Adult fluke can produce 1,000–4,000 eggs per day for at least 6 months. The fluke can survive in the biliary tract for as long as 20–25 years (Figs 11.8A and 11.8B).

Egg

The eggs are flask-shaped, measure 28–35 μm × 12–19 μm and are characterized by a distinct operculum with a prominent shoulders and a tiny knob (a comma-shaped appendage) at the posterior pole. Embryonated eggs are excreted in the stool (Figs 11.8C and D).

Larva

Metacercaria is the infective form of the parasite. It is found in the flesh of the fresh water fish. Other larval stages are cercaria (Fig. 11.8E), redia, sporocyst and miracidium.

Life Cycle (Fig. 11.9)

Hosts: Man and other domestic or wild animals (like dogs, pigs, cats, minks, weasels and rats) act as definitive hosts. It requires two intermediate hosts—first, fresh water snails (*Parafossarulus* and *Bithynia*) and second, fresh water fish of family Cyprinidae.

Mode of transmission: Man acquires infection by eating undercooked fresh water fish harboring metacercariae.

Development in Man

The metacercariae excyst in the duodenum and penetrate the intestine to reach the liver. They enter the biliary capillaries, mature into adult worms and start laying operculated eggs. The fully embryonated eggs are released into the duodenum and excreted in the feces. Human cycle takes around 3 months.

Development in Snail

In contrast to other trematodes, *Clonorchis* egg hatches out inside the snail (not in water) to release miracidium which then penetrates the intestine of snail and reaches the vascular space. Miracidium multiplies and passes through single generation of sporocyst and two generations of rediae and finally converts into cercaria.

Development in Fish

Cercariae escape from the snail host and infect the fresh water fish. After 3 weeks, cercariae transform into metacercariae. When the infected fishes are ingested by definitive hosts, the life cycle is repeated.

Pathogenesis

In light worm burden: People are usually asymptomatic
In chronic infection with heavy worm burden:
- Mechanical obstruction of the bile duct and irritation due to toxin released by the flukes leads to cholangitis, dilatation of the bile duct and bile retention
- There is marked ductal epithelial hyperplasia, periductal inflammation and fibrosis
- In some cases adenomatous hyperplasia of the ductal epithelium is seen

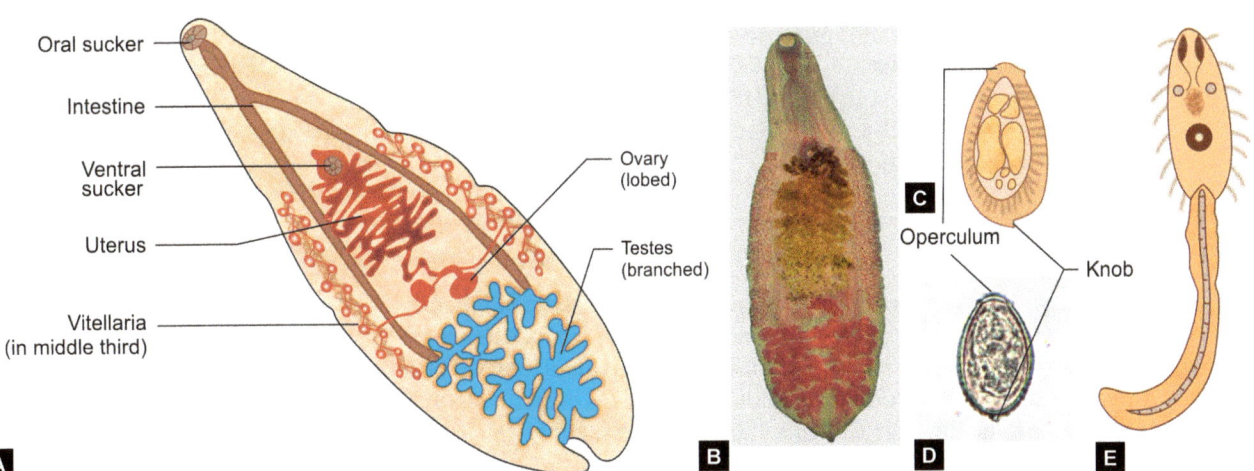

Figs 11.8A to E: *Clonorchis sinensis*: (A) Adult worm (schematic); (B) Adult worm (carmine-stained); (C) Egg (schematic); (D); Egg (saline mount) showing the small knob at the abopercular end (flask-shaped appearance); (E) Cercaria larva
Source: B and D—DPDx Image Library, Centers for Disease Control and Prevention (CDC), Atlanta (*with permission*).

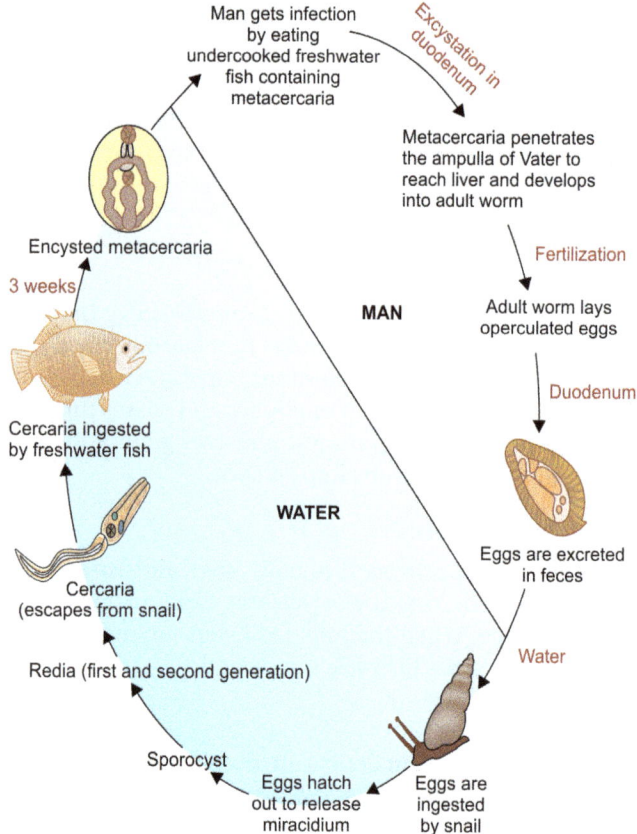

Fig. 11.9: Life cycle of *Clonorchis sinensis*

- **Bile duct carcinoma:** Chronic irritation of the bile duct for long periods can lead to **cholangiocarcinoma**. *C. sinensis* is a promotor but not an initiator for cholangiocarcinoma.
  - Risk factors for the bile duct carcinoma include elderly people (60–80 years old) and pre-existing primary sclerosing cholangitis
  - Inhibition of tumor suppressor genes (P53) and release of cytokines such as IL-6 and TNF-α are the factors associated with carcinogenesis.

Laboratory Diagnosis

Stool Microscopy

Demonstration of the characteristic flask-shaped eggs in the stool establishes the diagnosis. Microscopy of the duodenal aspirate is more sensitive than stool microscopy. Entero-test can be done to take duodenal sampling similar to that is done for *Giardia*. Formalin-ether concentration should be done when egg burden is low. However, the eggs of *C. sinensis* are morphologically similar to that of *Opisthorchis*, *Heterophyes*, and *Metagonimus*.

Serodiagnosis

- **Antibody detection:** ELISA using recombinant propeptide of cathepsin L proteinase (rCsCatL-propeptide) is available for detection of specific IgG4 antibodies. It has minimal cross-reactions and acceptable sensitivity. It is used to evaluate the level of infection and for monitoring the treatment response
- **Antigen detection:** ELISA is also available for detection of circulating antigen in the serum. Detection of antigen is more useful as it indicates current infection. Its sensitivity ranges from 75–93%.

Molecular Methods

- A **multiplex PCR** has been developed to detect *Clonorchis* and *Opisthorchis* simultaneously. It is rapid with high sensitivity and specificity
- **Real-time PCR** is developed targeting mitochondrial NADH dehydrogenase subunit 2 (nad2) DNA elements. The detection limit is as low as single *C. sinensis* egg and two *O. viverrini* eggs in 100 mg of fecal sample.

Treatment	*Clonorchis sinensis*
Praziquantel (25 mg/kg, three doses in 1 day) is the drug of choice for clonorchiasis.	

Prevention

Clonorchiasis can be prevented by: (i) avoidance of eating raw or undercooked fresh water fish, (ii) sanitary disposal of stool and sewage, and (iii) control of snail hosts.

OPISTHORCHIS VIVERRINI

Epidemiology

O. viverrini has been reported from Southeast Asia, mainly from Laos, Thailand and Cambodia.

More than 10 million people are infected globally with a prevalence of 35%. In certain places, prevalence is up to 90%. It commonly affects people of >10 years age.

Morphology

Adult Worm

It is elongated and dorsoventrally flattened similar to that of *C. sinensis* except that it is smaller (8–12 mm in length). It has a lifespan of 20 years (Figs 11.10A and B). Adult worm of *Opisthorchis* differs from adult worm of *Clonorchis*, in the shape of the testes and in distribution of vitelline glands.

Eggs

Eggs measure 27 μm × 15 μm in size, flask shaped with an operculum and a knob, similar to that of *C. sinensis*.

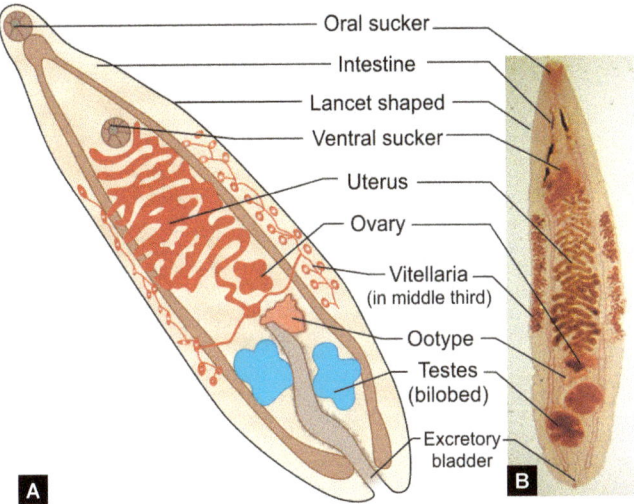

Figs 11.10A and B: *Opisthorchis viverrini*: (A) Adult worm (schematic); (B) Adult worm (carmine-stained)
Source: B—DPDx Image Library, Centers for Disease Control and Prevention (CDC), Atlanta (*with permission*).

Larvae

Metacercaria is the infective form of the parasite. It is found in the flesh of the fresh water fish. Other larval stages are cercaria, redia, sporocyst and miracidium.

The life cycle, pathogenesis, laboratory diagnosis and treatment are similar to that of *Clonorchis sinensis*.

In addition to cholangiocarcinoma, it also causes hepatocellular carcinoma; mainly from the Northeastern Thailand.

OPISTHORCHIS FELINEUS

Opisthorchis felineus is also known as **cat liver fluke**
- Infection is limited to Central and Eastern Europe, Russia and Kazakhstan
- **Morphology:** Similar to that of *O. viverrini*, its adult worm measures 7–12 mm long, eggs are operculated and measure 30 µm × 11 µm size
- Man and other feline animals (cat and dog) act as **definitive host**. Snail (Genus-*Bithynia*) is the **first intermediate host**, while fresh water fishes of crab family serve as second **intermediate host**
- Clinical disease, diagnosis, and treatment similar to that of *O. viverrini*.

LESS COMMON LIVER FLUKES

Dicrocoelium dendriticum, Dicrocoelium hospes, and *Eurytrema pancreaticum* are the less common liver flukes infecting man.
- **Epidemiology:** Mostly, they infect sheep and other animals. True human infection is rare
  - *D. dendriticum* infection in humans has been reported from Europe, Egypt, Iran, Nigeria and China
  - *D. hospes* has been reported Congo, Ghana, Nigeria, and Sierra Leone (30 human cases)
  - *E. pancreaticum* in humans has been reported in China and Japan.
- **Host:** Definitive host is sheep and accidentally man. First intermediate host is land snail. Ants *(Formica fusca)* are the second intermediate host for *D. dendriticum* and grasshoppers for *E. pancreaticum*
- **Habitat:** Adult worm of *D. dendriticum* resides in bile duct, whereas *E. pancreaticum* inhabit in the pancreatic duct
- The life cycle, clinical manifestations, laboratory diagnosis and treatment are similar to *F. hepatica*, but less severe in nature. Eosinophilia is characteristically absent
- **Diagnostic form:** The eggs are the diagnostic form; are operculated, and deep golden brown in color and measure 38–45 µm × 22–30 µm. Eggs of these two flukes cannot be differentiated from each other.

INTESTINAL FLUKES

FASCIOLOPSIS BUSKI

It is also known as **giant intestinal fluke**. It is the largest and the most common intestinal fluke infecting man. It was first noted by Busk in 1843 in the duodenum of an East Indian sailor.

Habitat

It is found in the mucosa of duodenum and jejunum of man and pig.

Epidemiology

F. buski is mainly endemic in Southeast Asian countries such as India, China, Pakistan, Bangladesh, Thailand and Malaysia.
- Risk factors include poverty, unhygienic sociocultural practices, food habits and availability of open type of pig farms
- **India:** In India, most of the cases have been reported from Eastern Uttar Pradesh, Bihar, West Bengal and Assam and Maharashtra. Sporadic cases were also reported from Odisha, Manipur, Tamil Nadu and Karnataka
- **Phulwaria endemic foci:** There is an emergent endemic focus of fasciolopsiasis in Phulwaria village, Bihar; 118 cases were detected during 2015.

Morphology

Adult Worm

The adult worm measures 2–7.5 cm in length, 0.8–2 cm in breadth and 0.5–3 mm in thickness.
- It is fleshy with broad anterior end but does not have cephalic cone which is present in *F. hepatica* (*see* Table 11.5)

Table 11.5: Differences between adult worm of *Fasciola hepatica* and *Fasciolopsis buski*

Properties	Fasciola hepatica	Fasciolopsis buski
Size	Smaller (3 cm)	Bigger (2–7.5 cm)
Anterior end (shoulder)	Bears cephalic cone	Does not have cephalic cone
Oral and ventral suckers	Well separated	Lie close to each other
Intestinal caeca	Bear lateral branches	Do not have lateral branches

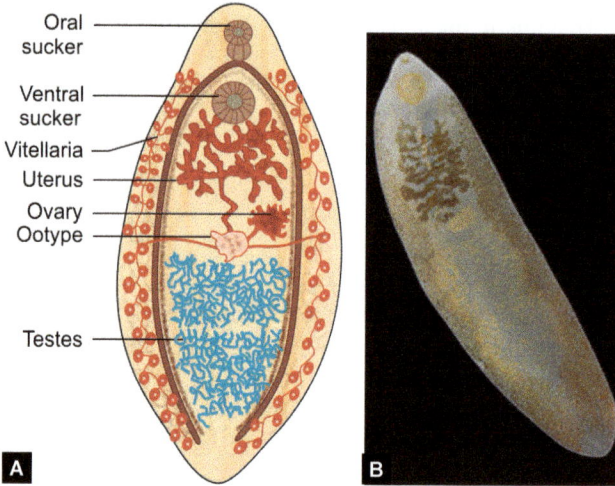

Figs 11.11A and B: Adult worm of *Fasciolopsis buski* (A) Schematic diagram; (B) Carmine-stained

Source: B—DPDx Image Library, Centers for Disease Control and Prevention (CDC), Atlanta (*with permission*).

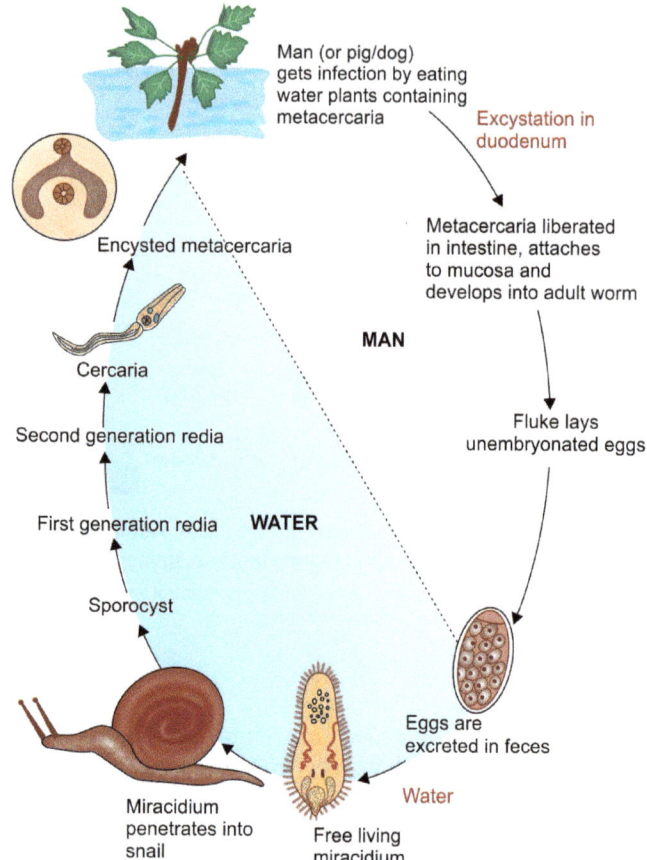

Fig. 11.12: Life cycle of *Fasciolopsis buski*

- It has two suckers, ventral and oral, present close to each other (Figs 11.11A and B)
- It is a hermaphrodite.

Eggs

Eggs are large (130–140 μm × 80–85 μm size), operculated and bile stained eggs, similar to that of *F. hepatica*.

Larvae

Metacercaria is the infective form to man and pig.

Life Cycle (Fig. 11.12)

The life cycle of *F. buski* is similar to that of *F. hepatica*.
- **Host:** It completes its life cycle in one definitive host (pig or man) and two intermediate hosts (first—snail of Genera *Segmentina* and *Hippeutis*, second—aquatic plants)
- **Modes of transmission:** Humans acquire infection by eating contaminated water plants, carrying the infective form, the metacercaria larvae

- **Development in man/pigs:** The larvae develop into adult worm in the intestine, which then lay unembryonated eggs that are excreted in feces
- **Development in water:** The eggs mature and hatch to release miracidia which infect the snails
  - *Development in snails:* The miracidia larvae undergo various stages of developments such as sporocysts, rediae (two generations) and cercariae
  - *Development in aquatic plants:* The cercaria larvae escape from snails and encyst to form metacercariae on the surface of water plants. On ingestion of plants by man or pig, the cycle is repeated.

Pathogenesis

The main pathogenesis is due to the traumatic and obstructive damage to the intestine.
- **Light infection:** It may be asymptomatic or its attachment to intestinal mucosa leads to local inflammation, ulcerations with mucus and blood in stool
- **In severe infection:** There may be partial obstruction of intestinal tract

- Malabsorption and protein losing enteropathy may be seen with profuse yellowish green stool
- Marked eosinophilia and leukocytosis are commonly observed.

Laboratory Diagnosis

Detection of large number of operculated eggs in the stool sample gives probable diagnosis of *F. buski*.
- Sedimentation methods are recommended for stool concentration when worm load is less
- However, the operculated eggs of *F. hepatica*, *Echinostoma* and *Gastrodiscoides* are morphologically similar to that of *F. buski*
- Definitive diagnosis can be done only after identification of the adult worm (see Table 11.5).

Treatment	*Fasciolopsis buski*
❑ Praziquantel is the drug of choice. It is given as 25 mg/kg, three doses in 1 day ❑ Niclosamide is given alternatively.	

OTHER LESS COMMON INTESTINAL TREMATODES

Gastrodiscoides hominis

It was discovered from India by Lewis and McConnell in 1880.
- **Habitat:** The adult worm lives in the cecum and ascending colon of pigs, monkeys and also man
- **Epidemiology:** *G. hominis* is reported mainly from India, China and Vietnam. Recently cases from Africa are also reported. In India, it has been reported from Assam (Kamrup district) and other states like Bihar and Odisha
- **Morphology:**
  - **Adult worms** are bright pink and measure 8–14 mm long and 4–5 mm wide, pyriform-shaped, with a conical anterior portion and hemispherical posterior portion. Oral sucker is near the anterior end while the ventral sucker is located at the posterior end. A large excretory bladder is located near the midline behind the ventral suckers (Fig. 11.13A)
  - **Eggs** are greenish-brown operculated similar to that of *F. buski*, measure 60–70 × 150 μm size.
- **Life cycle:** It is similar to *F. buski*. Humans are the **definitive hosts**. Snails (Genus: *Helicorbis coenosus* in India) are the **first intermediate hosts** and aquatic plants serve as **second intermediate host**. The duration of cycle is about 20 days in humans and 30–150 days in snail
- **Clinical feature:** Light infection is asymptomatic where as heavy infection may cause mucus diarrhea and other intestinal symptoms
- **Laboratory diagnosis:** Stool microscopy is done to demonstrate of operculated eggs in stool
- **Treatment:** Praziquantel is the drug of choice.

Watsonius watsoni

Watsonius watsoni is mainly a parasite of monkeys; human infection is rare.
- Few cases have been reported from West Africa.
- Adult worms are located in the small intestine. They measure 8–10 mm long and 4–5 mm wide. Ventral sucker is located posteriorly
- Eggs are operculated, measure 125–130 μm × 75–80 μm size
- Life cycle is not known. Infection probably occurs by ingestion of plants containing metacercariae
- Clinical feature, diagnosis and treatment of *W. watsoni* are similar to that of *G. hominis*.

Heterophyes heterophyes

H. heterophyes was first reported by Bilharz in 1851.
- **Habitat:** The adult worm lives in the small intestine (jejunum and upper ileum) of man and many fish eating mammals like dogs, cats and birds

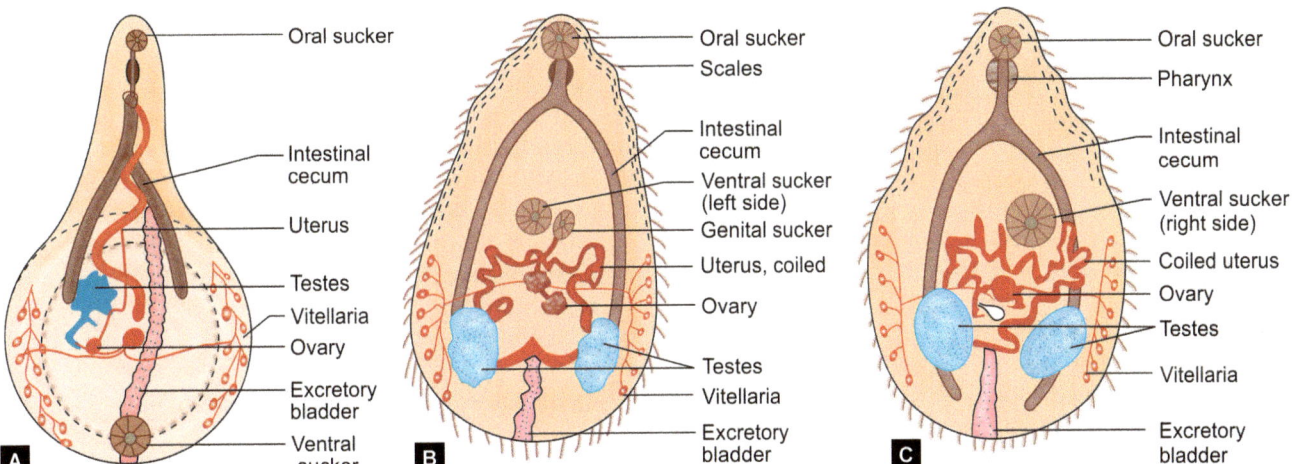

Figs 11.13A to C: Adult worms of (schematic): (A) *Gastrodiscoides hominis*; (B) *Heterophyes heterophyes*; (C) *Metagonimus yokogawai*

- **Epidemiology:** *Heterophyes heterophyes* is reported mainly from China, Egypt, India, Japan, Korea, and Sudan
- **Morphology:**
  - **Adult worm** measures 1–1.7 mm, gray with a round broad posterior end and possesses three suckers—oral, ventral (situated left side) and a genital sucker surrounding the genital pore (Fig. 11.13B)
  - **Eggs** are operculated and smaller, measure 27–30 µm × 15–17 µm size.
- **Life cycle:** It is similar to that of any intestinal trematode. Humans (or other mammals) are the **definitive host**. Snails (*Pironella* species) are the **first intermediate host** and brackish water fishes (Genus: *Mugil capito*) serve as **second intermediate host.** Man becomes infected by eating raw, pickled or poorly cooked fish containing metacercaria. Prepatent period is about 9 days
- **Clinical feature:** Light infection is asymptomatic where as heavy infection may cause mucus diarrhea, intestinal ulcers and abdominal pain. Myocarditis (in Philippines) and neurologic manifestations have also been reported
- **Laboratory diagnosis:** It is done by demonstration of operculated eggs. However, the eggs of *H. heterophyes* are morphologically similar to that of *M. yokogawai* and *C. sinensis*. The eggs of *H. heterophyes* have very inconspicuous opercular shoulders and, unlike *C. sinensis*, they lack the "seated" operculum and knob at the abopercular end
- **Treatment:** Praziquantel is the drug of choice.

Metagonimus yokogawai

- **Epidemiology:** *M. yokogawai* is considered as the most common intestinal fluke in Far East; most of the cases are reported from China, Japan, Indonesia, Israel and Taiwan
- **Habitat:** The adult worm lives in the small intestine
- **Morphology:**
  - Adult worms are similar to that of *H. heterophyes* except slightly larger in size (1–2.5 mm long), ventral sucker is situated on the right side of the midline and there is no genital sucker (Fig. 11.13C)
  - Eggs are operculated and smaller, measure 26–28 µm × 15–17 µm size.
- **Life cycle:** It is similar to that of any intestinal trematode. Humans (fish eating mammals like dogs, cats and birds) are the definitive hosts. Fresh water snails (*Semisulcospira* species) are the first intermediate host and freshwater fishes (Genus *Mugil*) serve as second intermediate host
- Clinical features, diagnosis and treatment are similar to that of *H. heterophyes* except that *M. yokogawai* is more invasive; causing more extraintestinal manifestations than *H. heterophyes*.

Echinostoma ilocanum

- **Habitat:** The adult worm lives in the small intestine of rats and dogs. Human infection is rare
- **Epidemiology:** It is mainly reported from China, Indonesia, Thailand, Taiwan and Philippines
- **Morphology:**
  - **Adult worms** are reddish gray and measure less than 1 cm long and the oral sucker is surrounded by a distinctive horseshoe-shaped collar of spines present near the anterior end
  - **Eggs** are ellipsoidal and operculated and measure 86–116 µm × 58–69 µm size. There is no opercular shoulders.
- **Life cycle:** It is similar to that of any intestinal trematode
- Clinical feature, diagnosis and treatment are similar to that of *H. heterophyes*.

Nanophyetus salmincola

It is an intestinal trematode found in North America. It commonly infects people eating salmon fish. Operculated eggs of *N. salmincola* often gets confused with that of *D. latum* and *Paragonimus*; can be differentiated as described in Table 10.3 and Fig. 10.8C.

LUNG FLUKE

PARAGONIMUS WESTERMANI

Paragonimus westermani is also known as **oriental lung fluke**. It causes endemic hemoptysis in man. Naterer was the first to describe the parasite in 1828.

Epidemiology

More than 40 species of *Paragonimus* are recognized as parasites of mammals; however, only 10 species infect humans with a global prevalence of 22 million.
- It is endemic in many parts of the world, except North America and Europe
- *P. westermani* is the most important species infecting humans, found in the Far East, principally Korea, Japan, Taiwan, China, and Philippines
- The other species are *P. miyazaki* (Japan), *P. skrjabini* and *P. hueitungensis* (China), *P. heterotremus* (China, Southeast Asia), *P. uterobilateralis*, *P. africanus* (Central and West Africa), *P. mexicanus* (Central and South America), and *P. kellicotti* (North America)
- **India:** Paragonimiasis is endemic in Northeast states of India. Many cases are reported from **Manipur** with a prevalence of 6.7%. Earlier, *P. westermani* was thought to be the causative agent of paragonimiasis in Manipur. However, according to the recent studies, *P. heterotremus* may be the responsible for paragonimiasis in Manipur. The first true case of, *P. westermani* infection in India was reported in 2015 from Manipur.

Habitat

The adult worm lives in the parenchyma of lung.

Morphology

Adult Worm

It is thick, fleshy (plump) and reddish brown in color.

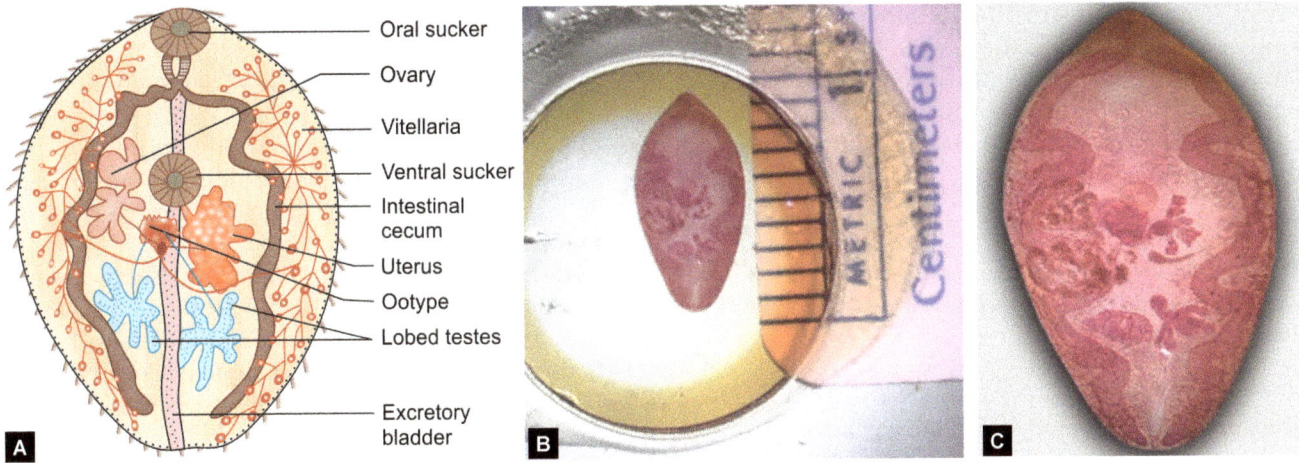

Figs 11.14A to C: *Paragonimus westermani* adult worm (A) Schematic diagram; (B) Carmine-stained; (C) Higher magnification of adult worm seen in Fig. 11.14B

Source: B and C—DPDx Image Library, Centers for Disease Control and Prevention (CDC), Atlanta (*with permission*).

- It measures up to 16 mm in length, 8 mm in breadth
- The fluke is oval in shape with broader anterior end
- Tegument is covered throughout by spines like scale
- The oral sucker is situated anteriorly and ventral sucker situated in the middle of the body (Figs 11.14A to C)
- The excretory bladder is large and divides the body of worm into two equal halves
- The parasite is hermaphrodite with two irregularly deep lobed testes at posterior end
- **Life span:** Most worms die after about 6 years; some may live up to 20 years.

Eggs

The eggs are oval, operculated and golden-brown in color and measures 80–120 μm × 45–65 μm. They are unembryonated when laid (see Figs 11.16A and B).

Larvae

Metacercaria is the infective form of the parasite. It is present in the flesh of second intermediate host (crab or crayfish).

Other larval stages are cercaria, redia, sporocyst and miracidium.

Life Cycle (Fig. 11.15)

Host: *P. westermani* completes its life cycle in one definitive host (man, or dogs and cats) and two intermediate hosts: first—snail (Genus: *Melania* or *Semisulcospira* and *Brotia* species), second—crabs or crayfishes.

Mode of transmission: Man acquires infection by eating uncooked, partially cooked, salted, or pickled crab or crayfish (second intermediate host) containing metacercariae.

Development in Man

In the small intestine, the larvae (metacercariae) escape out and penetrate the intestinal wall to reach peritoneal

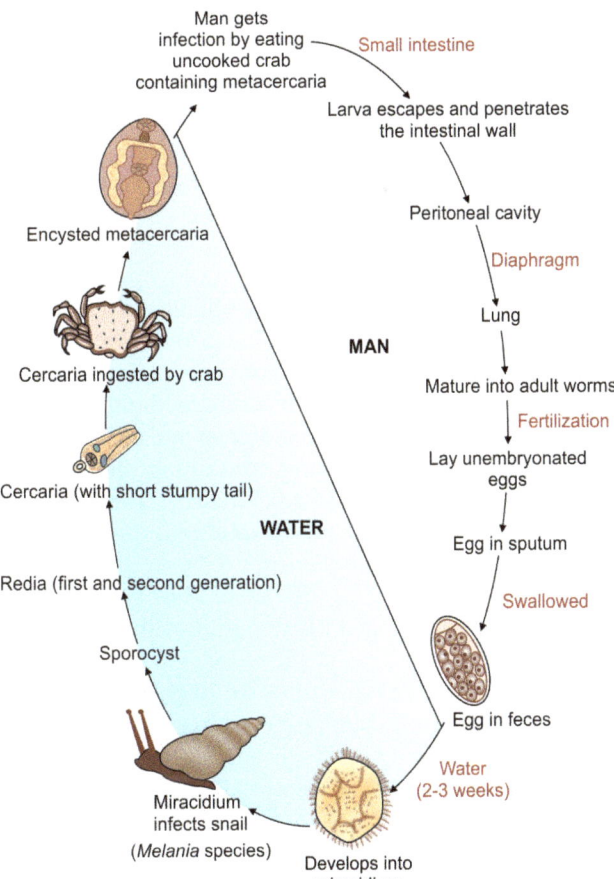

Fig. 11.15: Life cycle of *Paragonimus westermani*

cavity. Then they pierce the diaphragm to reach the lung parenchyma and settle near to the bronchus. The larvae mature into adult worms, which start laying unembryonated eggs that are coughed out in sputum. The eggs are swallowed and excreted in feces in 5-6 weeks after the onset of infection.

Development in Water

The further development of eggs takes place in the water where miracidia hatch out from the eggs in 2-3 weeks at 29-31°C.

Development in snail

The miracidium released from each egg infects the snail, undergoes asexual multiplication to produce sporocysts. The sporocysts through two generations of rediae give rise to stumpy-tailed cercariae in 3-5 months

Development in crab or crayfish

The mature cercariae escape from snail host and are ingested by crabs or crayfishes. Cercariae encyst to from metacercariae which when ingested by man, the cycle is repeated.

Pathogenesis

Metacercariae penetrate the intestinal wall and migrate into the abdominal cavity. This may cause abdominal tenderness, nausea and vomiting. Then they migrate to lungs and develop to adult worms that cause pulmonary paragonimiasis.

Pulmonary Paragonimiasis

The adult worm initially causes eosinophilic granulomatous inflammation in the lungs which leads to the formation of encapsulating fibrotic capsules or cysts surrounding the worms. The cysts are commonly found on the right lung.

- ❖ The cysts are about 1 cm in diameter and contain blood mixed thick purulent fluid containing one or more flukes and golden brown eggs. When cysts break up into bronchioles, the blood mixed sputum is expectorated
- ❖ Symptoms appear with moderate to heavy infection. The common presenting features are productive cough with brownish blood tinged rusty sputum with an offensive fishy odor
- ❖ Sometimes, frank hemoptysis occurs along with peripheral blood eosinophilia
- ❖ In chronic cases, bronchitis, bronchiectasis, pneumonia or lung abscess may be seen.

Extrapulmonary Paragonimiasis

The worms migrate from the ruptured cysts to various sites such as liver, spleen, abdominal wall and less commonly in brain.

- ❖ Extrapulmonary infections are usually associated with *P. mexicanus*, *P. heterotremus*, *P. skrjabini*, *P. hueitungensis* and occasionally with *P. westermani*
- ❖ **Cerebral paragonimiasis:** It is the most severe form of paragonimiasis. Encapsulated cysts in the brain parenchyma present as space-occupying lesions. Symptoms include fever, headache, vomiting, motor weakness or epilepsy
- ❖ **Cutaneous paragonimiasis:** Migratory subcutaneous nodules may be seen in 20-60% of *P. skrjabini* and 10% of *P. westermani* infected patients. They form tender nodules which vary from few milimeters to 10 cm
- ❖ **Larva migrans:** In China, *P. skrjabini* does not develop to the adult worm stage, but migrates to various places such as skin, brain and liver causing trematode larva migrans.

Laboratory Diagnosis	*Paragonimus westermani*
☐ **Sputum microscopy**—detects operculated eggs ☐ **Serological tests**—antibody detection (DIGFA, ELISA, western blot), antigen detection (Dot ELISA) ☐ **Imaging methods**—MRI, CT scan, X-ray can detect lesions in lungs and other organs ☐ Peripheral blood eosinophilia.	

Laboratory Diagnosis

Sputum Microscopy

Early morning, deeply coughed sputum sample is collected for microscopy. The saline mount of sputum sample (particularly blood-tinged flecks) is examined for characteristic operculated eggs. Histopathological stains can also be used (Figs 11.16A and B)

If the egg burden is less, then:

- ❖ Multiple sputum examination (up to seven samples) should be done

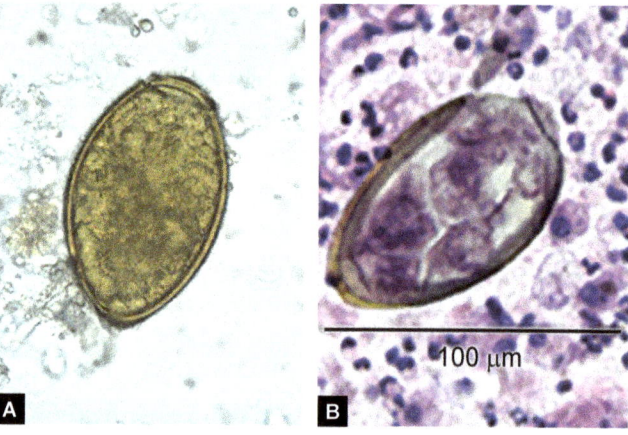

Figs 11.16A and B: Eggs of *Paragonimus* species (A) In sputum—wet mount; (B) In lung biopsy—stained with hematoxylin and eosin

Source: DPDx Image Library, Centers for Disease Control and Prevention (CDC), Atlanta (*with permission*).

- Sputum can be concentrated by formalin-ether sedimentation technique
- Mucoid sputum can be liquefied by mucolytic agents like sodium hydroxide
- Eggs of *Paragonimus* is often confused with *D. latum* and can be differentiated from the latter by the presence of opercular shoulders and a marked thickening at the aboperculan end, unlike *D. latum* eggs (Refer Table 10.3).

Stool microscopy may be done in children as the collection of sputum is difficult in them.

Serological Tests

Serological tests are useful in the early part of the disease, where the microscopy has failed to detect eggs in sputum and stool and also for epidemiological purpose.

Antibody detection

Serum antibodies to *P. westermani* can be detected by:
- **Rapid test:** Dot-immunogold filtration assay (**DIGFA**) has been developed in China, by using crude extracts of adult worms of *P. westermani*. It is rapid, gives result in 10 min. It shows 99% sensitivity and 92% specificity
- ELISA using purified adult excretory-secretory antigen to detect parasite specific IgG or IgE has shown a high sensitivity, especially with pleural fluid than serum
- Western blot test using adult worm homogenate is also highly sensitive and specific.

Antigen detection

Dot ELISA format has been developed to detect species specific and stage specific antigens by using monoclonal antibodies. Detection of antigens indicates active infection.

Other Tests

- Peripheral blood eosinophilia
- **Radiological tests:** MRI and CT scan are preferred to locate the cysts in the CNS or other sites. Even Chest X-ray may demonstrate the characteristic pulmonary lesions, including patchy densities, cavities, pleural effusion.

Treatment	*Paragonimus westermani*
□ Praziquantel (25 mg/kg/dose, three doses per day for 2 days) is the drug of choice for treatment of paragonimiasis □ Bithionol and niclofolan can also be used with 100% cure rate without any side effect □ Triclabendazole is also recommended □ Surgical management may be needed for pulmonary or cerebral lesions.	

Prevention

Paragonimiasis can be prevented by: (i) sanitary disposal of sputum, (ii) control of snails, (iii) treatment of cases and (iv) health education.

EXPECTED QUESTIONS

I. Write essay on:
  a. A 46-year-old man from Africa came to the OPD with abdominal pain, hematuria and dysuria. Urine culture was found as sterile. Urine wet mount examination revealed oval non-operculated elongated eggs with terminal spine.
  1. What is the etiological diagnosis?
  2. Write briefly about the life cycle of the etiological agent.
  3. What are the various diagnostic modalities?
  4. How will you treat this condition?

  b. A 8-year-old boy from Manipur presented with productive cough with blood tinged rusty sputum with offensive fishy odor. Sputum microscopy (wet mount) revealed large operculated oval eggs, golden brown in color, measuring 80–120 µm × 45–65 µm in size.
  1. Identify the disease and the causative agent.
  2. Write briefly about the life cycle of the etiological agent.
  3. What are the various diagnostic modalities?

II. Write short notes on:
  a. Cercarial dermatitis (swimmer's itch).
  b. *Clonorchis sinensis*.
  c. *Fasciola hepatica*.

III. Multiple choice questions (MCQs):
  1. Which of the following is the largest trematode?
     a. *Fasciola hepatica*
     b. *Fasciolopsis buski*
     c. *Clonorchis sinensis*
     d. *Schistosoma haematobium*
  2. Which of the following is called as lung fluke?
     a. *Clonorchis sinensis*
     b. *Ascaris lumbricoides*
     c. *Strongyloides stercoralis*
     d. *Paragonimus westermani*
  3. Carcinoma of urinary bladder is associated with which of the following parasites?
     a. *Schistosoma japonicum*
     b. *Schistosoma mansoni*
     c. *Schistosoma haematobium*
     d. *Schistosoma intercalatum*
  4. In which of the following trematode, the sexes are separate?
     a. *Schistosoma haematobium*
     b. *Clonorchis sinensis*
     c. *Fasciolopsis buski*
     d. *Paragonimus westermani*
  5. Chinese liver fluke is the common name of:
     a. *Fasciola hepatica*
     b. *Fasciola gigantica*
     c. *Clonorchis sinensis*
     d. *Fasciolopsis buski*

Answer
1. b   2. d   3. c   4. a   5. c

Nematodes—I (Intestinal Nematodes)

CHAPTER 12

CHAPTER OUTLINE

- Classification
- General description
- Large intestinal nematodes
- *Trichuris trichiura*
- *Enterobius vermicularis*
- Small intestinal nematodes
- Hookworm
- *Strongyloides* species
- *Ascaris* species

Nematodes are probably the most widespread animal group occurring in the world. Many of them are non-pathogenic and exist as free living forms in fresh or marine water and soil, while few of the species can be pathogenic and exist as parasitic form in both animals and plants.

CLASSIFICATION

Systemic Classification

Systemic classification is based on Anderson et al. (1974) classification. Phylum Nematoda has two classes Adenophorea and Secernentea which are different in many ways (Tables 12.1 and 12.2).

Classification Based on Habitat

Most of the nematodes inhabit in the intestine while some (e.g. filarial worms) reside in various tissues (Table 12.3).

Table 12.1: Differences between class Adenophorea and Secernentea

Characteristics	Class Adenophorea	Class Secernentea
Sensory structure (phasmids)	Absent	Present
Esophagus	Modified with presence of: • Gland cells (stichocytes) or • Reserve organ (trophosome)	Normal appearance
Excretory organs	Without lateral canals	Lateral canals present
Caudal papillae	Absent	Present
Infective form to the definitive host	First stage larva (*Trichinella*) or embryonated eggs (*Trichuris, Capillaria*)	Third stage larva or embryonated eggs (e.g. all other nematodes)

Classification Based on They Lay Egg or Larva

Nematodes can be classified into three groups based on they lay eggs or larvae after fertilization:

1. **Oviparous:** Following fertilization, the female worms produce eggs that take some time to hatch out to form larvae in the environment
   - Most of the intestinal nematodes are oviparous except *Strongyloides*. Examples include hookworm, *Ascaris*, *Trichuris*, *Enterobius*, etc.
   - Here, the diagnosis is made by detection of eggs in feces.
2. **Viviparous:** Female worms directly give birth to larvae; there is no egg stage.
   - Most of the somatic nematodes are viviparous. Examples include filarial worm, *Trichinella* and *Dracunculus*
   - Here, the diagnosis is made by detection of larva in tissues or blood.
3. **Ovoviviparous:** Here, the female worms lay eggs containing larvae; which immediately hatch out
   - Example includes *Strongyloides* species
   - The larvae are the diagnostic form detected in stool examination.

GENERAL DESCRIPTION

Nematodes pass through six developmental stages (Fig. 12.1) adult worm, egg stage and four larval stages (L_1–L_4). Each larval stage transforms to the next by shedding of the cuticle (called as **molting**).

Adult Worm

- **Shape:** Nematodes are elongated, cylindrical or filariform in shape with both the ends pointed. They are unsegmented without any appendages

CHAPTER 12 ◆ Nematodes—I (Intestinal Nematodes)

Table 12.2: Systemic classification of phylum nematoda (Anderson et al. 1974)

Superfamily	Family	Genus
Class: Adenophorea		
Trichinelloidea	Trichinellidae	Trichinella
	Trichuridae	Trichuris, Capillaria
Class: Secernenatea		
Oxyuroidea	Oxyuridae	Enterobius
Ascaridoidea	Ascarididae	Ascaris, Toxocara, Baylisascaris, Lagochilascaris
	Anisakidae	Anisakis
Ancylostomatoidea	Ancylostomatidae	Ancylostoma, Necator
Rhabditoidea	Strongyloididae	Strongyloides
Strongyloidea	Chabertiidae	Oesophagostomum, Ternidens
	Syngamidae	Mammomonogamus
Gnathostomatoidea	Gnathostomatidae	Gnathostoma
Metastrongyloidea	Angiostrongylidae	Angiostrongylus
Trichostrongyloidea	Trichostrongylidae	Trichostrongylus
Filarioidea	Onchocercidae	Wuchereria, Brugia, Loa loa, Onchocerca, Mansonella, Dirofilaria
Dracunculoidea	Dracunculidae	Dracunculus
Thelazioidea	Thelaziidae	Thelazia
Dioctophymatoidea	Dioctophymatidae	Dioctophyme

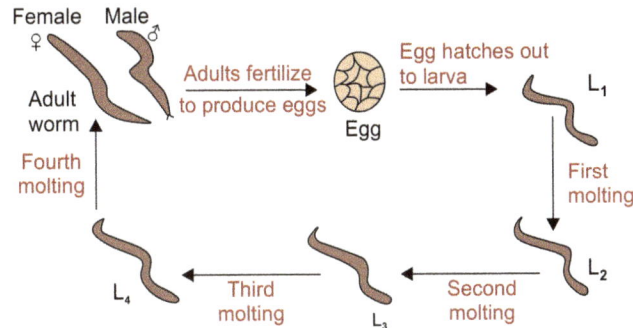

Fig. 12.1A: Developmental stages of nematodes

- **Size:** Variable, ranging from less than 5 mm (hookworm, *Trichinella* and *Strongyloides*) to as long as one meter (*Dracunculus*). Female worms are longer than male worms
- **Symmetry:** Body is bilaterally symmetrical (one plane) while head is radially symmetrical (multiple plane)
- **Body wall:** Made up of outer layer of tough acellular cuticle and inner layer of longitudinal muscle
- **Locomotion:** Nematodes move by contraction of the longitudinal muscles
- **Alimentary canal:** It is well developed and consists of mouth at the anterior end followed by a muscular and glandular esophagus, intestine and rectum that leads to subterminal anus at the posterior end. In some species (e.g. hookworm) mouth bears the teeth (cutting plate). The esophagus (or pharynx) may bear posterior bulb

Table 12.3: Classification of nematodes based on habitat

Intestinal human nematodes	Somatic human nematodes	Animal nematodes that rarely infect man	
		Larva migrans	Other animal nematodes
Small intestine *Ascaris lumbricoides* (common roundworm) *Ancylostoma duodenale* (old world Hookworm) *Necator americanus* (American or new world Hookworm) **Large intestine** *Trichuris trichiura* (whipworm) *Enterobius vermicularis* (threadworm or pinworm)	**Filarial worm** (1) **Lymphatics** *Wuchereria bancrofti* *Brugia malayi* *Brugia timori* (2) **Skin** *Loa loa* (also eye) *Onchocerca* (also eye) *Mansonella streptocerca* *Mansonella ozzardi* (Serous cavity) (3) **Serous cavity** *Mansonella perstans* **Other human somatic nematodes** *Trichinella spiralis* *Dracunculus medinensis* (Guinea worm)	**Visceral larva migrans** *Toxocara* (Liver) *Angiostrongylus cantonensis* (CNS) *Angiostrongylus costaricensis* (abdomen) *Anisakis* *Gnathostoma* *Baylisascaris* **Cutaneous larva migrans** *Ancylostoma braziliensis* *Ancylostoma caninum* *Ancylostoma ceylanicum* *Gnathostoma* species *Uncinaria stenocephala* *Bunostomum* species	**Zoonotic filariasis** *Dirofilaria* **Intestine** *Capillaria philippinensis* *Trichostrongylus* species *Strongyloides fuelleborni* *Oesophagostomum* *Ternidens* species **Conjunctiva** *Thelazia* species **Liver** *Capillaria hepatica* **Kidney** *Dioctophyma* species **Respiratory tract/lungs** *Mammomonogammus* *Capillaria aerophila* *Ascaris suum*

Abbreviation: CNS, central nervous system.

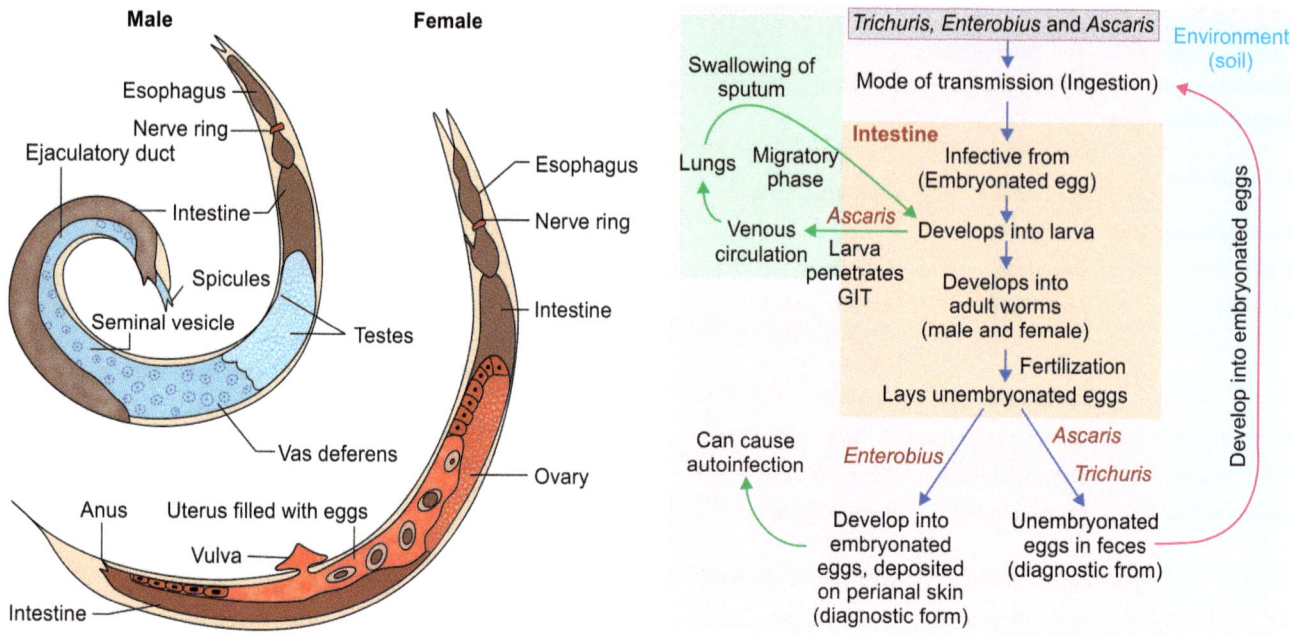

Fig. 12.1B: Adult male and female nematode (schematic diagram)

Fig. 12.2A: Life cycles of *Trichuris*, *Enterobius* and *Ascaris*

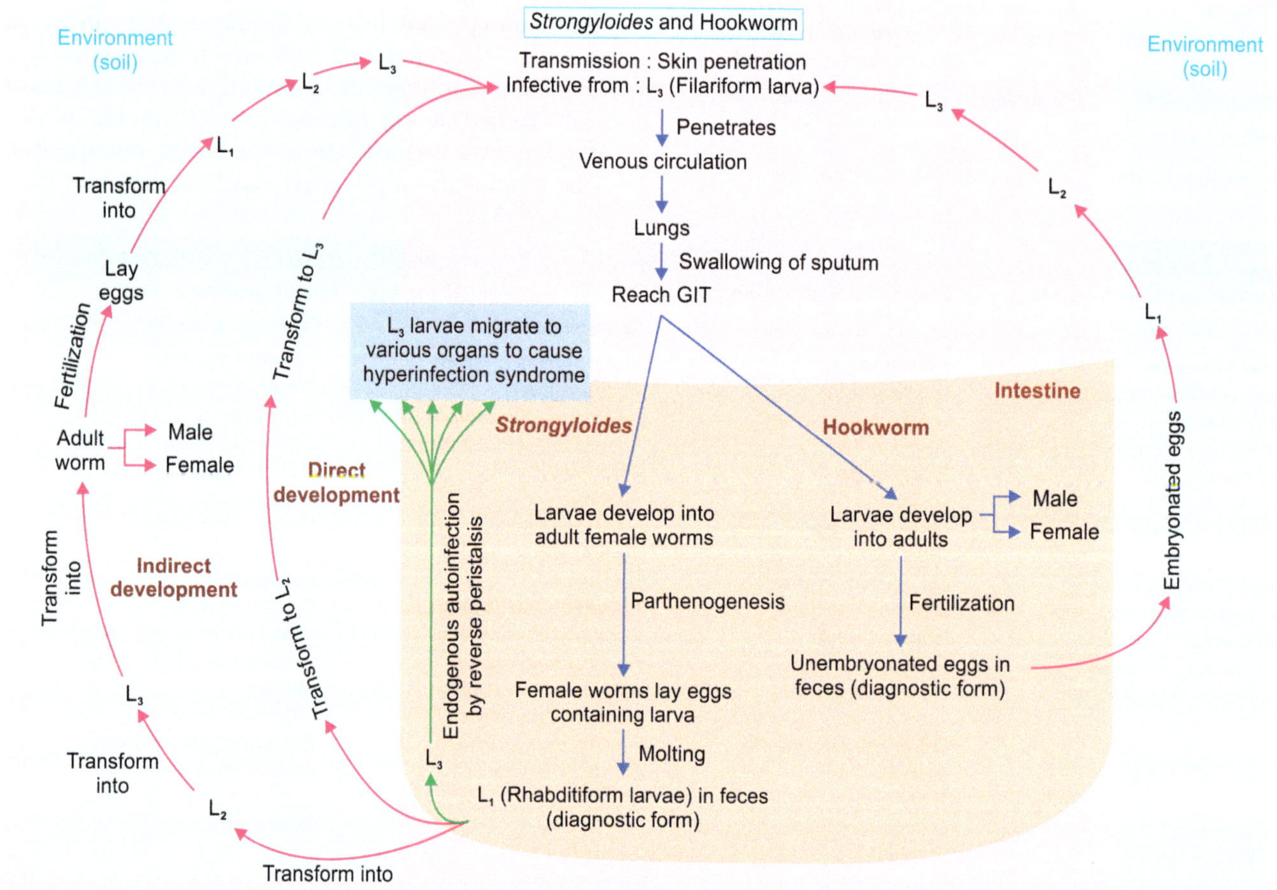

Fig. 12.2B: Life cycles of Hook worm and *Strongyloides*

(as in *Enterobius*). The intestine or midgut is lined by a single layer of columnar cells
- **Body cavity:** They possess a body cavity or a pseudocele (space between body wall and alimentary canal) with high hydrostatic pressure which is filled with body fluid secreted by intestine and genital organs
- **Sexes:** Nematodes are diecious (bisexual), i.e. sexes are different
- **Male reproductive system:** It consists of a long convoluted tube which can be differentiated into testes, vas deferens, seminal vesicle and ejaculatory duct. Some worms also bear accessory copulatory organs like a copulatory bursa with two spicules (rod like protrusible organ present at the posterior end) and gubernaculum (an elevation of cloaca that guides the spicule during copulation). The ejaculatory duct opens subterminally at the posterior end into a common passage along with the rectum (known as cloaca) (Fig.12.2)
- **Female reproductive system:** It consists of two (common) or one convoluted tube. Each tube is differentiated into an ovary, oviduct, seminal receptacle, and uterus and then both the tubes joined to form a common vagina that opens outside through vulva (genital pore) either in the middle of the body or near the mouth (Fig. 12.2)
- **Nervous system:** It is rudimentary and consists of circular nerve ring (brain) surrounding the esophagus and six longitudinal nerve trunks (one dorsal, one ventral and four lateral). The dorsal nerve is responsible for motor control, while the lateral nerves are for sensory and the ventral one combines both the functions. Some species possess sensory structure like sensory papilla and phasmid (chemoreception organs) over the cuticle
- **Excretory system:** It is also rudimentary. Unlike cestodes, they do not have flame cells. Various ways of waste disposal are:
  - Through anus
  - Excretion of nitrogenous waste in the form of ammonia through the body wall
  - In some species, H-shaped canal along each side of body regulates nutrients and waste content
  - In few other species; An excretory gland is situated near esophagus.

Life Cycle

Nematodes complete their life cycle in one host (man) except in filarial worms (need two hosts—definitive host-man and intermediate host—mosquito) and *Dracunculus* species (need two hosts—definitive host man and intermediate host cyclops).

The life cycles of intestinal nematodes have been summarized as flowcharts in Figs 2A and 2B; the detail has been discussed under each topic subsequently in this Chapter. The pathogenesis, diagnosis and treatment are discussed in detail under individual nematodes.

LARGE INTESTINAL NEMATODES

TRICHURIS TRICHIURA

It is also called as **whipworm** as the adult worm resembles to a handle of a whip. It is one of the soil-transmitted helminth (see the highlight box at the end of this Chapter for detail).
- It was first described by Linnaeus in 1771
- About 71 species of *Trichuris* are recorded so far. However, human infection is mostly confined to *T. trichiura* and very rarely *T. suis* (pig whipworm) and *T. vulpis* (dog whipworm).

Habitat

T. trichiura resides in the large intestine of man (mainly cecum and appendix).

Epidemiology

Trichuriasis is worldwide in distribution, mainly in warm and moist climate similar to ascariasis.
- Children are commonly affected
- Global prevalence in humans is approximately 604 million.

Morphology

Similar to other nematodes, *T. trichiura* exists in three forms: adult, larvae (four stages) and egg.

Adult Worm

The adult worm is whip shaped. Anterior three-fifth is thin, hair like, coiled (like rope of a whip) and posterior two-fifth is short and thick.
- The coiled anterior part contains the esophagus and is attached to the gastrointestinal tract (GIT) mucosa whereas the posterior thick part bears the genital organs and intestine and lie free in the human intestine
- The esophagus is glandular, surrounded by a gland called as **stichosome**
- Male is whitish, 30–45 mm long and bears a coiled posterior end
- Female is longer (35–50 mm) and its posterior part is either shaped like a comma or arc (resembles a handle of a whip) (Figs 12.3 and 12.4B).

Egg

Eggs of *T. trichiura* are barrel-shaped; surrounded by a shell, bear mucus plug at both the poles.
- Elongated, measure 50–54 µm long and 22–23 µm wide
- Unembryonated when freshly passed in feces; become embryonated later in environment

- Bile stained; yellowish-brown in color (in saline mount)
- Float in saturated salt solution.

Note: Eggs of *T. vulpis* is similar to that of *T. trichiura* but it is larger (70-80 μm × 30-42 μm) with smaller mucus plug.

Life Cycle (Fig. 12.3)

Host: Humans are the only host.
Infective form: Embryonated eggs serve as infective form.
Mode of transmission: Man (usually children) acquires infection by ingestion of contaminated food and water containing embryonated egg.

Egg-Larva-Adult Transformation

Eggs hatch out in the small intestine releasing the second stage larva, migrate to large intestine where they undergo further moltings to transform into adult worms. Adult female worms have a life span of 5-10 years.

Adults Laying Unembryonated Egg

Within 2-3 months (prepatent period), the female worms following fertilization start laying unembryonated eggs. Each female worm can lay 14,000-20,000 eggs per day for 1-3 years.

Embryonation

The unembryonated eggs passed in the feces are not infective. It takes about 10-14 days to become embryonated (it undergoes two molts to produce second stage larva within the egg shell). Embryonation occurs at 25°C in warm and moist condition. Such embryonated eggs are infective to man.

Pathogenicity and Clinical Feature

Incubation period varies from 70 to 90 days. Most infected individuals are asymptomatic, with or without having eosinophilia.

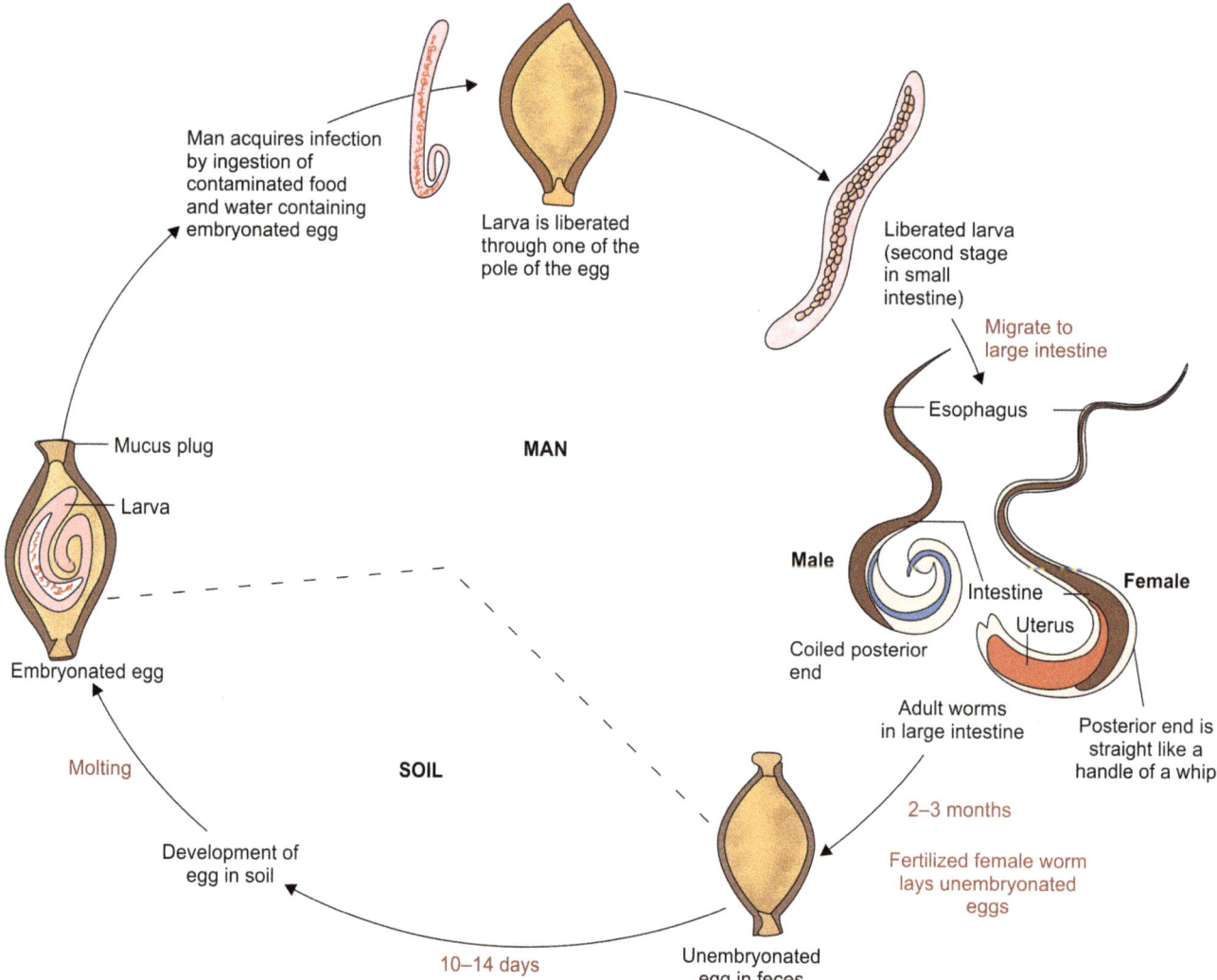

Fig. 12.3: Life cycle of *Trichuris trichiura*

In people with heavy infections: Adult female worm gets buried in the large intestinal mucosa that leads to:
- Mechanical distortion: Leading to inflamed, edematous, and friable mucosa
- Allergic response by the host: Large number of macrophages infiltrate in the lamina propria that produce tumor necrosis factor-α (TNF-α).

Common manifestations include:
- Abdominal pain, anorexia, etc.
- *Trichuris dysentery syndrome*—bloody or mucoid diarrhea resembling inflammatory bowel disease
- Iron deficiency anemia occurs as a result of blood loss; not due to blood ingestion as seen in hookworm
- Recurrent rectal prolapse (due to heavy worm load in the rectum and malnutrition)
- Growth retardation and impaired cognitive function (due to the release of anti-inflammatory cytokines induced by the secretory molecules of *Trichuris* species).

Laboratoy Diagnosis

Stool Examination

Because the level of egg output is high (approximately 200 eggs/g of feces per worm pair), microscopic examination of a single fecal smear is sufficient for diagnosis of symptomatic cases (Figs 12.4A and B).
- The characteristic 50 × 22 μm barrel-shaped, bile-stained *Trichuris* eggs (with mucus plugs at the ends) are readily detected on stool examination either by direct wet mount or following concentration of the stool (Fig. 12.4A)
- Preservative: Formalin is preferred to preserve the stool samples

- Whip shaped adult worms of 3–5 cm long, are occasionally seen on proctoscopy (Fig. 12.4B).

Other Findings
- Peripheral blood eosinophilia (<15%)
- Increased serum IgE level.

Treatment	*Trichuris trichiura*
□ Mebendazole (500 mg once) or albendazole (400 mg daily for three doses) is safe and moderately effective for treatment, with cure rates of 70–90% □ Ivermectin (200 mg/kg daily for three doses) is also safe but is less effective.	

Trichuris suis Therapy

Eggs of *Trichuris suis* are used for treatment of active ulcerative colitis. They induce a shift from T_H1 to T_H2 immune response counteracting the T_H1-mediated pathogenesis of active ulcerative colitis.

Prevention

Trichuriasis can be prevented by improved personal hygiene, proper disposal of feces and improved nutrition with dietary iron.

ENTEROBIUS VERMICULARIS

Enterobius vermicularis is also called as **pinworm** or **threadworm.**
- It is described first by Leuckart, in 1865
- *E. vermicularis* is the only species. The second species *E. gregorii* is identical to *E. vermicularis* (except the basal portion of spicule) and now it is considered as the younger stage of *E. vermicularis*.

Habitat

The adult worm remains attached to the large intestine (cecum, appendix and adjacent portion of colon) by their mouth end.

Epidemiology

Global prevalence in humans: Globally, around 209 million people are infected by pinworms:
- The prevalence is maximum in school children between the age of 5 and 14 years
- People carry the infection for years together due to auto infective cycles
- **It has been said that:** "*You had the infection as a child, you have it now and you will again get it when you have children*"
- **Factors promoting infection:** Overcrowding and impaired hygiene, poor personal care (nail biting or inadequate hand washing).

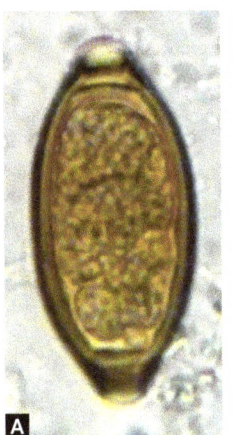 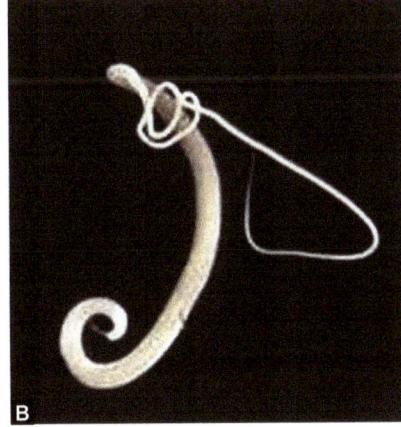

Figs 12.4A and B: *Trichuris trichiura* (A) Egg in saline mount; (B) Adult female

Source: A—Dr Anand Janagond, Associate Professor of Microbiology, S. Nijalingappa Medical college, Bagalkot, Karnataka (*with permission*); B—DPDx Image Library, Centers for Disease Control and Prevention (CDC), Atlanta (*with permission*).

Morphology

The life cycle of *Enterobius* passes through three forms: adult, larvae (four stages) and egg; similar to other nematodes.

Adult Worm

Adult worm of *Enterobius* is small, white and thread-like (hence named as threadworm).

- **Cervical alae:** The adult worm bears a wing-like expansion of the cuticle near the anterior end
- **Double bulb esophagus:** The posterior end of the esophagus is dilated to form globular bulb
- Male worm is smaller (2–5 mm long × 0.1–0.2 mm wide) and the posterior one-third is tightly curved and bears a copulatory bursa with spicules at the posterior end. Males die soon after fertilization
- Female worm is longer (8–13 mm long × 0.3–0.5 mm wide), and the posterior one-third is tapering, straight, thin and pointed (looks like a pin, hence called as pinworm).

Eggs

- **Shape:** Oval or planoconvex (one side is convex and the other side is flat because it is compressed laterally)
- **Size:** 50–60 μm long × 20–30 μm wide (Fig. 12.5)
- **Surrounded by:** Double layered egg shell
- Non bile-stained, colorless in saline mount
- Embryonated egg when freshly passed contains a tadpole shaped larva inside
- Floats in saturated salt solution.

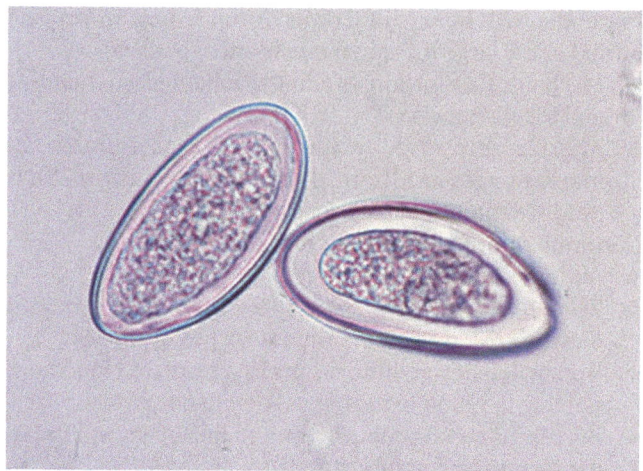

Fig. 12.5: Egg of *Enterobius vermicularis* (saline mount)
Source: DPDx Image Library, Centers for Disease Control and Prevention (CDC), Atlanta (*with permission*).

Life Cycle (Fig. 12.6)

Host: Humans are the only host.
Infective form: Embryonated eggs are infective to man.
Mode of transmission: Man (usually children) acquires infection by:

- Ingestion of eggs contaminated with fingers due to inadequate hand washing or nail biting habit
- **Autoinfection:** Autoinfection is of two types:
  1. Endogenous autoinfection—it occurs by retrograde migration of the larva hatched from the eggs in the perianal skin.
  2. Exogenous autoinfection—through contaminated finger.
- Infection can rarely occur through inhalation of the air-borne eggs.

Development in Man

Eggs usually contain the fully developed larvae. Larvae hatch out from eggs in the cecum and then develop into adult worms.

- Adult worms undergo maturation within 1 month. After fertilization with female worms, the male worms usually die. Gravid female worms fully filled with eggs migrate to large intestine (rectum, colon) and start laying eggs on the perianal skin. Adult female worms usually lay 10,000 eggs/day (Figs 12.7C and D)
- The eggs are embryonated and are the infective stage to man. The prepatent period is about 3–4 weeks
- Female worm lives for about 2 months but because of the autoinfection the cycle continues.

Pathogenicity and Clinical Features

- **Asymptomatic:** Most of the infections are asymptomatic
- **Symptomatic patients:**
  - **Age and sex:** Females, children and young adults are often symptomatic than males and older people
  - **Cardinal symptoms:** Perianal pruritus often worse at night as a result of the nocturnal migration of the female worm
    - The worms may be found in undergarments and can also be found lying in the buttock area of infected children
    - Repeated scratching is the main reason of contaminated finger; which causes auto-infection.
  - Excoriation of the perianal skin and bacterial super-infection may occur (due to continuous scratching of the skin)
  - Abdominal pain and weight loss (may be seen in heavy infections).
- **Migration of the worm:** Rarely, pinworms invade the female genital tract, causing vulvovaginitis and pelvic

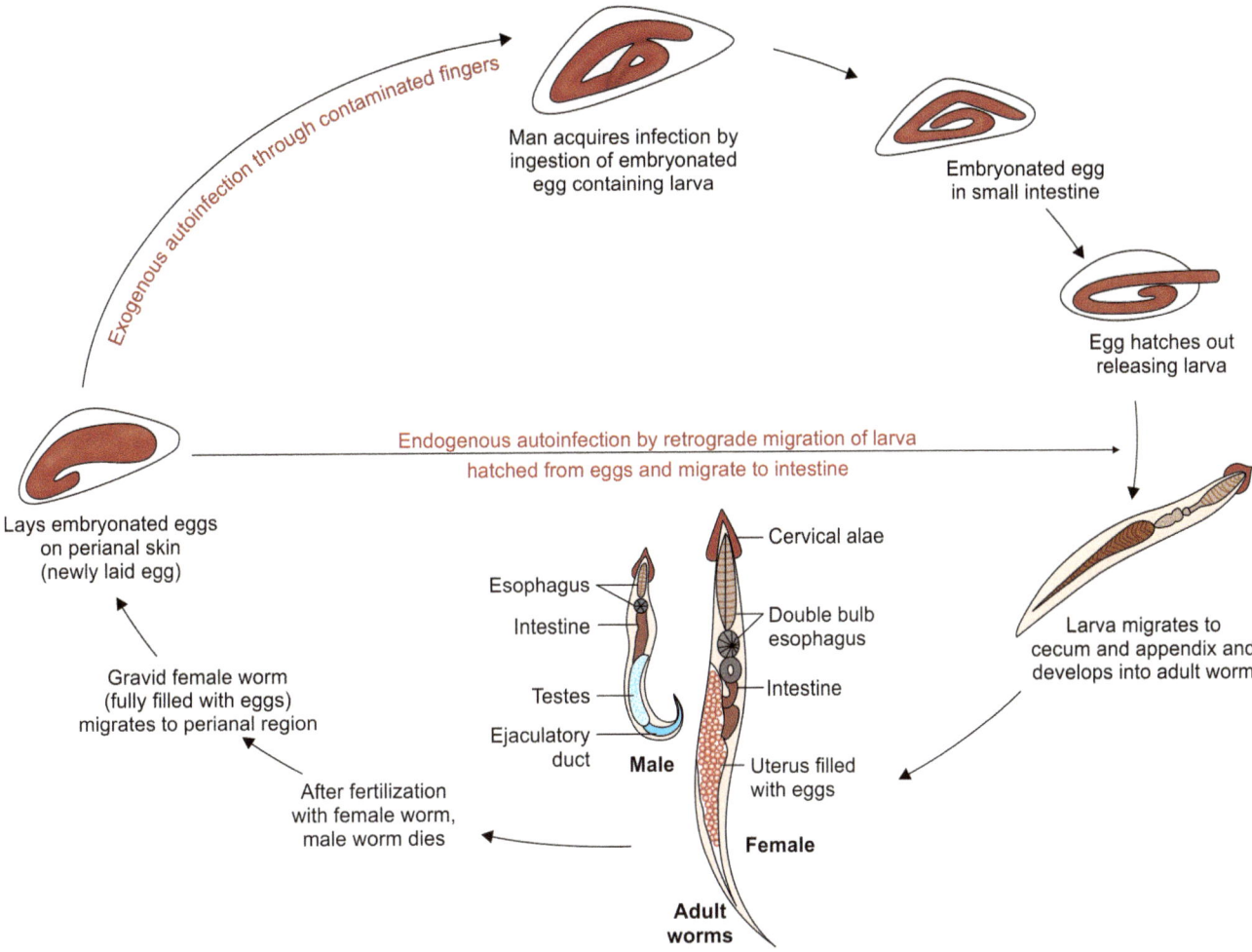

Fig. 12.6 Life cycle of *Enterobius vermicularis*

or peritoneal granulomas. Other sites involved are urinary tract, peritoneal cavity, lungs and liver
❖ Eosinophilia is inconsistent.

Laboratory Diagnosis

The female worms lay eggs in the perianal area; not in the rectum. Hence, eggs are rarely detected by stool examination; around 5% of cases.
❖ The eggs deposited in the perianal skin are collected by applying cellophane tape or its modification called, NIH swab. Eggs are non bile-stained, plancoconvex in shape, containing a larva inside (Fig. 12.5)
❖ The adult female worms may occasionally be found in the feces or crawling to the perianal skin (Fig. 12.7B)
❖ **Number of specimens:** A series of 4–6 consecutive tapes may be necessary as the female worms migrate intermittently
❖ **Timing:** Samples should be collected when the chance of egg deposition is more such as late in the evening, when the patient has been sleeping for several hours, or first thing in the morning.

Cellophane Tape Method

Eggs are detected by the application of clear cellulose acetate tape to the perianal region in the morning before the child goes for bath. The tape is then applied on the clear glass slide. The slide is observed under microscope for the detection of pinworm eggs (Fig. 12.7A).

NIH Swab Method

It is devised in National Institute of Health, USA (Fig. 12.7E).
❖ It consists of a glass rod attached to a cellophane tape by a rubber band
❖ The other end of the glass rod is fixed by a rubber stopper and kept in a test tube
❖ The cellophane part of the glass rod is rolled over the perineal and perianal skin area to collect the sample

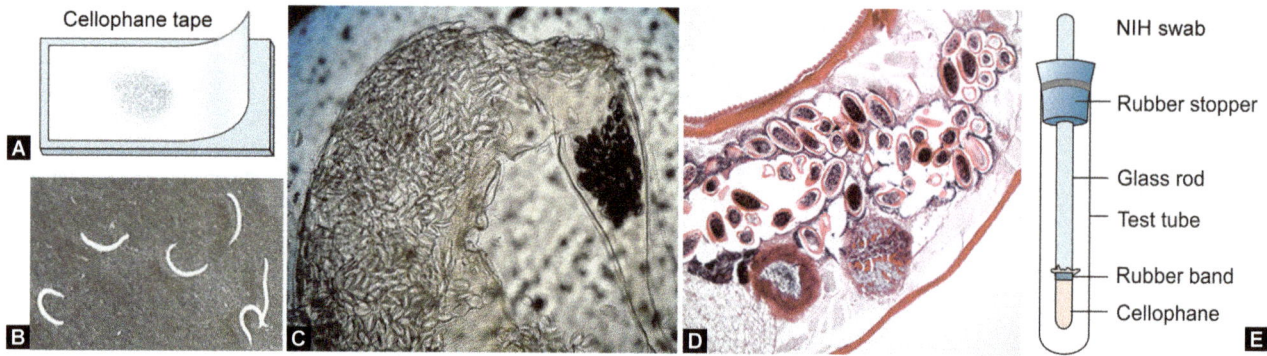

Figs 12.7A to D: *Enterobius vermicularis* (A) Cellophane tape; (B) Adult worms (actual size); (C) Adult female worm containing numerous eggs; (D) Longitudinal section of an adult female worm shows many planoconvex eggs; (E) NIH swab method (schematic)
Source: B and C—Head of Department, Microbiology, Meenakshi Medical College, Chennai; D—DPDx Image Library, Centers for Disease Control and Prevention (CDC), Atlanta (*with permission*).

❖ After the tape is transferred to a slide, microscopic examination will detect *Enterobius* eggs, which are planoconvex, flattened along one side, measure 50-60 µm × 20-30 µm, containing a larva inside.

Treatment	*Enterobius vermicularis*
❑ One of the following drugs can be given: ➢ Mebendazole (100 mg once) ➢ Albendazole (400 mg once) or ➢ Pyrantel pamoate (11 mg/kg once; maximum, 1 g) ❑ The same treatment should be repeated after 2 weeks ❑ Treatment of household members is advocated to eliminate asymptomatic reservoirs of potential reinfection.	

Prevention

Total prevention is neither realistic nor possible as the transmission is so common; aided by autoinfection. Improving personal hygiene such as proper washing of bed clothes, keeping nail short and clean, frequent hand washing are the key measures to contain the transmission.

SMALL INTESTINAL NEMATODES

HOOKWORM

Hookworm is one of the important causes of iron deficiency anemia in both tropics and temperate countries. It is so named because the anterior end of adult worm is bent. It is one of the soil-transmitted helminth (see the highlight box at the end of this Chapter for detail).

Classification

Hookworm belongs to the family Ancylostomatidae which consists of two species infecting humans. *Ancylostoma duodenale* and *Necator americanus*. The word *Ancylostoma* is derived from hooked mouth (*Ancylos*—hooked, *stoma*—mouth). Hookworm comprises of several species, which infect humans and animals.

❖ Human parasite:
  ▪ *A. duodenale* or old world hookworm
  ▪ *N. americanus* or new world hookworm or American hookworm.
❖ Animal parasites that rarely infect man, causing cutaneous larva migrans
  ▪ *Ancylostoma braziliensis*
  ▪ *Ancylostoma caninum* (more common than other animal species)
  ▪ *Ancylostoma ceylanicum*
  ▪ *Uncinaria stenocephala*.

History

❖ *A. duodenale* was first detected by an Italian physician Dubini in 1843 and life cycle and pathogenesis was described by Arthur Loss in 1898
❖ *N. americanus* was first described by Stiles in 1902 in Texas, USA, hence called as **American hookworm or the American murderer.**

Epidemiology

World

Hookworm infection is widespread. Globally, nearly 900 million people are infected. *N. americanus* infection (835 million) is more common than *A. duodenale* (135 million).

❖ *A. duodenale* is prevalent in southern Europe, North Africa, and northern Asia
❖ *N. americanus* is the predominant species in the Western world, found throughout Central and South Africa, Central and South America
❖ In Southeast Asia including India, both the species coexist

❖ Hookworm infection is almost eradicated from Europe and USA
❖ Males and young adults (15–25 years) are commonly affected; but the anemia due to iron loss is more severe in children and pregnant women.

India

Hookworm infection is widely prevalent in India. More than 200 million people are estimated to be infected in India.
❖ *N. americanus* is predominant in South India and *A. duodenale* in North India
❖ *Necator* is seen in all the states except in Punjab and Uttar Pradesh
❖ Recently, another species, *A. ceylanicum* has been reported from a village near Kolkata
❖ Heavily infected areas are: Assam (tea gardens), West Bengal, Bihar, Odisha, Andhra Pradesh, Tamil Nadu, Kerala and Maharashtra.

Endemic Index

Chandler's index is used in the epidemiological studies of hookworm disease to estimate the morbidity and mortality in the community due to hookworm infection (which depends much upon the worm load).

Morphology

Hookworm has three morphological forms: adult, larvae (four stages) and egg; similar to other nematodes.

Adult Worm (A. duodenale)

❖ **Size:** Male worm is smaller (7–11 mm) than the female (9–13 mm)
❖ **Shape:** Straight except the anterior end which is bent dorsally (in the same direction of body curvature), hence called as **hookworm**
❖ **Color:** Adult worm is pink or grayish-white but may look reddish due to ingested blood
❖ **Mouth:** It is present at the anterior end, directed dorsally. It contains the buccal capsule which is lined by a hard substance bearing six teeth (four hook-like teeth on ventral surface and two knob like teeth dorsally) (Fig. 12.8A)
❖ **Glands:** The digestive system is attached with five glands, one of them is the esophageal gland secreting a substance that prevents clotting
❖ **Copulatory bursa:** Presence of copulatory bursa in the caudal end of males differentiates it from the female worms of *A. duodenale* (Table 12.4) (Fig. 12.8B)
  ■ It is the umbrella like expansion of the posterior end of male worm bearing two spicules, consists of three lobes (one-dorsal and two-lateral)

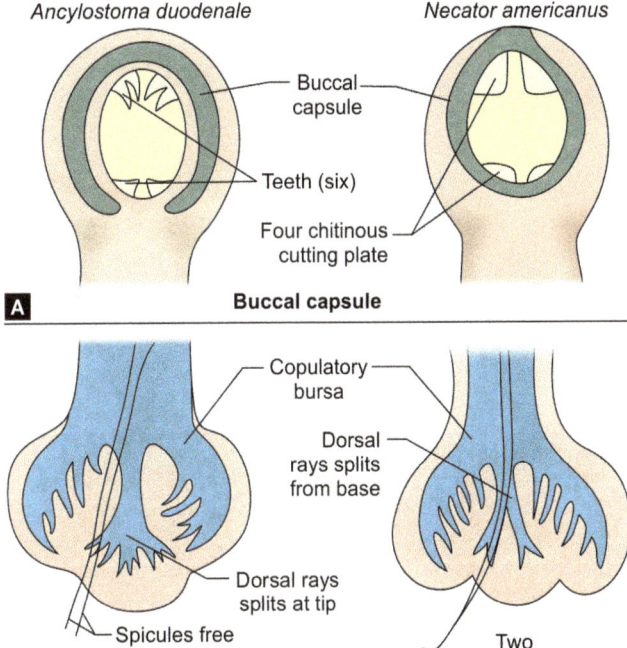

Figs 12.8A and B: (A) Buccal capsule and (B) Copulatory bursa of *Ancylostoma duodenale* and *Necator americanus* (schematic)

Table 12.4: Differences between male and female worms of *Ancylostoma duodenale*

Features	Male worm	Female worm
Size	Smaller (5–11 mm)	Longer (9–13 mm)
Copulatory bursa	Present posteriorly	Absent
Posterior end	Expanded due to copulatory bursa	Tapering and straight pointed tail
Genital opening	Opens in cloaca along with anus	Opens separately in the middle

  ■ All the three lobes again split in a tripartite fashion. Dorsal lobe contains three dorsal rays; each lateral lobe contains five rays (two-ventral and three lateral rays). So total numbers of rays are 13 (Fig. 12.8B).
❖ Other features are similar to any nematode described at the beginning of the chapter
❖ Adult worm of *N. americanus* is different from *A. duodenale* (Table 12.5).

Egg

Hookworm eggs are:
❖ Oval-shaped, measures 60 × 40 μm
❖ Not bile stained, appear colorless in saline mount
❖ Surrounded by thin, hyaline, translucent egg shell
❖ Ovum (embryo) is segmented; comprises of 4 to 32 blastomeres (Figs 12.9A and B)

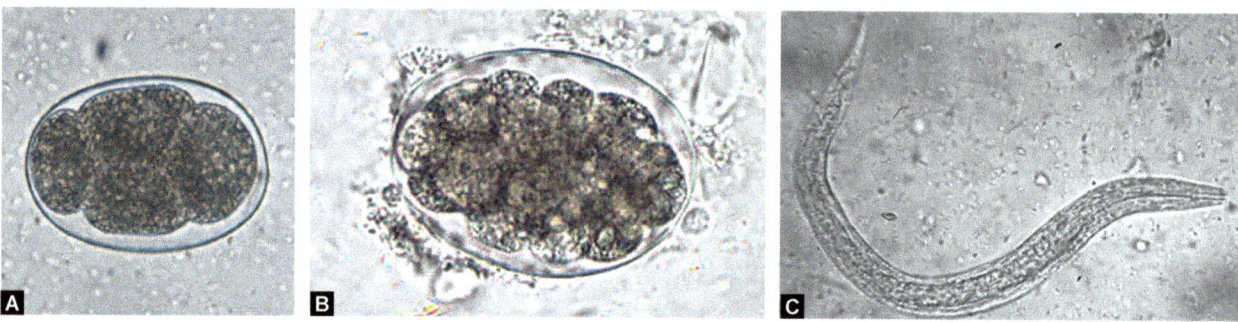

Figs 12.9A to C: Hookworm (A) Egg with four blastomeres; (B) Egg with many blastomeres; (C) Rhabditiform larva

Source: A to C—DPDx Image Library, Centers for Disease Control and Prevention (CDC), Atlanta (*with permission*).

Table 12.5: Differences between adult worm of *Ancylostoma duodenale* and *Necator americanus*		
Adult worm	***Ancylostoma duodenale***	***Necator americanus***
Size	Large and thick	Smaller and more slender
Bending of anterior end	Bends in the same direction of body curvature	Bends in the opposite direction of body curvature
Buccal capsule	Bears six teeth • Four hook-like ventral teeth • Two knob-like dorsal teeth	• Four chitinous cutting plates present • Two ventral and two dorsal • Dorsomedian teeth are present
Copulatory bursa	• Bifurcation is tripartite • Total number of rays 13 • Dorsal ray splits at the tip • Two spicules are present freely	• Bifurcation is bipartite • Total number of rays 14 • Dorsal ray splits from the base • Both spicules are fused at the tip
Posterior end of female worm	Bears a spine	No spine present in females
Vulva opens at	Behind the middle of the body	In front of middle of the body
Pathogenicity	More pathogenic because of: • Larger size, armed with teeth and more migratory • Blood loss 0.15–0.26 mL/worm/day	Less pathogenic • **Except:** Ground itch and dermatitis (more severe) • Blood loss 0.03 mL/worm/day

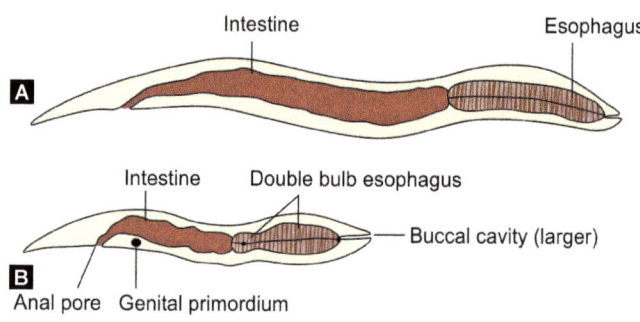

Figs 12.10A and B: Hookworm (*Acylostoma duodenale*) (A) Filariform larva; (B) Rhabditiform larva

❖ First stage larva is called as rhabditiform larva (Figs 12.9C and 12.10B)
❖ L_3 stage larva is called as filariform larva and is the infective form to man
❖ Filariform larva is longer (660–720 μm) than the rhabditiform larva (100–150 μm), the esophageal bulb extends to about one-third of the body length and the posterior end is more acutely tapered (Fig. 12.10A)
❖ The rhabditiform larva of *A. duodenale* and *N. americanus* is morphologically similar but they differ in the morphology of their filariform larva (Table 12.6).

Life Cycle (Fig. 12.11)

Host: Hookworm involves only one host (man).
Infective stage: Third stage filariform (L_3) larva acts as the infective form.
Mode of transmission: Through penetration of skin by the third stage larva (by walking bare foot in dampen soil). Though rare, but other routes of transmission of the larva has been reported through oral, in utero and transmammary routes.

Migratory Phase

Following penetration, the L_3 larvae enter into the small subcutaneous venules and through venous circulation, reach to the right side of heart and finally to the lungs.

❖ There is a clear space between the egg shell and the embryo
❖ Floats on saturated salt solution
❖ Eggs of both *A. duodenale* and *N. americanus* are morphologically indistinguishable.

Larva

There are four stages of hookworm larva (L_1 to L_4)

CHAPTER 12 ◆ Nematodes—I (Intestinal Nematodes)

Table 12.6: Differences between filariform (L3) larva of *Ancylostoma duodenale* and *Necator americanus*

Filariform (L$_3$) larva	Ancylostoma duodenale	Necator americanus
Size	720 μm	660 μm
Shape	Head end is blunt and tail is pointed	Same as *Ancylostoma*
Cuticle	Bears faint transverse striations	Bears prominent transverse striations
Buccal capsule	Shorter (10 μm), lumen larger and bound by two thin chitinous wall	Larger (15 μm), lumen short and bound by two thick chitinous wall
Esophagus-intestinal junction	No gap between esophagus and intestine	Gap between esophagus and intestine due to prominent anterior dilatation of intestinal lumen
Intestine	Posterior end of intestine has a refractile body	Refractile body absent

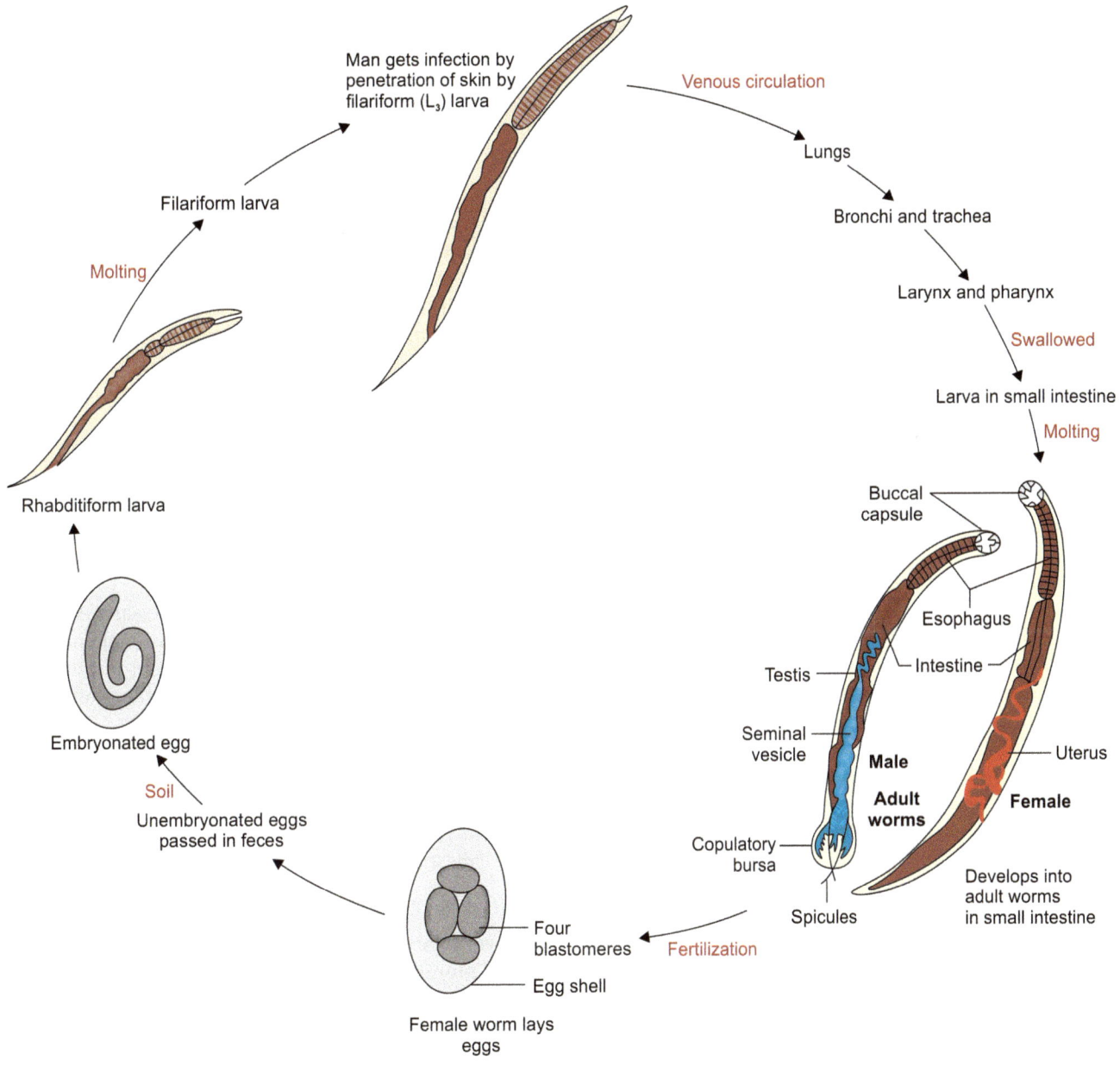

Fig. 12.11: Life cycle of hookworm

Here, they enter into the alveolar space and migrate up to bronchi, trachea and finally by swallowing of sputum, they enter GIT.

Intestinal Phase
Develop into Adults

The L_3 larvae undergo third molt (either in the migratory phase or on reaching esophagus) to form L_4 larvae that reach the small intestine where they undergo the final molt to develop into adult worms.

Laying Eggs

The adult worms attach to the intestinal mucosa by their teeth in buccal capsule. In about 5 months following infection, the adult worms mature and then following fertilization, the female worms start laying the eggs (with segmented ovum), which are excreted in the feces.

A gravid female of *A. duodenale* can lay 25,000-35,000 eggs/day, where as that of *N. americanus* can lay 6,000-20,000 eggs/day. The female worm survives for about 1-3 years (for *A. duodenale*) and 3-10 years (for *N. americanus*).

Development in Soil

Embryonation takes place in moist, shady, warm soil (sandy loam). The first stage (rhabditiform) larvae hatch out from eggs which then molt twice and finally the infective stage, i.e. L_3 larvae are developed within 5-8 days and they remain viable in soil for several weeks.

Pathogenicity

Hookworm has ability to suck blood from the intestinal vessels by:
- Attaching and making cuts in the intestinal wall by buccal capsule and teeth followed by sucking the blood through contraction of their muscular esophagus
- Secreting hydrolytic enzymes
- Releasing anticoagulants like factor Xa or VIIa/tissue factor inhibitor, helps to maintain continuous oozing of blood from the attachment site
- It is a habitual blood-sucker; produces active suction impulses 120-200 times/min.

It can also penetrate the skin which is facilitated by proteolytic enzymes (like aspartyl proteases) and hyaluronidase secreted by hookworm; leading to degradation of collagen types I, III, IV, and V, fibronectin, laminin, and elastin.

It is postulated that, hookworm infection can protect the individual from asthma and malaria but predispose to HIV, tuberculosis and other intestinal helminthic infections.

There is an increased T_H2 response leading to increased antibodies such as IgG4 or IgE levels.

Clinical Features
Affect due to Migrating Larva

- **Local lesion (in previously sensitized persons):**
    - Infective larvae may provoke pruritic maculopapular dermatitis and rashes **("ground itch")** at the site of skin penetration and
    - **Serpiginous tracks** may be formed due to subcutaneous migration of the larva similar to those of cutaneous larva migrans (described later).
- **Mild transient pneumonitis:** Migrating larva through the lungs occasionally cause mild transient pneumonitis, asthma and bronchitis; but the severity and frequency of lung manifestation is less compared to ascariasis.

Affect due to Adult worm in Intestine

Clinical spectrum produced by adult hookworm depends upon the worm load.

- **Asymptomatic:** Most hookworm infections are asymptomatic
- **Early intestinal phase (less worm load):** Infected persons may develop epigastric pain (often with postprandial accentuation), inflammatory diarrhea, or other abdominal symptoms, accompanied by eosinophilia
- **Late intestinal phase** (chronic hookworm infection with heavy worm load): Patients develop iron deficiency anemia and protein energy malnutrition resulting from blood loss. Other features are weakness and shortness of breath and rarely impaired intellectual power and behavioral changes
- **Wakana disease:** When L_3 larvae of *A. duodenale* are ingested by the oral route, both gastrointestinal (due to larva developing in to adult worm in intestine) as well as pulmonary symptoms (due to larva migrating through pharynx) are observed
    - Common symptoms include nausea, vomiting, pharyngeal irritation, cough, dyspnea, and hoarseness
    - This is not seen with *N. americanus* as their L_3 stage fails to develop after ingestion.

Arrested Development and Vertical Transmission

Hookworm larvae may undergo an arrested development up to 8 months, which facilitates the parasite to survive during the dry climatic season in the host. There is a strong evidence of vertical transmission in hookworm during the arrested phase leading to possibility of congenital infection.

Laboratory Diagnosis — Hookworm

- **Stool microscopy**—detects non bile stained oval segmented and non bile-stained eggs with 4–32 blastomeres. Eggs of *Acylostoma* and *Necator* are indistinguishable.
- **Stool culture**—eggs develop into filariform larvae, which help in differentiating *Acylostoma* from *Necator*
  - Harada-Mori filter paper tube method
  - Petri dish (slant culture) technique
  - Baermann funnel technique
  - Charcoal culture method
  - Agar plate technique (more sensitive)
- **Molecular method**—detects genes such as mitochondrial cytochrome oxidase I gene, ITS-1 and ITS-2 regions of ribosomal DNA
- **Other findings**— hypochromic microcytic anemia.

Table 12.7: Differences between rhabditiform larva of hookworm and *Strongyloides stercoralis*

Rhabditiform larva	Hookworm	Strongyloides
Size	100–150 µm long × 16 µm width	108–380 µm long × 14–20 µm width
Mouth (buccal cavity)	Three times longer	Shorter
Genital primordium	Less prominent and small	Prominent and large
Anal pore (subterminal)	80 µm from the posterior end	50 µm from the posterior end

Table 12.8: Classification of intensity of infection based on WHO guidelines (eggs per gram of stool)

	Light	Moderate	Heavy
Trichuris	1–999	1000–9999	≥10000
Ascaris	1–4999	5000–49999	≥50000
Hookworm	1–1999	2000–3999	≥4000

Laboratory Diagnosis

Stool Microscopy

The diagnosis is established by finding of characteristic oval segmented hookworm eggs in the feces (Fig. 12.9A).

- Stool concentration procedures may be required to detect lighter infections
- Eggs of *A. duodenale* and *N. americanus* are indistinguishable
- In a stool sample that is not fresh, the eggs may hatch out to release rhabditiform larvae, which need to be differentiated from those of *Strongyloides* (Table 12.7 and Fig. 12.9C)
- **Egg counting:** Number of eggs per gram of stool can be counted to estimate the disease burden in the individual as well as in the community. The WHO has classified the intensity of infection based on egg count which is directly related to the associated morbidity (Table 12.8). Various methods (described in detail in Chapter 15) are:
  - Kato Katz technique
  - Direct smear method of Beaver
  - Modified Stoll's dilution egg count method
  - FLOTAC technique and McMaster technique.

Stool Culture

Since the eggs of *A. duodenale* and *N. americanus* are indistinguishable, so freshly passed stool samples can be cultured where the eggs hatch out to develop to L_3 stage filariform larva in 5–7 days.

- The filariform L_3 larva of *A. duodenale* is different from *N. americanus* (see Table 12.6)
- The rhabditiform and filariform larva of hookworm and *Strongyloides* should also be differentiated (see Tables 12.7 and 12.10 and Figs 12.10 and 12.12)
- Various culture techniques used are (described in detail in Chapter 15):
  - Harada-Mori filter paper tube method
  - Petri dish (slant culture) technique
  - Baermann funnel technique
  - Charcoal culture method
  - Agar plate technique (more sensitive).

Molecular Diagnosis

PCR and real-time PCR based assays have been developed targeting genes such as mitochondrial cytochrome oxidase I genes (585-bp fragment) and ITS-1 and ITS-2 regions (internal transcribed spacer) of ribosomal DNA. Molecular methods have the advantages such as: (i) species specific; can differentiate between *Ancylostoma* and *Necator*; (ii) more sensitive, can detect as low as one copy per 200 mg of stool; (iii) can distinguish hookworm from *Oesophagostomum*, whose eggs are morphologically similar to hookworm.

Other Findings

Other findings include: (i) hypochromic microcytic anemia, (ii) eosinophilia and (iii) hypoalbuminemia.

Treatment — Hookworm

Antiparasitic

- Antiparasitic drugs like albendazole (400 mg once), mebendazole (500 mg once), and pyrantel pamoate (11 mg/kg for 3 days) can be given
- However, due to the widespread use of the drugs, their efficacy is decreased compared to the past. Resistance to albendazole and mebendazole has also been reported

Symptomatic treatment

- Mild iron-deficiency anemia can often be treated with oral iron with folic acid
- Severe hookworm disease with protein loss and malabsorption warrants nutritional support and oral or parenteral iron replacement

Prevention

General preventive measures include:
- Improved personal hygiene
- Proper disposal of feces
- Improved nutrition with dietary iron
- Treatment of infected persons.

Vaccine

No vaccine has been licensed yet for hookworm infection; however several vaccine trials are going on using vaccine candidates such as:
- *N. americanus* 24 kDa glutathione-S-transferase (Na-GST-1)
- *N. americanus* aspartic protease recombinant (Na-APR)-1
- Alhydrogel combined with an glucopyranosyl lipid A (GLA).

Ancylostoma Ceylanicum

A. ceylanicum is the second most common hookworm species infecting humans, comprising 6–23% of total hookworm infections.
- *A. ceylanicum* is endemic in South-east Asia; primarily infecting dogs and cats
- Clinically, it produces ground itch (**Cutaneous larva migrans**)
- It is the only zoonotic hookworm species that can develop into adult worm in man. A recent case of intestinal infection has also been reported from Solomon Islands in 2017.

STRONGYLOIDES STERCORALIS

History

Strongyloides stercoralis was known as the **"military worm"** as it was first found by Lois Normand in 1876 in the feces of French soldiers in Cochin-China
- The life cycle and pathogenicity were described later during early 1900s
- The name was coined by Stites and Hassall in 1902.

Classification

Strongyloides belongs to superfamily Rhabditoidea and family Strongyloididae. It comprises of 53 species but human infection is mainly caused by *S. stercoralis* and rarely by *S. fuelleborni*.

Epidemiology

S. stercoralis is distributed in hot, humid tropical areas.
- It is particularly common in South-east Asia (including India), Sub-Saharan Africa, and South America (Brazil)
- In the Western world, the parasite is found in immigrants, refugees, travelers, mental asylum, prisoners, and military personnels who have lived in endemic areas.

Habitat

The parasitic female worms reside in the human intestine (duodenum and upper jejunum) whereas the free-living female worms multiply in the environment.

Male worms are always free-living. The existence of parasitic male worm is debatable for many years. Most believe that parasitic male worms do not exist. However some school of thought believes that they may exist and fertilization may occur but they do not have penetrating power.

Morphology

Similar to other nematodes, *S. stercoralis* exists in three forms: adult, larvae (four stages) and egg.

Adult Worm

Only female worms are seen in the human intestine, male worms are rarely encountered.
- **Size:** The parasitic female worm (in human intestine) measures 2–3 mm long and 30–50 μm broad, whereas the free-living female worm is smaller and thicker (1 mm × 80 μm) (Figs 12.12A and B)
- **Alimentary tract:** Anterior portion is thicker bearing the mouth with three small lips, esophagus (with a posterior bulb and three esophageal glands) followed by the intestine with a midventral anus

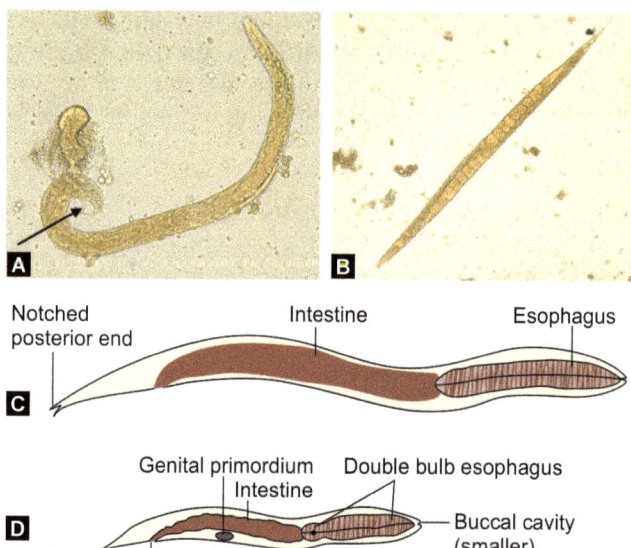

Figs 12.12A to D: *Strongyloides stercoralis* (A) Adult male (arrow shows spicules); (B) Adult female (containing single row of eggs); (C) Filariform larva (schematic); (D) Rhabditiform larva (schematic)

Source: B—DPDx Image Library, Centers for Disease Control and Prevention (CDC), Atlanta (*with permission*).

- Female reproductive organs consist of paired ovaries, oviducts and uteri which joined to form the vagina that leads to vulval opening at the junction of middle and posterior third of the body (Fig. 12.12B)
- The free living male worms are slightly smaller, having two spicules at the posterior end (Fig. 12.12A)
- Other features are similar to any nematode described at the beginning of the chapter.

Eggs

Eggs are conspicuous within the gravid female worm and arranged anteroposteriorly in a single row of 5–10 eggs in each uterus.
- They are oval and measure 50–58 × 30–34 μm in size
- Eggs of *Strongyloides* are ovoviviparous, i.e. they immediately hatch out to larvae.

Larva

There are four stages of *Strongyloides* larva (L_1 to L_4).
- **First stage or rhabditiform larva (L_1):** Eggs hatch out to form L_1 larvae in the human intestine. They measure 108–380 μm long × 14–20 μm width. They have a short mouth (buccal cavity), a double bulb esophagus and prominent, large genital primordium. It is the diagnostic form found in human feces (Fig. 12.12D)
- **Third stage or filariform larva (L_3):** In the environment, the L_1 larva molts twice to form filariform larva. It measures 630 μm long × 16 μm width and bears a long cylindrical esophagus and a notched tail. It survives few days in the environment and is the infective stage to human (Fig. 12.12C).

Life Cycle (Fig 12.13)

Host: *S. stercoralis* involves only one host (man). Rarely, domestic pets are recognized as reservoir of infection.

Infective stage: L_3 larva (filariform).

Mode of transmission:
- Penetration of skin by the L_3 larva (by walking bare foot). Larva releases hydrolytic enzymes that helps in penetration
- Autoinfection (internal autoinfection)

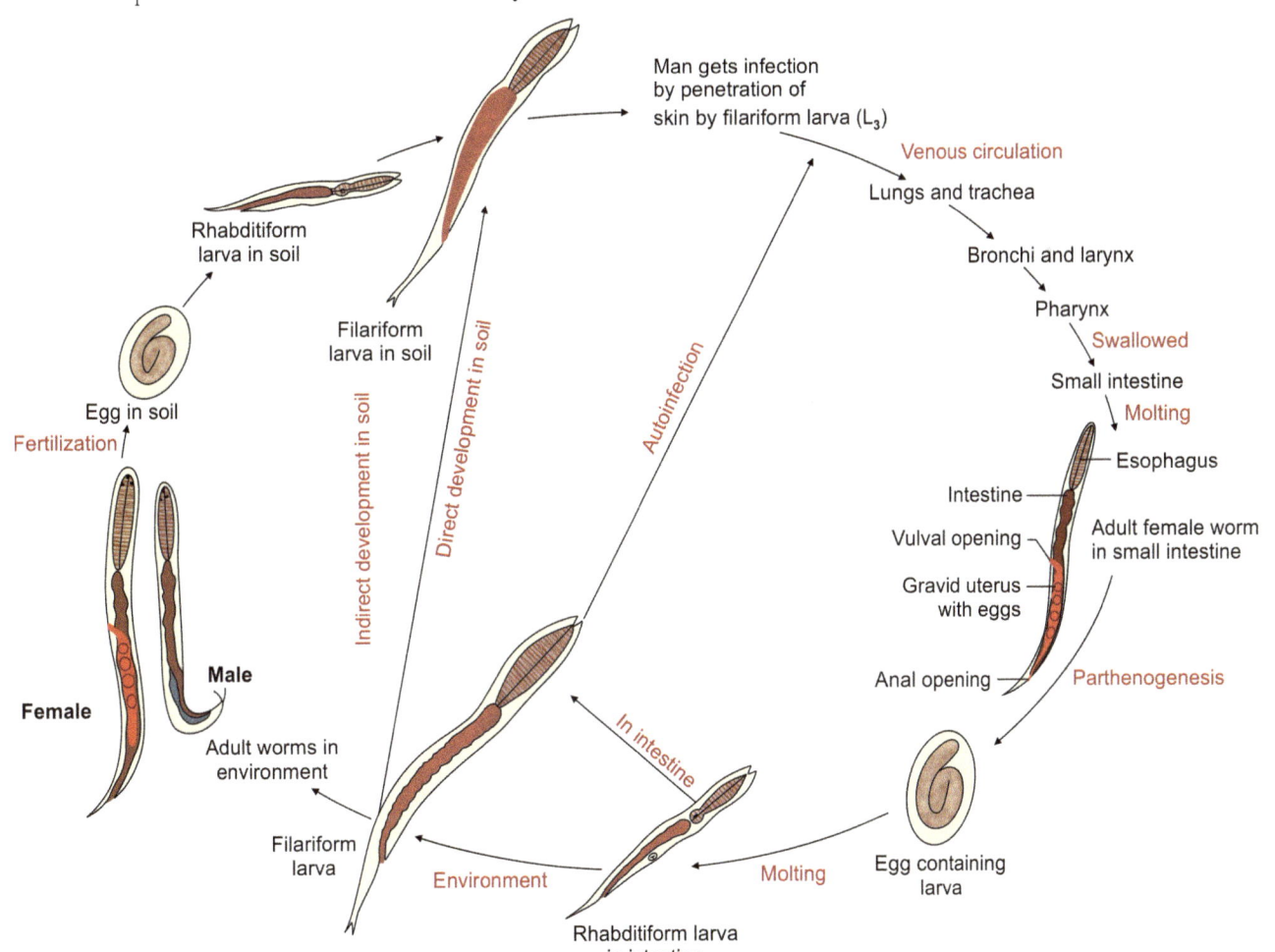

Fig. 12.13: Life cycle of *Strongyloides stercoralis*

- Though rare, but other routes of transmission of the larva has been reported like in utero, transmammary routes or zoonotic transmission.

Migratory Phase

Following penetration, the L_3 larvae enter the subcutaneous small venules through the venous circulation, they reach to the right side of heart and finally to the lungs. Here, they enter into the alveolar space and migrate up to bronchi, trachea and finally by swallowing of sputum, they enter GIT.

Intestinal Phase

Develop Into Adults

The L_3 larvae undergo third molt (mostly in the lungs or on reaching esophagus) to form L_4 larvae that reach the small intestine where they undergo the final molt to develop into adult females. However, adult males are not found in human intestine.

Laying Eggs

Only the female worms are seen buried in the intestinal mucosa. They can directly lay eggs without fertilization (called as **parthenogenesis**—a process by which the females produce offspring without fertilization with males).
- Eggs produced following fertilization with male worms have been postulated by some school of thoughts, but have never been confirmed
- Eggs soon hatch out liberating the rhabditiform (L_1) larvae into the intestinal lumen and are passed in the feces
- **Autoinfection:** Some times, the L_1 larvae released in the human intestine do not pass in the feces but develop into filariform larvae that eventually penetrate the intestinal wall or perianal skin, enter the venous circulation and reach lungs. Autoinfection is responsible for maintaining the infection as long as 30–40 years and can cause disseminated infection.

Development in Environment

In moist and warm soil, the rhabditiform (L_1) larva molts twice to form the L_3 larva. Then there are two types of development which takes place: (direct and indirect), depending on the environmental condition sensed by the chemosensory neurons present in the anterior end of the larva. Tropical climate favors indirect free-living cycle, whereas the direct parasitic cycle occurs more commonly in temperate climate.

Direct Development

The L_3 larva acts as the infective form and infects man through the penetration of skin. This cycle usually occurs in temperate climate.

Indirect Development

The L_3 larvae molt twice to develop into the adult worms (male and female) in the tropical environment. The free-living adult worms become sexually matured; fertilization takes place to lay eggs that hatch out soon to L_1 larvae which molts twice to form the infective L_3 filariform larvae.

Pathogenesis and Clinical Feature

Effect due to Migrating Larva

- **Asymptomatic infection:** More than 50% of chronically infected people may be asymptomatic
- **Rashes:** Some people develop recurrent maculopapular or urticarial rashes that involve primarily the buttocks, perineum, and thighs
- **Cutaneous larva migrans:** Migrating larvae may produce the pathognomonic serpiginous urticarial rash (commonly on thigh) called as **larva currens** (or racing larva), that advances as fast as 10 cm/hour
- Pulmonary symptoms are uncommon compared to ascariasis and hookworm. It occurs only secondary to underlying chronic obstructive lung disease.

Effect due to Adult Worm and Filariform Larva

- **Mild to moderate worm load:** Adult worms and larvae traversing the upper small bowel mucosa may produce epigastric pain (resembling peptic ulcer), nausea, diarrhea, constipation, and blood loss
  - Infection is associated with decreased expression of HLA-DR in epithelial cells
  - Radiologically, it mimics Crohn's disease.
- **Heavy larva load:** Hyperinfection syndrome and disseminated strongyloidiasis are the important complications (Table 12.9).

Laboratory Diagnosis — *Strongyloides stercoralis*

- **Microscopy** [stool or duodenal aspirate (by Entero-test), rarely sputum]—detects rhabditiform larvae
- **Stool culture**—
  - Harada-Mori filter paper tube method
  - Petri dish (slant culture) technique
  - Baermann funnel technique
  - Charcoal culture method
  - Agar plate technique (more sensitive)
- **Antibody detection**—ELISA (CrAg-ELISA), luciferase immuno-precipitation assay
- **Coproantigen** in stool—capture ELISA detecting excretory/secretory (E/S) antigen
- **Molecular diagnosis**—real time PCR detecting cytochrome C oxidase subunit I gene, 18S rRNA, or 28S RNA gene sequences.

Laboratory Diagnosis

Microscopy

The rhabditiform larvae can be demonstrated in stool by direct microscopy or following concentration techniques (Fig. 12.14A).

CHAPTER 12 ❖ Nematodes—I (Intestinal Nematodes)

Table 12.9: Complications of strongyloidiasis

Hyperinfection syndrome
The underlying cause of hyperinfection syndrome is the repeated autoinfection cycles; which leads to generation of large number of filariform larvae. The larvae penetrate the GIT and migrate to various organs.
- **Risk factors:** Impaired host immunity favors larva multiplication
  - Glucocorticoid therapy is the main risk factor
  - Other risk factors include immunosuppressive conditions such as transplant recipients, hematologic malignancies, and intake of immunosuppressive drugs
  - Hyperinfection syndrome is common in patients coinfected with human T cell lymphotropic virus type (HTLV-1)
  - Coinfection of *Strongyloides* with HIV is common. However, it is not associated with disseminated strongyloidiasis.
- **Features:** Colitis, enteritis, or malabsorption, and in severe cases disseminated strongyloidiasis may develop
- **Disseminated strongyloidiasis:**
  - Larvae may invade the GIT and migrate to various organs including CNS, peritoneum, liver, and kidneys
  - Moreover, the passage of enteric flora through disrupted mucosa lead to gram-negative bacterial sepsis, pneumonia, or meningitis which may dominate the clinical course
  - CNS invasion, brain abscess and meningitis are common. Larvae can be seen in the CSF occasionally. CSF examination shows pleocytosis, elevated protein, normal glucose and negative for bacterial culture.
- Eosinophilia is often absent in severely infected patients
- The mortality rate in untreated patients approaches 100% and even with treatment it may exceed 25%.

❖ Sometime, the hookworm eggs may hatch in the stool releasing the rhabditiform larva which has to be differentiated from that of *S. stercoralis* (see Table 12.7 and Figs 12.10B and 12.12B)

❖ Single stool examination is less sensitive (30%) due to irregular and low output of larvae. Hence repeated stool examination (four samples) is required

❖ **Entero-test:** Sometime duodenal aspirate can be collected by entero-test (described in Chapter 4) and examined for the presence of larva. *Stronglyoides* eggs are rarely seen stool; however they may be recovered from duodenal content

❖ Disseminated strongyloidiasis can be readily diagnosed by examining stool, sputum, other body fluids, and tissue biopsies, which typically contain high numbers of filariform larvae. In stool, numerous rhabditiform larva and occasional adult worms and eggs may also be seen (Fig. 12.14B).

Stool Culture

Freshly passed stool samples should be cultured.
❖ L_3 stage filariform larvae are formed within 2 days which should be differentiated from that of hookworm (Table 12.10, Figs 12.10A and 12.12C)
❖ Various culture techniques can be used (described in detail in Chapter 15). They are:
  - Harada-Mori filter paper tube method
  - Petri dish (slant culture) technique
  - Baermann funnel technique

Table 12.10: The differences between filariform larva of hookworm and *Strongyloides stercoralis*

Filariform larva	Hookworm	Strongyloides
Size	720 µm long	630 µm long × 16 µm width
Esophagus	Shorter	Long and cylindrical
Tail	Long pointed tail	Blunt and notched

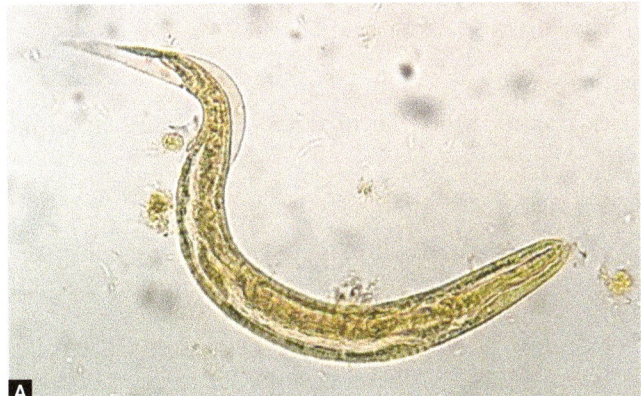 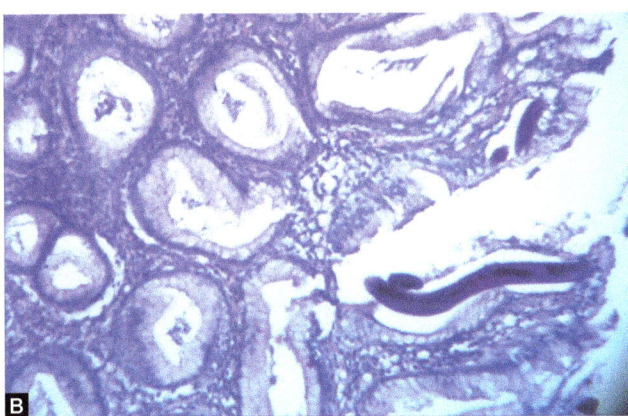

Figs 12.14A and B: Rhabditiform larva of *Strongyloides stercoralis* (A) Iodine mount; (B) Histopathology from Intestinal biopsy (hematoxylin and eosin stain)

Source: Meenakshi Medical College, Chennai; A—Department of Microbiology; B—Department, Pathology (*with permission*).

- Modified Baermann technique
- Charcoal culture method
- Agar plate technique (more sensitive).

Serology

ELISA using crude larval antigens (CrAg-ELISA) has a greater sensitivity (95%) and should be used when microscopic examinations are negative.

- However, it is less specific because of cross-reactivity with other helminthic infection
- More so, antibody detection cannot differentiate recent and past infection
- It can also be used for monitoring the treatment response; however antibodies disappear slowly following 6–12 months of clinical cure.

Newer antibody detection assays include:
- Luciferase immunoprecipitation system assay (LIP assay): It has been developed using a 31-kDa recombinant antigen (called NIE) and/or the recombinant *S. stercoralis* immunoreactive antigen (SsIR)
- ELISA using NIE antigen has also been developed.

Coproantigen Detection in Stool

Antigen capture ELISA has been developed using polyclonal rabbit antiserum raised against *Strongyloides ratti* excretory/secretory (E/S) antigen. It does not show cross-reactivity with other intestinal helminthic infections.

Molecular Diagnosis

Real-time PCR assays are available targeting various genes of *S. stercoralis* such as cytochrome C oxidase subunit I gene, 18S rRNA, or 28S RNA gene sequences in fecal samples. They showed 100% specificity with variable sensitivity (low in asymptomatic patients with very low levels of larval output).

Treatment	*Strongyloides stercoralis*
☐ Even in the asymptomatic stage, strongyloidiasis must be treated because of the potential for subsequent fatal hyperinfection
☐ Ivermectin (200 mg/kg daily for 2 days) is more effective than albendazole (400 mg daily for 3 days)
☐ For disseminated strongyloidiasis: Prolonged course of Ivermectin should be given at least 5–7 days or until the parasites are eradicated.	

Prevention

Prevention of strongyloidiasis is same as for hookworm and other intestinal nematodes.

Strongyloides Fuelleborni

It is a zoonotic parasite affecting monkeys and apes. Occasionally, it causes human infection.

- **Swollen belly syndrome:** It is a serious life-threatening condition characterized by diarrhea, respiratory distress and protein losing enteropathy, leading to hypoalbuminemia and edema
- *S. fuelleborni* infection in humans is seen in tropical forest regions of Central and East Africa
- A non-zoonotic infection of *S. fuelleborni* occurs in forest areas of Western Papua New Guinea; affecting infants of 2–4 months age. It is possibly transmitted through breast milk. Previously, it was named as *S. fuelleborni kellyi*; recent molecular studies suggest that this is not a separate subspecies
- It is diagnosed by detecting the eggs (50–70 μm long) but not larvae in the stool (different from *S. stercoralis*).

Treatment: Thiabendazole is used for treatment of swollen belly syndrome.

ASCARIS LUMBRICOIDES

Ascaris lumbricoides is the largest nematode parasitizing the human intestine. The name is derived from *Askaris* means intestinal worm and *Lumbricus* means resembling with common earthworm. It is commonly called as **roundworm**. It is one of the soil-transmitted helminth (see the highlight box at the end of this Chapter for detail).

Epidemiology

A. lumbricoides is cosmopolitan in distribution, mainly affecting tropical countries including India.

- It is estimated that, 1470 million people are infected globally out of which around 120–250 million of people are symptomatic
- Transmission typically occurs through fecally contaminated soil and is due to either lack of sanitary facilities or use of human feces as fertilizer
- Clay soils are the most favorable for the development of *Ascaris* egg (in contrast to moist porous soil required for hookworm)
- **Risk factors:** Children (most important disseminator of the disease) and malnutrition.

Morphology

Ascaris exists in three forms: adult, larvae (four stages) and egg.

Adult Worm

- **Appearance:** It is pinkish-creamy in color when freshly passed from intestine, but gradually fades color and looks whitish
- **Size:** Female worms (20–35 cm) are longer than male worms (15–31 cm). Adult worms life span is 1–2 years
- **Shape:** Cylindrical (hence called as round-worm); with tapering ends (tapering is more anteriorly)

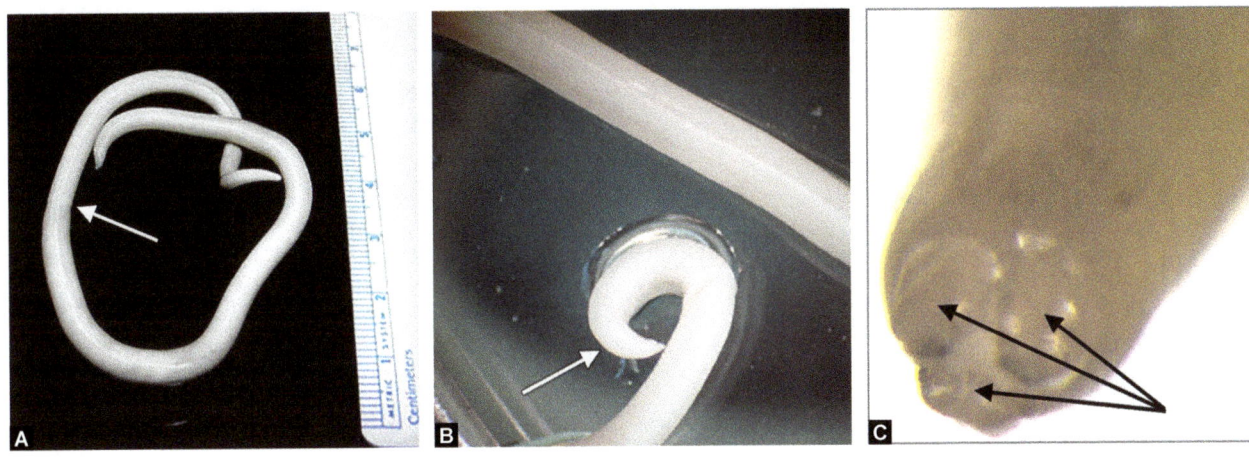

Figs 12.15 A to C: Adult worm of A. *lumbricoides* (A) Adult female with vulvar waist (arrow showing); (B) Posterior end of adult male showing the curled tail (arrow showing); (C) Close-up of the anterior end of an adult showing the characteristic three 'lips' (arrows showing)

Source: A to C—DPDx Image Library, Centers for Disease Control and Prevention (CDC), Atlanta (*with permission*); C—Orange County Public Health Laboratory, Santa Ana, CA.

Table 12.11: Differences between fertilized and unfertilized eggs of *Ascaris* species

	Fertilized eggs	**Unfertilized eggs**
Shape	Round to oval	Elongated
Size	45–75 µm × 35–50 µm	85–95 µm × 43–47 µm
Covering (egg shell)	Surrounded by a thick mamillated, albuminous coat	Albuminous coat is thin, distorted and scanty
Crescentic space at poles	Present	Absent
Bile staining	Yes, golden brown in saline mount	Yes, golden brown in saline mount
Saturated salt solution	Floats	Does not float
Ovum	Egg contains a large unsegmented ovum of granular mass with clear space at both the end	Egg contains an unsegmented, small atrophied ovum with a mass of disorganized highly refractile granules

- **Mouth part:** The mouth opens anteriorly and bears three characteristic toothed lips (one dorsal and two ventral) (Fig. 12.15C). The character of the toothed lip is used to differentiate *A. lumbricoides* and *A. suum*
- **Body cavity:** It is filled with a characteristic fluid called as **ascaron** or **ascarase** in which the intestine and genital organs float. This fluid is irritant in nature and if leaked, then can cause allergic manifestations
- **Male:** The posterior end of the male worm is curved and pointed bearing two spicules. Rectum and genital duct open together at cloaca near the posterior end (Fig. 12.15B)
- **Females:** Posterior end is straight and pointed. Anus is subterminal and situated posteriorly while the vulva is situated at the junction of anterior and middle third of the body (on the ventral surface). This portion of the worm is narrower and referred to as **vulvar waist** (Fig. 12.15A)
- Other features are similar to any nematode adult worm, described in the beginning of the chapter.

Egg

Two types of eggs are liberated from the female worm of *A. lumbricoides*—(1) fertilized and (2) unfertilized eggs (Table 12.11 and Figs 12.17A and B). Sometimes, the fertilized eggs may lose the thick mamillated albuminous coat. Such types of eggs are called as decorticated eggs (Fig. 12.17C).

Larva

There are four stages of *Ascaris* larvae (L_1 to L_4).

Life Cycle (Fig. 12.16)

Host: Involves only one host (man).
Infective stage: Embryonated eggs containing the L_2 larvae.
Mode of transmission: Ingestion of embryonated eggs from the contaminated soil, food and water.

Migratory Phase

Following ingestion, the eggs hatch out to liberate the L_2 larvae (250 µm long) in the duodenum.
- The L_2 larvae molt once to form L_3, which penetrate the intestine, reach right side of heart via portal circulation and finally enter the lungs via pulmonary capillaries
- Within 6–10 days in lungs, the larvae mature to become 550 µm long, molt to form next stage larvae (L_4)
- The larvae break up into the alveoli, migrate via bronchi, trachea and pharynx and finally swallowed to reach intestine.

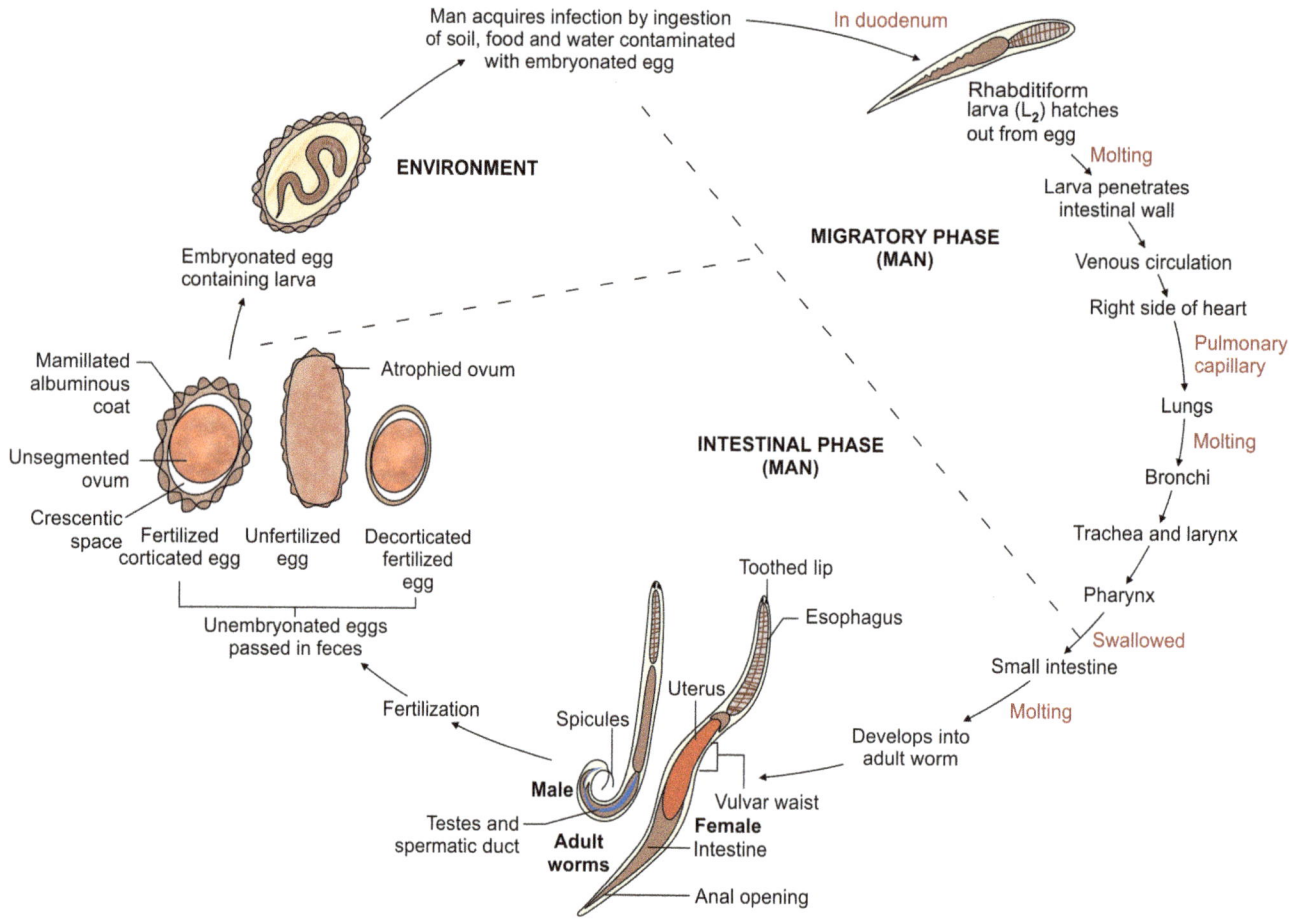

Fig. 12.16: Life cycle of *Ascaris lumbricoides*

Intestinal Phase

The larvae undergo final molt to develop into adult worms in the small intestine. Adult worms become sexually mature, fertilize and the female worms start laying the fertilized eggs which are passed in the feces. Sometime, before mating, the female worms may directly lay the unfertilized eggs. If the unfertilized eggs alone are detected in stool, it indicates the presence of only female worms in the intestine.

- **Pre-patent period:** It is the time from ingestion of egg to egg passage in the feces and is around 2 months
- A gravid female can lay 2.4 lakh eggs/day. The female worm survives for 1–2 years.

Development in Soil

The fertilized eggs become embryonated in 2 weeks under suitable conditions such as warm and clay soil, 22–30°C and 40% humidity. The unfertilized eggs cannot develop further.

- Rhabditiform larvae (L_1) are produced inside the eggs which then molt to produce L_2 larvae. Embryonated eggs containing the L_2 larva are the infective stage
- *Ascaris* embryonated eggs survive for as long as 15 years as they are highly resistant due to the characteristic thick egg shell. *Ascaroside*, a lipoprotein present in the egg shell is responsible for its resistant to disinfectants
- The unfertilized eggs are not infective, they disintegrate in sometime.

Pathogenesis and Clinical Feature

Pathogenesis caused by *Ascaris* infection is attributed to (i) the host immune response, (ii) migration of larva (iii) mechanical obstruction by the adult worms, and (iv) nutritional deficiencies due to presence of the adult worms. Incubation period is about 60–70 days; however the pulmonary symptoms can be seen 4–6 days after the infection.

Effect due to Migrating Larva

- **Pulmonary symptoms:** Observed in the second week after ingestion of eggs. Migrating larvae in lungs provoke an immune-mediated hypersensitivity response. Common symptoms include a non-productive cough, chest discomfort and fever

❖ **Eosinophilic pneumonia (Loeffler's syndrome):** In severe cases, patients develop dyspnea and an transient patchy infiltrates seen on chest X-ray along with peripheral eosinophilia. The pulmonary stage in ascariasis is short-term with rapidly falling eosinophilia, which should be differentiated from that of *Toxocara* larva migrans; where the pulmonary infection is long-term with persistent eosinophilia.

Effect due to Adult Worm

❖ **Asymptomatic:** Most people with mild *Ascaris* infections are asymptomatic
❖ **Malnutrition and growth retardation:** Robbing the nutrition from the host may result in chronic malnutrition and growth retardation (in children <5 years). It is observed that helminthic infection is often associated with impairment of educational performance, language learning, social, gross motor, and fine motor skills in children
❖ **Intestinal complications:** A large bolus of entangled worms can cause acute pain abdomen due to small-bowel obstruction, rarely perforation, **intussusception**, or volvulus. Mortality may occur occasionally (0–8.6%). A single worm can also cause intestinal obstruction as a result of worm migration; induced by stimuli such as fever. Intestinal obstruction is usually seen in age group >5 years
❖ **Extraintestinal complications:** Larger worms can enter and occlude the biliary tree, causing biliary colic, cholecystitis, pancreatitis, or (rarely) intrahepatic abscesses. Wandering worms may migrate to pharynx and can cause respiratory obstruction or may block the eustachian tube
❖ **Allergic manifestations** like fever, urticaria, angio-neurotic edema and conjunctivitis may occur due to toxic fluid (ascaron or ascarase) released by the adult worm.

Laboratory Diagnosis — *Ascaris lumbricoides*

- **Stool examination** (saline and iodine mount)—detects three types of eggs
  - Fertilized egg—round to oval with outer thick albumin coat
  - Unfertlized eggs—rectangular and elongated, surrounded by thin albumin coat
  - Decorticated eggs—it is a fertilized egg with albumin coat lost
- **Adult worm detection**—X-ray (Trolley car lines), USG and Barium meal of GIT
- **Larva detection** (sputum/gastric aspirate)
- **Serology** (antibody detection)—ELISA, IFA, IHA test
- **Other findings** such as eosinophilia and Charcot-Leyden crystals in sputum and stool.

Laboratory Diagnosis

Detection of the Parasite

Egg Detection (Stool Examination)

Both fertilized and unfertilized eggs can be detected by stool examination by saline and iodine wet mount. (Refer Table 12.11). Concentration techniques by sedimentation method should be done if direct stool microscopy is negative. Floatation method for stool concentration is not preferred as unfertilized eggs do not float on saturated salt solution (Figs 12.16 and 12.17). Histopathological staining of intestinal biopsy tissues may also reveal eggs (Fig. 12.18).

Adult Worm Detection

Occasionally, adult worms may be detected in stool or sputum of the patients by naked eye. Barium meal X-ray of the GIT may demonstrate the adult worms in the intestine. When two worms are lying parallel, gives *trolley car lines* appearance in X-ray. Ultrasound (USG) or cholangiopancreatography should be done to detect the adult worms in extraintestinal sites.

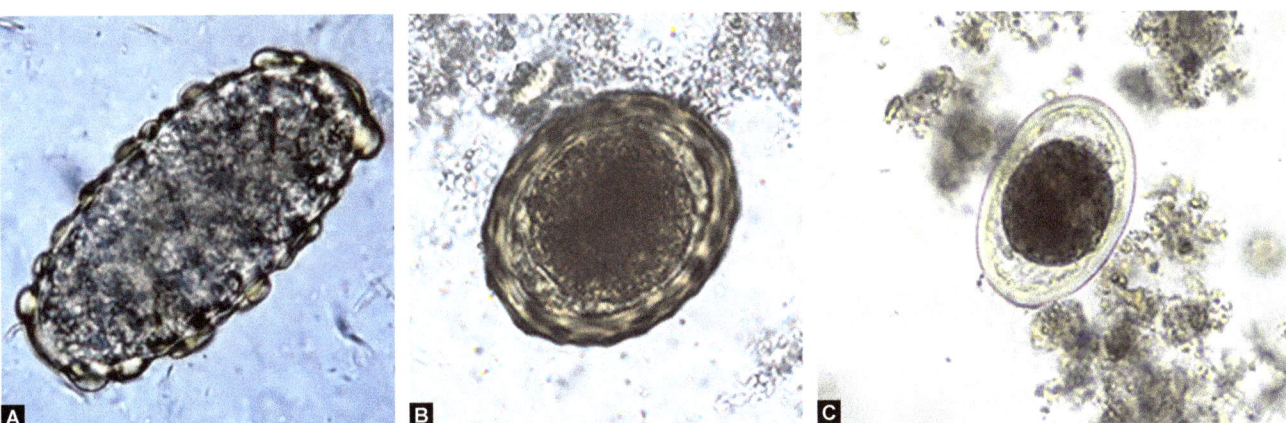

Figs 12.17A to C: Eggs of *Ascaris lumbricoides* (saline mount) (A) Unfertilized egg; (B) Fertilized egg; (C) Decorticated fertilized egg

Source: DPDx Image Library, Centers for Disease Control and Prevention (CDC), Atlanta (*with permission*).

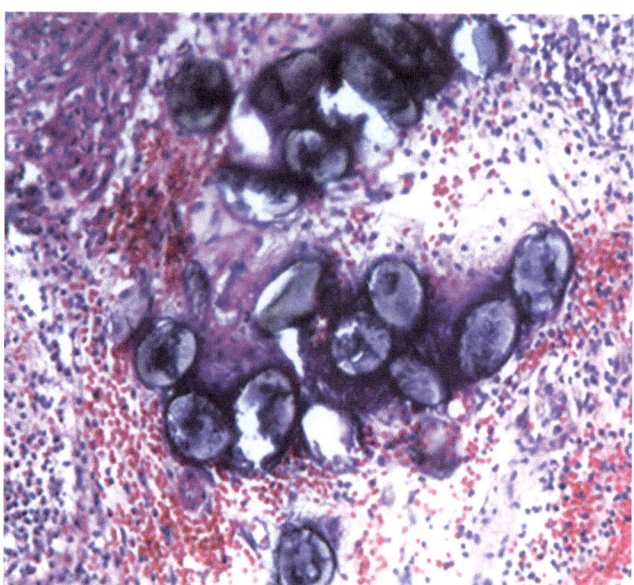

Fig. 12.18: Eggs of *A. lumbricoides* in an appendix biopsy, stained with H&E. This image was taken at 200x magnification

Source: DPDx Image Library, Centers for Disease Control and Prevention (CDC), Atlanta (*with permission*).

Larva Detection

During the early pulmonary migratory phase, larvae can be found in sputum or gastric aspirates before the eggs appear in the stool.

Serology

Antibody detection (by ELISA and other formats) though sensitive; cannot differentiate between recent and past infection. It also cross-reacts with other helminthic infections. It is mainly useful for seroepidemiological purposes and for assessing transmission in areas aiming for elimination.

Molecular Method

PCR assay has been developed targeting internal transcribed spacer region (ITS1) or cytochrome oxidase-1 of *Ascaris* egg in stool. Multiplex PCR can simultaneously differentiate *Ascaris*, *Trichuris* and hookworm. Real time PCR can be used for quantitation of the parasite load in stool.

Other Methods

- **Eosinophilia** is prominent during the early lung stage, but disappears later
- Presence of **Charcot-Leyden crystals** in sputum and stool, a nonspecific finding seen in ascariasis
- **Biomarkers** such as fatty acid products of *Ascaris* may be detected in urine by gas-liquid chromatography, and it is observed that their levels correlate well with worm burden. It is not commercially available yet.

Treatment — *Ascaris lumbricoides*

Antiparasitic drugs

Ascariasis should always be treated early to prevent potentially serious complications.
- Albendazole (400 mg once), mebendazole (100 g twice daily for 3 days or 500 mg once) is recommended. It effectively kills the adult worm, but has limited effect on larval migration phase
- Alternate drugs like ivermectin (150–200 mg/kg once) and nitazoxanide are also effective
- In pregnancy, pyrantel pamoate is safe

Symptomatic treatment

Partial intestinal obstruction should be managed with nasogastric suction, intravenous (IV) fluid administration but complete obstruction and its severe complications like intussusception require immediate surgical intervention.

Prevention

Same as for other soil transmitted helminths like hookworm and *Trichuris*. The use of human feces, or "night soil," for fertilization of crops should be avoided as it is an important source of *Ascaris* (mainly) and other helminthic infections.

Soil-transmitted helminths

Soil-transmitted helminths (STH) refer to the intestinal worms infecting humans that are transmitted through contaminated soil such as *Ascaris*, *Trichuris* and hookworm.
- **Global situation:** Worldwide >1.5 billion people (i.e. 24% of the world's population) are infected with STH infection. Infections are widely distributed in tropical and subtropical areas, with the greatest numbers occurring in sub-Saharan Africa, the America, China and East Asia
- **High risk group** for contracting GTH infection include preschool children, school-age children, women of childbearing age (including pregnant women) and adults in certain high-risk occupations such as tea-pickers or miners
- **Presentation:** Infected children are nutritionally, intellectually and physically impaired and suffer from malabsorption of nutrients, anemia, diarrhea and dysentery, depending upon type of helminths infected
- **Deworming:** It is a periodic prophylactic measure to prevent high-risk people from worm infestation; initiated by World Health Organization (WHO)
- **The National Deworming Day:** Every year, 10th February and 10th August are celebrated as National Deworming Day in India
    - Deworming should be done once in a year if the prevalence of STH infection is >20% in the community and twice a year if >50%
    - In this day, single dose albendazole (400 mg) is given to all children aged 1–19 years.
- **Elimination:** The WHO's global target is to eliminate morbidity due to STH infection in children by 2020. This will be obtained by regularly treating at least 75% of the children in endemic areas.

Ascaris suum

Ascaris suum, also known as large **roundworm** of pig, causes **ascariasis** in pig. Some authors believe that *A. lumbricoides* is the ancestor, from which it is derived.

- **Life cycle:** The human (or pig) ingests the egg with an L$_2$ larva inside. Life cycle is similar to that of *A. lumbricoides*
- **Clinical feature:** Human infection is rare
  - Most of the infections are asymptomatic
  - Rarely, the adult worms penetrate into the intestinal mucosa leading to intestinal manifestations
  - Migration to lungs can cause *Ascaris* pneumonitis.
- **Laboratory diagnosis:** It is done by detection of eggs by stool examination which is morphologically identical to that of *A. lumbricoides*. Only the adult worms are slightly different by the characteristic toothed lip at the anterior end.

EXPECTED QUESTIONS

I. **Write essay on:**
  a. A 8-year-old girl came to the pediatric OPD for school health check-up. On examination, she had pallor. Peripheral blood smear revealed microcytic, hypochromic anemia. Stool microscopy (saline mount) showed round to oval non-bile stained egg with segmented ovum (four blastomeres).
    1. Identify the disease and the causative agent.
    2. Write briefly about the life cycle of the etiological agent.
    3. What are the various diagnostic modalities?
    4. What is deworming strategy?
  b. A 9-year-old girl was brought to the OPD with history of epigastric pain, nausea, diarrhea, and blood loss. On examination, a serpiginous urticarial rash was observed in her lower limb. The stool specimen was sent for wet mount examination which revealed larvae of 250 μm × 16 μm in size, with short buccal cavity and prominent large genital primordium.
    1. Identify the disease and the causative agent.
    2. Write briefly about the life cycle of the etiological agent.
    3. What are the various complications seen?
  c. A 3-year-old boy came to the OPD with history of severe acute abdominal pain associated with nausea and vomiting. On examination, the child was malnourished. The stool microscopy revealed passing of bile-stained eggs which were round to oval in shape having a thick albumin coat.
    1. Identify the disease and the causative agent.
    2. Draw a labeled diagram of the ova of the causative agent.
    3. Which is the infective stage and mode of transmission?
    4. How will you diagnose this condition in the laboratory?
    5. Mention two complications caused by the adult worm.

II. **Write short notes on:**
  a. Trichuriasis.
  b. *Enterobius vermicularis*.
  c. Hyperinfection strongyloidiasis.
  d. Ascariasis.

III. **Multiple choice questions (MCQs):**
  1. **All of the following nematodes are oviparous, *except*:**
     a. Roundworm
     b. *Strongyloides*
     c. Hookworm
     d. *Enterobius*
  2. **Common name of *Trichuris trichiura* is:**
     a. Pinworm
     b. Roundworm
     c. Hookworm
     d. Whipworm
  3. ***Ascaris* infects humans by:**
     a. Penetration of skin by infective larvae
     b. Ingestion of unembryonated eggs present in contaminated food and water
     c. Ingestion of embryonated eggs present in contaminated food and water
     d. Autoinfection
  4. **Larva currens is caused by:**
     a. Ascariasis
     b. Cutaneous larva migrans
     c. Strongyloidiasis
     d. *Toxocara canis*
  5. **Number of eggs laid down by a female *Ascaris lumbricoides* in a day is about:**
     a. 5,000
     b. 20,000
     c. 1,00,000
     d. 2,40,000

Answer
1. b   2. d   3. c   4. c   5. d

Nematodes—II (Nematodes of Lower Animals that Rarely Infect Man)

CHAPTER 13

CHAPTER OUTLINE

- Classification
- Larva migrans
  - General properties
  - Toxocariasis
  - *Angiostrongylus* species
  - *Baylisascaris* species
  - *Lagochilascaris* species
- Anisakiasis
- *Gnathostoma* species
- Other animal nematodes
  - *Capillaria* species
  - *Trichostrongylus* species (Pseudo hookworm)
  - *Dioctophyme renale*
- *Oesophagostomum* species
- *Ternidens deminutus*
- *Mammomonogamus laryngeus*
- *Thelazia* species

CLASSIFICATION

This chapter reviews the less common zoonotic infections in humans caused by nematodes of lower animals. Humans are not the natural host for these parasites. Human infections are accidental; they are not able to complete their life cycle in humans as they do in the animal host. The disease process differs accordingly which may not resemble that of the animal host. The classification is given in Table 13.1. Filarial zoonotic infection is discussed in Chapter 14.

LARVA MIGRANS

GENERAL PROPERTIES

The life cycle of most of the human nematodes involve penetration of the skin by the larval stage followed by migration of the larvae to intestine, lungs or other organs. However, the larvae of lower animal nematodes when accidentally infect man, they are not able to complete their normal development (because humans are the unusual host for them) and their life cycle gets arrested. The larvae wander around aimlessly in the body. This is called as **larva migrans (LM)**.

Two types of larva migrans exists:

- **Cutaneous larva migrans:** Also called as **creeping eruption**. Larva migration occurs in skin and subcutaneous tissue
- **Visceral larva migrans:** Larva migration takes place in viscera.

Cutaneous Larva Migrans

Etiology

Cutaneous larva migrans (CLM), also called creeping eruption is mainly caused by filariform larvae of nonhuman hookworm species such as *Ancylostoma brasiliensis*, *A. caninum* and *A. ceylanicum*. Others can rarely cause CLM (Table 13.2).

Arrested Life Cycle and Pathogenesis

Host: Felines act as natural hosts. Humans are abnormal accidental host.
Infective stage: Filariform larva (L_3)
Mode of transmission: Penetration of skin by filariform larva (L_3) present in moist and warm soil contaminated with animal feces.

Man being the unnatural host, they can neither develop further nor migrate to intestine. Instead, they wander in the superficial layers of the skin of feet, legs, thigh, buttock and back and provoke allergic reaction in previously sensitized patients that leads to:

- **Ground itch:** Pruritic maculopapular dermatitis and rashes (ground itch) at the site of skin penetration of hookworm larva
- **Larva currens:** Migrating *Strongyloides* larvae produce the pathognomonic serpiginous urticarial rash called as **larva currens** near the legs.

Laboratory Diagnosis

Diagnosis is made mainly by clinical feature (presence of the linear tracks) and history of exposure. Larvae are usually not detected in skin biopsy. Recently, PCR has been

CHAPTER 13 ◆ Nematodes—II (Nematodes of Lower Animals that Rarely Infect Man)

Table 13.1: Nematodes of lower animals that rarely infect humans

Genus	Species	Primary host	Localized in man	Infective form	Disease in man
Toxocara	T. canis (Dog roundworm)	Dog	Liver or other viscera	Eggs (ingestion)	Visceral larva migrans (hepatomegaly)
	T. cati (Cat roundworm)	Cat			
Anisakis	A. simplex	Sea mammals	Intestine	L_3 larva (ingestion)	Eosinophilic granuloma of bowel
Angiostrongylus	A. cantonensis	Rat	CNS	L_3 larva (ingestion)	Eosinophilic meningitis
	A. costaricensis	Rat	Ileocecum	L_3 larva (ingestion)	Abdominal angiostrongyliasis
Baylisascaris	B. procyonis	Raccoon	CNS	Eggs (ingestion)	Eosinophilic meningoencephalitis
Lagochilascaris	L. minor	Feline	Skin	Ingestion of larva	Subcutaneous lesions
Ancylostoma	A. braziliensis	Dog and cat	Skin	L_3 larva (skin penetration)	Cutaneous larva migrans
	A. caninum	Dog			
	A. ceylanicum	Cat			
Gnathostoma	G. spinigerum	Dog and cat	Skin, CNS and eye	L_3 larva (ingestion of fish)	Cutaneous larva migrans, cerebral and ocular infection
Capillaria	C. philippinensis	Fish eating bird	Intestine	L_3 larva (ingestion of fish)	Malabsorption
	C. hepatica	Rodent	Liver	Eggs (ingestion)	Hepatitis and hepatomegaly
	C. aerophila	Carnivores	Trachea and bronchus	Eggs (ingestion)	Tracheobronchitis
Thelazia	T. callipaeda	Dog	Conjunctiva	L_3 larva (insect bite)	Lacrimation and itching of eye
Trichostrongylus	T. colubriformis T. orientalis	Sheep, goat and camel	Intestine	L_3 larva (ingestion)	Mild anemia
Oesophagostomum	O. bifurcum O. aculeatum	Monkey	Intestine	L_3 larva (ingestion)	Nodular lesions of the intestinal wall
Mammomonogamus	M. laryngeus	Cattle	Larynx and trachea	L_3 larva (ingestion)	Chronic cough and hemoptysis
Ascaris	A. suum	Pig	Lungs and Intestine	Egg ingestion	Pulmonary and intestinal symptoms
Strongyloides	S. fuelleborni	Monkey	Intestine	L_3 larva (skin penetration)	Swollen belly syndrome
Ternidens	T. deminutus	Ape and monkey	Intestine	L_3 larva (ingestion)	Anemia, pseudotumors and abscess of bowel
Dioctophyma	D. renale	Carnivorous (mink)	Kidney	L_3 larva (ingestion)	Hematuria

Abbreviations: CNS, central nervous system; L_3, filariform larva

developed for detection of larval DNA in human tissues. Elevated eosinophilia may be seen in peripheral blood or sputum. Charcot-Leyden crystals in sputum may be seen.

Treatment	Cutaneous larva migrans
☐ Oral and topical thiobendazole is effective ☐ Freezing the advancing end of creeping eruption in ethyl chloride is useful.	

Visceral Larva Migrans

In visceral larva migrans (VLM) migration of the infective larva and arrest of life cycle takes place in visceral organs.

- ❖ It is caused primarily by infection with *Toxocara* but less frequently caused by other helminths (Table 13.2)
- ❖ The further discussion of VLM is done for toxocariasis. Other rare agents of VLM are described later.

TOXOCARIASIS

Toxocara species belong to family ascarididae which also includes *Ascaris*, *Baylisascaris* and *Lagochilascaris*.
- ❖ **Species:** Two important species are *T. canis* (dog roundworm) and *T. cati* (cat roundworm)
- ❖ **Epidemiology:** Toxocariasis is prevalent wherever dogs or cats are found and *Toxocara* eggs are able to survive

Table 13.2: Etiology of larva migrans (LM)	
Causes of cutaneous larva migrans (CLM)	
Important causes (nonhuman *Ancylostoma* species): • *A. brasiliensis* • *A. caninum* • *A. ceylanicum*	**Rare causes:** Occasionally human nematodes may cause LM: • *Strongyloides stercoralis* • *Ancylostoma duodenale* • *Necator americanus*
Other rare nematodes: • *Gnathostoma spinigerum* • *Uncinaria stenocephala* • *Bunostomum phlebotomum*	**Due to non-helminthic agents:** • *Hypoderma* species • *Gasterophilus* species
Causes of visceral larva migrans (VLM)	
Important causes: *Toxocara* species (*T. canis* and *T. cati*)	
Other agents: • *Angiostrongylus* species • *Gnathostoma spinigerum* • *Anisakis* species	• *Baylisascaris procyonis* • *Hexametra leidyi* • *Lagochilascaris minor*

❖ **Risk Factors:** (i) children younger than 6 years, (ii) exposure to contaminated soil and (iii) rural area.

Morphology

❖ Male and female worms measure 9-13 cm and 10-18 cm, respectively. Anterior end bears lateral cervical alae. Males have a curved caudal end (Fig. 13.1A)
❖ Eggs are oval to spherical with a pitted surface and measure from 72-85 µm (Fig. 13.1B).

Life Cycle (Arrested) and Pathogenesis

Host: Felines are the natural host. Humans act as abnormal host.
Infective stage: Embryonated eggs are the infective form (Fig. 13.1B).
Mode of transmission: Ingestion of embryonated eggs contaminated in soil is the most common mode. In felines, other modes of transmission include (i) ingestion of larvae encysted in tissues of small mammals (e.g. rabbits) and (ii) vertical transmission of larvae through infected placenta and/or breast milk.

Development in Humans/Felines

Larvae hatch out from the eggs in intestine, penetrate the intestinal wall and carried via the portal circulation to the liver. If transmission occurs via larvae ingestion, they are directly carried to liver. The larvae may remain in liver or migrate to other organs like lungs or eye

❖ **In humans:** Since humans are the unusual host for these animal nematodes, further development of the larvae does not take place. Instead, the larvae get encapsulated in dense fibrous tissue in liver (most common site) or lungs or may continue to wander around the body producing granuloma
❖ **In dogs and cats**, the adult worms lay eggs, which are passed in stool
  ▪ In addition in older felines (females), the larvae undergo encystment in tissues; which later get reactivated during late pregnancy and infect their offsprings by the transplacental (dogs only) and transmammary (dogs and cats) routes
  ▪ In off springs, larvae develop into adult worms which subsequently mature in intestine and lay eggs. The immature eggs passed in feces take 2-3 weeks to transform to embryonated eggs (infective form).

Clinical Features

❖ **Visceral larva migrans (VLM):** The liver is the most frequently involved organ (hepatosplenomegaly). Usually younger children (around 3 years) are affected. But any organ can be affected. Other features include lymphadenopathy, lung involvement, skin lesions (urticaria and nodules) and seizures
❖ **Ocular larva migrans (OLM):** The most common cause of OLM is *Toxocara* larva; usually older children (around 8 years) are affected
  ▪ Unilateral painless chorioretinal granuloma in the posterior pole is the most common presentation
  ▪ But in some cases, diffuse panuveitis, retinal detachment and unilateral visual loss may occur.

Laboratory Diagnosis

Diagnosis is often difficult and mainly stay on:
❖ **Serology:** Enzyme-linked immunosorbent assay (ELISA) employing excretory secretory antigen of larva of *T. canis* is highly sensitive and specific
  ▪ Titers of 1:32 and 1:8 are considered diagnostic for VLM and OLM respectively
  ▪ It showed 91% sensitivity and 86% specificity
  ▪ It can confirm the infection but may also be elevated in asymptomatic patients.
❖ Biopsy of the tissue from liver, lungs, brain may occasionally reveal the larvae; however biopsy is usually not recommended
❖ Blood eosinophilia
❖ Increased gamma globulin level.

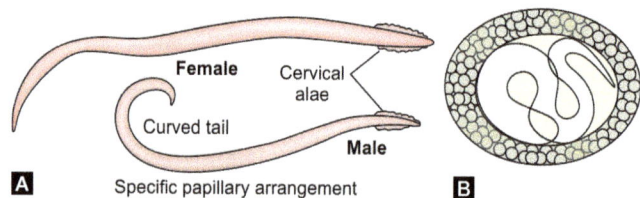

Figs 13.1A and B: *Toxocara* species (schematic diagram): (A) Adult worms; (B) Embryonated egg

Treatment	Toxocariasis
The recommended regimen includes albendazole for 5 days or mebendazole for 21 days with glucocorticoid.	

ANGIOSTRONGYLUS SPECIES

Various *Angiostrongylus* (recently renamed as *Parastrongylus*) species infecting man are:
* *A. cantonensis* causes **eosinophilic meningitis**
* *A. costaricensis* causes **abdominal angiostrongyliasis**
* *A. malaysiensis* rarely infect man, causes **abdominal angiostrongyliasis**.

Eosinophilic Meningitis

A. cantonensis; also called as the rat lung worm is the causative agent of eosinophilic meningitis.

Epidemiology

This infection occurs principally in South-east Asia, Mainland China and the Pacific Basin but has also been reported from other areas of the world.

Life Cycle

Host: Rat is the natural definitive host. Humans are accidental definitive host.
Intermediate hosts are land snails and slugs.
Mode of transmission: Man (or rat) acquires infection by ingestion of L_3 larvae in raw or undercooked intermediate host, or in contaminated water.

Development in man

The infective larvae penetrate the intestine and through the blood circulation, they migrate to the central nervous system (CNS). Here, they molt twice to become adult worms. As man is an abnormal host, adult worms die soon and cause a serious condition known as **eosinophilic meningitis**.

Development in rodents

In rodents, from CNS the adults migrate to lungs via blood. Adult worms lay eggs in the lungs, which are swallowed and are expelled in the feces. Eggs are ingested by intermediate host (molluscs-like land snails and slugs), where they develop into infective third-stage larvae.

Clinical Features

A. cantonensis infection occurs in three forms; eosinophilic meningitis (most common), encephalitis and ocular form. Eosinophilic meningitis is characterized by the following features.
* Migrating larvae cause marked local eosinophilic inflammation and hemorrhage, with subsequent necrosis and granuloma formation around the dying worms
* The adult worms within the brain tissue measure 2 mm long; in contrast to their ex-vivo size of 17–25 mm
* Clinical symptoms develop 20–40 days after the ingestion of larvae
* Patients usually present with headache, neck stiffness, nausea and vomiting, and paresthesia
* Fever, cranial nerve palsies, and seizures are the less frequent findings.

Laboratory Diagnosis

The diagnosis is generally based on the clinical presentation with epidemiologic history.
* Examination of cerebrospinal fluid (CSF) can reveal: increased CSF pressure, protein and WBC count, eosinophilic pleocytosis of more than 20%, and normal glucose level
* Larvae or young adult worms can often be recovered in the CSF
* Peripheral blood eosinophilia may be mild
* **Antibody detection:**
    * ELISA is available using purified young adult or larval antigens to detect antibodies in serum (more sensitive) and CSF
    * Western blot is available; detects antibody against 31-kDa antigen, but it may cross react with *Toxocara*.

Treatment	Eosinophilic meningitis
❑ Specific chemotherapy is not beneficial because larvicidal agents like albendazole may exacerbate inflammatory brain lesions ❑ Management consists of supportive measures, including the administration of analgesics, sedatives and in severe cases- glucocorticoid is given to reduce inflammation.	

Abdominal Angiostrongyliasis

A. costaricensis (or rarely *A. malaysiensis*) are the agent of abdominal angiostrongyliasis.
* **Epidemiology:** Infection has been recognized commonly in Central and South America (most common in Costa Rica), occasionally the Caribbean and Africa
* **Transmission** is through accidental ingestion of vegetable salads contaminated with snails, slugs or molluscs infected with L_3 larvae
* **Life cycle:** Similar to *A. cantonensis* except that the adults migrate to arteries and arterioles of ileocecal region and lay eggs
* Both eggs and adult worms provoke an inflammatory response in the ileocecal arteries and arterioles which results in occlusion of vessels, accompanying vasculitis and an eosinophilic granulomatous abdominal mass.

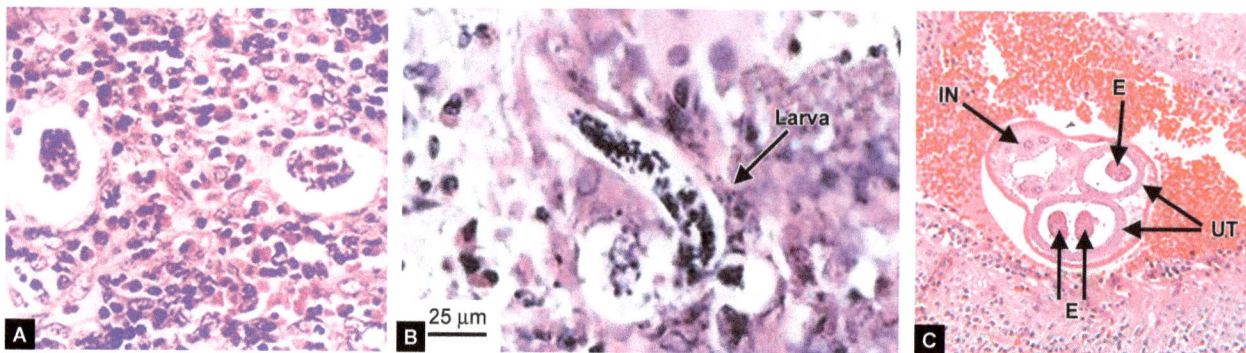

Figs 13.2A to C: *Angiostrongylus costaricensis* in intestinal biopsies hematoxylin and eosin (H&E): (A) Eggs; (B) L1 larva; (C) Adult worm showing intestine (IN) and eggs (E) within the uterus (UT)

Source: DPDx Image Library, Centers for Disease Control and Prevention (CDC), Atlanta (*with permission*).

- ❖ **Clinical Features:** Characterized by abdominal pain, vomiting, and a right lower quadrant mass commonly in children
- ❖ **Laboratory diagnosis:** Histology of intestinal biopsies may reveal eggs or L1 larvae or young adults within the tissues (Figs 13.2A to C).

BAYLISASCARIS PROCYONIS

Baylisascaris procyonis belongs to the superfamily Ascaridoidea, named after HA Baylis.
- ❖ **Life cycle:** The life cycle is similar to that of *Toxocara*
- ❖ **Transmission:** Human infection occurs after ingestion of eggs excreted in raccoon feces that subsequently contaminates soil and the environment (Fig. 13.3)
- ❖ **Clinical features:** Although the clinical manifestations are similar to those caused by dog and cat ascarids, severe and commonly fatal eosinophilic meningoencephalitis occurs in more than half of the cases (neural larva migrans). 20 cases have been reported so far, with 18 deaths. Eye involvement can occur, causing diffuse unilateral subacute neuroretinitis
- ❖ **Laboratory diagnosis:** The diagnosis is established by detecting typical larvae in tissues. Serological diagnosis by ELISA, IFAT (immunofluorescent antibody test) and western blot have been available; detecting antibodies in serum and CSF.

Treatment	Baylisascaris
There is no proven therapy. Albendazole with corticosteroids are tried commonly.	

LAGOCHILASCARIS MINOR

L. minor belongs to the superfamily Ascaridoidea:
- ❖ **Morphology:** Females (15 mm) are longer than the males (9 mm). Eggs are similar to that of *Toxocara*
- ❖ **Epidemiology:** It has been reported from Mexico, Central and South America. More than 100 cases have been reported from Amazon region
- ❖ **Life cycle:** Felines and leopard (and rarely men) act as **definitive host** and wild rodents are the **intermediate hosts**. Humans get infection by ingestion of either uncooked or lightly cooked rodent meat containing encysted larvae
- ❖ **Clinical features:** Symptoms vary from mild subcutaneous purulent lesions or abscesses on the side of the neck (or over mastoid) to more severe manifestations involving the CNS
- ❖ **Diagnosis:** Recovery of eggs, larvae and adult worms from the lesions is the mainstay of diagnosis.

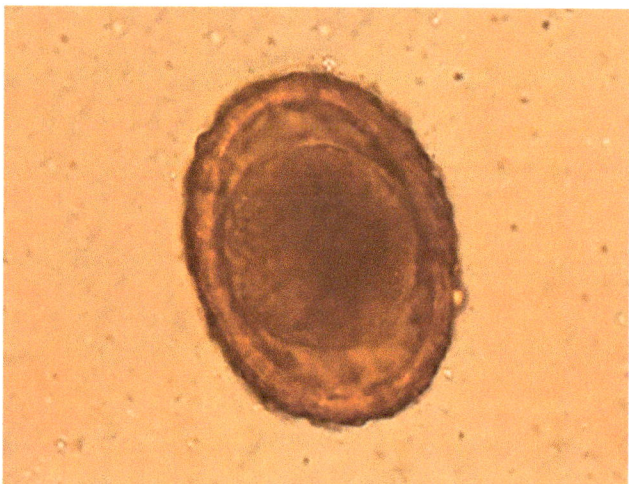

Fig. 13.3: Unfertilized egg of *Baylisascaris procyonis* (under microscope)

Source: DPDx Image Library, Centers for Disease Control and Prevention (CDC), Atlanta (*with permission*).

Treatment	Lagochilascaris
Definite treatment is surgery. Levamisole is found to be affective.	

ANISAKIASIS

Anisakiasis in man is caused by accidental ingestion of larvae found in saltwater fish. The usual definitive hosts are the marine mammals.

- ❖ **Epidemiology:** The disease is first reported from Netherlands. Now cases have been reported from the USA because of increased ingestion of raw fish, particularly Pacific salmon
- ❖ **Etiology:**
  - *Anisakis simplex:* It is most common cause of Anisakiasis; acquired from saltwater
  - **Other agents:**
    - ◆ *Pseudoterranova* species
    - ◆ *Contracaecum* species
    - ◆ *Hysterothylacium* species
    - ◆ *Porrocaecum* species.
- ❖ **Life cycle:** Following accidental ingestion, the larvae make burrows in the stomach or intestine. Then the life cycle is arrested as they do not develop further
- ❖ **Clinical feature:** It is characterized by upper or lower abdominal symptoms, or both (eosinophilic gastroenteritis)
- ❖ **Laboratory diagnosis:** The diagnosis is suggested by a history of ingesting raw, salted, pickled, smoked, or poorly cooked fish
  - Definitive diagnosis can be established by demonstration of the larva by endoscopy, radiographic studies, or pathologic examination of tissues
  - Serological diagnosis by ELISA or western blot and molecular diagnosis by PCR have been described.

Treatment	Anisakiasis
By removing worms lodged in the stomach during endoscopy.	

GNATHOSTOMA SPECIES

Gnathostoma spinigerum belongs to the order Spirurida and superfamily Gnathostomatoidea.

Epidemiology

G. spinigerum is endemic in South-east Asia (Thailand) and parts of China, Mexico and Japan. A second species named *G. doloresi* has been reported from Japan from a case of nodular lesions in colon.

Morphology

- ❖ Adult males and females are 11–25 mm and 25–54 mm long respectively. Head bulb bears 8–11 rows of cuticular hooklets. Anterior half has leaf-like spines whereas the posterior half is smooth. Esophagus is surrounded by four salivary glands (Figs 13.4A)

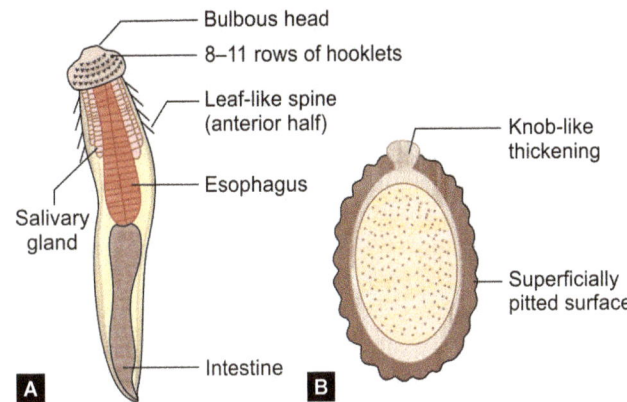

Figs 13.4A and B: *Gnathostoma spinigerum* (schematic diagram) (A) Adult worm; (B) Egg

- ❖ Eggs are oval, 69 µm × 38 µm size, superficially pitted and bear a knob-like thickening at one pole (Fig. 13.4B)
- ❖ L_3 **larva:** 3-4 mm long, covered by cuticular spines and the bulbous head bears four rows of hooklets.

Life Cycle

Host: There are two types of hosts:
1. **Definitive host:** Cat, dogs, and humans act as **accidental definitive host.**
2. **Intermediate host:** First intermediate host- crustaceans (cyclops) and **second intermediate host**- fresh water fish.

Modes of transmission: Humans (or carnivores) usually acquire infection by ingestion of fish (or rarely cyclops) containing L_3 larva.

Development in Man

Humans are abnormal host, so the larvae do not develop further; instead they penetrate the intestine and wander aimlessly into cutaneous, visceral, neural, or ocular tissues.

Development in Cats and Dogs

In cats and dogs, the larvae develop into adult worms that form nodules (tumor-like mass) in the stomach. Adult worms lay eggs; which are passed in feces and hatch out to form L_1 larva, which again molts to form L_2 larva in the environment.

Development in Intermediate Hosts

L_2 larva is ingested by cyclops where it molts to form L_3. Freshwater fishes eat cyclops containing L_3, but they behave as **paratenic host**, i.e. only maintain the larva without any development and can be infective to humans or carnivores.

Clinical Features

The migrating larvae of *G. spinigerum* can cause:
- ❖ Migratory cutaneous swellings (creeping eruption)

- Invasive masses of the eye and visceral organs (lungs)
- Eosinophilic meningoencephalitis.

Diagnosis

- **Clinical diagnosis:** Cutaneous migratory swellings with marked peripheral eosinophilia, supported by an appropriate geographic and dietary history
- **CNS involvement:** CSF shows eosinophilic pleocytosis, but worms are never recovered from CSF
- Surgery-guided biopsy may reveal the worms or advanced L_3 larvae from subcutaneous or ocular tissues. Identification can be done based on the number of hooklets in each row of bulbous head
- CT scan or MRI may reveal characteristic pathology
- No serological test is available except immunoblot technique.

Treatment	Gnathostoma
Both ivermectin (200 μg/kg for one dose) and albendazole (400 mg/day for 21 days) give cure rates of more than 90%.	

OTHER ANIMAL NEMATODES

CAPILLARIA SPECIES

Capillaria and *Trichuris* belong to the same family Trichuridae. Their eggs are morphologically similar and often get confused.

It has more than 200 species but only three species infect humans:
1. *C. philippinensis* causes intestinal capillariasis
2. *C. hepatica* causes hepatic capillariasis
3. *C. aerophila* causes pulmonary capillariasis.

Capillaria philippinensis

This parasite was first reported from Philippines by Chitwood in 1963.

Epidemiology

It is widespread in Philippines (Northern Luzon area) and Thailand. Recent cases are also reported from Japan, Taiwan, Iran and Egypt.

Morphology

Adult worm

It is similar to *Trichuris* except that it is a smaller whip worm; female worm is is 2.5–4.3 mm long and male worm is 2.3–3.17 mm long. They reside in the small intestine.

Egg

Eggs also resemble with *Trichuris* eggs except (Fig. 13.5):
- **Size:** smaller (36–45 μm long × 20 μm wide)
- **Shape:** Peanut-shaped (less barrel-shaped)
- Surrounded by striated thick shell
- Mucous plugs present but they are less prominent and do not protrude out like in *Trichuris*.

Life Cycle

Host: There are two types of hosts:
1. **Definitive host:** Fish eating birds are the natural definitive host and reservoir of infection. Humans act as the accidental definitive host.
2. **Intermediate host:** Fresh and salt water fish containing the larval stage.

Mode of transmission: Humans acquire infection by (i) ingestion of undercooked or pickled fishes, crab, shrimp or snails containing the infective larvae; (ii) internal autoinfection.

Development in man/birds

Larvae mature into adult worms in 10–11 days and live burrowed into the mucosa of small intestine (jejunum).

Adult worms fertilize to lay unembryonated eggs, which are passed in the feces. Eggs require 10–14 days in the soil to become embryonated.

Some of the eggs become embryonated in the intestine and develop into larval stage that can cause **autoinfection**. Heavy worm load can lead to hyperinfection.

Developmen in fish

Embryonated eggs in soil are infective to fishes. Following ingestion of the eggs, in the intestine of the fishes eggs hatch out into larval forms, which are infective to man and birds.

Pathogenesis and Clinical Features

Pathogenesis is related to worm load in intestine.
- Mild-to-moderate worm load cause nonspecific abdominal pain and watery diarrhea

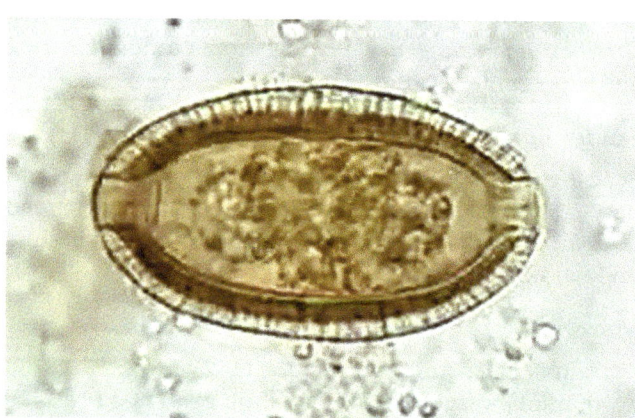

Fig. 13.5: Egg of *Capillaria philippinensis* (under microscope)
Source: DPDx Image Library, Centers for Disease Control and Prevention (CDC), Atlanta (*with permission*).

- Severe worm load can cause intestinal inflammation, loss of villi, crypt proliferation and eosinophilic granuloma
- This leads to severe malabsorption that in turn can cause protein-losing enteropathy and severe weight loss (wasting syndrome)
- Autoinfection is responsible for maintaining the worm load
- Heavy worm load sometime can cause superinfection syndrome (like strongyloidiasis).

Laboratory Diagnosis

By identification of the characteristic peanut-shaped eggs on stool examination (Fig. 13.5).

Capillaria hepatica

C. hepatica is a parasite of rodents and other small mammals. Human infection is rare. Cases have been reported from Zaire, Nigeria and other parts of West Africa where people eat rodents.

- **Life cycle:**
    - **Host:** It passes its life cycle in only one host (usually rodents, rarely humans)
    - **Mode of transmission:** It is transmitted through accidental ingestion of eggs infected in soil
    - **Development in man/rodents:** Eggs hatch out into larvae that penetrate the intestine and reach the liver via portal circulation where they develop into adult worms. After 4 weeks, the female worms start laying the eggs following fertilization. Eggs become embryonated and encapsulated in the liver parenchyma.
- **Clinical feature:** Ranges from hepatitis, hepatomegaly, peritonitis and eosinophilia
- **Laboratory diagnosis:** Depends on the detection of characteristic eggs, larvae or adult worms in the liver parenchyma
    - Eggs are similar to *C. philippinensis* except that they are larger (51–68 μm long × 30–35 μm wide) (Fig. 13.6)
    - IFAT (indirect fluorescent antibody test) is available for detection of antibodies in serum.

Capillaria aerophila

C. aerophila commonly infects carnivores, human infection is quite rare. Cases have been reported from Russia, Morocco, and Iran

- **Life cycle:** The adult female worms reside in the respiratory tract (both upper and lower) where they lay eggs, that are swallowed, passed in the feces, get embryonated outside and infect another host
- **Clinical feature:** Heavy infection can cause tracheobronchitis and hemoptysis

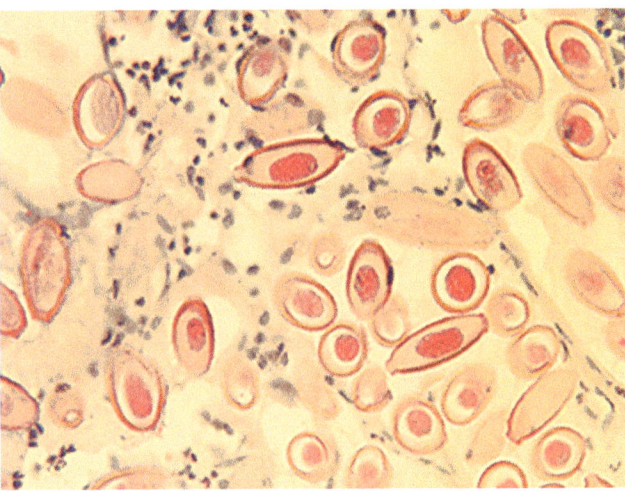

Fig. 13.6: Egg of *Capillaria hepatica* in liver stained with hematoxylin and eosin

Source: DPDx Image Library, Centers for Disease Control and Prevention (CDC), Atlanta (*with permission*).

- **Laboratory diagnosis:** Depends on the demonstration of eggs in the sputum. Eggs are similar to *C. philippinensis* except they are larger (59–80 μm long × 30–40 μm wide).

Treatment	Capillaria species
❑ Prolonged treatment with albendazole (200 mg twice daily for 10 days) is required ❑ Severely-ill patients require fluid replacement and supportive therapy.	

TRICHOSTRONGYLUS SPECIES

Trichostrongylus species, also called as "pseudo-hookworm," are normally parasites of herbivorous animals (sheep, goat, camel, etc.)

Epidemiology

Occasionally infect humans, particularly in Middle-east (Iran), Asia, and North Africa. *Trichostrongylus orientalis*, *T. axei* and *T. colubriformis* are the common species infecting man.

Life Cycle

- **Host:** It involves single host usually herbivorous animals, but rarely man
- **Mode of transmission:** Humans acquire the infection by accidentally ingesting *Trichostrongylus* L_3 larvae, present on the contaminated leafy vegetables
- **Development in Herbivorous animals/man:** The larvae mature directly into adult worms in the small bowel in 3–4 weeks
    - The adult worms penetrate the intestinal mucosa and ingest blood (far less than hookworms).

Adult worms are larger than hook worm and lack distinct buccal capsule with teeth and cutting plates
- Adult worms lay eggs that are passed in the feces. In moist and warm soil, the eggs hatch out to form L_1 larva that molts twice to form infective L_3 larva. Unlike hookworm, there is no migration of larvae in lungs.

Clinical Features

Most infected persons are asymptomatic, but heavy infections may give rise to abdominal pain, diarrhea, mild anemia and eosinophilia.

Laboratory Diagnosis

- **Stool examination:** Eggs are morphologically similar to those of hookworms but are larger (75-95 × 40-50 µm). It contains segmented ovum with four or more blastomeres surrounded by an egg shell (Fig. 13.8A)
- **Stool culture (Harada-Mori technique):** Eggs hatch out in the culture to form rhabditiform larva that can be differentiated from that of hookworm (Table 13.3 and Fig. 13.7).

Table 13.3: Differences between *Trichostrongylus* species and hookworm

Features	Trichostrongylus	Hookworm
Mode of transmission	Ingestion of L_3 larva	Skin penetration by L_3 larva
Lung migration phase	Absent	Present
Natural host	Herbivorous animals	Humans
Eggs	Longer and thinner, Pointed at one pole 73–95 µm long × 40–50 µm wide Four blastomeres, egg shell present	Smaller Blunt poles 60 µm long × 40 µm wide Four blastomeres, egg shell present
Rhabditiform larva	No distinct buccal cavity; Tail end has a bead-like swelling or knob	Prominent buccal cavity Pointed tail end
Blood loss	Sucks less blood	Sucks more blood
Epidemiology	Middle-east (Iran), Asia and North Africa	Throughout tropics and temperate regions

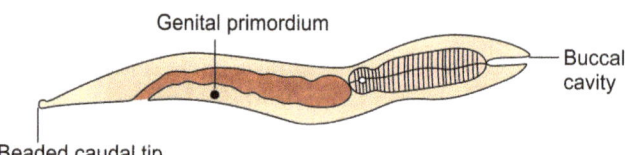

Figs 13.7: Rhabditiform larva (schematic) of *Trichostrongylus* species

Treatment	Trichostrongylus
Patients respond well to mebendazole or albendazole.	

DIOCTOPHYME RENALE

Dioctophyme renale is commonly known as **"giant kidney worm"** because of its large size and ability to infect the kidneys.
- **Epidemiology:** *D. renale* is distributed commonly in the temperate region, affecting fish eating mammals. Human infection are quite rare. Only few cases (23 cases, including 3 cases from India) have been reported so far, mainly from region surrounding Caspian Sea (Iran), Africa and Oceana
- **Morphology:** Adult worms measure 14–20 cm × 46 mm. It lives in right kidney or in body cavities.

  Eggs are oval-shaped, measure 60–80 µm × 40 µm size, contain an embryo surrounded by characteristic thick sculptured egg shell (i.e. surface appears to be pitted except at the poles) (Fig. 13.8B)
- **Life cycle:**
  - **Host:** The hosts are as follows:
    1. Definitive hosts: Carnivorous mammals (mink). Humans are accidental definitive host.
    2. Intermediate hosts: annelids, including earthworms.
    3. Paratenic hosts: includes fish and amphibians.
  - **Mode of transmission:** Transmission to definitive host occurs by ingestion of paratenic or intermediate hosts infected with larva of *D. renale*
  - **Development in definitive host:** Larva penetrates the intestine and reach the kidney (right kidney affected commonly) and transform into adult worms. Adult worms are larger in size and can block the kidney and ureter. Adult worms lay eggs that are passed in urine which further infect freshwater fishes or frog
  - **Development in intermediate host:** Eggs hatch into larvae which molts twice to develop L3 larva
  - **Paratenic host:** Fish or frogs eat intermediate host containing L3 larvae. The larvae get encysted, do not develop further.
- **Clinical features:** It includes hematuria and renal colic. Extensive destruction of kidney parenchyma may occur
- **Laboratory diagnosis:** Condition is diagnosed by demonstration of characteristic eggs in urine
- **Prevention:** Proper cooking of fish prior to consumption.

Treatment	Dioctophyme renale
Surgical excision of either adult worms or the infected kidney is the only mean of treatment. Ivermectin has been tried in one case.	

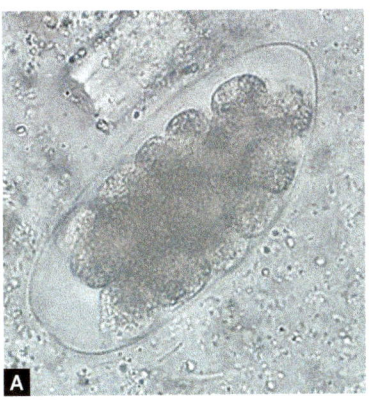 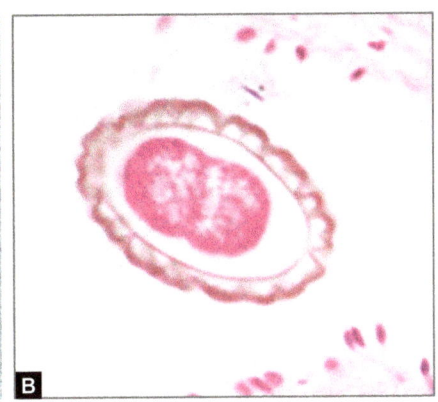 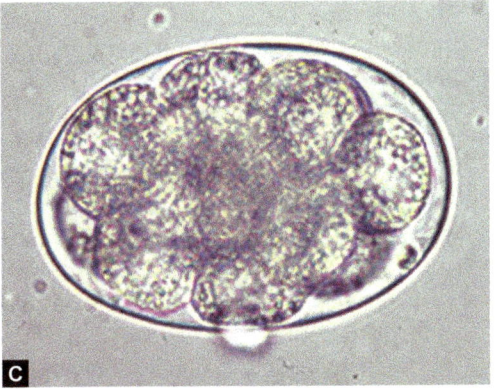

Figs 13.8A to C: Eggs of (A) *Trichostrongylus* species; (B) *Dioctophyme renale*; (C) *Oesophagostomum* species
Source: DPDx Image Library, Centers for Disease Control and Prevention (CDC), Atlanta (with permission).

OESOPHAGOSTOMUM SPECIES

Oesophagostomum species is a parasite of the large intestine of ruminants, swines and monkeys. It is found in Africa (Togo and Ghana), Asia and South America

- Human infection is very rare
- *O. bifurcum* is common in Africa where as *O. aculeatum* infection occurs in South-east Asia
- It belongs to the superfamily Strongyloidea
- **Transmission:** Ingestion of L_3 larva
- The larvae develop into adult worms. Both larvae and adult worms form nodular lesions in the intestinal wall
- **Diagnosis:** The eggs of *O. bifurcum* are nearly identical to hookworm eggs. Eggs tend to be shed in greater numbers in oesophagostomiasis than in hookworm infection. However. finding an intact worm during surgery or in a biopsy specimen can provide a definitive diagnosis. PCR can also help in differentiating.

Treatment	*Oesophagostomum*
Pyrantel pamoate and albendazole are effective.	

TERNIDENS DEMINUTUS

Ternidens deminutus (or African colon worm) is a small nematode belonging to superfamily Strongyloidea.
- **Epidemiology:** It usually affects apes and monkeys in South Africa and Asia including India. Human infections are are, reported from South Africa
- **Life cycle:**
  - **Host:** There is only one definitive host (Man, cat babbon, etc.)
  - **Mode of transmission:** Hosts become infected by ingestion of infective filariform larvae in contaminated food. L_3 larva has paired sphincter cells at esophageal-intestinal junction
- **Development in definitive host:** Larvae develop into adult worms and attach to the large intestinal mucosa by their mouths. Adult worms lay eggs in 30–40 days of infection. Eggs hatch out in the soil and become rhabditiform larvae and then develop into filariform larvae (infective form).
- **Clinical feature:** Asymptomatic. Rarely, it can produce iron deficiency anemia, pseudotumors and abscesses of the bowel
- **Laboratory diagnosis:** By demonstration of eggs and adult worms in the feces. Both eggs and adult worms are morphologically similar to hookworm (hence called as **false hookworm**) except that eggs are larger in size (84 μm × 51 μm). Adult worm can be differentiated by the presence of double crown of 22 stout bristles. PCR can also be done for specific diagnosis.

Treatment	*Ternidens deminutus*
Albendazole is found to be effective.	

MAMMOMONOGAMUS LARYNGEUS

Mammomonogamus laryngeus is a parasite of cattle and other ruminants.
- **Epidemiology:** Human infection is rare. Around 100 human cases have been reported so far, mainly from Caribbean island (Martinique)
- It belongs to the family Syngamidae; hence the disease is sometime called as **syngamiasis**
- **Transmission:** By ingestion of third stage larva (or egg containing larva)
- **Life cycle** in human is not fully understood. Probably, the larvae penetrate the intestinal wall and reach lungs via blood and then ascend to reach trachea and larynx

- **Main symptoms** are chronic cough, hemoptysis and other upper respiratory tract symptoms
- **Diagnosis:**
  - Adult worms can be demonstrated by endoscopy. The unique aspect of this species is that the smaller male worm is attached in permanent copula to the female and found as y shaped; where the short arm and ling arm of y represent the male and female worms respectively. Adult worm has a thick buccal capsule, armed with 8 small teeth; appear reddish brown as they ingest blood
  - Occasionally, eggs may be seen in sputum samples. Eggs are ellipsoidal, measure 78–95 μm × 42–54 μm in size.

Treatment	*Mammomonogamus laryngeus*
Treatment is by removal of worm by endoscopy or through forceps or surgery followed by treatment with thiabendazole and ivermectin.	

THELAZIA SPECIES

Thelazia species have been recovered from human conjunctiva. They can cause lacrimation, itching, foreign body sensation in the eye and keratitis.
- **Species:** Three species are known to cause human infection:
  1. *T. callipaeda* (the Oriental eyeworm)
  2. *T. californiensis* (the California eyeworm)
  3. *T. gulosa* (the cattle eyeworm).
- **Host:** Dogs, cattle, and horses are the definitive host, whereas the intermediate host are the flies (*Musca* and *Fannia*). Men act as accidental definitive host
- **Transmission:** The infected flies when feed on lacrimal secretion of humans, transmit the infective

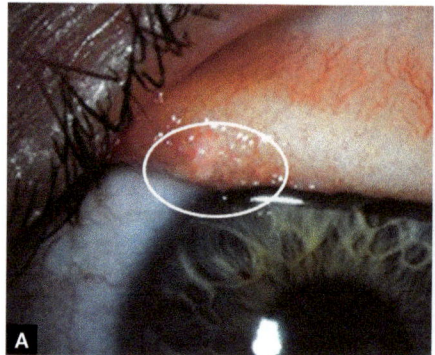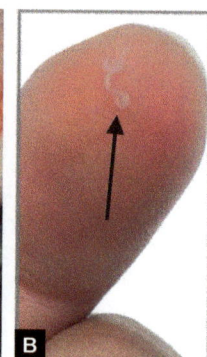

Figs 13.9A and B: *Thelazia gulosa* (A) In conjunctival surface (circle) and; (B) Removed from the eye and placed on finger (arrow showing)

Source: DPDx Image Library, Centers for Disease Control and Prevention (CDC), Atlanta (*with permission*).

L_3 larvae which transform to adult worms in human eyes
- **Epidemiology:** Cases of ocular infection have been recorded from the United States, Nepal, China, Thailand, Taiwan, Russia, Italy, France, India, and Japan. In India, less than 10 cases have been reported from places such as Assam, Karnataka, Haryana, etc.
- **Laboratory diagnosis:** Includes recovery of adult worm from eyes. The worms are 1–1.5 cm long and 250–800 μm wide and are thread-like (Figs 13.9 A and B).

Treatment	*Thelazia*
□ For the treatment of human cases, removal of the worm is the mainstay of treatment □ Topical treatment with cocaine or thiabendazole have also been reported to kill the worms □ Sanitary practices for control of flies can reduce the spread of thelaziasis.	

EXPECTED QUESTIONS

I. **Write short notes on:**
   a. Cutaneous larva migrans.
   b. Visceral larva migrans.
   c. Eosinophilic meningitis.
   d. Anisakiasis.
   e. *Gnathostoma spinigerum*.

II. **Multiple choice questions (MCQs):**
   1. **Eosinophilic meningoencephalitis is caused by:**
      a. *Toxocara canis*
      b. *Naegleria fowleri*
      c. *Acanthamoeba*
      d. *Angiostrongylus cantonensis*
   2. **Oval shaped eggs with thick sculptured egg shell can be demonstrated in urine of patients infected with?**
      a. *Schistosoma mansoni*
      b. *Schistosoma haematobium*
      c. *Dioctophyme renale*
      d. *Enterobius vermicularis*
   3. **True about anisakiasis is:**
      a. Transmitted by ingestion of larvae found in saltwater fish and squid
      b. Transmitted by Ingestion of adult worm
      c. Marine mammals serve as intermediate host
      d. Transmitted by Ingestion of meat containing eggs
   4. **Cutaneous larva migrans is mainly caused by:**
      a. *Ancylostoma brasiliensis*
      b. *Necator americanus*
      c. *Ancylostoma duodenale*
      d. *Strongyloides stercoralis*
   5. **Visceral larva migrans is caused by:**
      a. *Ancylostoma duodenale*
      b. *Necator americanus*
      c. *Ancylostoma caninum*
      d. *Toxocara canis*

Answers
1. d 2. c 3. a 4. a 5. d

Nematodes—III (Somatic Nematodes)

CHAPTER 14

CHAPTER OUTLINE

- Filarial nematode
- Lymphatic filarial nematodes
  - *Wuchereria bancrofti*
  - *Brugia* species
- Other filarial nematodes
  - *Loa loa*
  - *Onchocerca volvulus*
  - *Mansonella* species
- *Dirofilaria* species
- Other Somatic nematodes
  - *Dracunculus medinensis*
  - *Trichinella spiralis*

Somatic nematodes inhabit in the extraintestinal sites. They can be grouped into filarial and non-filarial nematodes (Table 14.1).

FILARIAL NEMATODE

Habitat: Filarial worms reside in the lymphatic system, skin, subcutaneous tissue and rarely body cavity. They are viviparous; exist in two morphological forms: adult worm and larvae. There is no egg stage.

- **Adult worm:** The adult worms are slender, round measuring 2–10 cm in length (except the female *Onchocerca* 35–50 cm). Some adult filarial worms can survive for many years in humans causing a number of chronic obstructive and inflammatory conditions including elephantiasis and hydrocele—a condition, known as lymphatic filariasis
- **Microfilariae:** The female worm produces large number of L_1 larvae called as **microfilariae,** which are highly motile thread like larvae. They are usually non pathogenic, but sometimes hypersensitivity reactions can occur against the microfilarial antigen, resulting in tropical pulmonary eosinophilia (TPE).

Classification

Filarial nematodes belong to class Secernentea, superfamily Filarioidea and family Onchocercidae. They can be differentiated by a number of properties such as (Table 14.2 and Fig. 14.1):

- **Habitat:** Whether they reside in lymphatics or subcutaneous tissues or body cavities
- Geographical distribution
- Vector responsible for transmission

Table 14.1: Somatic nematodes

Filarial nematodes	Other somatic nematodes
Lymphatics • *Wuchereria bancrofti* • *Brugia malayi* and *Brugia timori*	Skin and subcutaneous tissue • *Dracunculus medinensis* (guinea worm) Muscle • *Trichinella spiralis*
Skin and subcutaneous tissue • *Loa loa* (eye also) • *Onchocerca volvulus* (eye also) • *Mansonella streptocerca*	Somatic animal nematodes (Described separately in chapter 13) • *Toxocara* • *Angiostrongylus* • *Anisakis* • *Gnathostoma*
Serous cavity • *Mansonella ozzardi* • *Mansonella perstans*	
Zoonotic filariasis: *Dirofilaria*	

- Structure of their larvae (microfilariae) (Fig. 14.1) such as presence of sheath and nuclei at the tail tip region
- **Microfilarial periodicity:** It is defined as the time when most of the microfilariae are found in the peripheral blood
  - Microfilariae of various filarial worms exhibit different periodicity and are found in the peripheral blood in different time of the day (Table 14.3)
  - Periodicity occurs due to biological and evolutionary co-adaptation of the microfilariae to the feeding habit of the mosquito (*Culex* bites in night, *Aedes*- bites in daytime)
  - However, other factors like sleeping pattern of the individual, temperature and other climatic conditions also contribute
  - When not in peripheral blood, the microfilariae are found in the pulmonary blood vessels.

Table 14.2: Differences between various filarial nematodes

Parasite	Location of adult	Location of microfilaria	Microfilaria periodicity	Vector	Epidemiology
Lymphatic filariasis					
Wuchereria bancrofti	Lymphatic tissue	Blood, rarely hydrocele fluid and chylous urine	Nocturnal (mostly)	Culex—Worldwide Anopheles in rural Africa	Cosmopolitan, (South America, Africa, South Asia)
			Subperiodic (Rare)	Aedes	Pacific islands Andaman and Nicobar
Brugia malayi	Lymphatic tissue	Blood	Nocturnal (mostly)	Mansonia Anopheles	South-East Asia, Indonesia and India
			Subperiodic (rare)	Coquillettidia and Mansonia	South-east Asia
Brugia timori	Lymphatic tissue	Blood	Nocturnal	Anopheles barbirostris	Indonesia
Subcutaneous filariasis					
Loa loa	Subcutaneous tissue and conjunctiva	Blood Eyes (adult worm)	Diurnal	Chrysops (deerflies)	West and Central Africa
Onchocerca volvulus	Subcutaneous tissue	Skin	None	Simulium (blackflies)	South and Central America and Africa
Mansonella streptocerca	Subcutaneous tissue	Skin	None	Culicoides (midges)	West and Central Africa
Serous cavity					
Mansonella perstans	Body cavities and mesentery	Blood	None	Culicoides (midges)	South and Central America and Africa
Mansonella ozzardi	Subcutaneous tissue Body cavities	Blood	None	Culicoides (midges) Simulium (blackflies)	South and Central America Caribbean islands

Table 14.3: Periodicity of filarial nematodes

Periodicity	Microfilaria in blood	Examples
Nocturnal	Peak at night (9 pm to 4 am)	Wuchereria, Brugia
Diurnal	Present throughout the day and night, peaks at mid-day (12 noon–2.00 pm)	Loa loa
Subperiodic	Present throughout; with (i) slight increase in the afternoon (3–5 pm, diurnal sub-periodic) or (ii) slight increase in the night (7–9 pm, nocturnal sub-periodic)	Wuchereria transmitted through Aedes
Nonperiodic	No periodicity is noticed	Onchocerca Mansonella

LYMPHATIC FILARIAL NEMATODES

Lymphatic filariasis is caused by *Wuchereria bancrofti*, *Brugia malayi* and *B. timori*.

WUCHERERIA BANCROFTI

History

The existence of lymphatic filariasis has been recorded in ancient Indian, Chinese, Persian and Egyptian writings. Indian physician Sushruta was the first to describe elephantiasis.

❖ Microfilaria of *W. bancrofti* was first discovered by Demarquay (1863) in hydrocele fluid from a patient in Cuba
❖ Wucherer (1868) had detected the microfilaria in urine and Lewis (in Kolkata, 1872) in blood
❖ Bancroft was the first to describe the female worm in 1872, followed by the discovery of adult male by Bourne (1888)
❖ Manson (1899) had described the periodicity of the microfilaria and the role of insect vector
❖ **India:** The disease was narrated by Sushruta in his famous book **Sushruta Samhita**, in 6th century BC. Madhavakara in 7th century AD, described the disease in his treatise **'Madhava Nidhana'**. In 1709, Clarke called elephantoid legs in Cochin as **Malabar legs**.

Epidemiology

World

W. bancrofti, is the most widely distributed filarial parasite of humans

❖ Approximately two billion people residing in 83 countries are at risk; while an estimate of nearly 120 million people are infected

Microfilaria	Head end	Tail end	Features*
Wuchereria bancrofti	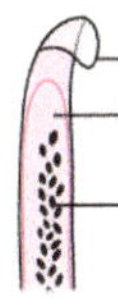 Sheath; Cephalic space (1:1); Coarse nuclei well seprated	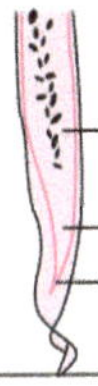 Terminal nuclei elongated; No nuclei in the tail tip; Pointed tail tip	A: 260 (244–296) μm B: Nocturnal C: Sheathed D: Blood
Brugia malayi	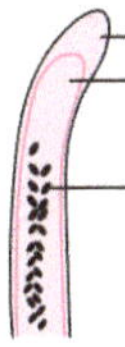 Sheath; Cephalic space (2:1); Darkly stained large coarse overlapping nuclei	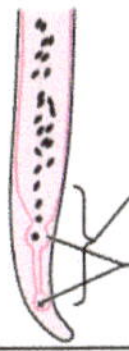 Four to five nuclei in the tail region; Two widely spaced round nuclei in tail tip	A: 220 (177–230) μm B: Nocturnal C: Sheathed D: Blood
Loa loa	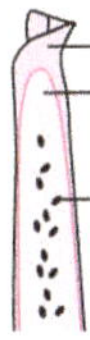 Sheath; Cephalic space (1:1); Coarse nuclei	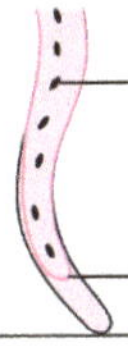 Column of nuclei extend into tail tip; Blunt tail tip	A: 275 (250–300) μm B: Diurnal C: Sheathed D: Blood
Onchocerca volvulus	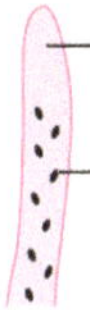 Cephalic space (large); Coarse and well-separated nuclei	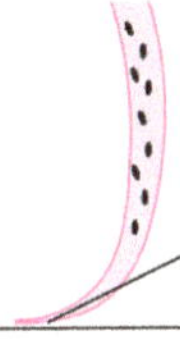 Pointed tail tip with no nuclei	A: 254 (221–287) μm B: Non-periodic C: Unsheathed D: Skin, eye
Mansonella perstans	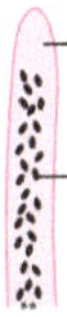 Cephalic space; Nuclei overlapping	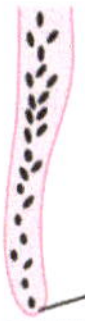 Blunt tail tip with nuclei	A: 195 (190–200) μm B: Nonperiodic C: Unsheathed D: Blood
Mansonella streptocerca	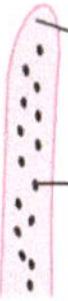 Cephalic space; Fine and well-separated nuclei	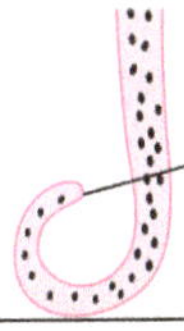 Blunt, curved tail tip with nuclei (Shepherd's crook appearance)	A: 210 (180–240) μm B: Nonperiodic C: Unsheathed D: Skin
Mansonella ozzardi	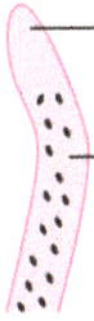 Cephalic space (large); Fine and well-separated nuclei	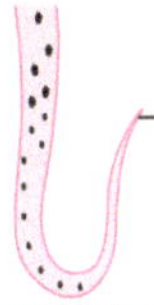 Hooked and pointed tail tip with no nuclei	A: 200 (173–240) μm B: Nonperiodic C: Unsheathed D: Blood

*A, Size; B, Periodicity; C, Sheath; D, Habitat

Fig. 14.1: Comparison of microfilariae of various filarial worms

- Southeast Asia accounts for highest burden; comprises of 50% of globally infected lymphatic filariasis (LF) cases; followed by Sub-Saharan Africa, Pacific Island, some areas of South America and the Caribbeans
- In general, *W. bancrofti* is nocturnally periodic, except in Pacific Islands; where it is subperiodic
- Globally, 90% of lymphatic filariasis are caused by *Wuchereria bancrofti* and the remainder by *Brugia* species and in India, the ratio is 99.4 and 0.6% respectively.

India
It is estimated that about 650 million people are at risk, residing in 256 districts of 21 states in India; accounting for 40% of global burden.
- Highly endemic states are Uttar Pradesh, Jharkhand, Bihar and West Bengal, which account for two-thirds of the lymphatic filariasis burden in India
- Prevalence is low in North-eastern states, Jammu and Kashmir and Punjab

❖ Subperiodic *W. bancrofti* (transmitted by *Aedes*) has been reported from Nicobar Island.

Morphology

Adult Worm

Adult worms are located in the lymphatic vessels and lymph nodes.
- ❖ They are long, slender, creamy-white thread like, filariform shaped with tapering ends
- ❖ Adult males (4 cm × 0.1 mm) are smaller than females (8–10 cm × 0.2–0.3 mm) (Fig. 14.2A)
- ❖ Male worms can be differentiated from female worms by their small size, cork-screw like tail and presence of two spicules (helps in copulation) at posterior end
- ❖ Both adult male and female remain coiled together
- ❖ Females are **viviparous** and they directly discharge larvae without any eggs.

Larva

Like other nematodes, there are four larval stages. The first stage larva is called as **microfilaria**. The third stage larva is called as **filariform larva**; which is the infective form to humans.

Microfilaria

Microfilariae are the diagnostic forms, found in the blood vessels (Fig. 14.2B).
- ❖ It measures 260 (244–296) μm × 7.5–10 μm covered by a long hyaline sheath (360 μm) within which it moves
- ❖ The head end is blunt while the tail end is pointed
- ❖ In unstained film, microfilariae are transparent and colorless. But when stained with Giemsa or other Romanowsky stains they look pink with a column of violet nuclei
- ❖ It also contains excretory pore (or anterior V spot), cloaca or anal pore (posterior V spot) and genital cells (G1 to G4). From anterior V spot to G1 cells is known as **central body of Manson**, that represents rudimentary alimentary system
- ❖ The nuclei are present throughout the body except near the head and the tail end. Nuclei are also absent in few places which represent various primordial organs like nerve ring, excretory pore, anal pore and genital cells
- ❖ Based on the structure of microfilaria, different filarial nematodes can be differentiated (*see* Fig. 14.1).

Cultivation

Limited success has been achieved to cultivate the filarial worms.

Cell line: *W. bancrofti* and *B. malayi* can be cultivated in mosquito cell line (like *Aedes togoi* and *Anopheles maculatus*) grown in modified RPMI-1640 medium or medium-TC199 supplemented with 20% newborn calf serum and LLC-MK2 cells. Human embryonic kidney cell line is also used as a feeder layer
- ❖ Microfilariae ex-sheath and molt twice to L_3 stage larvae in 12–16 days
- ❖ However, culture methods are not employed in diagnosis. They are used for the maintenance of the parasite for:
  - Preparation of antigen for immunological tests
  - Antifilarial drug susceptibility testing
  - Research purpose.

Laboratory animals: African green leaf monkeys (*Presbytis melalophos*) are highly susceptible to subcutaneous

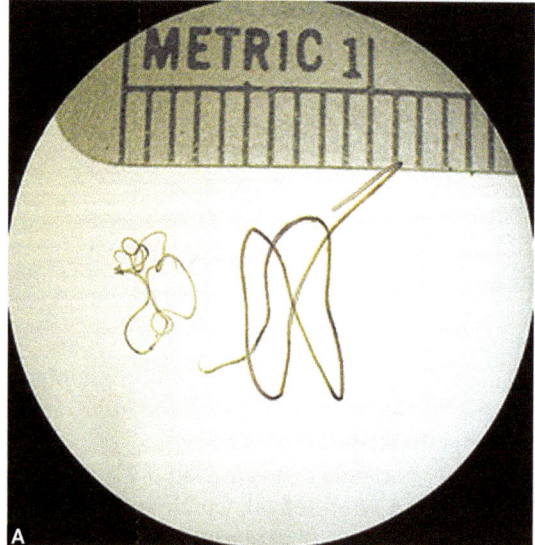
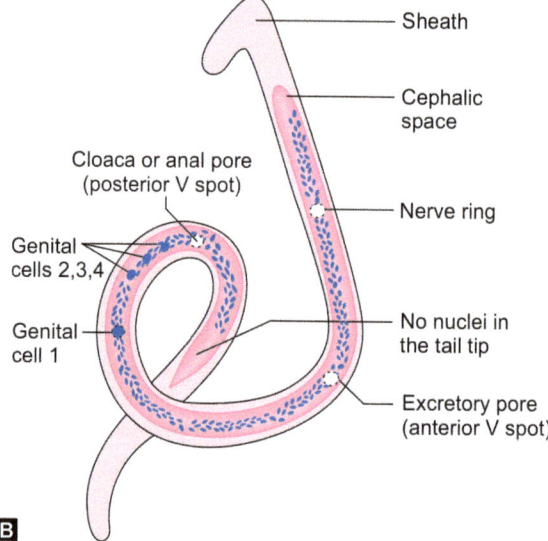

Figs 14.2A and B: *Wuchereria bancrofti* (A) Adult worms: male (left) and female (right); (B) Microfilaria (schematic diagram)
Source: DPDx Image Library, Centers for Disease Control and Prevention (CDC), Atlanta (*with permission*).

inoculation of L_3 larva that transform to microfilaria in 4–6 weeks.

Life Cycle (Fig. 14.3)

Host: *W. bancrofti* completes its life cycle in two hosts.
1. **Definitive host:** Man is the definitive host and also the only reservoir host.
2. **Intermediate host:**
   - Mosquito named *Culex quinquefasciatus* is the principle vector worldwide.
   - Rarely *Anopheles* (rural Africa) or *Aedes* (Pacific Island) can serve as a vector.

Infective form: Third stage filariform larvae are the infective form found in the proboscis of the mosquito.

Mode of transmission: L_3 filariform larvae get deposited in skin by the mosquito bite. Residents living in the endemic areas are exposed to about 50–300 L_3 larvae every year.

Note: Transmission through blood transfusions and congenital transmission have been reported in few cases; however such transmissions are not clinically significant as life-cycle does not proceed and microfilariae die in few weeks.

Human Cycle

- **Develop into adults:** Larvae penetrate the skin, enter into lymphatic vessels and migrate to the local lymph nodes where they molt twice to develop into adult worms in 6–12 months (4–6 weeks for *B. malayi*)
- **Adults lay L_1 larvae (microfilariae):** Adult worms reside in the afferent lymphatics or cortical sinuses of the lymph nodes where they mate and start laying the first stage larvae (microfilariae). Male worms die after mating, whereas the female worms live up to 20 years. A gravid female can discharge 50,000 microfilariae/day. Microfilariae have a life span of up to 1 year
- **Prepatent period:** It is the time period between the infection (entry of L_3 larvae) and diagnosis (detection of microfilariae in blood). This is variable ranging from 82–142 days.

Mosquito Cycle

- **Transmission:** When the mosquito bites an infected man, the microfilariae are ingested. *Culex* bites at night, whereas *Aedes* bites in daytime
- **Exsheathing:** Microfilariae come out of the sheath within 1–2 hours of ingestion
- **Migration to thoracic muscle:** L_1 larvae penetrate the stomach wall and migrate to thoracic muscle in 6–12 hours where they become sausage shaped (short and thick)
- **Develop to infective L_3 larvae:** L_1 larvae molt twice to develop L_2 (long and thick form) followed by L_3 (long and thin form). The highly active L_3 larvae migrate to the labella (distal part of proboscis) of the mosquito and serve as the infective stage to man
- **Extrinsic incubation period:** Under optimum conditions, the mosquito cycle takes around 7–21 days.

Pathogenesis and Pathology

The pathologic changes occur as a result of inflammatory damage to the lymphatics which in turn is due to summation of many effects such as:
- Tissue alterations related to migration of live adult worms such as lymphatic dilatation and thickening of the vessel walls
- Tissue alterations related to antigen and toxic metabolites released from dead adult worm
- Secondary bacterial and fungal infections
- Host's inflammatory response to both live and dead parasite
  - Infiltration of plasma cells, eosinophils, and macrophages in the infected vessels, along with endothelial and connective tissue proliferation
  - This leads to tortuosity of the lymphatics and damage to lymph valves resulting in lymph edema of limbs and brawny edema on the overlying skin.
- As long as the worm remains viable, the lymphatic vessels though damaged, still remains patent

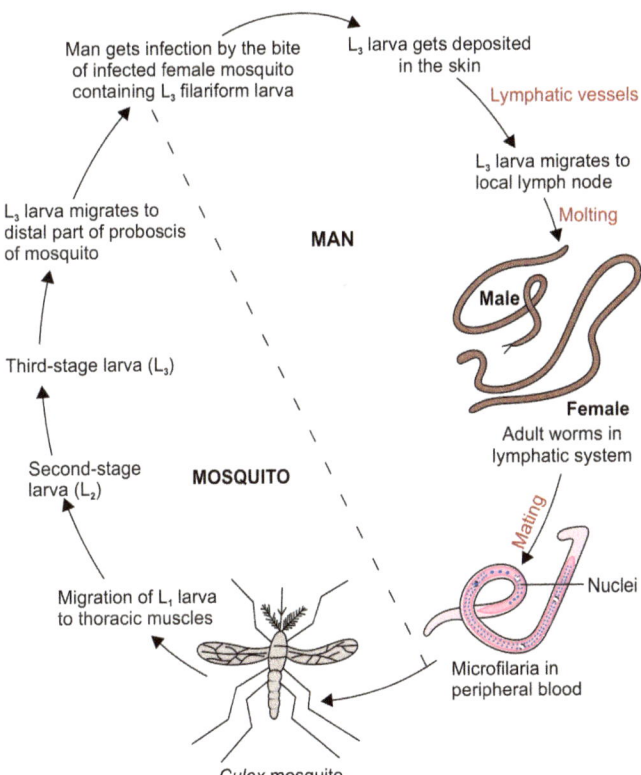

Fig. 14.3: Life cycle of *Wuchereria bancrofti*

- However, the death of the worm leads to enhanced granulomatous reaction, thrombi formation and fibrosis of the lymph vessels with extensive perilymphangitis
- This results in severe lymphatic obstruction. The lymphatic function is severely compromised
- **Endosymbiosis:** Pathogenic *W. bancrofti* is found to be infected with a *Rickettsia* group of bacteria called *Wolbachia* and maintain an endosymbiotic relationship. It is proved that this symbiosis is essential for the parasite survival, fertility and larval development
    - Filarial and *Wolbachia* antigens together induce release of inflammatory cytokines, vascular endothelial growth factor which causes vascular leakage and angiogenesis and thereby promoting lymphedema and hydrocele
    - They also induce scarring and fibrosis in lymphatic filariasis and skin thickening and corneal scarring in onchocerciasis.
- **Age and gender:** Microfilaremia increases with age; starts at 5 years and peaks at >30 years. Males are more commonly affected than females. Hormonal factors in females may be attributed to their higher resistance to infection.

Host Immune Response

Both cellular and humoral immune response are altered. Antigens of both adult worms and microfilariae are processed by the antigen presenting cells (macrophages) and presented to T helper cells (T_H cells). T_H cells are stimulated and differentiated into T_H1 cells and or T_H2 cells.

In Early Infection (Amicrofilaremic Individuals)

There is activation of parasite specific delayed type of hypersensitivity response
- Parasite specific T_H cell proliferation occurs and both T_H1 cells and T_H2 cells are stimulated
- This leads to a mixed cytokine response. Both T_H1 cytokines such as interleukin-2 (IL-2) and interferon-γ (IFN-γ) and T_H2 cytokines (IL-4 and IL-5) are elevated
- There is profound eosinophilia and higher titers of immunoglobulin (IgE) antibody level.

Microfilaremic Individuals (Asymptomatic and Acute Stage)

At this stage, diminished parasite specific T cell proliferation occurs
- Predominant T_H2 cells response is seen that leads to:
    - Elevation of IL-4, IL-5, IL-13 and IL-10
    - Low production of IFN-γ and IL-2.
- Profound eosinophilia

- Increased parasite specific IgG-4 antibodies is observed; level of which decreases with successful therapy
- **Hyper IgE levels:** Total IgE level is maximum in acute filariasis, whereas the parasite specific IgE level is maximum in amicrofilaremic individuals and in occult filariasis, suggestive of the protective role of parasite specific IgE in containing the disease.

In Chronic Filariasis

- There is increased production of T_H2 cells induced cytokines like IL-4, IL-5 and IL-13
- Elevation of parasite specific IgG-1, IgG-2 and IgG-3.

Clinical Features

Incubation period is about 8–16 months. Clinical manifestations can be categorized into:
- Lymphatic filariasis
- Tropical pulmonary eosinophilia (TPE)/(Occult filariasis)
- Immune complex mediated manifestations.

Lymphatic Filariasis

Endemic normal

These are the normal people residing in endemic area. Their prevalence ranges from 0 to 50%. They are not infected by the parasite. This might be due to:
- Insufficient exposure
- Immunological resistance
- May be in prepatent period at the time of study.

Asymptomatic microfilaremia

In endemic area, many infected individuals do not exhibit any symptoms of filarial infection.
- These people have a down regulated T_H1 cells response (low IFN-γ) and elevated T_H2 cells response ($\uparrow$IL-4)
- However, it is observed that most of the asymptomatic people have some degree of evidence of subclinical infection like:
    - Microfilaremia demonstrated in their peripheral blood
    - Microscopic hematuria and/or proteinuria
    - Dilated and tortuous lymphatics (visualized by imaging)
    - Filarial dance sign (ultrasound showing motile adult worm in scrotal lymphatics).

Acute filariasis (acute adenolymphangitis)

It is characterized by recurrent episodes of:
- Filarial fever (high-grade fever)
- Lymphatic inflammation (lymphangitis and lymphadenitis):
    - Lower extremities are more commonly affected than the upper limbs

- Lymph nodes most often affected are the epitrochlear, axillary, femoral or inguinal
- The nodes are firm, discrete, tender and enlarged, while the lymph vessels are inflamed and indurated. The overlying skin is erythematous and edematous with occasional abscess formation
- In addition, lymphatics of the male genital organs are frequently involved that leads to funiculitis, epididymitis and orchitis (not seen in brugian filariasis).

❖ **Transient local edema:** Early pitting edema; reversible on limb elevation
❖ **Dermatolymphangitis:** Plaque like lesion is formed over the affected skin with fever, chill and lymphatic inflammation
❖ In brugian filariasis, the episodes are more frequent and abrupt in onset.

Chronic filariasis

It develops 10–15 years after infection.

❖ Chronic host immune response against the dead worm leads to enhanced granuloma, thrombi formation and fibrosis of the lymph vessels leading to severe lymphatic obstruction and pedal edema
❖ **Grading of lymphedema:** Early pitting edema (grade-1) becomes nonpitting and irreversible on limb elevation (grade-2) followed by brawny lymphedema with thickening of the skin (grade-3), finally lead to fibrosis and fissuring (grade-4)
❖ The manifestations in descending order of occurrence are:
  - **Hydrocele** (most common manifestation): Accumulation of clear straw colored fluid in the cavity of tunica vaginalis of testes (Fig. 14.4B)
  - Elephantiasis (swelling of lower limb or less commonly arm, vulva or breast) (Fig. 14.4A)
  - Chronic funiculitis and epididymitis
  - **Chyluria:** Excretion of chyle, a milky white fluid in urine may occur rarely, in the form of episodes lasting for weeks. It is more pronounced in the morning or after a fatty meal. This is due to rupture of lymph vessels into the urinary system.

Occult Filariasis or Tropical Pulmonary Eosinophilia (TPE)

Also called as **Weingarten's syndrome:** It is a distinct syndrome that develops in some infected individuals of endemic places.

Pathogenesis

It represents a hypersensitivity reaction to microfilaria antigen. Microfilariae are rapidly cleared from the blood stream and filtered, lodged and destroyed in the lungs initiating an allergic response. Hence, microfilariae are not detected in peripheral blood.

Epidemiology

The majority of cases have been reported from India, Pakistan, Sri Lanka, Brazil, Guyana, and Southeast Asia. Males are affected more than females (4:1), mainly in the third decade of life.

Clinical features

Common features include nocturnal paroxysmal cough and wheezing weight loss, low-grade fever (Table 14.4).

Occasionally, microfilariae are entrapped in other organs like spleen, liver and lymph node leading to hepatosplenomegaly and lymphadenopathy. This is sometimes called as **Meyers Kouwenaar Syndrome**.

Laboratory Diagnosis

Occult filariasis is diagnosed by:
❖ Blood eosinophilia (absolute eosinophil count more than 3000/μL)

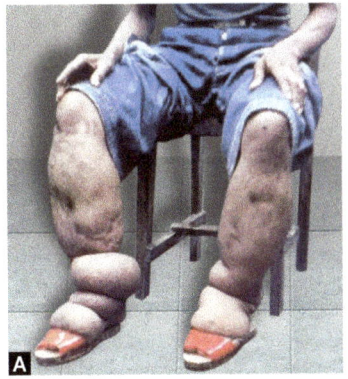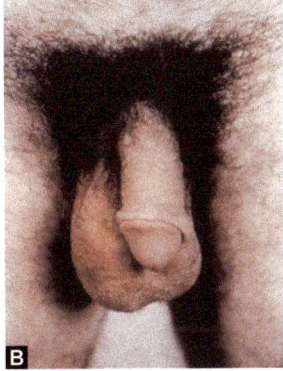

Figs 14.4A and B: Clinical features of filariasis: (A) Elephantiasis; (B) Hydrocele of scrotum

Source: A—ID#-373; B—ID# 354, Public Health Image Library, Centers for Disease Control and Prevention (CDC), Atlanta (*with permission*).

Table 14.4: Differences between classical filariasis and occult filariasis

Characters	Classical filariasis	Occult filariasis
Probable etiology	Inflammatory changes to adult worm	Hypersensitivity reaction to microfilaria antigen
Diagnostic form	Microfilaria in blood and in fluid	Microfilaria absent in blood
Organs affected	Lymph nodes and lymphatic vessels	Lungs, liver and spleen
Pathology	Lymphangitis and lymphadenitis	Eosinophilic granuloma
Serology	Antibody detection is not diagnostic	IgE antibody detection is diagnostic

- **Chest X-ray:** Shows diffuse infiltration
- Elevated serum IgE levels
- Pulmonary function test shows obstructive changes in lungs.

Treatment

It responds well to diethylcarbamazine (DEC), 4-6 mg/kg for 14 days. Relapse may occur in 12-25% of cases.

Immune Complex Mediated Manifestations

Circulating immune complexes containing microfilarial antigens are found to be deposited in various organs such as:
- Kidney (causes nephrotic syndrome, hematuria and proteinuria)
- Joints (causes filarial arthritis of knee or ankle).

> **Laboratory Diagnosis** — *Wuchereria bancrofti*
>
> - **Demonstration of microfilariae** by thin or thick smear stained with Giemsa or by QBC examination—blood collected during night hours (or day time after DEC provocation test)
>   - *W. bancrofti*—tail tip pointed, free of nuclei
>   - *B. malayi*—tail tip blunt, nuclei extended upto tail tip
> - **Antigen detection** (ELISA, ICT)— detects Ag by using mAb to Og4C3 Ag and AD12 Ag.
> - **Antibody detection**
>   - Flow-through assay using WbSXP-1 Ag
>   - Luciferase immunoprecipitation system using Wb123 Ag
> - **Imaging methods**—filarial dance sign in USG, indicates serpentine movement of adult worms in lymphatics
> - **Molecular methods**—real-time PCR detecting genes such as *SspI* repeat, *pWb12* repeat, *pWb-35*, etc.
> - **Other methods**—eosinophilia, elevated IgE.

Laboratory Diagnosis

Microscopy (To Detect Microfilariae)

- **Sample:** Microfilariae can be found in blood, and occasionally in hydrocele fluid, urine or other body fluids. Blood is collected from finger prick, ear lobes or peripheral veins using EDTA vials
- **Direct wet mount:** Demonstrates serpentine movement of microfilariae
- **Thick and thin smears:** Leishman's, Giemsa or hematoxylin and eosin staining can be performed to observe the sheath and nuclei of microfilaria (Fig. 14.5)
- Microfilaremia ranges from 1-1,000 or some time up to 10,000/mL of blood.
- **Concentration techniques:** Blood can be examined after concentration techniques to increase sensitivity (detail is given in Chapter 15)
  - Membrane filtration technique
  - Knott's centrifugation technique.
- **Collection time:** It is critical and should be based on the periodicity of the microfilariae. For nocturnal periodicity, blood should be collected between 9 pm and 4 am
- **DEC provocation test:** This test is done to collect the blood in the day time
  - Patient takes a tablet of DEC orally (2 mg/kg) so that the nocturnal microfilariae are stimulated and come to peripheral blood within 15 minutes to 1 hour
  - Remember that, in case of subperiodic *W. bancrofti*, the microfilariae level falls rather rise after DEC provocation
  - This test is contraindicated in *Onchocerca* and *Loa loa* infection.
- **QBC (Quantitative buffy coat examination):** It involves centrifugation of blood, staining with acridine orange stain and examination under fluorescent microscope. This technique is more sensitive than smear microscopy
- Microfilariae may not be found in blood because of many reasons such as:
  - Occult filariasis

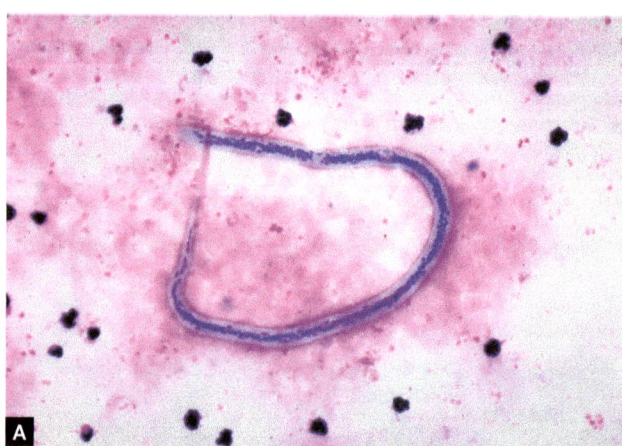
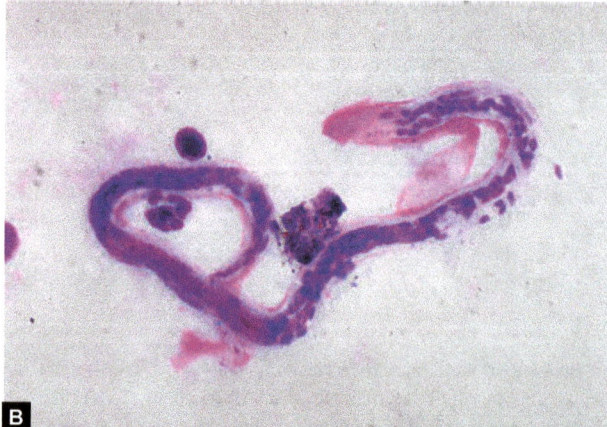

Figs 14.5A and B: Thick blood smears stained with Giemsa showing microfilaria of (A) *Wuchereria bancrofti*; (B) *Brugia* species
Source: A—ID# 3009/, B—ID# 3003, Dr. Mae Melvin, Public Health Image Library, Centers for Disease Control and Prevention (CDC), Atlanta.

- Chronic filariasis and endemic normal people
- Wrong time of blood collection.

Antigen Detection

Circulating antigens of *W. bancrofti* can be detected by using monoclonal antibodies against Og4C3 and AD12 antigens.

- Both enzyme-linked immunosorbent assay (ELISA) and rapid immunochromatographic test (ICT) are commercially available
- ELISA is 100% sensitive and 99–100% specific, whereas ICT card test (Alere) is 96–100% sensitive and 95–100% specific. Recently, an ICT strip test (Alere) has been developed which showed better result than ICT card test
- No antigen detection methods are available for *Brugia* infection
- **Advantages of antigen detection:**
  - More sensitive than microscopy
  - Can be detected in day time
  - Can differentiate the current and past infection. Antigen disappears after clinical cure
  - Can be detected in urine.

Antibody Detection

In endemic area, most people have a positive serologic response (total IgG antibodies) due to prior exposure to non-human filarial worms and cross-reaction to other helminths. Therefore, antibody detection tests are useful only for epidemiologic purposes (seroprevalence studies). In non-endemic area, it may be of diagnostic value.

In contrast, detection of parasite-specific antibodies (e.g. IgG4) has a better diagnostic value, as described below:

- Parasite-specific IgG4 is increased in active filariasis and is less cross-reactive
- IgG2 level appears to be elevated in patients with elephantiasis
- The young people who are resistant to filarial infection in endemic areas, often express protective anti-sheath antibodies
- In TPE, marked IgE response is observed in addition to elevated eosinophilia.

Though most tests lack both sensitivity and specificity, some newer methods as described below, have showed promising results.

- **Flow-through assay:** It is a rapid test, based on flow-through immunofiltration method for detection of total IgG antibodies to recombinant filarial antigen WbSXP-1 through colloidal gold-protein A.
  - It is a rapid, user-friendly test, applicable for field use as an initial screening method
  - It showed sensitivity of 91.4% and 90.8%, for bancroftian and brugian filariasis respectively
  - It is also recommended for epidemiologic monitoring.
- **Luciferase immunoprecipitation system:** It is another rapid test using *W. bancrofti* Wb123 antigen, developed in North America; found to be 100% sensitive and specific.

Imaging Methods

Ultrasound

High-frequency ultrasound with Doppler techniques are employed to detect:

- It can demonstrate anatomical abnormalities of lymphatics, dilated and tortuous vessels
- **Filarial dance sign:** Serpentine movement of adult worms within the lymphatic vessels of scrotum—positive in 80% of cases.

Lymphoscintigraphy

Lymphoscintigraphy of the limbs reliably demonstrates the functional abnormalities of lymphatics (like flow abnormalities) and lymphangiectasia (dilatation) even in asymptomatic microfilaremic persons.

X-Rays

It can detect:
- Dead and calcified worms
- Pulmonary infiltrates in patients with TPE.

Molecular Methods

Molecular methods have the following advantages: (i) can detect low level of parasitemia, (ii) can differentiate past and present infection, (iii) can distinguish between filarial parasites, (iv) for monitoring treatment response, (v) to detect parasite in carriers.

- **Various methods** include DNA hybridization, PCR and its modification such as semi-nested PCR (for speciation), real-time PCR (for quantification), PCR-ELISA and PCR-RFLP (restriction fragment length polymorphism)
- **Parasite-specific primers** used are:
  - *W. bancrofti*: SspI repeat, pWb12 repeat, pWb-35 repeat and LDR repeat
  - *B. malayi*: HhaI repeat, glutathione peroxidase gene and mitochondrial DNA.

Other Methods

- Eosinophilia (absolute eosinophil count >3000/μL)
- Elevated serum concentrations of IgE (>1000 ng/mL)
- Cellular assays: Filarial skin test and lymphocyte response to filarial antigen, both are less specific

- Biopsy of enlarged lymph node to demonstrate adult worm
- Urine examination reveals microscopic hematuria and proteinuria.

Treatment	Wuchereria bancrofti
Diethylcarbamazine (DEC) □ It is the drug of choice for the treatment of filariasis □ It is given 6 mg/kg daily for 12 days □ It can kill both adult worms and microfilariae. However, adult worms are cleared slowly **Albendazole:** It is given as 400 mg twice daily for 21 days. It has also demonstrated efficacy against adult worms and microfilariae **Ivermectin:** 400/kg single dose, can kill microfilariae but has no effect on adult worms. High rate of recurrence occurs, hence not used in India (used only in Africa) **Doxycycline:** It is given to target the intracellular *Wolbachia*. It also shows significant microfilaricidal activity as DEC **Penicillin:** Secondary infections due to bacteria such as streptococci can be treated with systemic antibiotics like penicillin till the infection subside.	

Prevention

Vector Control

Antilarval measures

Antilarval measures are highly expensive hence mainly restricted to urban areas. Chemicals can be used like:
- Mosquito larvicidal oil
- Pyrethrum-based oil (pyrosene oil-E)
- Organo-phosphorus larvicides like fenthion, temephos.

Antiadult measures

Antiadult measures like pyrethrum spray can be used. However, DDT and hexachlorocyclohexane (HCH) are not effective.

National Vector Borne Disease Control Program

The National filariasis control program in India is active since 1955; which was integrated with National Vector Borne Disease Control Program (NVBDCP) in 2006.

Hathipaon Mukt Bharat: India (under NVBDCP) has launched a massive campaign in 2015 for achieving filaria free India named *"Hathipaon Mukt Bharat"*. It aims at assisting the filariasis elimination program of India.

Elimination of Lymphatic filariasis (ELF)

Global program to eliminate lymphatic filariasis (LF) was launched by WHO in 2000 aiming at global elimination by the year 2020
- **Strategy:** WHO recommends yearly mass drug administration (MDA) to all people at-risk in the endemic areas. Single dose of DEC + albendazole is the agent of choice for MDA in all endemic areas of the World except:
  - In onchocerciasis endemic areas where ivermectin+ albendazole is given
  - In *Loa loa* endemic area (albendazole twice per year given)
  - Recently in 2018, WHO recommended IDA regimen (combination of ivermectin, DEC and albendazole) under elimination program. It is yet to be implemented.
- **Global LF elimination status:** To date, 11 countries achieved the LF elimination status including Egypt added latest in 2018. Of 73 endemic countries, 39 have completed MDA and are in the process of conducting surveillance to validate elimination. The remaining 33 countries have not achieved MDA coverage yet
- **Anti-Filaria** Day is observed on 5th June globally. In addition, the **National filariasis day** in India is celebrated on 11th November every year.

ELF in India

In India, ELF is in operation since 2004 in parallel with global strategy. It is conducted through NVBDCP.
- **Twin Strategies** employed: Comprises of (1) annual mass drug administration **(MDA)** of DEC + albendazole; (2) Home based management for lymphedema cases and up scaling of hydrocele operations.
- **Dosage:** DEC is given at a single dose of 100 mg, 200 mg and 300 mg for the age groups of 2–5 years, 6–14 years and ≥15 years respectively and albendazole is given 400 mg for all age group of >2 years
- **Indication:** MDA is indicated in all high-risk population of 256 endemic districts of India; except in children <2 years, pregnant women and severely ill.
- **Duration:** MDA should be continued annually for minimum **five years**; with a target of >65% coverage of at risk population
- **Three visits per MDA:** Each MDA activity includes household enumeration about ELF program in first visit, followed by mass drug administration (MDA) 15 days later in second visit and then mopping up in two subsequent days of MDA in third visit, to cover up absentees
- **Microfilaria (mf) survey:** The impact of the MDA is measured by mf survey. It is conducted every year; one month prior to the next MDA, targeting 500 people per site for eight sites per endemic district. Blood is collected during night time (8.30 pm–12.00 am) and are subjected to thick smear examination. (Table 14.5)
- **Transmission assessment survey (TAS):** The districts which achieve a sustained mf rate of <1% at the end of 5 years of MDA are proceeded for transmission assessment survey.
  - *Rapid test:* Here, ICT detecting circulating antigens is performed for school going children of 6–7 years (see Table 14.5). Detection of circulating antigen indicates on-going transmission
  - If the ICT result is satisfactory, the area will be qualified for stoppage of MDA and initiate post-MDA surveillance. Otherwise, the MDA activity should be continued.
- **Post-MDA surveillance:** The following strategies will be carried out under post-MDA surveillance for a period of four years.
  - Entomological data collection
  - Annual mf survey in 5–9 years children,

Contd...

Contd...

- Activities to manage morbidity to prevent disability through home-based management for lymphedema cases and up scaling of hydrocele operations
- Screening of high-risk population such as migrants
- Treatment and follow up of positive cases and
- Vector control measures.
- ❑ **Filariasis elimination:** After four years of post-MDA surveillance, the area is declared as having achieved elimination status
- ❑ **Elimination status:** As of 2018, five states (Assam, Tamil Nadu, Goa, Puducherry, Daman and Diu) stopped MDA after achieving elimination status and observing post-MDA surveillance activities.

BRUGIA MALAYI

History

- Microfilariae were described first by Lichtenstein in blood films from natives in Indonesia
- Brug had described it as a new species (1927)
- Rao and Maplestone (India) were the first to describe the adult worm (1940).

Epidemiology

There is considerable overlapping in the geographical distribution of brugian filariasis and bancroftian filariasis.
- *B. malayi* occurs primarily in eastern India, Indonesia, Malaysia, Thailand and Philippines
- It also shows two types of periodicity of microfilaremia. The nocturnal form is more common, transmitted in areas of coastal rice fields, while the subperiodic form is rare, found in the forests of Malaysia and Indonesia
- In India, the major states involved are Kerala, Odisha, Assam and West Bengal.

Morphology

The adult worms are essentially similar to that of *W. bancrofti* except they are smaller in size; males (3.5 cm × 0.1 mm) and females (5–6 cm × 0.1 mm).

Microfilariae measure 220 (177–230) µm × 5–6 µm in size. Like that of *W. bancrofti*, the microfilaria of *B. malayi* is also sheathed with some minor differences (Table 14.6).

Table 14.5: Tests employed under filariasis elimination program

Target detected	Field assay	Confirmatory*	Indication
Microfilariae	Blood film by thick smear	PCR	Microfilaria survey
Filarial antigen of *W. bancrofti*	ICT	Og4C3 ELISA (antigen detection)	Transmission assessment survey
Filarial antibody for *Brugia***	Brugia Rapid™	Bm14 ELISA (antibody detection)	Transmission assessment survey

*Laboratory-based assays
**In *Brugia* endemic area, tests for both *W. bancrofti* (antigen) and *Brugia* (antibody) are performed.

Life Cycle

The life cycle is similar to *W. bancrofti* except:
- **Vector:** *Mansonia* (*M. annulifera* and *M. uniformis*) is the main vector for the nocturnal strains, *Anopheles* and *Aedes* can also transmit the infection. The subperiodic strains are transmitted by *Coquillettidia* and *Mansonia*
- **Reservoir:** Humans are the main reservoir; except for the subperiodic strains of *B. malayi* where monkeys, cats and dogs are the animal reservoirs
- Shorter pre-patent period: 3–4 months
- Shorter life cycle in mosquito (external incubation period).

Clinical Features

Both lymphatic filariasis and tropical pulmonary eosinophilia syndrome are observed in brugian filariasis. Clinical features are similar to bancroftian filariasis except:
- More frequent episodes of acute adenolymphangitis, adenitis (femoral nodes), and filarial abscesses
- Chronic manifestations (lymphedema and elephantiasis) occur less frequently
- The genital involvement is not seen
- Elephantiasis: Swelling is limited to leg below the knee
- Chyluria does not occur.

Laboratory Diagnosis

As in bancroftian filariasis, the diagnosis of brugian filariasis depends on:
- **Microscopy:** Microfilaria in blood can be detected by Giemsa stained peripheral blood smear examination (*see* Table 14.6, Fig. 14.5B). Giemsa stains the sheath of *B. malayi*; but not that of *W. bancrofti* and *B. timori*
- **Antibody detection methods:** ICT (*Brugia Rapid*) is available detecting parasite-specific IgG-4 antibodies

Table 14.6: Microfilariae of *Wuchereria bancrofti* and *Brugia malayi*

Microfilariae	Wuchereria bancrofti	Brugia malayi
Appearance	Graceful and sweeping curves	Crinkled with secondary curves
Size	260 (244–296) µm	Smaller, 220 (177–230) µm
Cephalic space	Length to width ratio is 1:1	Longer (length to width ratio is 2:1)
Excretory pore	Not prominent	Prominent
Nuclei column	Large, coarse and well separated	Darkly stained, large, coarse, overlapping and extended till the tail tip
Tail	• Pointed tail tip • No nuclei in the tail region	• Pointed tail tip • Four to five nuclei are present in the tail region • Two widely spaced nuclei at the tail tip—terminal and sub terminal

against recombinant BmR1 antigen of *B. malayi*. It shows good sensitivity and specificity. ELISA employing recombinant *B. malayi* antigen (Bm-14) is available. Both the tests are currently used under filariasis elimination program
- However, there is no antigen detection method is available
- Imaging methods like ultrasound can be employed
- **Molecular methods:** As described earlier, PCR and other molecular methods can differentiate between *B. malayi* and *W. bancrofti*.

Treatment

Treatment for brugian filariasis is same as for bancroftian filariasis. Except that frequency of adverse effects following DEC medication is more; therapy should be started with lower dose.

Prevention

Same as for bancroftian filariasis (i.e both chemoprophylaxis and vector control).

Removal of pistia plants: In South India and Sri Lanka where the *Mansonia* is the main vector, breeding is best controlled by removing the supporting plant *Pistia stratiotes* from all water collections and converting ponds to fish or lotus cultures. Herbicidal agents like phenoxylene 30 and shell weed killer-D may be used to destroy the plants.

BRUGIA TIMORI

B. timori was first detected by David and Edeson on 1965.
- Its distribution is limited to the Timor islands of Southeastern Indonesia
- Morphologically microfilariae are similar to that of *B. malayi* except (Fig. 14.6):
  - **Longer:** Measures 310 (290–325) μm long
  - Cephalic space—length to width ratio is 3:2
  - About 5–8 nuclei are present in the tail region (with two nuclei in tail tip)
  - Sheath does not stain with Giemsa stain.
- Transmitted by *Anopheles barbirostris*
- Clinical feature, laboratory diagnosis, treatment are similar to that of *B. malayi*.

OTHER FILARIAL NEMATODES

LOA LOA

History

Loa loa (also called as African eye worm) was first reported in West Indies in 1770.

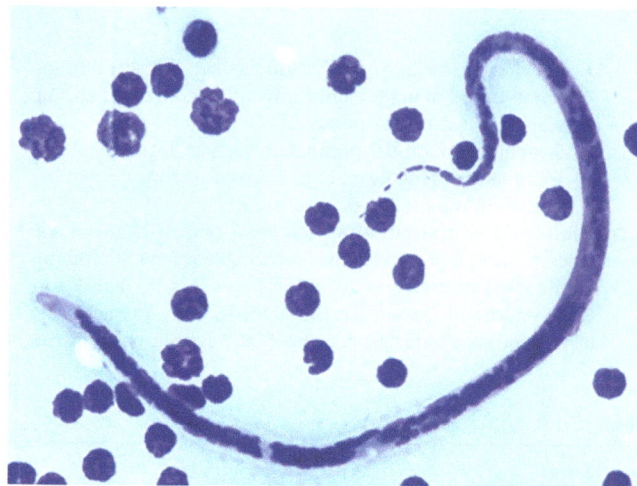

Fig. 14.6: Microfilariae of *Brugia timori* (stained with Giemsa)
Source: DPDx Image Library, Centers for Disease Control and Prevention (CDC), Atlanta (*with permission*).

Later in 1895, Argyll-Robertson described the adult worm from the subcutaneous swelling of the eye of a woman residing in Calabar from West Africa. Hence, this condition is named as **Calabar swelling**.

Epidemiology

Loa loa is restricted to the rain forests of West and Central Africa. Approximately, 13 million people are infected.

Morphology

Adult worms (females, 50–70 mm long and 0.5 mm wide; males, 30–35 mm long and 0.3 mm wide) live in subcutaneous tissues.

Microfilariae circulate in the blood with a diurnal periodicity that peaks about midday; between 12:00 noon and 2:00 p.m. They are sheathed, measure 275 (250–300) μm long and bear a column of nuclei extending till the tail tip (*see* Figs 14.1 and 14.7).

Life Cycle

Life cycle is similar to that of *W. bancrofti* except the vector is female *Chrysops* species (deer flies, mango flies, red flies or tabanid flies)
- **Mode of transmission** infective (L_3) larvae are transmitted by the bite of female *Chrysops* species during the blood meals in the daytime
- Larvae transform into adult worms over 6–12 months and migrate to subcutaneous tissues and eyes. Adult female worms have a life-span of 17 years. Microfilariae released from gravid female worms migrate to the blood and exhibit a diurnal periodicity
- Microfilariae are ingested by the deer flies during the blood meal, loose sheath, penetrate the gut wall,

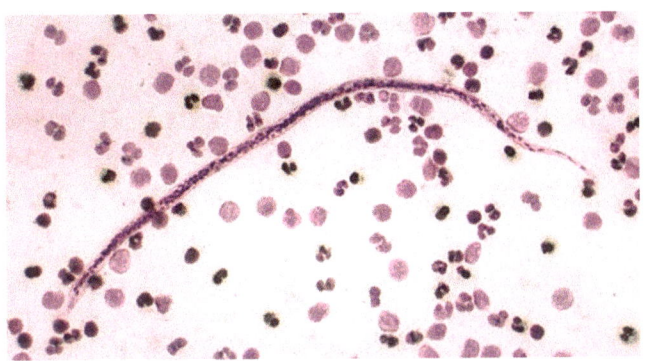

Fig. 14.7: *Loa loa* microfilaria (under microscope)
Source: Public Health Image Library, ID# 914/ Dr Lee Moore, Centers for Disease Control and Prevention (CDC), Atlanta (*with permission*).

then migrate to fat body and molt twice to become the infective L_3 larvae in about 10–12 days of time.

Pathogenesis and Clinical Feature

Calabar Swellings

This is the most common form of loiasis, also called as **fugitive swelling.**

- It is a subcutaneous swelling developing on the extremities (knee or wrist) and less frequently at other sites
- Swelling develops rapidly in few hours, preceded by localized pain, pruritus and urticaria, which lasts for 3–4 days
- It occurs due to host inflammatory response to the migrating adult worm (at a speed of 1 cm/minute) or its metabolic products. Microfilariae are not pathogenic.

Ocular Manifestations

It includes conjunctival granuloma, edema of the eye lid leading to proptosis (bulging).

Complications

Meningoencephalitis is the most severe complication and is frequently fatal.

- It occurs in DEC treated patients with higher microfilaremia. It can be prevented by administration of anti-inflammatory drugs along with DEC
- DEC should be stopped if any neurological symptoms appear.

Nephropathy and cardiomyopathy are the other rare complications noted.

> **Native vs travelers to the endemic zone**
>
> Manifestations are more severe and frequent in the visitors going to the endemic areas of Africa. Eosinophilia and increased levels of antifilarial antibodies are characteristic. However, microfilaremia is less common
>
> The native people of endemic areas are often asymptomatic with microfilaremia (90%) or may show episodic Calabar swellings (10%), moderate eosinophilia and variable levels of antibodies.

Laboratory Diagnosis

Microscopy

Definite diagnosis of loiasis requires:

- Detection of microfilariae in the peripheral blood: Blood is collected between 10 am to 3 pm. Sheathed microfilariae may be demonstrated with nuclei extended to the tail tip (*see* Figs 14.1 and 14.7, Table 14.2)
- Isolation of the adult worm from the eye or biopsy of subcutaneous swelling
- However, microfilariae usually appear in blood after few years of infection and travelers are often negative for microfilaremia.

Molecular Methods

Nested PCR-based assays for the detection of *L. loa* DNA in blood are available in specialized laboratories and are highly sensitive (95%) and specific.

Antibody Detection

Lateral flow assay (ICT) is recently developed which detects antibodies to Ll-SXP-1 antigen. It is found as 94% sensitive and 100% specific.

Other Methods

Other findings in the travelers include:

- Hypergammaglobulinemia
- Elevated levels of serum IgE
- Elevated leukocyte and eosinophil counts
- Characteristic history and clinical presentation.

> **Treatment** — *Loa loa*
>
> - **Diethylcarbamazine (DEC)** is the drug of choice—multiple courses are necessary to resolve loiasis completely
>   - **Dose:** DEC is given in a dose of 8–10 mg/kg per day for 21 days
>   - It is effective against both the adult and the microfilarial forms of *L. loa*
> - **Glucocorticoids:** It is required in heavy microfilaremia, to reduce inflammatory reactions against microfilariae and thereby preventing neurological complications
> - **Albendazole or ivermectin** is effective in reducing microfilarial loads, but ivermectin is contraindicated in heavily infected patients with loiasis
> - **Surgical removal** of the adult worms is rarely required if they migrate through the bridge of the nose or through the conjunctiva

Prevention

The preventive measures for loiasis are same as that for bancroftian filariasis.

ONCHOCERCA VOLVULUS

Onchocerca volvulus is the causative agent of **"river blindness"** in man. *O. gutturosa* is a cattle parasite, rarely infects man causing skin nodules.

History

O'Neill was the first to describe about the microfilaria in 1875; Leuckart in 1893 described the adult worm from skin nodules in Africa. Robies (1917) from Guatemala had suggested the role of the vector—Black flies for transmission. Dr Satoshi Omura and Dr William C Campbell discovered ivermectin, the life-saving drug used for onchocerciasis; for which they were awarded Nobel prize in 2015.

Epidemiology

Worldwide, about 37 million individuals from 38 countries are infected with >1 million people suffering from blindness.

Endemic area: The majority of individuals infected with *O. volvulus* live in the rural poor region of Sub-Saharan Africa, particularly West Africa. The infection is also found in Yemen and in part of central and South America.

Morphology

Adult Worm

The adult worms are long, thin, tapering at both the ends.
- Cuticle: They bear transverse striations on the cuticle with annular and oblique thickening. This helps in differentiating from other filarial worms
- Female worms are longer (35–50 cm × 300 μm) than males (2.5–5 cm × 125–200 μm). The female worms of *O. volvulus* are much longer than any other filarial worms (2–10 cm)
- Adult worms are mainly found coiled within the subcutaneous nodules.

Microfilaria

They are usually found in skin dermis (90%) or rarely in the subcutaneous nodules, blood, sputum or urine.
- They measure 254 (221–287) μm long, pointed tail tip without any nuclei (Fig. 14.1)
- They are unsheathed, nonperiodic.

Life Cycle

Life cycle is similar to that of *W. bancrofti*, except the vector is *Simulium* (black flies).
- **Mode of Transmission:** Infective form (i.e. L_3/filariform larva) is transmitted by *Simulium* (blackflies or buffalo gnats) flies during the blood meals
- Within the dermis, the L_3 larvae molt twice to transform to adult worms over 12 months and then the adult worms migrate in subcutaneous tissues and eyes
- Microfilariae are released from gravid female worms (1,000–3,000/day) within 15 months after infection (prepatent period). Microfilariae may have a life-span of up to 15 years in humans.
- Microfilariae are ingested by the black flies during the blood meal. Then they penetrate the gut wall, migrate to the flight muscles and molt twice to become the infective larvae (L_3) in about 6–12 days of time (extrinsic incubation period).

Clinical Features

Patients are asymptomatic when the worm load is less. However, in heavy infections the major manifestations include skin (dermatitis), subcutaneous fibrous nodule (onchocercoma), lymphadenitis and ocular changes. Except for the skin nodules (occurs due to adult worms), the other manifestations are due to hyperreactive immune response to the microfilarial antigens.

Skin (Dermatitis)

Intense pruritus and generalized papular rashes are the most common manifestations.
- Prolonged infection results in loss of elastic fibers and epidermal atrophy which can lead to loose, redundant wrinkling of skin
- **Leopard skin:** Skin may be hypo to hyperpigmented. The spots of repigmentation within a depigmented area are known as **leopard skin**
- Lichenoid changes and hyperkeratosis may occur in late stages
- **Sowda:** It is a chronic hyperreactive form of dermatitis, results from formation of autoantibodies against defensins. It occurs in a subset of individuals from Arabica, Sudan, Guatemala and West Africa.

Onchocercoma (Subcutaneous Nodules)

Subcutaneous nodules are firm, nontender, variable in size containing the coiled adult worms and rarely microfilariae.

In African patients, nodules are common over the trunk (sacrum and hip area), while in patients from South and Central America, they tend to develop on the head, neck and shoulders.

Ocular Involvement

- **Bilateral blindness (river blindness)** is the most serious complication of onchocerciasis. Lesions may develop in all parts of the eye
- **Conjunctivitis with photophobia:** It is the most common early finding
- **Punctate keratitis:** It is a self-resolving, acute inflammatory reactions to surrounding dying microfilariae seen in younger patients and presented as **"snowflake opacities"**
- **Sclerosing keratitis** occurs in 1–5% of infected persons and is the leading cause of **Onchocercal blindness** in Africa

- **Other manifestations:** Anterior uveitis and iridocyclitis (Africa), retinal pigmentation, secondary glaucoma (seen in Latin America).

Lymph Nodes

Lymphadenopathy in the inguinal and femoral areas is commonly noted.

The enlarged nodes may hang down ("*hanging groin*") and may predispose to hernia.

Host Immune Response

Symptomatic patients especially with Sowda have a marked T_H2 response and increase in interleukin-4 (IL-4) and IL-5 that leads to increase in the levels of IgE, IgG4 and eosinophilia.

Laboratory Diagnosis

Detection of the Microfilariae

Detection of microfilariae in a skin snip smear is the gold standard method for diagnosis of onchocerciasis. Microfilariae are found either in the skin (90%) or in the nodules (10%).

- **Skin snips technique:**
    - **Most common sites:** Both iliac crests or sometimes from calves and the shoulders
    - **Procedure:** Skin is lifted by a needle and a small piece (1 to 3 mm) is excised with a sterile scalpel blade.
- After incubating the biopsy tissue in saline, microfilariae emerge from the skin (60% within 30 minutes, 75% in 24 hours)
- The movement can be seen by direct microscopy. However, differentiation from other microfilariae can be done following Giemsa or hematoxylin and eosin (H & E) staining (*see* Figs 14.1 and 14.8A)
- Quantification of microfilariae can be done (number of microfilariae per mg of skin); which is an accurate tool to measure the endemicity of infection in the community.

Detection of the Adult Worm

It can be done from the biopsy of the subcutaneous nodules but it is less sensitive (Fig. 14.8B).

Serology

Cocktail of recombinant antigens of *O. volvulus* can be used to detect specific antibodies which show better specificity and do not cross react with other nematodes. However, it cannot differentiate the current from the past infection.

However, currently developed IgG4 specific dip stick assay detecting Ov16 antigen may indicate active infection. There is no licensed antigen detection method is available.

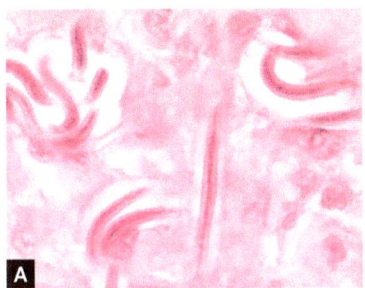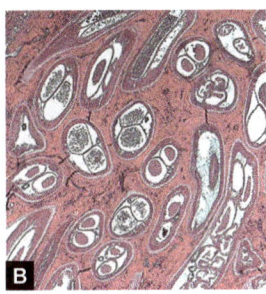

Figs 14.8A and B: *Onchocerca volvulus* from a skin nodule stained with hematoxylin and eosin stain (H & E) (A) Microfilariae; (B) Adult worms—transverse section

Source: DPDx Image Library, Centers for Disease Control and Prevention (CDC), Atlanta (*with permission*).

Molecular Methods

PCR detecting onchocercal DNA in skin snips or even from skin scrapings is available in specialized laboratories and is highly sensitive and specific. It can differentiate the *Onchocerca* species and also the various strains of *O. volvulus*. Real-time PCR is available, which can detect and quantify *O. volvulus* O-150 DNA sequence.

Other Methods

- Eosinophilia and elevated serum IgE can be demonstrated
- **Slit lamp examination:** Sitting with head placed between the knees for 10 minutes may help the microfilariae to concentrate in anterior chamber of eyes behind the cornea; which may be visualized by slit lamp examination.

Mazzotti Skin Test (DEC Patch Test)

Topical application of DEC on the skin leads to local reaction (erythema and itching) to the dead worm. Sometime, the reaction is much severe in heavy infection. Hence, this is done only in light infection without eye involvement.

Treatment	*Onchocerca volvulus*
Ivermectin is the drug of choice for onchocerciasis. ❏ It is active against the microfilariae but not against the adult worms ❏ It is given orally in a single dose of 150 µg/kg, either yearly or biannually ❏ It is contraindicated in areas of Africa co-endemic for *O. volvulus* and *L. loa*. Surgical excision is recommended when nodules are located on the head	

Prevention

Vector control is useful in highly endemic areas. Insecticide spraying can be carried to destroy the breeding sites.

Mass administration of ivermectin every 6–12 months is being used to interrupt the transmission in endemic areas.

MANSONELLA SPECIES

Mansonella species are named after Patric Manson. They rarely infect humans and are either nonpathogenic or asymptomatic in most of the individuals.

Mansonella Perstans

Mansonella perstans is found mainly in the Central Africa and in Central and South America

- ❖ **Transmission:** It is transmitted by *Culicoides* (midges)
- ❖ **Life cycle:** It is similar to other filarial worms. Adult worms reside in serous cavities, mesentery and perirenal tissues. Microfilariae circulate in the blood without periodicity. Man, gorilla and monkey are the reservoir host
- ❖ **Clinical features:** Usually nonpathogenic, but occasionally, it can cause manifestations like angioedema, urticaria, pruritus and **calbar-like swelling** similar to that of *Loa loa*. It also produces acute periorbital inflammation; known as **bung-eye** or **bulge-eye**
- ❖ **Laboratory diagnosis:** Microfilariae in peripheral blood are nonperiodic, nonsheathed, measures 195 (190–200) μm long with a straight tail with blunt end. Body nuclei are extended till the tail tip (*see* Figs 14.1 and 14.9A).

Treatment	*Mansonella perstans*
DEC or albendazole are found to be effective; lowering the level of microfilaremia.	

Mansonella Streptocerca

M. streptocerca is found mainly in tropical forest area western and central sub-Saharan Africa such as Congo (incidence may reach up to 90%) and Uganda.

- ❖ **Transmission:** It is transmitted by the biting midges (*Culicoides grahami*)
- ❖ **Life cycle** is similar to other filarial worms. Monkeys serve as reservoir host
- ❖ **Clinical feature:** Many infected individuals are asymptomatic, although some people may develop inguinal lymphadenopathy, pruritus, dermatitis with hypopigmented macule similar to leprosy except that there is no sensory loss
- ❖ **Laboratory diagnosis:** The diagnosis is made by detection of the characteristic microfilariae in skin snips
    - It is nonperiodic, nonsheathed, measures 210 (180–240) μm with a curved tail (looks like **Shepherd's crook**). Nuclei are extended till the blunt tail tip. (*see* Figs 4.1 and 14.9B)
    - Microfilariae of *M. streptocerca* must be differentiated from that of *O. volvulus* by (i) its length (it is two-thirds that of *O. volvulus*) (ii) thinner than *O. volvulus*, (iii) presence of Shepherd's crook at posterior end of *M. streptocerca* (*see* Figs 14.1 and 14.9B).

Treatment	*Mansonella streptocerca*
DEC is effective for streptocerciasis.	

Mansonella Ozzardi

M. ozzardi infection was first noted by Ozzard in an Indian patient in South America and then it was described by Manson.

- ❖ **Epidemiology and transmission:**
    - *M. ozzardi* is found mainly in Central and South America and transmitted by *Culicoides* (midges)
    - Rarely, it is also found in certain Caribbean islands and transmitted by *Simulium amazonicum* (blackflies).
- ❖ **Life cycle:** It is similar to other filarial worms. Adult worms are rarely recovered from humans. Microfilariae circulate in the blood without periodicity. Man is the only reservoir host.

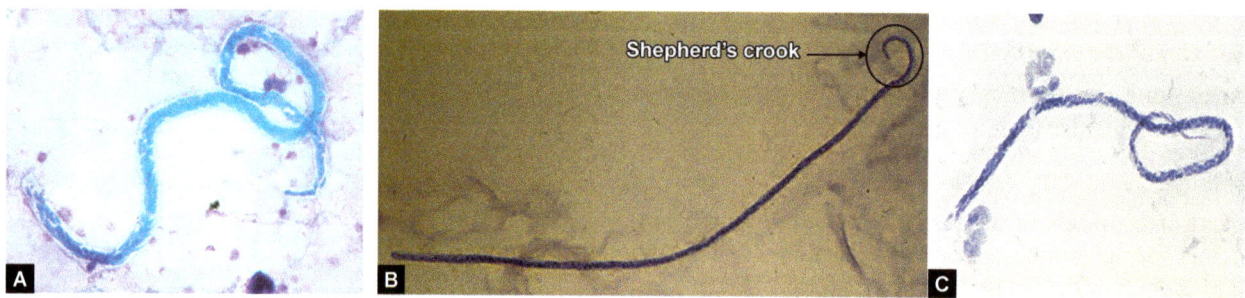

Figs 14.9A to C: (A) Microfilariae of *Mansonella perstans* (stained with Giemsa); (B) Microfilaria of *Mansonella streptocerca* (stained with hematoxylin); (C) Microfilaria of *Mansonella ozzardi* (Giemsa stain)

Source: A and B—DPDx Image Library, Centers for Disease Control and Prevention (CDC), Atlanta (*with permission*); C—Public Health Image Library, ID# 909/ Centers for Disease Control and Prevention (CDC), Atlanta (*with permission*).

- **Clinical features:** Most infections are asymptomatic, but occasionally cause lymphadenopathy, urticaria, pruritus, pulmonary symptoms, arthralgia and keratitis
- **Diagnosis:** Microfilariae can be detected in peripheral blood; which are nonperiodic, nonsheathed, measures 200 (173–240) µm long with a fine attenuated hooked and pointed tail tip without any nuclei (*see* Figs 14.1 and 14.9C). Microfilariae of *M. ozzardi* may be confused with those of *M. perstans*; however, the tail of *M. ozzardi* tends to be pointed and slightly flexed with a longer caudal space.

Treatment	*Mansonella ozzardi*
Ivermectin is effective in lowering the level of microfilaremia. Use of DEC is controversial.	

Zoonotic filariasis

Several zoonotic filarial worms are known to transmit to man via accidental mosquito bites.
- Zoonotic *Brugia* infections (American brugian filariasis): Around 50 cases have been reported so far. Usually systemic manifestations are not seen. Most of the patients present with a tender lymphadenopathy
  - *B. beaveri* is transmitted from raccoon, human cases have been reported from Northeast USA
  - *B. leporis*—infects swamp rabbits and eastern cottontails; human cases have been reported from Malaysia
  - *B. guyanensis*—infects the raccoon; human cases, reported from South America
  - *Brugia pahangi*: It is a common parasite of dogs and cats in Malaysia. It has been reported to cause lymphangitis and lymphadenitis in men
  - Subperiodic strains of *B. malayi*—infects the monkeys and cats; human cases, reported from Southeast Asia
- **Others:** Other zoonotic filarial species include, *Dirofilaria* (explained subsequently in the chapter), *Onchocerca*, *Dipetalonema*, *Loaina*, and *Meningonema*.

DIROFILARIA SPECIES

Dirofilaria species are parasites of lower animals. Humans are unusual hosts. Hence, the parasite undergoes an incomplete development in humans either in the lungs, eyes and or subcutaneous tissue
- **Transmission:** Man acquires infection by the bite of mosquito (*Aedes, Culex, Anopheles*, or *Mansonia*) containing L3 filariform larvae. Larvae undergo only partial development and immature adults are lodged in subcutaneous tissue from which they may migrate to other organs
- **Various species** are:
  - Infection with *D. repens* (from dogs) or *D. tenuis* (from raccoons) or *D. ursi* (bears) can cause local subcutaneous nodules in humans

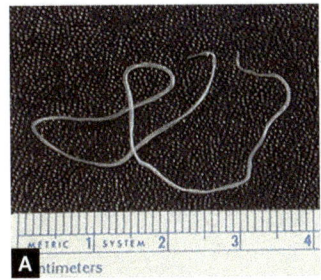 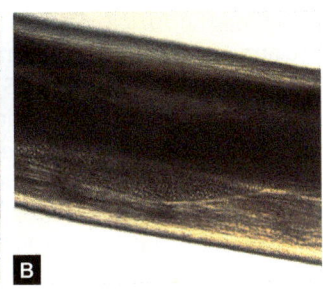

Figs 14.10A and B: Dirofilaria species: (A) Adult worm surgically removed from eye; (B) Higher magnification shows thick laminated cuticle

Source: DPDx Image Library, Centers for Disease Control and Prevention (CDC), Atlanta (*with permission*).

  - *D. immitis* (dog heart worms) can cause pulmonary infection in humans
  - *D. conjunctivae* can cause ocular manifestations in sclera and conjunctiva
  - Humans have also been infected with *D. subdermata* (porcupines), and *D. striata* (wild cat).
- **Epidemiology:** Less than 1,000 cases have been reported so far, mainly from Italy, Sri Lanka and Ex Soviet union. In India, about 10–20 human cases have been reported; mainly from Kerala, Karnataka, Assam and Odisha
- **Diagnosis:** By identification of the adult worms by surgery or autopsy. Microfilariae are not found in blood or tissue
  - Adult worm measures 230–310 mm long by 350 µm wide; is identified by their thick laminated cuticle, large muscle cells and broad lateral ends (Figs 14.10A and B)
  - *D. immitis* can be differentiated from *D. repens* by the absence of ridges
  - Calcofluor white stain can be used to demonstrate the chitinous wall (Fig. 14.10B).

Treatment	*Dirofilaria*
Surgical removal of the worm is the only treatment available. No drugs are found to be effective.	

OTHER SOMATIC NEMATODES

DRACUNCULUS MEDINENSIS

Dracunculus medinensis causes **Guinea worm disease** or **dracunculiasis**.

Epidemiology

Currently, dracunculiasis is endemic to only three countries namely Chad, Ethiopia and Mali; all located in

Sub-Saharan Africa. About 187 countries including India are already declared free of transmission.
- In 1986, an estimated 3.5 million new cases occurred globally. After the initiation of control program, there was a dramatic fall of cases
- In 2017, only 30 cases were reported, 15 each from Chad and Ethiopia. Mali reported zero human cases for two consecutive years
- However, infection in dogs may be worrying factor for maintaining the parasite and its re-emergence.

Life Cycle (Fig. 14.11)

Host: There are two types of hosts:
1. **Definitive host:** Man
2. **Intermediate host:** Copepods (*Cyclops*)

Infective form: Third stage filariform larvae.
Mode of transmission: Man gets infection by drinking water from stagnant pools containing minute fresh water crustaceans (*Cyclops*) infected with L_3 larvae.

Development in Man

- **Migration to thoracic muscle:** Cyclops are digested in stomach releasing the L_3 larvae. They penetrate the wall of the small intestine and migrate to the thoracic musculature. Larvae molt twice to form adult worms [(male (2 cm) and female (1 meter)]; which later sexually mature in deep connective tissue
- Gravid female worms mature over 10 to 14 months, migrate throughout the body, and ultimately reach the skin, particularly over the ankles, feet, and lower legs
- When skin comes in contact with water, the female worm induces a local blister that eventually ruptures. Large numbers of L_1 larvae are released into the water when prolapsed loops of the uterus of female worm contracts.

Development in Cyclops

The motile free-swimming L_1 larvae infect *Cyclops*. They molt twice to form L_3 larvae which are infective to man over a period of 2 weeks.

Pathogenesis and Clinical Feature

Signs and symptoms appear approximately 1 year after the infection; when gravid adult female worm emerges near the surface of the skin.

- The initial presentation is a painful papule that enlarges over hours to days to form a blister from which the worm emerges (Fig. 14.12A)
- The blister may be accompanied by local erythema, urticaria, fever, nausea and pruritus. The entire worm may emerge over a period of several weeks (Fig. 14.12 B)
- Complications include secondary bacterial infections that may lead to sepsis, local abscesses and pyogenic arthritis
- The most common site—lower leg, ankle and foot
- The prevalence of dracunculiasis is a strong indicator of poor socioeconomic development of the community such as inadequate treatment of drinking water and improper separation of bathing and drinking water facilities
- The manifestations are seasonal (June to September); due to appearance of stagnant water pools (containing *Cyclops*).

Laboratory Diagnosis

Dracunculiasis is diagnosed by:
- **Detection of adult worm:** This is possible when the gravid female worms appear in the blisters. The calcified adult worms from the deeper tissue can be detected by X-ray
- **Detection of L_1 larvae:** When the leg with ulcer is placed in a container with cold water, a large number of motile larvae are discharged which can be examined under microscope

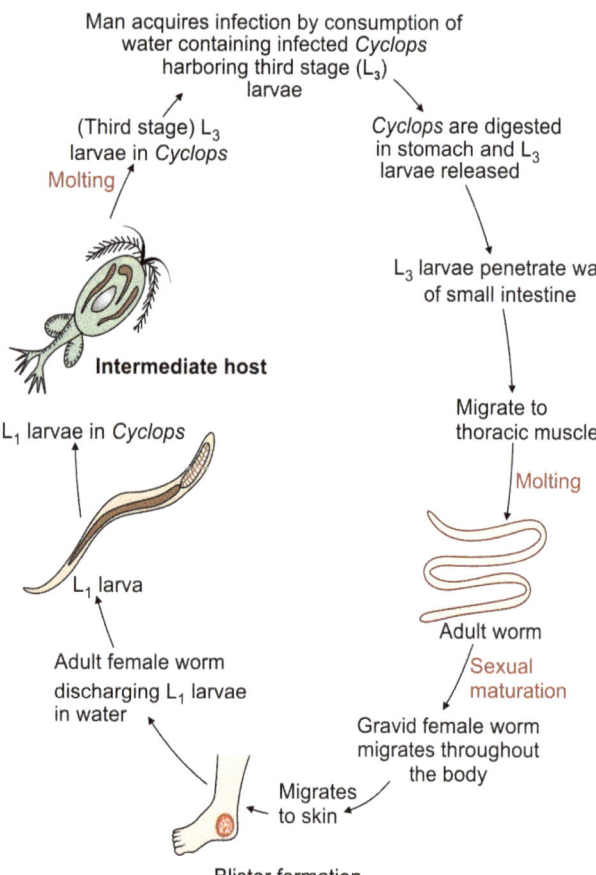

Fig. 14.11: Life cycle of *Dracunculus medinensis*

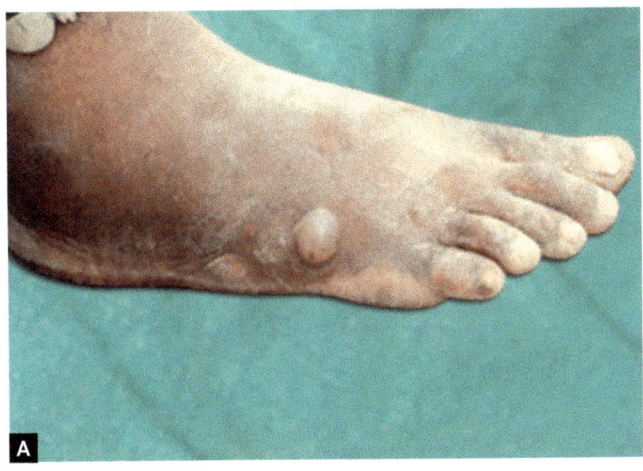
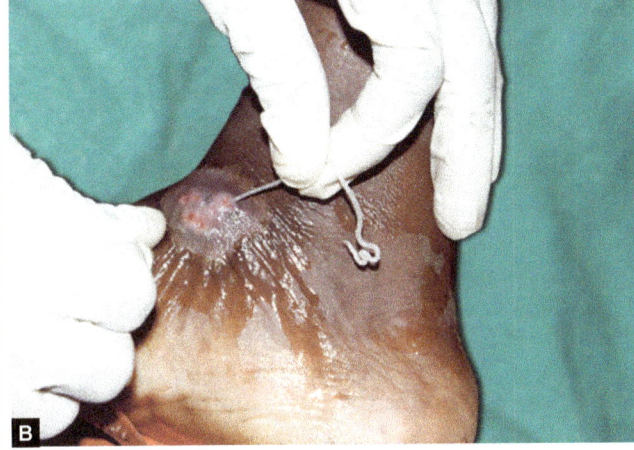

Figs 14.12A and B: Dracunculiasis (A) Blister formed; (B) Adult female worm of *Dracunculus medinensis* emerging from the blister
Source: DPDx Image Library, Centers for Disease Control and Prevention (CDC), Atlanta *(with permission).*

- **Antibody detection:** Antibodies to *D. medinensis* can be detected by ELISA
- Peripheral blood *Eosinophilia*.

Treatment	*Dracunculus medinensis*

- **Worm removal:** Worms are slowly and gently extracted over a period of 15–20 days using a small stick and wounding out daily with small traction. Heavy pressure should be avoided because breaking the worm can lead to allergic reactions and secondary bacterial infection
- There are no anti-helminthic drugs known to be effective against *D. medinensis*
- **Symptomatic treatment:** Includes application of wet compresses to the affected skin, administration of analgesics and prevention of secondary bacterial infection by the use of topical antibiotics

Reasons for Eradication of Guinea Worm Disease from India

The national Guinea worm eradication program was launched in 1984 with technical assistance from World Health Organization (WHO).
Simple and cost-effective measures were taken to eradicate the disease such as:
- **Provision of safe drinking water:** Filtration of drinking water, installing hand pumps and pipes
- ***Cyclops* control:** Killing copepods ins sources of drinking water by application of abate (temephos) larvicide
- Provision of clean drinking water from boreholes or wells
- Health education about boiling or filtering of drinking water
- Treatment of cases.

TRICHINELLA SPIRALIS

Trichinella spiralis causes **trichinellosis** (or trichinosis) which is a zoonotic infection acquired from domestic pigs or other carnivores.

History

T. spiralis was first detected by James Paget and Richard Owen (1835) from a cadaver muscle. Later on, in 1859 Virchow had described the life cycle.

Classification

Trichinella belongs to the class Adenophorea, superfamily Trichinelloidea and family Trichinellidae.
- DNA analysis had shown that *Trichinella* comprises of 9 species which are further divided into 12 genotypes (T1-T12). *T. spiralis* has one genotype (T1). It is the predominant species distributed worldwide affecting humans
- Other species usually infect animals. However, some of them rarely infect humans: *T. pseudospiralis, T. nativa, T. nelsoni, T. britovi, T. murrelli, T. papuae, T. zimbabwensis* and *T. patagoniensis*.

Epidemiology

Human trichinellosis is widely prevalent in the pork eating countries (more in temperate zone than tropics) like Europe, South America and North America including the USA. More so, meats of horses and wild boars have also been implicated to cause disease.

In India

Few cases of animal trichinellosis have been reported. Human infection is very rare. The first case was reported from the Punjab. In 2010, an outbreak of human trichinellosis had occurred in Uttarakhand affecting 18 people eating roasted wild boar meat called **kachmoli.**

Morphology

Adult Worm

It is one of the smallest intestinal nematode. Female worm (3 mm long) is longer than male worm (1.5 mm long)
- **Shape:** Thread like just visible to naked eye
- Esophagus occupies one-third to half of the body and bears a row of esophageal glands (stichocytes). Esophagus leads to intestine and ending at anus
- **Male worm:** Identified by presence of pair of copulatory organs (papillae) at the tail end called as **claspers**, but there is no copulatory bursa
- **Female worm:** Females have single ovary, uterus, vagina and vulva opened in the middle. They are viviparous, i.e. they directly lay larvae; there is no egg stage.

Larva

There are four larval stages (L_1–L_4)
- The newborn larva (L_1) measures 80 μm long, its esophagus has a stylet (a sphere like organ that helps to enter into the cells)
- The infective L_1 larva in muscle measures 1 mm long. Inside the muscle cyst, the larva remains coiled; hence, the species name is given as "*spiralis*" (Fig. 14.13).

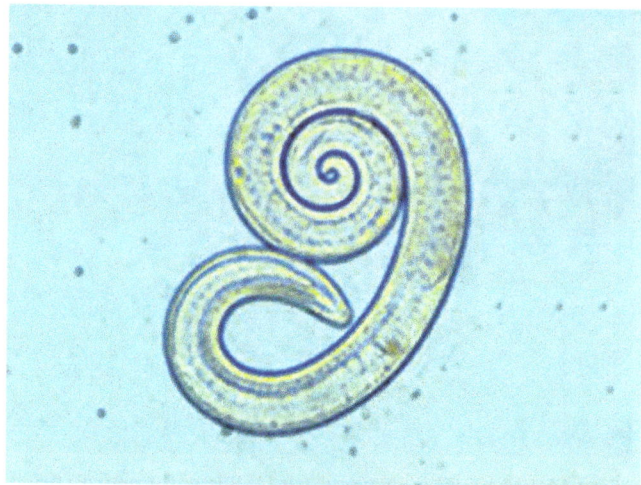

Fig. 14.13: Larvae of *Trichinella* liberated from bear meat (microscopic view)

Source: DPDx Image Library, Centers for Disease Control and Prevention (CDC), Atlanta (*with permission*).

Life Cycle (Fig. 14.14)

Host:
- Pig is the **optimum host** and is the principal reservoir of infection
- Animals-like rats horses or other carnivores can also serve as the host
- Transmission usually occurs in nature from one flesh eating animal to other. Common cycles are pig to pig, rat to rat, pig to rat
- Man is an **accidental host** and acts as dead end

Infective form: First stage (L_1) larvae are the infective form.
Mode of transmission: By ingestion of raw or uncooked pork or other animal meat containing L_1 larvae. It is estimated that 100–300 larvae are required to initiate the infection.

Intestinal Phase

- **L_1 larvae transform to adults:** Ingested L_1 larvae are immediately freed from the animal flesh by digestive enzymes in stomach. Then, they are carried to the small intestine (upper two-thirds). They penetrate the intestinal mucosa where they undergo four molts to develop into adult worms in 48 hours

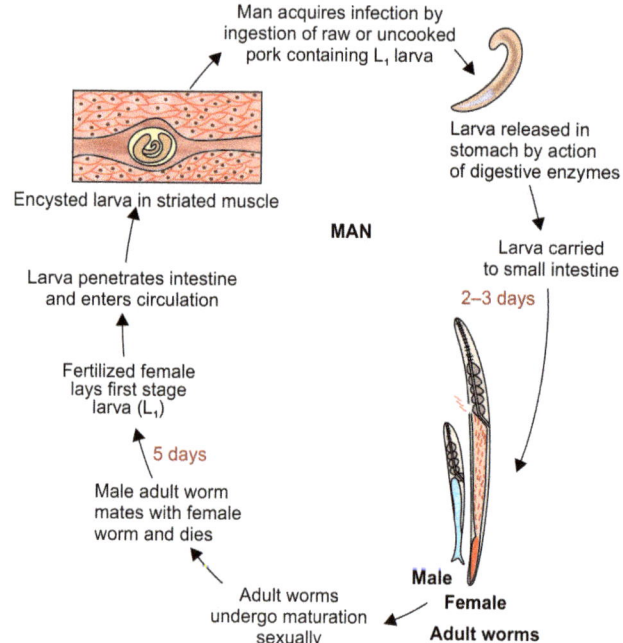

Fig. 14.14: Life cycle of *Trichinella spiralis*

- **Female worms lay L_1 larvae:** Male worms mate with female worms on second day and die soon. Females are viviparous. By the 5th day of infection, they start laying the first stage larvae. Each female worm produces 1500 larvae in its life span in nonimmune host.

Migration Phase

The L_1 larvae penetrate the intestine and carried to skeletal muscle via intestinal lymphatics and mesenteric venous circulation.

Encystment

L_1 larvae enter inside the skeletal (striated) muscle cells and behave as obligate intracellular anaerobic parasite.
- The secretion of esophageal glands modulates the host DNA to alter the hostile environment
- The muscle cells are modified within 2-3 weeks; to form **nurse cells,** surrounded by blood vessels which provide the required environment for the nourishment and containment of the parasite for years. *T. pseudospiralis, T. papuae,* and *T. zimbabwensis* do not produce nurse cells.

Only skeletal muscle cells are infected, encystment does not occur in cardiac and smooth muscles.

Organization

After some years, the nurse cell-larva complex undergo Encystment.
- The cyst measures 400 X 260 μm in size, containing the coiled L_1 larva which measures 800 to 1,000 μm in length. It is the infective form; survives in muscle cells for up to 20-40 years. However, men are the dead end
- The cyst undergoes fibrosis and calcification after weeks to years
- The parasite inside the cyst remains metabolically active by acquiring nutrition and discharging metabolic waste products into blood vessels present on the surface of cyst.

Pathogenicity and Clinical Feature

Clinical symptoms of trichinellosis depend on the phase of parasitic invasion—intestinal invasion, larval migration, and muscle encystment.

Intestinal Stage

Most of the light infections are asymptomatic; however, heavy infections can be life-threatening. Symptoms start appearing during the first week of infection
- Invasion of the gut by large number of parasites can provoke watery diarrhea (most common feature) during the first week after infection
- Abdominal pain, constipation, nausea or vomiting may also be seen.

Stage of Larval Migration (Parenteral Stage)

Symptoms appear in the second week after infection
- Hypersensitivity reaction: The migrating *Trichinella* larvae provoke a marked local and systemic hypersensitivity reaction, with fever and hypereosinophilia
- Periorbital and facial edema is common
- Hemorrhages are seen in the subconjunctiva, retina and nail beds ("splinter" hemorrhages)
- Maculopapular rash
- Migration to heart, CNS and lungs may occur—leading to myocarditis (5-20%), encephalitis, or pneumonia that become severe after 4-8 weeks. Myocarditis is transient as the larvae do not encapsulate in cardiac muscle.

Stage of Muscle Encystment

Occurs 2-3 weeks after infection
- Common symptoms are myositis with myalgia, muscle edema, and weakness
- **Most commonly involved muscles:** Extraocular muscles followed by biceps, muscles of the jaw, neck, lower back, and diaphragm
- Death may occur between 4th to 8th week of infection. As few as five larvae/g of body muscle can cause death.

Laboratory Diagnosis

Demonstration of Larvae

Definite diagnosis by demonstration of larvae in muscle biopsy:
- **Sample:** Muscle biopsy is obtained from gastrocnemius, deltoid, and biceps. It is useful only after 2-3 weeks of onset of illness
- **Direct slide technique:** The fresh muscle tissue should be compressed between glass slides and examined under low power microscope
- **Histopathologic study:** Can be done using H & E stain but larvae may be missed by examination of routine histopathologic sections alone (Fig. 14.15)
- **Artificial digestion technique:** Involves enzymatic digestion of muscle mass by pepsin with conc. HCl and mounting the digested tissue, which may yield better result
- "Squash" preparation: Larvae of *Trichinella* species do not form the capsule; however, the unencapsulated larvae can still be seen in a "squash" preparation of biopsy material.

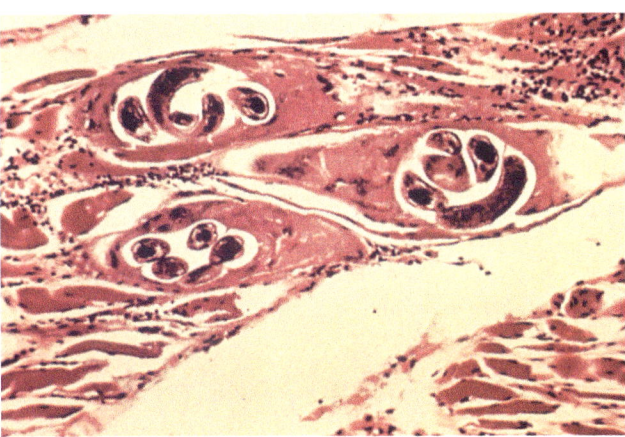

Fig. 14.15: *Trichinella* cysts within human muscle tissue (hemotoxylin and eosin stain)

Source: Public Health Image Library, ID# 5234/ Centers for Disease Control and Prevention (CDC), Atlanta (*with permission*).

Antibody Detection

ELISA is available detecting parasite specific IgG antibody against excretory secretory antigen of muscle larvae.
- It is 93% sensitive and 85% specific
- Cross reactivity with filarial worms and *Strongyloides* is common
- Positive after 2–4 weeks of infection
- It confirms the diagnosis but cannot differentiate past and present infection.

Coproantigen Detection

- A modified double sandwich ELISA has been developed using polyclonal antibodies raised in rabbit to detect larval somatic antigens in stool. It is detectable from first day of infection up to third week
- Another ELISA format detecting cathepsin B-like protease antigen of *T. spiralis* is under development.

Bachman Intradermal Test

Intradermal injection of Bachman antigen (prepared from *Trichinella* larva obtained from rabbit muscle) causes an immediate small induration surrounded by erythema of 5 cm diameter in 15–20 minutes. It becomes positive in 2–3 weeks of infection and persists for life, hence cannot differentiate past infection present infection.

Animal inoculation

Rats are fed with muscle tissue of suspected patients and after appropriate time, they are examined for *T. spiralis* larvae in the diaphragm.

Other Tests

- **Blood eosinophilia:** Elevated in more than 90% symptomatic patients and levels may peak at 2–5 weeks after the infection and remains elevated for 4–8 weeks
- Increase in WBC count is seen
- **Elevated muscle enzymes:** Elevated serum creatine phosphokinase
- History of consumption of pork or wild animal meat
- **X-ray** to detect the calcified muscle cyst.

Treatment	*Trichinella spiralis*

- **Mild infection:** Symptomatic treatment is required with bed rest, antipyretics, and analgesics
- **Moderate infection:** Mebendazole and albendazole are active against enteric stages of the parasite, but their efficacy against encysted larvae has not been conclusively demonstrated
- **Severe infection:** Glucocorticoid is added which is beneficial for severe myositis and myocarditis.

Prevention

Trichinellosis can be prevented by the following measures.
- Direct inspection of pork and microscopic examination of small tissue samples of pig diaphragm before commercial use
- Maintenance of strict standards for freezing, cooking, and curing of pork and pork products is necessary
- All parts of pork muscle tissue must be heated to >58.3°C. Microwaving might not kill the parasite
- Sanitary disposal of dead animals.

EXPECTED QUESTIONS

I. Write essay on:
  a. A 35-year-old female from a village of Bihar came to the hospital with history of fever on and off for the past one year and recently developed unilateral swelling of the left lower limb. Her blood sample was sent for peripheral blood smear examination which revealed microfilariae, 240 µm in length, tail tip pointed free of nuclei.
  1. What is the etiological diagnosis?
  2. Write briefly about the life cycle of the etiological agent.
  3. What are the various diagnostic modalities?
  4. How will you treat this condition?
  5. Write a note on elimination program going on for this disease?
  b. Classify somatic nematodes. Describe the life cycle, pathogenesis and laboratory diagnosis of *Brugia malayi*.

II. Write short notes on:
  a. Onchocerciasis.
  b. Loiasis.
  c. Guinea worm infection.

III. Multiple choice questions (MCQs):
  1. Causative agent of Calabar swelling is:
     a. *Dracunculus medinensis*   b. *Wuchereria bancrofti*
     c. *Brugia malayi*   d. *Loa loa*
  2. Which of the following infection is eradicated from India?
     a. *Wuchereria bancrofti*   b. *Brugia malayi*
     c. *Dracunculus medinensis*   d. *Ascaris lumbricoides*
  3. Which of the following microfilariae is sheathed?
     a. *Mansonella perstans*   b. *Onchocerca volvulus*
     c. *Brugia malayi*   d. *Mansonella streptocerca*
  4. Microfilaria of *Brugia malayi* differs from that of *Wuchereria bancrofti* by all, *except*:
     a. Coarse, overlapping and darkly-stained nuclei
     b. Tail-tip free from nuclei
     c. Cephalic space longer   d. Possesses secondary kinks
  5. Which of the following microfilaria comes to peripheral blood in the day time?
     a. *Wuchereria bancrofti*   b. *Brugia malayi*
     c. *Loa loa*   d. *Brugia timori*

Answer
1. d 2. c 3. c 4. b 5. c

SECTION 4

MISCELLANEOUS

Section Outline

15. Laboratory Diagnosis of Parasitic Diseases   *233*
16. Medical Entomology   *258*

Appendices
1. Appendix 1: Relative size of morphological forms of parasites   *265*
2. Appendix 2: Clinical syndromes in parasitology   *267*

Laboratory Diagnosis of Parasitic Diseases

15 CHAPTER

CHAPTER OUTLINE

- Introduction
- Morphological identification techniques
- Culture techniques in parasitology
- Immunodiagnostic methods
- Molecular methods
- Intradermal skin tests
- Xenodiagnostic techniques
- Animal inoculation methods
- Imaging techniques

INTRODUCTION

Laboratory diagnosis plays a vital role in the diagnosis of parasitic infections. Following diagnostic techniques are used for diagnosis of parasitic infections:

- ❖ Morphological identification techniques either macroscopically or microscopically
- ❖ Culture methods
- ❖ Immunodiagnostic methods
- ❖ Molecular methods
- ❖ Intradermal skin tests
- ❖ Xenodiagnostic techniques
- ❖ Animal inoculation methods
- ❖ Imaging techniques.

MORPHOLOGICAL IDENTIFICATION TECHNIQUES

The parasites can be identified by their morphology either macroscopically or microscopically. Various morphological forms of different parasites can be seen in different specimens (Table 15.1).

Microscopically, they can be visualized directly by wet mount (saline/iodine) for stool specimen or either by different staining techniques.

EXAMINATION OF FECES

Specimen Collection

Stool specimens should be collected in a wide-mouthed, clean, leak-proof, screw capped containers and should be handled carefully to avoid acquiring infection from organisms present in stool (Fig. 15.1).

- ❖ **Timing:** Specimen should be collected before starting antiparasitic drugs and closer to the onset of symptoms

Table 15.1: Various morphological forms of parasites seen in different specimens

Specimen	Morphological form	Parasite
Feces	Trophozoite	Entamoeba histolytica Giardia lamblia Balantidium coli Trichomonas hominis
	Cyst	E. histolytica G. lamblia B. coli
	Adult worm	Ascaris lumbricoides Enterobius vermicularis Fasciolopsis buski
	Adult worm segments	Taenia solium T. saginata Diphyllobothrium latum
	Egg	Schistosoma species Fasciola hepatica Fasciolopsis buski Clonorchis sinensis Opisthorchis felineus Heterophyes heterophyes Metagonimus yokogawai Diphyllobothrium latum Taenia species Hymenolepis nana H. diminuta Dipylidium caninum Ascaris lumbricoides Ancylostoma duodenale Necator americanus Enterobius vermicularis Trichuris trichiura Capillaria species Trichostrongylus

Contd...

Contd...

Specimen	Morphological form	Parasite
Peripheral blood smear	Ring form, schizont and gametocyte	*Plasmodium* species
	Amastigote	*Leishmania* species
	Trypomastigote	*Trypanosoma* species
	Microfilaria	*Wuchereria bancrofti* *Brugia malayi* *Loa loa* *Mansonella* species
Bone marrow, liver, lymph node, spleen aspirate	Tachyzoite	*Toxoplasma gondii*
	Amastigote	*Leishmania donovani*
Liver aspirate	Trophozoite	*Entamoeba histolytica*
Lymph node aspirate	Trypomastigote	*Trypanosoma* species
Lymph node biopsy	Adult worm	*Wuchereria bancrofti* *Brugia malayi*
Cerebrospinal fluid (CSF)	Trypomastigote	*Trypanosoma* species
	Larva	*Angiostrongylus* species
	Trophozoite	*Naegleria fowleri* *Acanthamoeba*
Urine	Trophozoite	*Trichomonas vaginalis*
	Microfilaria	*Wuchereria bancrofti*
	Egg	*Schistosoma haematobium* *Dioctophyma renale*
Sputum	Adult worm	*Paragonimus* species
	Egg	*Paragonimus* species *Capillaria aerophila*
	Larva (migrating)	*Ascaris lumbricoides* *Strongyloides stercoralis* *Ancylostoma duodenale* *Necator americanus*
	Trophozoite	*Entamoeba histolytica*
Duodenal aspirate	Trophozoite	*Giardia lamblia*
	Larva	*Strongyloides stercoralis*
Corneal scrapings	Trophozoite	*Acanthamoeba* species
Skin	Amastigote	*Leishmania* species
	Microfilaria	*Onchocerca volvulus*
	Larva in skin ulcer fluid	*Dracunculus medinensis*
Muscle tissue	Encysted larva	*Trichinella spiralis*
	Cysticercus cellulosae	*Taenia solium*
Perianal area	Egg	*Enterobius* species *Taenia saginata*

- **Frequency:** At least three stool specimens collected on alternate days (within 10 days) are adequate to make the diagnosis of intestinal parasitic diseases (if no loose stool is present, then a third specimen should be obtained after purgatives). For intestinal amoebiasis, six specimens may be recommended, which ensures detection of approximately 90% of infections

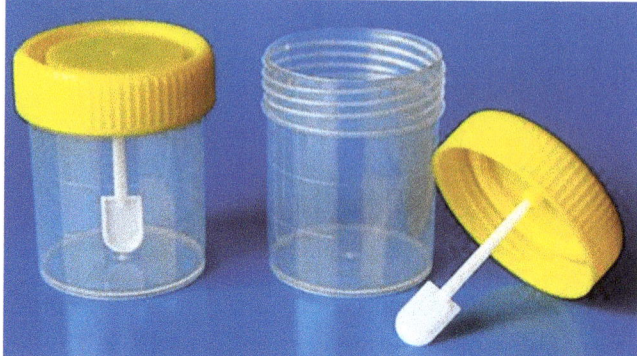

Fig. 15.1: Sample container for stool

- **When to examine:** Liquid stool specimens should be examined within 30 minutes, semisolid stools within 1 hour and formed stools up to 24 hours after collection. On prolonged storage, trophozoites may disintegrate, become nonmotile and may appear as artifacts
- **For monitoring response to therapy:** Repeat stool examination can be done 3 to 4 weeks after therapy for intestinal protozoan infection, and 5–6 weeks for *Taenia* infection
- **If delay in transport:** Fecal specimens should be kept in room temperature; never be incubated or frozen prior to microscopic examination. However for molecular and in some immunoassays, frozen specimen(s) can be used. Preservatives (e.g. 10% formalin) can be used to maintain the morphology of the parasitic cysts and eggs
- **Specimens other than stool:**
  - **Perianal swabs (cellophane tape or NIH swab):** Useful for detecting eggs of *Enterobius vermicularis* deposited on the surface of perianal skin. It is also used for eggs of *Schistosoma mansoni* and *Taenia* species
  - **Duodenal contents:** It is very useful for the detection of small intestine parasites like, *Giardia intestinalis*, *Clonorchis sinensis* and *Strongyloides stercoralis*. Duodenal fluid can be collected by intubation or by entero-test (discussed in Chapter 4).

Macroscopic Examination

- **Mucoid bloody stool:** Found in acute amoebic dysentery, intestinal schistosomiasis, and invasive balantidiasis
- **Color:** Dark red stool indicates upper gastrointestinal tract (GIT) bleeding and a bright red stool is suggestive of bleeding from lower GIT

❖ **Frothy pale offensive stool** (containing fat) is usually found in giardiasis.

Stool consistency

In liquid stool, trophozoites are usually found whereas in semi-formed stool both trophozoites and cysts are found and the cysts are mainly found in formed specimens (Fig. 15.2). Exceptions to this general statement include:
- ❖ Coccidian oocysts, microsporidian spores, helminth eggs that can be found in any type of fecal specimen. In cryptosporidiosis, the oocysts load is higher in liquid stool. In liquid stool due to the dilution factor, the chance of detection of helminth eggs is lesser as compared to formed stool
- ❖ Tapeworm proglottids may be found on or beneath the stool on the bottom of the collection container
- ❖ Adult worms of *Enterobius* and *Ascaris* are occasionally found on the surface or in the stool.

Microscopic Examination

Direct Wet Mount (Saline and Iodine Mount)

Drops of saline and Lugol's iodine are placed on left and right halves of the slide respectively (Fig. 15.3). A small amount of feces (~2 mg) is mixed by a stick to form a uniform smooth suspension.
- ❖ A ~2 mg sample of stool forms a low cone on the end of a wooden applicator stick
- ❖ More fecal material makes the wet mount too thick and lesser material results in a thin suspension; in both cases, the chance of finding stool parasites decreases
- ❖ Cover slip is placed on the mount and examined under low power objective (10X) for detection of helminths eggs and larvae; followed by high power objective (40X) for protozoan cysts and trophozoites
- ❖ **Screening area:** The entire coverslip preparation should be examined under low power objective and at least one-third to one-half under high power before indicating the examination is negative. The coverslip should be examined in a zigzag fashion starting from left top corner (Fig. 15.4).
- ❖ **Motility:** If a finding is suspected to be a trophozoite, then at least 15 seconds should be allowed to detect motility. Motility can be stimulated by—application of heat by placing a hot penny on the edge of a slide or tapping on the coverslip or increasing the intensity of the light source.

Following structures can be visualized by microscopic examination of stool specimen, which may be confused with various protozoan trophozoites, cysts and helminthic eggs and larvae (Table 15.2 and Figs 15.5A to Y).
- ❖ **Normal constituents:** Such as plant fiber, starch cells (stains blue black with iodine), muscle fibers, animal hair, pollen grains, yeast cells, bacteria, epithelial cells, fat globules, and air bubbles are present
- ❖ **Cellular elements:** Like pus cells (in inflammatory diarrhea), red blood cells (RBC) (in dysentery) may be present
- ❖ **Charcot-Leyden crystals (diamond-shaped):** They are the breakdown products of eosinophils and may be seen in the stool or sputum of patients with parasitic diseases such as amoebic dysentery, ascariasis, and allergic diseases like bronchial asthma (sputum).

Saline mount

Useful in the detection of trophozoites and cysts of protozoa and eggs and larvae of helminths.

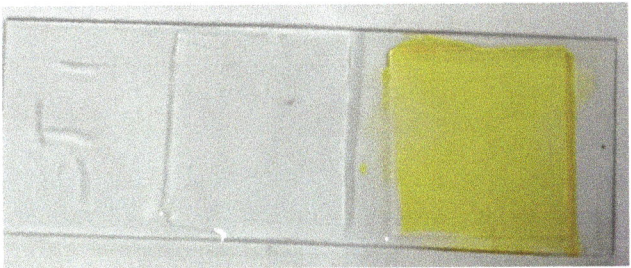

Fig. 15.3: Saline and iodine wet mount
Source: Department of Microbiology, JIPMER (with permission).

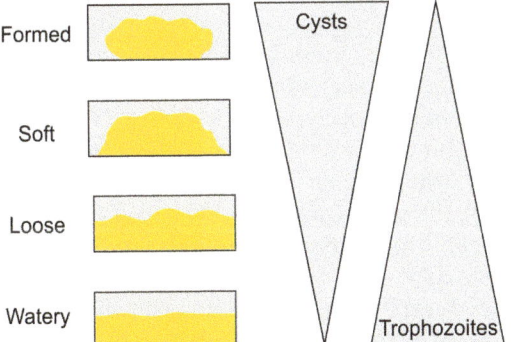

Fig. 15.2: Relative frequency of trophozoites and cysts in stool specimens with various consistencies

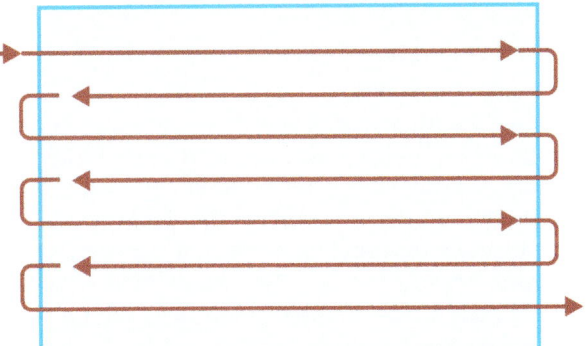

Fig. 15.4: Method of screening of slide during wet mount examination of stool

Table 15.2 Artefacts seen in wet mount or permanent stained smears of stool (Figs 15.5A to Y)

Artifacts	Morphologically resembling parasitic structures
Yeast cells	Protozoan cysts, *Cryptosporidium*, *Cyclospora*
Fungal spores	Helminth eggs, *Cystoisospora*
Bacteria	Microsporidian spores
Plant materials	
Vegetative cells	Protozoan cysts, helminth eggs
Pollen grains	Trophozoites, Helminth eggs (*Ascaris* or *Taenia*), *Blastocystis*
Root hairs	Nematode larvae
Pineapple juice or kiwi crystals	Charcot-Leyden crystals
Mite egg	Hookworm eggs
Diatoms	Do not resemble any parasites
Human cells	
PMNs	*Entamoeba* cyst
Macrophages	*Entamoeba* trophozoite
RBCs	*Cryptosporidium*, *Cyclospora*
Epithelial cells	*Entamoeba* trophozoite

- Motility of trophozoites and larvae can be demonstrated in acute infection
- Bile staining property can be appreciated—bile-stained eggs appear golden brown and nonbile-stained eggs appear colorless
- In stool specimen with preservatives, directly the wet mount can be prepared without using saline.

Iodine mount

Advantages

Nuclear details of cysts, helminthic eggs and larvae are better visualized compared to saline mount.

Disadvantages

- Iodine immobilizes and kills parasites, hence motility of the protozoan trophozoites and helminthic larvae cannot be appreciated
- Bile staining property cannot be appreciated.

Types of iodine stains

- **Lugol's iodine:** Stock solution contains potassium iodide (KI) 10 g + iodine crystals (5 g) + 100 mL of distilled water. This can be diluted (1:5) with distilled water for routine use (working solution)
- **D'Antoni's iodine:** Stock solution contains KI 1 g + iodine crystals (1.5 g) + 100 mL of distilled water. It is directly used as working solution, dilution is not required
- **Dobeil's iodine:** KI 2.0 g + iodine 1.0 g + 50 mL of distilled water.

Storage of iodine

A brown-stoppered container should be used. The solution should have strong tea color. The stock solution should be held in the dark, while the working solution is usually kept outside and have to be periodically replaced once the color fades (usually in 10–14 days).

Quality control in iodine stain

- In iodine mount, the protozoan cysts should appear to have yellow-gold cytoplasm, brown glycogen material, and paler refractile nuclei. The chromatoidal bodies are not clearly visible in iodine mount as compared to saline mount
- Human WBCs (buffy coat cells) mixed with negative stool can be used as a quality control specimen as they mimic protozoan parasites when stained.

Reporting of Wet Mount Examination

The wet mount examination report is preliminary and the result is given as 'presumptive identification'; which should be confirmed only after examination of permanent stained smear or immunoassay (*Cryptosporidium* and *Cyclospora*).

Permanent Stained Smear

Permanent stained smears are required for accurate diagnosis of protozoan cysts and trophozoites by staining their internal structures.

Commonly used methods are (described below):
- Trichrome stain
- Iron-hematoxylin stain
- Modified acid-fast stain.

Other less commonly used stains are:
- Polychrome IV stain
- Chlorazol black E stain
- Rapid safranin method for *Cryptosporidium* and *Cyclospora*
- Carbol fuchsin negative stain for *Cryptosporidium*
- Auramine O stain for coccidian parasites.

Trichrome Stain (of Wheatley)

Trichrome stain is the most widely used permanent staining method for protozoan parasites. It is not used for demonstration of helminth eggs and larvae. The Wheatley technique for fecal specimens is a modification of Gomori's original staining procedure for tissue.

- **Constituents:** It contains—(i) chromotrope 2R (0.6 g), (ii) light green SF (0.3 g), (iii) phosphotungstic acid (0.7 g), (iv) glacial acetic acid (1.0 mL) and (v) distilled water (100 mL). A properly prepared specimen appears purple color
- **Procedure:** It comprises of the following seven steps, which takes around 45 minutes
  1. **Smear preparation:** A thin smear of freshly collected fecal specimen is fixed in Schaudinn's

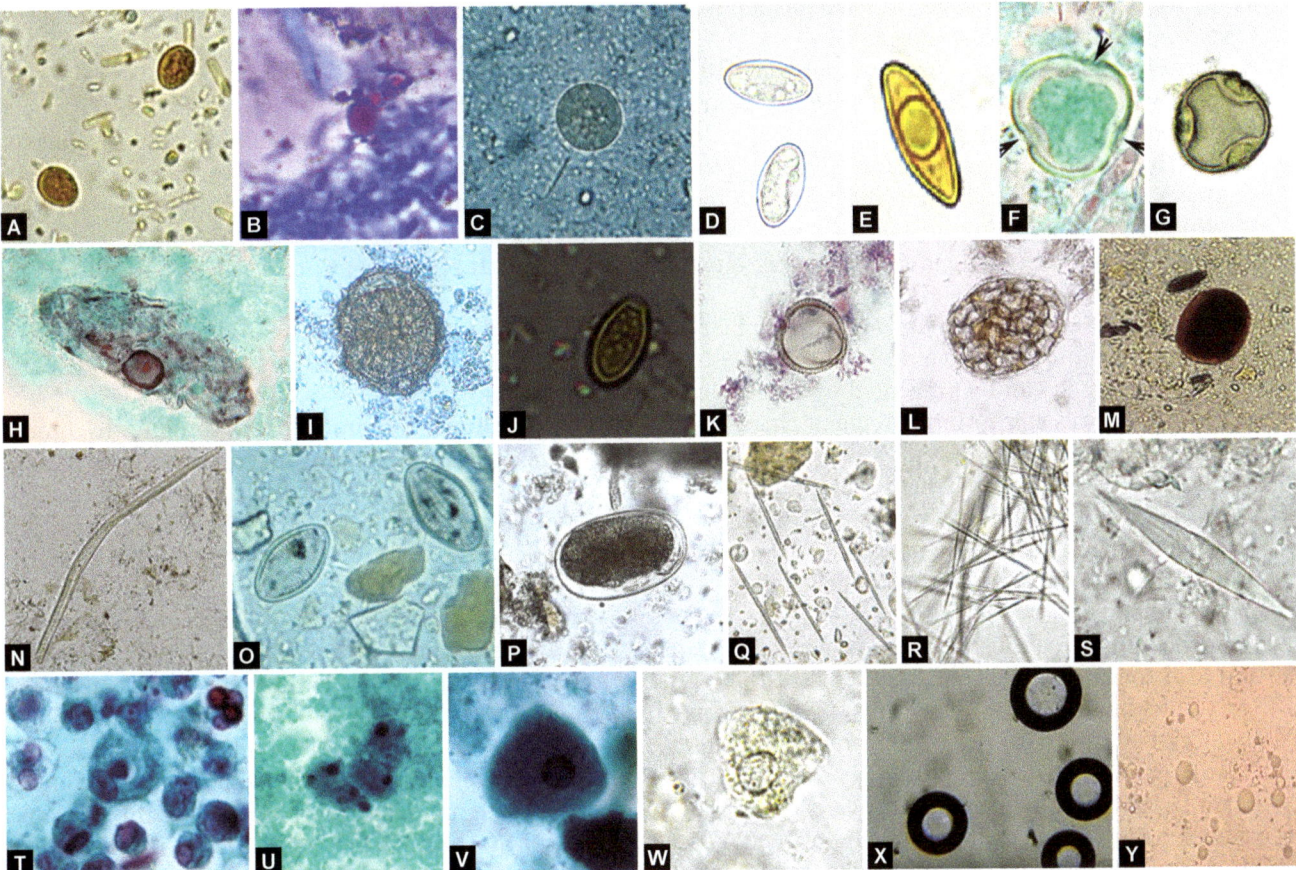

Figs 15.5A to Y: Normal constituents and artifacts found in stool in wet mount examination. **(A and B) Yeast cell** resembling: (A) Giardia cyst; (B) *Cryptosporidium* oocyst; **(C to E) Fungal spore** resembling: (C) Cyst of *Entamoeba*; (D and E) *Cystoisospora* oocyst; **(F to K) Pollen grain** resembling: (F) *Blastocystis* (Trichrome staining); (G) *Blastocystis* (saline mount); (H) Protozoan trophozoite; (I) *Ascaris* egg; (J) *Clonorchis* egg; (K) *Taenia* egg; **(L and M) Plant cell** resembling: (L) Helminth eggs; (M) Hookworm egg; **(N) Plant hair** resembling *Strongyloides* larva; **(O) Diatoms; (P) Mite egg** resembling hookworm egg; **(Q to S) Crystals:** (Q and R) Pineapple juice crystals and kiwi crystals; (S) Charcot-Leyden crystals; **(T to W) Human cells** resembling trophozoites: (T) White blood cells; (U) Macrophages; (V and W) Epithelial cell; **(X) Air bubbles; (Y) Fat globule**

Source: F to H, W—Swierczynski G, Milanesi B. "Atlas of Human Intestinal Protozoa Microscopic Diagnosis" (*with permission*); A to E, I to V—DPDx Image Library, Centers for Disease Control and Prevention (CDC), Atlanta (*with permission*); X and Y—Department of Microbiology, JIPMER, Puducherry (*with permission*).

solution immediately before drying (for 30 min or overnight). Usually two slides are prepared.

2. **Ethanol immersion:** Slide is immersed in 70% ethanol for 5 min.
3. **Mercuric chloride removal:** Slide is immersed in 70% ethanol for 5 min, then dipped in 70% ethanol containing iodine for 1 min to remove mercuric chloride from the smear. Then the slide is immersed in 70% ethanol for 5 min followed by 3 min to remove iodine residues. This step is not required if non-mercury based fixatives are used.
4. **Trichrome staining:** Then the slide is immersed in trichrome stain for 10 min
5. **Destaining step:** Then the slide is immersed in 90% ethanol plus acetic acid for 1-3 seconds, to remove the excess stain.
6. **Dehydration:** Then the slide is rinsed in 100% ethanol for several times and then immersed in 100% ethanol for 3 min two times. Stained smear is then placed in xylene for 5-10 min for two times.
7. **Mounting:** Finally, the slide is mounted by placing a coverslip on top of the smear, using a mounting medium (e.g. Permount) and then dried overnight at room temperature or 37°C for 1 hour. Coverslip use should not be avoided as the dry fecal material on the slide may scratch the surface of the lens. The slide is focussed under oil immersion. A waiting period of 10-15 min before is required which allows for the oil to sink into the film.

❖ **Interpretation:** When the procedure is performed correctly, the cytoplasm of protozoan trophozoites

appears blue-green, sometimes with a tinge of purple. Cysts tend to be slightly more purple
- Nuclei and inclusions (chromatoidal bars, RBCs, bacteria, and Charcot-Leyden crystals) are red, sometimes tinged with purple
- The background material usually stains green, providing a nice color contrast. This contrast is more distinct than that of iron hematoxylin stain, which tends to stain everything in shades of gray-blue to black
- Smears that are predominantly green may be due to the inadequate removal of iodine by the 70% ethanol; which can be prevented by lengthening the time of this step or more frequent changing of the 70% ethanol.

❖ **Quality control:** Stool specimen known to contain protozoa or spiked with buffy coat cells (PMNs) or cultured protozoa is generally used as quality control. It should be examined at least once a week or when new stain is prepared

❖ **Quantification:** Quantification is done for *Blastocystis* and also for human cells such as WBCs, RBCs and yeast cells. Quantitated as follows: few (≤2), moderate (3-9) and many (≥10) per 10 oil immersion field. Quantification is not done for other protozoa. Yeast quantification should be interpreted carefully as yeast cells keep multiplying in unpreserved specimen

❖ **Modified Trichrome stain:** There are several modifications of trichrome staining, which are available mainly for Microsoporidia
- *Weber—Green modification* method: It differs from Wheatley's trichrome method in various ways: (i) chromotrope 2R dye concentration is 10 times greater (6 g), (ii) the staining time with trichrome is much longer (90 min, compared to 10 min), (iii) fast green dye is used instead of light green SF and (iv) absolute methanol is used instead of ethanol in the second step. Microsporidian spore wall appears bright pinkish red. The majority of the bacteria and other debris (back ground) tend to stain green
- In *Ryan blue modification:* It differs from Weber-Green method in that aniline blue is used instead of fast green; which stains the back ground blue
- *Kokoskin—Hot Method:* Here, trichrome stain is used for 10 min at 50°C as compared to 90 min at room temperature as for Weber-Green method
- *Acid-fast trichrome stain:* This can be used for *Cryptosporidium* in addition to Microsporidia. This is especially helpful in patients with HIV/AIDS where both these infections are likely to coexist. Here following methanol fixation, acid fast staining is done first with carbol fuchsin for 10 min without heating followed by decolorization with 0.5% acid-alcohol with subsequent trichrome staining at 37°C for 30 min.

Iron-hematoxylin Stain

It is another method for permanent staining used for protozoan parasite. Three methods are available:
1. **Spencer-Monroe method:** This is the most common method of iron-hematoxylin staining used.
   - **Constituents:** Comprises of equal volume of solution 1 and 2. Solution 1 contains hematoxylin and ethanol (absolute); solution 2 contains ferrous and ferric ammonium sulfate with conc. HCl and distilled water
   - **Procedure:** The procedure is same for trichrome stain except that (i) iron-hematoxylin stain (for 4-5 min) is used instead of trichrome stain, (ii) there is no destaining step and (iii) in dehydration step, 70% and 95% ethanol are used followed by 100% ethanol and xylene
   - **Interpretation:** The cytoplasm of trophozoites appears blue-gray, sometimes with a tinge of black. Cysts tend to be slightly darker. Nuclei and inclusions are dark gray-blue, sometimes almost black. The background material usually stains pale gray or blue, providing lesser color intensity contrast with the protozoa as compared to trichrome stain.
2. **Tompkins and Miller method:** It is more time consuming; employs phosphotungstic acid to destain the protozoa, which gives excellent results.
3. A **modified Iron Hematoxylin staining method** is available incorporating the carbol fuchsin step for additional detection of coccidian parasites.

Modified Acid-fast Stain

Modified acid-fast stain is used for detection and identification of *Cryptosporidium parvum*, *Cyclospora* and *Cystoisospora belli*. Two methods are available—hot and cold. The constituent is described in Table 15.3 and the procedure is described below.

Kinyoun's cold method

The procedure of cold method is as follows.
❖ **Smear fixation:** Fecal smear is fixed with absolute methanol for 1 minute
❖ **Primary staining:** Then the slide is stained with Kinyoun's carbol fuchsin for 5 minutes
❖ **Decolorization:** The slide is rinsed with 50% ethanol for 3-5 seconds and then rinsed with water, followed by decolorization with 1% sulfuric acid for 2 minutes or till no more color runs from the slide
❖ **Counter staining:** Then the slide is rinsed with tap water and counterstained with alkaline methylene blue for 1 minute.

Table 15.3: Differences between hot and cold methods of acid-fast staining for parasites

Cold method	Hot method
Kinyoun's Carbol Fuchsin	**Carbol Fuchsin**
Solution A 4 g of basic fuchsin in 20 mL of 95% ethanol	Solution A 0.3 g of basic fuchsin in 10 mL of 95% ethanol
Solution B 8 g of phenol crystals in 100 mL of distilled water	Solution B 5 g of phenol crystals in 100 mL of distilled water
Loeffler alkaline methylene blue	**Methylene blue**
0.3 g of methylene blue in 30 mL of 95% ethanol added with 100 mL of dilute (0.01%) potassium hydroxide	0.3 g of methylene blue in 100 mL of distilled water.

Note: Solution A and B should be mixed to prepare the final carbol fuchsin.

Hot method

The procedure of hot method is as follows.
- **Smear fixation:** A thin smear of feces is made on a slide which is then heat fixed at 70°C for 5 min
- **Primary staining:** The slide is flooded with carbol fuchsin for 5 minutes. The slide is intermittently heated till carbol fuchsin starts steaming (do not allow to boil). If the slide dries, more stain is added without any more heating
- **Decolorization:** Then slide is washed with tap water and decolorized with 1–3 % sulfuric acid for 30 seconds, followed by washing with tap water
- **Counter staining:** It is done with methylene blue for 1 minute.

Interpretation

The acid-fast oocysts of *Cryptosporidium*, *Cyclospora* and *Cystoisospora belli* stain pink-red to deep purple and the non-acid-fast background stains blue. Formalin preserved control slide of *Cryptosporidium* should be included as quality control with each staining batch run.

Rapid Safranin Method for Cryptosporidium

Fecal smear made on a slide is air dried, heat fixed, followed by fixation with 3% HCl in methanol for 3 to 5 min. Slide is rinsed with water, then stained with 1% aqueous safranin for 1 min (heating is done until steam appears). Slide is again rinsed with tap water followed by counterstaining with 1% methylene blue for 30sec. Crystal violet can also be used as a counterstain, but malachite green is unsatisfactory.

Auramine O Stain for Coccidia

It is a low cost, rapid and simple staining method.

Constituents

- **Auramine O stain** is prepared by adding solution 1 (0.1 g auramine O in 10 mL of 95% ethanol) and Solution 2 (3g phenol crystals in 87mL of distilled water)
- **Destaining agent** (0.5% acid-alcohol): 0.5 ml of conc. HCl in 100 mL of 70% ethanol
- **Counterstain:** 0.5% Potassium permanganate (0.5 g in 100 mL of distilled water).

Procedure

- Fecal smear is prepared on a slide from the sediment of a concentrated stool specimen, and then it is is heat fixed or methanol fixed for 1 min
- Slide is cooled to room temperature and then flooded with the Auramine O stain for 15 min. Slide is rinsed with water and then flooded with the destaining solution for 2 min. and then counterstained with potassium permanganate solution for 2 min. The timing of this counterstain step is critical
- Slide is rinsed with water, air dried and examined under fluorescence microscope
- Advantage of this method is that the stained smear can be restained by modified acid-fast method to examine with light microscopy.

Interpretation

Cryptosporidium and *Cyclospora* oocysts fluoresce bright and have a regular round "starry sky" appearance. The fluorescence of oocysts is heterogeneously, in contrast to the fluorescent artifacts which stain homogeneously. *Cystoisospora* oocysts can also fluoresce brightly.

Concentration Techniques

If the parasite output is low in feces (egg, cysts, trophozoites and larvae) and direct examination may not be able to detect the parasites, then the stool specimens need to be concentrated. These methods are also useful in epidemiological analysis and for assessing the response to treatment. Eggs, cysts and larvae are recovered after concentration procedures; however, the trophozoites get destroyed.

Commonly used concentration techniques are:
- **Sedimentation techniques:** Eggs and cysts settle down at the bottom following centrifugation:
  - Formalin-ether concentration technique
  - Formalin-ethyl acetate concentration technique
  - Formalin-acetone sedimentation technique.
- **Floatation techniques:** The eggs and cysts float at the surface due to specific gravity gradient:
  - Saturated salt (sodium chloride) solution technique
  - Zinc sulfate floatation concentration technique

- Sheather's sugar floatation technique (useful for *Cryptosporidium*, *Cystoisospora* and *Cyclospora*).

Two commonly used concentration techniques are formalin-ether and saturated salt solution technique.

Sedimentation Techniques

Principle: It involves concentration of stool specimen by centrifugation. The protozoan cysts and helminthic eggs are concentrated at the bottom of the tube because they have greater density than the suspending medium.

Formol-ether sedimentation technique

Procedure (nine steps)

Step 1: About half teaspoonful (~ 4 g) of feces is transferred to a tube containing 10 mL of 5–10% formalin, mixed thoroughly and allowed to stand for 30 minutes.

Step 2: Then the mixture is filtered into a 15 mL conical centrifuge tube covered with two layers of gauze. About 8 mL of the filtrate is collected (3–4 mL for formalin preserved stool).

Step 3: 0.85% saline (or 5–10% formalin) is added almost to the top of the tube containing the filtrate and centrifuged for 10 minutes at 500 × g.

Step 4: The supernatant is discarded and 0.5–1 mL of the sediment is resuspended in saline or formalin (filled up to the top of the tube) and centrifuged again for 10 minutes at 500 × g.

Step 5: This step 4 may be repeated if the supernatant fluid is not clear after the first wash. Then the sediment is resuspended in 5–10% formalin filled half of the tube.

Step 6: 4–5 mL of ether (or ethyl acetate) is added and the tube is closed with a stopper and shaken vigorously for at least 30 sec to mix well. The tube should be held away from the face while shaking. The stopper is removed after a waiting period of 15–30 sec and the tube is centrifuged at 500 × g for 10 minutes.

Step 7: Four layers are formed. Top layer consists of ether, second is a plug of debris, third is a clear layer of formalin and the fourth is the sediment (Figs 15.6A to C).

Step 8: The debris is removed from the side of the tube with the help of a glass rod and supernatant is discarded.

Step 9: With a pipette, the sediment is removed and the saline or iodine mount is made and examined under the microscope.

> **Note**
> - Substitute for ether: Since ether is explosive; it can be replaced by ethyl acetate or acetone or clearing agent Hemo-De, which are much safer with equal efficacy
> - If the stool is formalin preserved, then the Step 1 is omitted
> - If stool contains lot of mucus, then following Step 1, the mixture is centrifuged for 10 minutes at 500 × g and the sediment is directly mounted
>
> *Contd...*

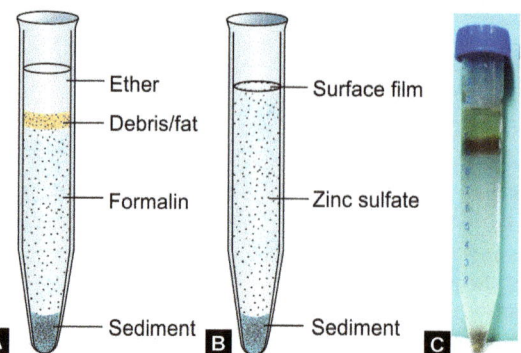

Figs 15.6A to C: (A) Formol-ether sedimentation technique (schematic diagram); (B) Zinc sulfate flotation concentration technique (schematic diagram); (C) Formol ether sedimentation technique (real image)

Source: C—Dr Anand Janagond, Associate professor, of Microbiology, S Nijalingappa Medical college, Bagalkot, Karnataka (*with permission*).

Contd...

> - If the stool is polyvinyl alcohol (PVA) preserved, then following Step 1, the saline or formalin mixed stool is filtered immediately. Then the procedure is same from Step 3
> - One should start monitoring the centrifugation time only after reaching the recommended speed by the centrifuge
> - The woven gauze should never be more than two layers.

Advantages

- The sensitivity of detecting the ova or cysts increases by 8–10 folds
- The size and shape of the parasitic structures are maintained
- Inexpensive, easy to perform
- Fecal odor is removed
- As formalin kills the fecal parasites, no risk of acquiring laboratory acquired infection.

Disadvantages and procedure limitations

- Trophozoite forms are killed and hence not detected in this method
- *Cryptosporidium* oocysts may be missed unless the centrifugation speed is 500 × g for a minimum of 10 min
- PVA preserved stool specimens are not suitable for sedimentation method especially for *Giardia*, *Trichuris*, *Strongyloides* and hookworm eggs and *C. belli* oocysts; which are better seen when performed with formalin-preserved stool.

Flotation Techniques

Principle: Flotation involves suspending the specimen in a medium of greater density than that of the helminthic eggs and protozoan cysts. The eggs and cysts float to the top and are collected by placing a glass slide on the surface of the meniscus at the top of the tube.

Saturated salt flotation technique

Procedure

About half tea spoon (~ 4g) of fresh stool is placed in a flat bottomed container of less than 1.5 inches diameter and 20 mL capacity (Fig. 15.7)

- Then, few drops of saturated salt solution (specific gravity 1.200) is added and stirred to make a fine emulsion
- More salt solution is added with stirring throughout to fill the container up to the brim, until a convex meniscus is formed
- A glass slide (3" × 2") is carefully laid on the top of the container so that the center is in contact with the fluid
- Preparation is allowed to stand for 20 minutes after which the glass slide is quickly lifted, and examined under the microscope after putting a coverslip.

Disadvantages

- Flotation technique is not useful for heavier eggs that do not float in the salt solution such as:
  - Unfertilized eggs of *Ascaris lumbricoides*
  - Larva of *Strongyloides*
  - *Taenia* eggs
  - Operculated eggs of trematodes.
- If left for more than 20 minutes, protozoan cysts and thin-walled nematode eggs get collapsed and become distorted due to high specific gravity of the solution.

Zinc sulfate flotation technique

Step 1–5: First five steps are same as that of formol-ether sedimentation technique.

Step 6: After the second wash, the clear supernatant is poured off and the sediment in the tube is suspended with 1–2 mL of 33% zinc sulfate (specific gravity 1.18). More zinc sulfate solution is added to fill the tube up to the top and the tube is centrifuged again at 500 × g for 2 minutes

Step 7: Two layers are formed (*see* Fig. 15.6B). Sample is taken from the surface film by a wire loop (make sure not to dip below the surface film), mounted on a glass slide. Then the supernatant is discarded and the sediment is also mounted and examined.

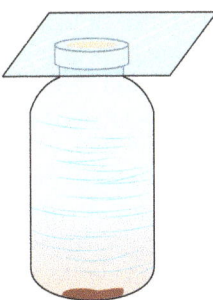

Fig. 15.7: Flotation technique (schematic diagram)

Note:

- The protozoan cysts and lighter helminth eggs are concentrated in the surface film whereas operculated and heavy eggs, larvae are deposited in the bottom
- Zinc sulfate of specific gravity 1.20 should be used for formalin preserved stool
- Sample should be taken from surface film within 5 min of centrifugation; otherwise cysts and eggs may get collapse due to prolonged contact with zinc sulfate.

Sheather's sugar centrifugal flotation technique

It is the recommended stool concentration method for coccidian parasites. Sheather's sugar solution contains table sugar (500 g), and phenol crystal (6.5 g) added with distilled water (320 mL). Specific gravity is adjusted to 1.27 using hydrometer. The procedure is as follows:

- One gram of feces is softened by adding water and then the aqueous suspension is strained through a wire sieve
- One part of aqueous suspension is mixed with 2 parts of Sheather's sugar solution
- The solution is poured into a tube and centrifugated at 500 × g for 10 minutes
- The supernatant is discarded and the Sheather's sugar solution is further added to bring the meniscus to the top
- A coverslip is put on the top touching the meniscus, waited for 10 minutes and then examined under microscope.

Alternatively, Sheather's technique can be performed by adding 1 gm of stool into 6mL of 10% formalin and kept for 30 min at room temperature → then subjected to gauze filtration → Sheather's solution is added to the filtrate up to the brim of the tube → centrifuged at 500 × g for 10 minutes → A coverslip is put on the top touching the meniscus, waited for 10 minutes and then examined under microscope.

Automated systems

- **Commercial fecal concentration devices:** A number devices are commercially available nowadays, which automates the fecal concentration method. Examples include MACRO-CON, SPINCON, SED-CONNECT, PARA-SED concentration systems
- **Automated workstation** for microscopic analysis of fecal concentrates: The FE-5 (Apacor Ltd, USA) is a commercially available workstation that automates various steps of microscopic analysis of fecal concentrates such as aspiration, resuspension, staining, transfer, presentation and disposal.

Preservation of Fecal Specimen

Preservation of fecal specimens is essential for following reasons:

- To maintain morphology of the parasitic cysts, eggs and larvae
- To prevent further development of some helminthic eggs and larvae
- For teaching purpose
- For epidemiological analysis
- Transport of specimen to a referral laboratory for further identification.

However, no motility will be visible (as organisms are killed by the fixatives).

Several preservation methods are available (Table 15.4):

- **Formalin fixative method:** About 5% formalin is recommended for protozoan cysts and 10% formalin for helminthic eggs and larvae
  - **Neutral formalin:** Formalin added with sodium phosphate buffer is known as neutral formalin; which helps in maintaining the organism morphology better than plain formalin
  - **Hot formalin:** As some thick-shelled eggs (e.g. *Ascaris*) continue to develop in room-temperature formalin, hot (60°C) formalin can be used as an alternative.
- **Sodium acetate formalin (SAF) fixative method:** Formalin buffered with sodium acetate and glacial acetic acid is used to maintain the morphology of the parasites
- **Merthiolate-iodine formalin (MIF) solution fixative method:** It contains formalin, Lugol's iodine, thimerosal and glycerin; acts both as fixative and stain
- **Schaudinn's fluid:** It is a mixture of mercuric chloride and ethyl alcohol with glacial acetic acid. It fixes and preserves the specimen for 1 year or more
- **Schaudinn's fluid with PVA:** PVA powder is incorporated to Schaudinn's fluid. PVA is a plastic resin serves as adhesive for stool specimen where as Schaudinn's fluid helps in fixation. Liquid stool is added to PVA at 1:3 ratio
- **Modified Schaudinnss's fluid with PVA:** It uses copper sulfate or zinc base instead of mercury chloride
- **Universal fixative (TOTAL-FIX):** It is a mercury-, formalin-, and PVA-free fixative that preserves parasite morphology and does not have disposal and monitoring problems.

Egg Counting Methods

The intensity of intestinal helminthic infection can be estimated using egg counting in the feces, used mainly for *Trichuris*, *Ascaris* and hookworm. It is also useful for treatment monitoring.

- However, egg counts do not always correlate with or accurately predict the parasite burden of the host
- The disease is considered as severe with clinically significant infection if the egg count is >10,000, 50,000 and 4000 per g of stool in case of *Trichuris*, *Ascaris* and hookworm infections respectively.

The following methods are available.

Direct Smear Counting Method of Beaver

Smear is made by using 2 mg of feces mixed in a drop of saline on a slide and examined under microscope (low power).

- Number of eggs in 2 mg feces is counted and then multiplied by factor 500 to calculate the number of eggs per gram of feces
- It is simple and accurate when performed by an experienced technologist.

Kato-Katz Thick Film

It is the recommended method by WHO for soil-transmitted helminthic eggs, and *Schistosoma mansoni* eggs in human stool. The procedure is as follows (Fig. 15.8A):

- **Filtering out of stool specimen:** Stool specimen is added with few drops of water to make it mushy. Then a filter-mesh is applied over the stool specimen and the filtered out part of the stool is scrapped off by an applicator stick
- **Metal template delivering 50 mg stool:** A slide with a metal template containing a hole calibrated to deliver 50 mg stool is taken. The scrapped-off stool on the applicator stick is placed over the hole to fil it up. Then the metal template is removed from the slide
- **Cellophane tape:** A cellophane tape of 22 × 30 mm size which was pre-soaked in glycerine malachite green solution (for at least 24 hours) is placed over the stool on the slide. Glycerine malachite green solution contains 10 mL of glycerine added with 1 mL of 3% malachite green in 100 mL of distilled water
- **Making the thick smear:** The slide containing stool specimen is turned upside down on a paper towel and then is pressed until the fecal film spreads to form a thick smear of 20 to 25 mm diameter
- **Clearing period:** The preparation is allowed to stand for 1 hour for clearing of the fecal material. The clearing period should not exceed 1 hour as hookworm eggs will collapse. For *S. mansoni* eggs, the clearing time can be extended up to 24 hours
- **Examination:** Then the slide is examined under low power. The number of eggs of seen in the entire smear (50 mg of stool) is counted and then multiplied by 20 to obtain the egg count per g of stool.

Stoll's Method or Dilution Egg Counting Method

It is the most widely used method for egg counting (Fig. 15.8B).

- About 4 g of feces is mixed thoroughly with 56 mL of N/10 NaOH in a calibrated Stoll's flask and a uniform suspension is made using glass beads

CHAPTER 15 ◆ Laboratory Diagnosis of Parasitic Diseases

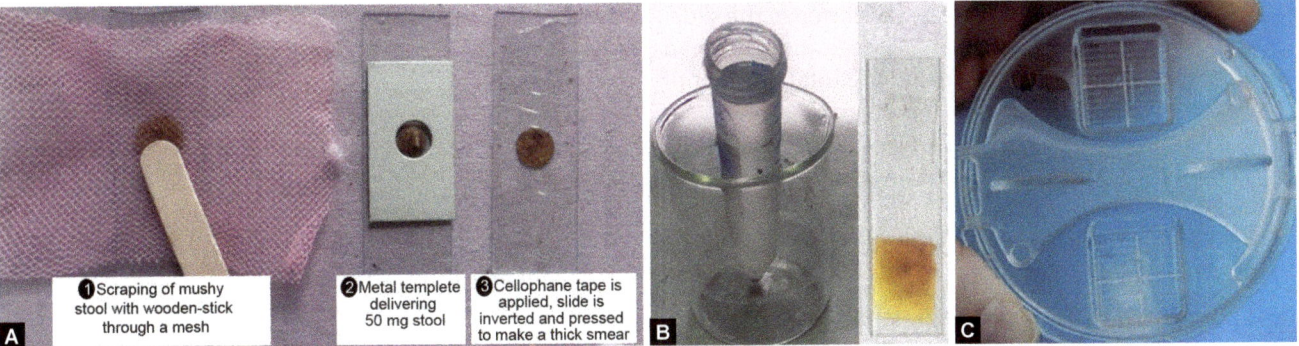

Figs 15.8A to C: Egg counting methods: (A) Kato-Katz method; (B) Stoll's dilution method; (C) FLOTAC technique
Source: A and B—Department of Microbiology, JIPMER, Puducherry (*with permission*); C—Veterinary parasitology Pvt. Ltd.

Table 15.4: Comparison of stool preservation methods		
Preservatives	*Advantages*	*Disadvantages*
Formalin	• Easy to prepare, long shelf life • Overall good for stool concentration • Can be used for fecal immunoassay kits*	• Not good for permanent smear • Carcinogenic and corrosive, have offensive odor
MIF (Merthiolate-iodine –Formalin)	• Both fixes and stains the stool sample, no need of a separate iodine mounting • Easy to prepare, long shelf life • Useful for the field study • Good for stool concentration	• Not so good as Schaudinn's fluid for permanent smear • Contains mercury compounds (disposal problem) • Not good for fecal immunoassay kits
SAF (Sodium acetate formalin)	Useful for: • Stool concentration • Permanent smear by iron hematoxylin • Fecal immunoassay kits* • Easy to prepare, long shelf life • It does not contain mercury	• Adheres poorly to the slide (albumin coated slide is recommended) • Not good for trichrome permanent smear
Schaudinn's fluid	• Fixative for the fresh stool • Excellent for preservation of stool • For many years, considered as the "gold standard"	• Contains mercury compounds • Not good for concentration • Not good for faecal immunoassay kits • Poor adhesive quality with liquid and mucoid specimen
Schaudinn's fluid with PVA (Polyvinyl alcohol)	• Best for trichrome stain • Long shelf life (in tight container at room temperature) • Excellent for stool preservation, specimens can be shipped to distant places	• Difficult to prepare • Not good to preserve *Giardia* cyst, *Trichuris* egg, *Cystoisospora* oocysts and *Strongyloides* larvae • Not good for fecal immunoassay kits • Contains mercury compounds • May turn white and gelatinous when it begins to dehydrate or when refrigerated
Modified Schaudinn's fluid- with PVA added with copper or zinc	• Permanent staining and concentration techniques can be performed • It does not contain mercury	• Morphology preserved poorly particularly in copper based fixative
Universal fixative (TOTAL-FIX)	• Permanent staining including modified trichrome stain can be performed • Concentration techniques can be performed • It does not contain mercury, PVA or formalin • Immunoassay can be performed • Molecular staining can be performed • Protozoan morphology preserved well	• Organism morphology lesser maintained than mercuric chloride

Note: Trophozoites are distorted in all types of stool preservatives.
*Fecal immunoassay kits for *E. histolytica* cannot be performed on any typed of preservative added stool specimen.

- About 0.15 mL of this mixture is transferred to the slide. The slide is kept over a mechanical stage and examined under a low power objective and the total number of eggs is counted (n)
- The number of eggs per gram of feces (N) is calculated by multiplying the count (n) with 100
- Estimated daily output of eggs is calculated by multiplying the number of eggs/gram with the weight of 24 hour fecal sample.

Note: The above mentioned calculation is applied for formed feces. However, the estimate (eggs per gram) will vary according to the consistency of the stool. If feces is not formed, then 'N' is multiplied by the correction factor as given below:
- Mushy formed: N × 1.5
- Mushy stool (pulpy or soft): N × 2
- Mushy diarrheic: N × 3.

Modified Stoll's Dilution Egg Counting Method

One mL of stool specimen is added to 14 mL of 0.1 N sodium hydroxide in a 15-mL centrifuge tube and mixed thoroughly with a applicator stick. If the stool is hard, the mixture is allowed to stand for several hours.
- About 0.15 mL is pipetted from the middle of the suspension and a wet mount is prepared and eggs are counted
- Multiply the egg count per preparation by 100 to give an uncorrected count of eggs per mL of stool. Corrections should be made for original stool consistency as in the Stoll dilution method.

McMaster Technique

This technique uses a counting chamber where a known volume of fecal suspension (2 × 0.15 mL) is added and examined microscopically. The fecal suspension is made by mixing known weight of feces and a known volume of flotation fluid so that fecal debris will sink while eggs will float to the surface. Then the number of eggs per gram of feces is calculated by multiplying the number of eggs under the marked areas of counting chamber by a simple conversion factor.

FLOTAC Technique

This is another method of egg counting similar to McMaster method where feces (2g) is homogenized with flotation fluid (38 mL, 1:20 dilution) and is filtered. Then the filtrate is filled onto the flotation chambers of FLOTAC apparatus and examined microscopically to count the number of eggs (Fig. 15.8C).

Search for tapeworm scolex

This is very useful for proper identification of species.
- 24 hours stool sample is mixed with water, make watery suspension
- The watery suspension is filtered through a double layered sieve
- The cleansed debris is examined with hand lens to look for scolices and proglottids
- If no scolices are found, then the filtration step is repeated and cleansed debris is examined with a magnifying hand lens against the background to increase the contrast
- Tapeworm segments are picked with an applicator stick, rinsed with saline and placed between two slides and observed under low power objective.

EXAMINATION OF BLOOD

Blood examination is useful in diagnosis of infection caused by blood parasites like *Plasmodium, Trypanosoma, Leishmania, Babesia, Wuchereria bancrofti, Brugia malayi, Loa loa* and *Mansonella*.

Various methods of examination of blood include:
- Direct wet mount examination
- Examination of blood smears after permanent staining
- Examination of buffy coat region (quantitative buffy coat)
- Concentration of blood.

Direct Wet Mount Examination

A drop of blood is collected by finger prick and placed on a glass slide. A coverslip is placed over the blood drop and examined under low power objective.
- It is useful for detection of microfilariae and trypanosomes by their motility
- Counting of microfilariae may be done by examining the blood on a Neubauer counting chamber.

Permanent Staining

Thick and thin blood smears are made from peripheral blood, stained with Romanowsky stains and examined under oil immersion field.
- Romanowsky's stains include Giemsa stain, Leishman's stain, Wright's stain. Field's stain and Jaswant Singh and Bhattacharya (JSB) stain
- These stains contain a combination of methylene blue (basic) which stains the nucleus and eosin (acidic) which stains the cytoplasm
- They also contain oxidation products of methylene blue called azures; which provide further contrast in the stained peripheral smears
- The differentness between various Romanowsky stains have been described in Table 15.5.

CHAPTER 15 ◆ Laboratory Diagnosis of Parasitic Diseases

Table 15.5: Differentness between various Romanowsky stains

Characteristics	Giemsa stain	Wright's stain	Leishman's stain	Field's stain	JSB stain
Color contrast of different structures					
RBCs	Pale red	Light tan, reddish, or buff	Pink	Gray to pale mauve pink	Pale grayish pink
WBCs					
Nucleus	Purple	Bright blue	Purple	Deep purple	Deep purple
Cytoplasm	Pale purple	Light blue	Light blue	Deep purple	Deep purple
Eosinophilic granules	Bright purple-red	Bright red	Pink	Red	Pink
Neutrophilic granules	Deep pink-purple	Pink or light purple	Purple	Deep purple	Deep purple
Malaria parasite					
Nucleus	Red to purple-red	Red	Red	Red	Red
Cytoplasm	Pale blue	Pale blue	Pale blue	Pale blue	Pale blue
Schüffner's dots	Red	Do not stain or stain very pale	-	-	-
Nuclei of microfilariae	Blue to purple	Pale to dark blue	Blue to purple	Deep purple	Deep purple
Advantages					
	Gold standard Provides good color contrast Works well over a range of temperatures	Provides good color contrast Works well over a range of temperatures	Provides good color contrast	Rapid, economical	Rapid, economical Extensively used in field conditions under NVBDCP
Disadvantages					
	Time consuming Expensive Less useful in field conditions	Time consuming Expensive Less useful in field conditions Stained thick smear is inferior to Giemsa stain.	Cannot be used in hot climatic field conditions	Water-based stain, so gives variable results Precipitation artifacts due to methanol evaporation are commonly seen	Requires expertise to achieve very good color contrast Less helpful in diagnosing other blood parasites

Romanowsky Stains

Giemsa stain

Composition

- Stock Giemsa stain contains Giemsa stain powder (0.6 g), absolute methanol (50 mL) and glycerine (50 mL)
- The working solution is prepared by diluting in phosphate buffer (pH 7.0 to 7.2). The dilution factor ranges from 1:10 for thin smear to 1:50 for thick smear. Some recommend phosphate buffer of pH 6.8 for better visualization of Schüffner's dots
- The stock solution is stable for many years if protected from moisture
- The aqueous working solution should be prepared daily as on exposure to oxygen in water, the oxidative staining reaction is initiated which destroys the stain.

Staining procedure

For thin blood smears

- The smear is fixed in absolute methanol for 1 minute and then the slide is allowed to air dry
- Smear is stained with Giemsa working solution (1:10) for 10 minutes. Note that the staining time is proportional to the dilution factor (i.e. 20 min staining for 1:20 dilution, 30 min staining for 1:30 dilution and so on)
- Then the slide is washed in phosphate buffer or tap water and air dried in vertical position.

For thick blood smears

- Slide is not fixed with methanol
- Slide is stained with working solution of 1:50 dilution for 50 min.

Note: Smears stained with Giemsa or other Romanowsky stains, that are mounted usually fade with time and eventually become pink. This can be prevented by adding an antioxidant(2,6-di-tert-butyl-p-cresol) to the mounting medium such as Permount medium.

Wright's stain

Composition

The stock solution contains Wright's stain powder (0.9 g) and absolute methanol (500 mL). It is diluted with phosphate buffer of pH 6.6 to 6.8 to prepare the working solution similar to as that for Giemsa stain.

Staining procedure (For Thin and Thick Smear)

- The slide is covered with the stain for 1–3 minutes
- Equal amount of phosphate buffered water is added to the slide and kept for 4–8 minutes
- The stain is flooded from the slide with phosphate buffer. Stain should not be poured off before washing; otherwise a precipitate will be deposited on the slide
- The bottom of the slide is wiped to remove excess stain and then the slide is air dried.

Leishman's stain

Composition

It contains Leishman's stain powder 150 mg and absolute methanol (100 mL). Leishman's stain powder is a mixture of "polychromed" methylene blue (i.e. demethylated into various azures) and eosin.
- The stain should be kept in a glass-stoppered brown bottle
- The bottle is kept under sunlight or in an incubator (37°C) for 1 hour for 3 days for maturation of the stain.

Staining procedure

For thin blood smear
- The smear is poured with about 10 drops of stain for 2 minutes
- Double the volume (20 drops) of distilled water is added and mixed by gently rocking the slide
- After 15 minutes, the slide is washed with buffered distilled water and air dried.

For thick blood smear
Thick blood smear should be dehemoglobinized before staining, by immersing the slide in water until red color disappears. Methanol fixation is not done. Other steps are same as that for staining a thin smear.

Field's stain

This is a quick method of staining of malarial parasites in thick films (without fixation).

Composition

- Field's solution A: contains methylene blue, azure, potassium phosphate, disodium hydrogen phosphate and distilled water
- Field's solution B: contains eosin, potassium dihydrogen phosphate, disodium hydrogen phosphate and distilled water

Staining method for thin smear

- The thin blood film is fixed with methanol for 1 min
- Slide is immersed in koplin jar with Field's stain A for 2–3 seconds and then washed in distilled water
- Slide is again stained with Field's stain B for 2–3 seconds and then washed in distilled water
- Slide is air dried in vertical position.

For thick smear, the procedure is same except that there is no methanol fixation.

Jaswant-Singh-Bhattacharya (JSB) Stain

Jaswant-Singh-Bhattacharya stain is a rapid Romanowsky's staining method for malarial parasites. This is the standard method used by the laboratories under the National vector borne disease control program in India (NVBDCP).

Composition

- Solution I contains methylene blue (0.5 g), potassium dichromate (0.5 g), sulfuric acid 1% (3 mL), potassium hydroxide 1% (10 mL) and distilled water (500 mL)
- Solution II contains eosin (1 g) and distilled water (500 mL).

Staining procedure

For thin blood smears
- Slide is immersed in methanol for 1 minute to fix the smear and then is air dried
- Slide is immersed in solution I for 30 sec and then washed with water
- Slide is immersed in solution II for 1 sec then washed with water
- Slide is immersed again in solution I for 30 seconds
- Then the slide is washed as above till the smear gives a pink background, then air dried.

For thick blood smears
Smear is not fixed with methanol. Other steps are same as that for staining a thin smear.

Quantitative Buffy Coat (QBC)

This involves collection of blood in a capillary tube coated internally with acridine orange stain, centrifugation at 12,000 rpm for 5 minutes and examination of the buffy coat region under ultraviolet (UV) rays.
- This extremely useful for the detection of the malaria parasites and microfilariae
- Detail is given in Chapter 6.

Concentration of Blood

Concentration techniques are useful for detection of microfilariae from blood specimen.

Various concentration methods are:
- Sedimentation technique
- Cytocentrifugation (cytospin)
- Knott's concentration
- Gradient centrifugation
- Membrane filtration
- Triple-centrifugation method for trypanosomes
- Delafield's Hematoxylin for microfilarial sheath.

Sedimentation Technique

About 5–10 mL of blood is collected and centrifuged at $500 \times g$ for 2 minutes. Supernatant is discarded and the sediment is used to prepare a wet mount and a smear. The smear is air dried, fixed and stained.

Cytocentrifugation Technique

It uses an apparatus (cytospin) to centrifuge blood (100 µL) and to produce a sediment smear of 6 mm circle on a microscope slide.
- A hemolyzing and isotonic saponin solution is used to lyse RBCs and platelets, which contains formalin as a fixative
- It is cost effective, detects many blood stage parasites in the same sediment. However, young trophozoites of *P. falciparum* do not concentrate well due to their small size.

Knott Concentration

About 10 mL of 2% formalin is mixed thoroughly with 1 mL of venous blood in a centrifuge tube and centrifuged at $500 \times g$ for 2 minutes. Sediment is collected to prepare a wet mount and a smear. The smear is stained and examined for microfilariae. Here the disadvantage is that as the microfilariae are killed by formalin, their motility cannot be demonstrated in wet mount.

Gradient Centrifugation

Heparinized venous blood (4 mL) is mixed with 4 mL of Ficoll-Hypaque solution and centrifuged at $400 \times g$ for 40 minutes. Three distinct layers are formed; lower most white blood cell (WBC) layer, middle Ficoll-Hypaque layer and upper most plasma layer. The middle layer is examined for presence of microfilariae.

Membrane Filtration

- Blood (1 mL) is lysed by shaking gently with 10 mL of distilled water in a syringe. Then the lysed blood is passed through 25 mm membrane filter of pore size 5 µm such as millipore or nucleopore membrane filters. The microfilariae are liberated from the blood on the filter. The filter is removed, stained and examined
- For detection of *Mansonella perstans* microfilariae, 3 µm size membrane filter is used.

Triple-Centrifugation Method for Trypanosomes

It is useful to detect trypomastigotes of trypanosomes in the peripheral blood, especially helpful when the parasitemia is light.
- Anticoagulated blood is centrifuged three times, each for 10 min at $500 \times g$
- The supernatant fluid is decanted and the sediment is examined as a wet preparation and thin smear preparation.

Delafield's Hematoxylin for Microfilarial Sheath

It is a special stain for demonstrating sheath and greater nuclear detail of microfilaria.

Blood Artifacts

- **Platelets:** Elongated and degenerating platelets in blood may be confused for trypomastigotes of *Trypanosoma*; platelet plug can be confused with different stages of malaria parasite
- **Nucleated RBCs** (e.g. immature RBCs) may be confused for schizonts of *Plasmodium*
- **Air-borne fungal spore contaminants** in blood may be mistaken with microfilariae
- **Howell-Jolly bodies** in a thin blood smear may be confused with ring stage of *Plasmodium*.

EXAMINATION OF OTHER SPECIMENS

Examination of Skin Snips

Examination of skin snips is the method of choice for detection of microfilariae of *O. volvulus* and *M. streptocerca*.
- **Sample collection:**
  - **Site:** Buttock region (above the iliac crest) is the preferred site in African onchocerciasis and shoulders (over the scapula) is preferred site for Central American onchocerciasis
  - **Thickness:** The thickness should be so much that it includes the outer part of the dermal papillae and while collecting, there occurs just a slight oozing of fluid without any bleeding
  - **How to collect:** Skin snips may be collected by— (i) skin fold is held between thumb and forefinger and snips are taken by razor blade, or (ii) a skin slice taken from a small "cone" of skin pulled up by a needle or corneal-scleral punch instrument. The procedure is easy to perform and is painless.

Corneal-scleral punch instrument produces skin snips of uniform size and depth and an average weight of 0.8 mg.
- **Wet mount:** Skin snips are placed immediately in a drop of normal saline or distilled water and may be teased with dissecting needles, which facilitates the release of microfilariae. Microfilariae tend to emerge within 30 min to 1 hour and can be viewed under a microscope
- **Staining:** This is required to observe morphologic details of the microfilariae. The snip preparation is dried, fixed in absolute methanol, and stained with Giemsa.

Examination of Cerebrospinal Fluid (CSF)

Direct wet mount examination of CSF is useful for the detection of motile free living amoebae, (*Naegleria* and *Acanthamoeba*), trypanosomes and larvae of *Angiostrongylus cantonensis*. CSF should not be diluted before examination.

Examination of Aspirates

- **Spleen, lymph node and liver aspirates** are subjected to Giemsa stain for demonstration of LD bodies (*Leishmania* amastigotes)
- **Aspirates from bone marrow** are collected and subjected to Giemsa staining to detect *Leishmania* amastigotes, *Trypanosoma cruzi* trypomastigotes, or *Plasmodium*
- **Duodenal aspirate** is evaluated for *S. stercoralis*, *Giardia*, *Cryptosporidium*, *Cyclospora* or microsporidia. They are collected by **Entero-test** (described in Chapter 4) and then subjected to concentration by centrifugation followed by wet mount examination and permanent staining
- **Aspirate from suspected amoebic liver abscess** is subjected to concentration by centrifugation, digestion followed by wet mount examination for trophozoites, culture and permanent staining (trichrome)
- **Cyst aspirates from suspected hydatid sand** (daughter cysts, small protoscolices, hooklets) can be examined as direct wet mount after centrifugation. Ryan blue modified trichrome stain can be used to visualize the hooklets
- **Bronchoalveolar lavage specimens** are concentrated by centrifugation followed by wet mount and permanent staining to detect *Toxoplasma gondii*, and *Cryptosporidium*.

Examination of Biopsy

In addition to standard histologic preparations of biopsy tissues, other preparations such as impression smears, teased and squashed preparations are also recommended. They are recommended for detection of the following tissue parasites.
- Lung biopsy—Microsporidia, *E. histolytica*, *Toxoplasma gondii* and *Cryptosporidium*
- Liver biopsy—*Toxoplasma*, *Leishmania*
- Brain biopsy—free-living amoebae, *Toxoplasma*, *E. histolytica* and microsporidia (*Encephalitozoon*)
- Skin biopsies—*Leishmania*, *Onchocerca volvulus*, *Mansonella streptocerca*, *Acanthamoeba* and *E. histolytica*
- Nasopharynx, sinuses—Microsporidia
- Intestine—Small intestine (*Cryptosporidium*, *Cyclospora*), Jejunum (microsporidia), duodenum (*Giardia*) and colon (*E. histolytica*)
- Cornea, conjunctiva—microsporidia, *Acanthamoeba*
- Muscle—*Trichinella* (squash preparation), microsporidia
- Balder biopsy—*Schistosoma haematobium*
- Rectal biopsy—*Schistosoma mansoni*.

Examination of Sputum

Examination of sputum is useful in demonstration of eggs of *Paragonimus* in cases of pulmonary paragonimiasis and trophozoites of *E. histolytica* in cases of pulmonary amoebiasis.

Examination of Urogenital Specimen

- **Examination of urogenital specimens** such as vaginal discharge, urethral discharge, prostatic secretions and urine sediment are useful in detection of *Trichomonas vaginalis* trophozoites by saline wet mount. The trophozoites can be identified by their typical jerky motility
- **Examination of urine** is useful for detection of microfilariae of *Onchocerca volvulus* by triple concentration technique and *Schistosoma haematobium* eggs by membrane filter technique using Nuclepore membrane of pore size of 14 µm.

CULTURE TECHNIQUES IN PARASITOLOGY

Culture Methods for Protozoa

The protozoa feed on bacteria, so the culture media are supplemented with bacterial growth. Accordingly there are four types of culture media which are used for protozoa:

1. **Axenic cultures:** If the parasites are grown as pure culture without any bacterial associate, the culture is referred as axenic culture
2. **Xenic cultures:** Cultures of parasite grown in association with an unknown microbe are referred as xenic cultures
3. **Monoxenic culture:** If the parasites are grown with a single known bacterium, the culture is referred as monoxenic culture, e.g. corneal biopsy specimens cultured with *E. coli* for recovering *Acanthamoeba*.

4. **Polyxenic culture:** It contains multiple bacterial supplements, starch and serum providing nourishment to amoeba.

Uses of Culture Media

Culture media are not routinely used in diagnostic parasitology. They are useful in research and teaching purpose.
- Polyxenic media is used for cultivation of protozoa from the suspected patients
- Axenic culture is useful when the bacterial flora interferes with the result such as:
  - Studying pathogenicity
  - Drug susceptibility testing
  - Preparation of antigen for serological tests.

Culture Media Used for Entamoeba histolytica

Culture media used for *E. histolytica* are given in Table 15.6.

Boeck and Drbohlav's Locke-Egg-Serum (LES) Medium

Boeck and Drbohlav's LES medium is the most commonly used culture medium for *E. histolytica*.

Composition:
- ***Locke's solution*** comprises of NaCl (9.0 g), $CaCl_2$ (0.2 g), KCl (0.4 g), $NaHCO_3$ (0.2 g), glucose (2.5 g), distilled water (1,000 mL). The solution should be autoclaved before storage
- ***Complete Medium:***
  - Four eggs are washed, the shells are wiped with 70% alcohol, and then the eggs are broken into a sterile flask containing glass beads
  - About 50 mL of Locke's solution is added and shaken until becomes homogenous
  - The medium is dispensed in screw capped tubes and then it is placed in a slant position in an inspissator at 70°C until the slant solidifies.
- One part of *sterile inactivated human serum* is added to 8 parts of sterile Locke's solution. The mixture is sterilized by filtration, and incubated at 37°C for 24 to 48 hours as a sterility check before use
- Locke's solution/serum mixture is added to a depth of <1 cm to the tube containing complete medium slant. Loopful of *sterile rice powder* is added.

Procedure

Stool specimen is inoculated into the tube, thoroughly mixed in the medium, and incubated at 37°C.
- The cultures should be checked on 2nd, 3rd and 4th day, by examining 0.1 mL of sediment under the microscope (high power field with low intensity light) for characteristic motility of trophozoites
- Although the initial cultures may appear to be negative, subcultures may reveal trophozoites.

Culture Media Used for Free-Living Amoebae

Nonnutrient agar

It is useful for the isolation of *Acanthamoeba* and *Naegleria*.
- **Composition**
  - **Page's saline** (10×): It comprises of NaCl (60 mg), hydrated $MgSO_4$ (2 mg), hydrated $CaCl_2$ (2 mg), Na_2HPO_4 (71 mg), KH_2PO_4 (68 mg), distilled water (500 mL). It is autoclaved at 121°C for 15 min and can be stored in a glass bottle at 40°C for up to 6 months
  - **Nonnutrient agar:** It comprises of Page's saline (10×) (100 mL), Difco agar (15 g) and double-distilled water (900 mL). The mixture is autoclaved at 121°C, at 15 lb/in.2 for 15 min. The molten agar is poured in petri dishes (20mL) which may be stored in the refrigerator for up to 3 months.
- **Monoxenic culture:** Before use, the plates should be removed from the refrigerator and placed at 37°C for 30 min
  - The sample is inoculated on the center of the nonnutrient agar plate coated with bacterial (*Escherichia coli*) overlay
  - After the fluid/specimen has been absorbed, the plates are sealed with strip of Parafilm; incubated

Table 15.6: Culture media used for *Entamoeba histolytica*

Culture medium	Type	Important ingredients
Boeck and Drbohlav's medium	Polyxenic	Solidified egg or solidified blood, Locke's solution, Inactivated human serum
Balamuth's medium	Polyxenic	Egg yolk-liver concentrate infusion medium
Robinson's medium	Polyxenic	Erythromycin, Bacto peptone, Phthalate solution, bovine serum, *E. coli* strain 0111 and R-medium*
Jones' medium	Polyxenic	Horse serum and yeast autolysate in phosphate buffered saline
Diamond's (TYM) medium	Axenic	Trypticase-yeast extract-maltose
TYI-S-33 medium	Polyxenic	TYI broth, heat-inactivated bovine serum, special 107 vitamin mix
TYSGM-9 medium	Polyxenic	Nutrient broth, 5% Tween 80 solution, phosphate-buffered saline, buffered methylene blue solution, added with antibiotic solution of penicillin G and streptomycin

*****R-medium:** Composed of sodium chloride, citric acid, potassium phosphate buffer, ammonium sulfate, magnesium sulfate and lactic acid.

in inverted position at 37°C (for CSF and other CNS specimens) or at 30°C (for contact lens solutions or other tissues)
- The plates are examined at low power for amoebic cysts or trophozoites daily for 10 days. Thin, linear tracks, which represent areas where amebae have ingested the bacteria will be seen
- *Balamuthia* species cannot be cultured by this method. They can be grown only by using tissue culture methods.

Other culture media used for free-living amoebae are as follows:
- **Peptone yeast extract glucose (PYG) liquid culture media:** Useful for cultivation of *Acanthamoeba* species
- **Nelson's liquid culture medium:** Useful for cultivation of *N. fowleri*. Nelson's medium comprises of ox liver digest, glucose, Page's saline, and double-distilled water added with heat inactivated fetal calf serum
- **Tissue culture techniques:** Various mammalian cell lines such as monkey kidney cell line, HEP2 and diploid macrophage cell line are used for cultivation of *Acanthamoeba, Naegleria* and *Balamuthia* species.

Culture Media Used for Giardia lamblia

Giardia can be cultivated in axenic media like Diamond's media used for cultivation of *E. histolytica* and in polyxenic medium such as Keister's Modification of TYI-S-33 medium.

Culture Media Used for Trichomonas vaginalis

- InPouch TV culture system—It is a commercially available system, considered as gold standard culture method for *T. vaginalis*
- Lash's cysteine hydrolysate serum media
- Cysteine peptone liver maltose (CPLM) media
- Diamond's trypticase yeast maltose (TYM) media
- Hollander's modification of TYM medium
- Diamond's complete medium (modified by Klass)
- Cell lines like McCoy cell line highly sensitive, can detect as low as three trophozoites/mL.

Culture Media Used for Leishmania and Trypanosoma

NNN medium

NNN medium is described by Novy, McNeal 1903 and Nicolle 1908. It supports the growth of flagellates causing leishmaniasis and Chagas' disease.
- **Composition:** It is biphasic media composed of two part salt agar and one part defibrinated fresh rabbit blood. The medium (4 mL) is dispensed and allowed to solidify in slanted position
- **Procedure:** Materials (blood, bone marrow aspirate, splenic pulp) are inoculated in water of condensation of the NNN medium and incubated at 37°C for 1–4 week

- **Observation:** The culture fluid is examined every day up to 10 days of inoculation for the presence of flagellates. On the solid medium, flagellates grow as thick, grayish-white mucoid spreading lawn.

Liquid medium for hemoflagellates:

Schneider's *Drosophila* medium (30% fetal calf serum) and Grace's insect tissue culture medium.
- Amastigote forms transform to promastigote forms and multiply by binary fission
- It is found to be more sensitive and rapid than NNN media.

Other media used are:
- Offutt's Modification of NNN Medium (leishmaniasis)
- Evan's Modified Tobie's Medium (leishmaniasis or Chagas' Disease)
- NIH Method for trypanosomes and leishmaniae
- 4N Medium for trypanosomes and leishmaniae
- Yaeger's LIT medium for Chagas' disease
- USAMRU blood agar medium for leishmaniasis.

Culture Techniques Used for Malaria Parasites

Culture techniques for malaria parasites are mainly used for preparation of malaria antigens.

Trager and Jensen technique using **RPMI 1640 medium** is most widely used method, in detail discussed in Chapter 6.

Culture Medium for Other Protozoans

- For *Blastocystis:* TYGM-9 (tryptone, yeast extract, glucose, methionine) Xenic medium
- For *Toxoplasma:* cell line such as complete human foreskin fibroblast, continuous cell lines (HeLa, LLC, and Vero)
- For *Dientamoeba fragilis:* Loeffler's serum slant containing inactivated horse serum overlaid with Earle's balanced salt solution
- For *Cryptosporidium*: Cell lines such as primary human intestinal epithelial cells, human colonic tumor cells (HCT-8, CCL-224), Madin Darby canine kidney cells (MDCK, CCL-34)
- For Microsporidia: Cell lines such as rabbit kidney cell line, RH-13, goldfish skin (GFSK-S1) and brain (GFB3C-W1).

Culture Methods for Nematode Larvae

Fecal culture methods (coproculture) are especially useful for specific identification of hookworm, *Strongyloides stercoralis* and *Trichostrongylus* species.
- Eggs hatch out into rhabditiform larvae in the culture medium which can be used to differentiate between hookworm, *Strongyloides stercoralis* and *Trichostrongylus* species

* Further rearing of nematode larvae leads to transformation into filariform larvae which can be used to differentiate *A. duodenale* and *N. americanus*.

The various methods are described below.

Harada-Mori Filter Paper Strip Culture (Fig. 15.9A)

Smear is made with 0.5 g to 1 g of fresh feces in the center of a narrow strip of filter paper (15 cm × 1.5 cm)
* The filter paper is placed in a conical centrifuge tube with sterile water in such a way that the lower end dips in water. The water level should be approximately half inch below the fecal spot
* This preparation is incubated for 10 days at room temperature after sealing the mouth of the tube loosely with cotton plug
* Larvae develop on the filter paper migrate and are liberated in water, which can be examined under a microscope.

Petri Dish/ Slant Culture Method (Little et al.) (Fig. 15.9B)

Fresh stool material is placed on the microscope slide shaped filter paper.
* The filter paper is then placed on the slanted glass slide, kept in a glass petri dish plate containing water
* This technique allows direct examination of the culture system with a dissecting microscope to look for nematode larvae in the fecal mass.

Charcoal Culture

About 20 g of fresh stool mixed in water to form thick suspension, which is then added to storage dish containing hardwood granulated charcoal. Water is added to provide moisture. The dish is covered, and placed in dark for 5-6 days.
* **Harvesting:** The larvae can be harvested by placing a round moistened gauze pad of 10-12 layer thick over the surface of the charcoal. A light source should be kept near the charcoal surface for 1 hour. Then the pad is removed and placed onto a surface of water in a beaker. Larvae migrate to the bottom of the beaker which should be pipetted after 1 hour and examined by wet mount
* The condition of this culture technique provides an environment that mimics natural condition, efficient to harvest large numbers of infective-stage larvae.

Baermann Technique (Fig. 15.9C)

This technique is useful for examining a stool specimen suspected of containing small numbers of *Strongyloides* larva.
* This technique exploits the property of the *Strongyloides* larva to migrate from cooler to warmer area
* It differs from Harada-Mori and Petri dish methods in that it uses more amount of stool, so has a better sensitivity in case of light infection. It can also be used for isolating larvae from soil.

Procedure

This method uses glass funnel fitted with a rubber tubing and clamp.
* A round wire screen is kept on the surface of the funnel, above which two layers of gauze are placed
* Five gram of feces is placed on the gauze
* Funnel is filled with warm water, left for 2 hours (or longer) to give time for *Strongyloides* larvae to emerge from the feces
* Clamp of the tubing is opened slowly and 10 mL of fluid is collected in a beaker. Larvae in the stool migrate downward to the bottom in the fluid
* After centrifugation (500 × g for 2 min), sediment is examined microscopically.

Modification of Baermann technique

Funnel used in the original version is replaced by a test tube with a rubber stopper, which is perforated to allow insertion of a plastic pipette tip. The tube containing the fecal suspension is inverted over another tube containing 6 mL of saline solution and incubated at 37°C for 2 hour. Centrifuged saline solution is screened for larvae.

Agar Plate Culture for Strongyloides Stercoralis

This is the best method for stool culture for *Strongyloides*. Agar plates are composed of 1.5% agar, meat extract (0.5%), peptone (1%) and NaCl (0.5%).
* Approximately, 2 g of fresh stool specimen is placed onto the center (1 inch area) of agar plates; the plates are sealed and held with right side up for 2 days at room temperature
* The plates are examined under the microscope for the presence of tracks (bacteria carried over agar by migrating larvae)

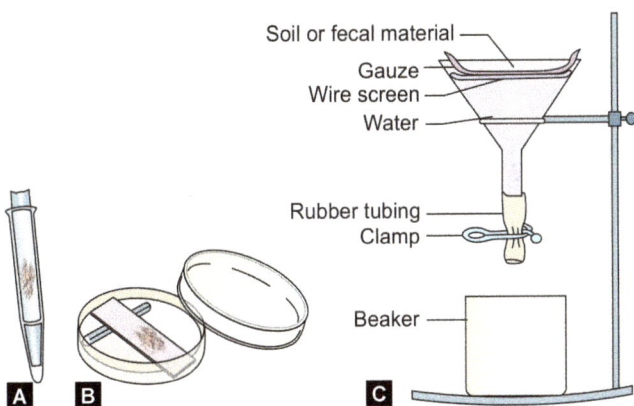

Figs 15.9A to C: Schematic diagram of techniques (A) Harada-Mori filter paper strip culture; (B) Petri dish/slant culture method; (C) Baermann technique

- A whole is made with a hot forceps on the petri dish lid through which 10 mL of 10% formalin is poured over the surface of the agar and is allowed to stand for 30 min
- Then the lid is opened, formalin is poured onto a tube, centrifuged for 5 min at 500 x g and the sediment is screened for the presence of nematode larvae
- Daily search for furrows on agar plates for up to 6 consecutive days results in increased sensitivity for diagnosis of both S. stercoralis and hookworm larvae.

Parasitic form vs free-living form of S. stercoralis

The larvae may be found any time after the fourth day or even on the first day in a heavy infection. Agar plate method is more sensitive, larvae can be seen on first or second day. The stool culture methods allow both parasitic and free-living forms of nematodes to develop.

- This is important if there is risk of contamination of specimens with soil or water containing free-living forms, which can be distinguished from the parasitic forms by adding with acid (concentrated HCl in 1:30 dilution)
- The parasitic form can live for about 24 hours of HCl treatment, while the free-living forms are killed immediately.

IMMUNODIAGNOSTIC METHODS

This method involves detection of parasite specific antibodies in serum, and detection of circulating parasitic antigen in the serum.

Immunodiagnostic methods are useful when:
- Parasites are detected only during the early stages of the disease
- Parasites occur in very small numbers
- Parasites reside in internal organs and morphological identification is not possible
- When other techniques like culture are time consuming.

Antibody Detection Tests

Antibodies are detected in various parasitic infections mainly from serum, sometime from other sites like CSF (neurocysticercosis) or pleural fluid (paragonimiasis). They various methods have been described in Table 15.7.

Table 15.7: Antibody detection tests

Disease	Test format	Target (antibody detected against)	Comments
Intestinal amoebiasis	ELISA (IgG)	170 kDa of lectin antigen	Sensitivity- early stage 75-85%, convalescent stage 90%
Amoebic liver abscess	ELISA (IgG)	170 kDa of lectin antigen	Sensitivity-90%, specificity-85%
Visceral leishmaniasis	Direct agglutination test (DAT)	Extract of L. donovani axenic amastigotes or promastigotes	Sensitivity-100%, specificity-100%
	ICT	rK-39, rKE16	Sensitivity-100%, specificity-98%
African trypanosomiasis	Card agglutination test for trypanosomes (CATT)	VSG antigen of T.b. gambiense	For field use and mass screening. Sensitive (87–98%), but less specific. Titer of >1:16 is considered significant
	ELISA	VSG antigen of T.b. gambiense Anti-TLTF antibodies	Can be used both for serum and CSF
Toxoplasmosis	Sabin-Feldman dye test	Complement mediated neutralization test that requires live tachyzoites	Most specific, but cannot differentiate recent and past infection
	IgG (ELISA, IFA)	Detects IgG antibodies	Four-fold rise indicates recent infection
	IgM and IgA (ELISA, IFA and ISAGA)	Detects IgM or IgA antibodies	Marker of acute infection and congenital infection
	IgG avidity test (ELISA, ELFA)	Detects low avidity IgG antibodies	Low avidity indicates recent infection
Cysticercosis	ELISA	Crude extract of cysticerci or vesicular fluid, can detect Ab in serum and CSF	Sensitivity—75–90%
	ELISA	Purified glycoprotein antigens	Better sensitivity, but low specificity
	Quick ELISA	Ab in serum against T24H Ag	Sensitivity-96%, specificity-99%
	Western blot	Uses highly specific 50–13 kDa lentil lectin-purified seven glycoprotein (LLGP) antigenic fractions	Presence of one to seven Gp bands confirms the diagnosis Sensitivity-98%, specificity-100%

Contd...

Contd...

Disease	Test format	Target (antibody detected against)	Comments
Hydatid disease	ELISA	Using B2t or 2B2t antigen	Sensitivity 91% and specificity 93% Indicator of cure in surgically treated patients
	DIGFA (Dot immunogold filtration assay)	Against four native antigens; cyst fluid (EgCF), AgB and protoscolex extract and Em2 antigen	Sensitivity is 80% and 93% for cystic and alveolar echinococcosis Specificity >90%
	Western blot	h-HCF-IB (human hydatid cyst fluid-immunoblot)	Sensitivity- 83%, specificity-98%
		Detecting antibody against antigen B fragment (produces 8–12 kDa band)	Sensitivity-92%, specificity-100%
Schistosomiasis	HAMA-FAST-ELISA	*S. haematobium* adult worm microsomal antigen	Sensitivity-95%, specificity-99%
Clonorchis sinensis	ELISA	Using recombinant propeptide of cathepsin L proteinase (rCsCatL-propeptide)	Used for monitoring the treatment response, minimal cross-reactions It has acceptable sensitivity
Paragonimus westermani	DIGFA	Crude extracts of adult worms of *P. westermani*	Sensitivity-99%, specificity-92% Rapid, gives result in 10 min
	ELISA	Purified adult excretory-secretory antigen	High sensitivity with pleural fluid
	Western blot	Using adult worm homogenate	Highly sensitive and specific
Strongyloides stercoralis	CrAg-ELISA	Using crude larval antigens	Sensitivity-95%
	LIP assay (Luciferase immuno-precipitation assay)	Using 31-kDa recombinant antigen (NIE) and/or the recombinant *S. stercoralis* immunoreactive antigen (SsIR)	It is a newer antibody detection assay
Lymphatic filariasis	Luciferase immunoprecipitation	Using *W. bancrofti* Wb123 antigen	Sensitivity and specificity-100%
	Flow-through assay*	Recombinant filarial antigen (WbSXP-1)	Sensitivity of 91.4% and 90.8%, for bancroftian and brugian filariasis
	Brugia Rapid*	Recombinant *B. malayi* Ag (Bm-14)	Shows good sensitivity and specificity

* Used under filariasis elimination program, in transmission assessment survey.

Abbreviations: TLTF, trypanosome-derived lymphocyte triggering factor; VSG, variant surface glycoprotein; ISAGA, immunosorbent agglutination assay, ELFA, enzyme-linked immunofluorescence assay, DIGFA, Dot immunogold filtration assay; ICT, immunochromatographic test; ELISA, enzyme-linked immunosorbent assay; FAST, Falcon assay screening test, Ag, antigen; Ab, antibody.

Antigen Detection Tests

The antigen detection methods available for various parasitic diseases have been described in Table 15.8.

MOLECULAR METHODS

Molecular methods most frequently used in diagnostic parasitology include: (i) DNA probes, (ii) Polymerase chain reaction (PCR) and its modifications such as multiplex and nested PCR, (iii) real-time PCR, (iv) LAMP assay (Loop mediated isothermal amplification), (v) Transcription based amplification, etc. Refer author's Essentials of Medical Microbiology for the principle of theses assays. The format of molecular tests for various parasitic diseases and the genes targeted have been described in Table 15.9. The commercial molecular systems approved for parasitic diseases have been depicted in Table 15.10.

INTRADERMAL SKIN TESTS

Skin tests are useful when a reliable antibody detection methods are not available. They are employed for research and epidemiological purpose. Positive intradermal skin tests are suggestive of pastexposure. As they remain positive for longer duration, so they cannot differentiate old and recent infection. More so, nonstandardized crude antigens are used, hence they lack sensitivity and specificity. There is always a danger of provoking an anaphylactic reaction in the patient (Table 15.11).

XENODIAGNOSTIC TECHNIQUES

Principle

Xenodiagnosis uses laboratory reared arthropod vectors to detect low levels of parasites during chronic stages of the disease, when their numbers in the blood will be very low.

Table 15.8: Antigen detection tests

Disease	Test format	Target* (antigen detected)	Comments
Amoebiasis	ELISA	170 kDa of lectin Ag (blood, stool)	Sensitivity—65%, Positive in early stage
	Immunochromatographic test (Triage parasite panel)	Simultaneous detection of 3 antigens: • *Giardia* (alpha-1 giardin antigen) • *E. histolytica/ E. dispar* (29 kDa Ag) • *Cryptosporidium* (isomerase Ag)	Sensitivity—83–96% Specificity—99–100%
Giardiasis	ICT (Triage parasite panel)	Same as for amoebiasis	Same as for amoebiasis
	ELISA	Cyst wall protein antigen	Sensitivity—90–100% Specificity—99–100%
Visceral leishmaniasis	Latex agglutination test	Heat stable low molecular weight carbohydrate antigen in urine	Sensitivity—40–80% Specificity—good
Malaria	ICT	Histidine rich protein-2 (Pf. HRP 2)— *P. falciparum* specific Parasite lactate dehydrogenase (pLDH) and aldolase—common to all species	Sensitivity—>90% (at parasite density >100/µL) pLDH—useful for monitoring response to treatment HRP-2—diagnose in pregnancy
Cryptosporidiosis	ICT (Triage parasite panel)	Same as for Amoebiasis	Same as for amoebiasis
Intestinal taeniasis	ELISA	Taenia specific antigen detection in stool by using polyclonal *Taenia* antibodies	Can detect *Taenia* carriers
Schistosomiasis	ELISA	Using soluble egg antigen (M Ab-SEA)	Sensitivity of 90% (serum) and 94% (urine)
	ELISA or dip stick assays	Circulating cathodic antigen (CCA), circulating anodic antigen (CAA) in serum and urine	Indicates recent infection Can be used for monitoring the treatment response
Clonorchis sinensis	ELISA	Circulating antigen in the serum	Sensitivity—75–93%. Indicates current infection
Strongyloides stercoralis	Coproantigen (Ag capture ELISA)	Against *Strongyloides ratti* excretory/secretory (E/S) antigen	No cross-reactivity with other intestinal helminthic infections.
Lymphatic filariasis	ELISA	Using monoclonal Ab against Og4C3 and AD12 antigens	Sensitivity—99%, specificity—99–100%
	ICT		Sensitivity—96–100%, Specificity—95–100%

* Antigen detected or monoclonal antibodies used against antigen.

Abbreviations: ICT, immunochromatographic test; ELISA, enzyme-linked immunosorbent assay; FAST, Falcon assay screening test; Ag, antigen; Ab, antibody.

- This technique is employed to diagnose Chagas' disease
- This technique may be useful in endemic areas, but not in routine diagnostic laboratories.

Xenodiagnosis in Chagas' Disease

Procedure

Laboratory reared *Triatomine* (reduviid) bugs are starved for 2 weeks and then fed on the patient's blood, suspected to have Chagas' disease.
- If Trypanosomes are present in the blood, they will multiply and develop into epimastigotes and trypomastigotes in about 30 days and are passed in the feces of the reduviid bug
- After 1–2 months, feces from the bugs are examined over a 3 month period for the developmental stages of the parasite, in the hind gut of the bug. The bugs may also be dissected and examined microscopically.

ANIMAL INOCULATION METHODS

Animal inoculation techniques are not routinely used in diagnosis of parasitic infections; but useful in some parasitic infections (Table 15.12).

IMAGING TECHNIQUES

Being noninvasive methods, imaging techniques such as the X-ray, ultrasound (USG), computed tomography (CT) and magnetic resonance imaging (MRI) are extensively used various space occupying parasitic infections (Table 15.13).

Table 15.9: Molecular detection tests

Disease /parasite	Test format	Target gene detected	Comments
Amoebiasis	Nested multiplex PCR	Small subunit rRNA Differentiates *E. histolytica, E. dispar* and *E. moshkovskii*	Sensitivity—90%, specificity—90–100%
	Real time PCR	18S rRNA	More sensitive than conventional PCR
	BioFire FilmArray	Refer the table 15.10	High sensitivity and specificity
Naegleria fowleri	Nested PCR	5.8S rRNA, ITS	High sensitivity and specificity
	Multiplex real time PCR	Three regions of small subunit 18S rRNA	For simultaneous detection of *Naegleria, Acanthamoeba* and *Balamuthia* in CSF
Acanthamoeba	PCR	18S rRNA	High sensitivity and specificity
Giardiasis	PCR	• glutamate dehydrogenase (*gdh*) • β-giardin (*bg*) • triosephosphate isomerase (*tpi*)	High sensitivity and specificity
	BioFire FilmArray	Refer the table 15.10	High sensitivity and specificity
Trichomoniasis	PCR	β-tubulin gene	Sensitivity—80–90%, Specificity—100%
Visceral leishmaniasis	Nested PCR	Kinetoplast DNA Others: 18S rRNA, SSU rRNA, gene coding for β-tubulins, cysteine protease, gp-63	Sensitivity—70–93%
	LAMP assay	Kinetoplast DNA	Useful in field setting.
Chagas' disease	PCR	Kinetoplast or nuclear DNA (e.g. 188 bp TCZ1-TCZ2 primer and 330 bp S35-S36 primer)	More sensitive than microscopy and serology
Malaria	Nested multiplex PCR	18S rDNA	Sensitivity—95–100%, Specificity—98–100%
	Real time PCR	*cox1* gene of *P. falciparum*, 18S rDNA, and mitochondrial DNA sequence	Highly sensitive and specific
	LAMP assay	Loop mediated amplification	Can differentiate *P. falciparum* with non-falciparum species
Cryptosporidiosis	PCR	18S rRNA and β-tubulin gene	More sensitive, can differentiate genotypes
	BioFire FilmArray	Refer the Table 15.10	High sensitivity and specificity
Intestinal taeniasis	PCR	Mitochondrial DNA followed by sequencing	Can distinguish between *T. saginata, T. asiatica*, and two genotypes of *T. solium*
Hydatid disease	PCR	Targeting mitochondrial DNA	High sensitivity and specificity
	PCR-RFLP	Targeting specific gene	Used to detect genotypes (G1 to G10)
Schistosoma japonicum	Pyrosequencing	Targeting specific gene	To differentiate *S. japonicum* from and *S. mekongi*
Clonorchis sinensis	Multiplex PCR	Targeting specific gene	Detects *Clonorchis* and *Opisthorchis* simultaneously
	Real-time PCR	Mitochondrial NADH dehydrogenase subunit 2 (nad2) DNA elements	High sensitivity and specificity
Hookworm	PCR and real-time PCR based assays	Mitochondrial cytochrome oxidase I genes (585-bp fragment) ITS-1 and ITS-2 regions of rDNA	Can differentiate between *Ancylostoma* and *Necator*
Strongyloides stercoralis	Real-time PCR	Cytochrome C oxidase subunit I gene, 18S rRNA, or 28S RNA	100% specificity with variable sensitivity
Ascaris lumbricoides	PCR	ITS1 or cytochrome oxidase-1	High sensitivity and specificity
	Multiplex PCR	Targeting specific gene	Can differentiate *Ascaris, Trichuris* and hookworm

Abbreviations: ITS-internal transcribed spacer gene; PCR, polymerase chain reaction, LAMP, loop-mediated isotheral amplification; rDNA, ribosomal DNA.

Table 15.10: Commercially available Molecular panels

Molecular panels	Used for	Test format/principle
BioFire FilmArray Gastrointestinal Panel	Simultaneously detect 22 enteric pathogens including 4 parasites such as—*E. histolytica, G. lamblia Cryptosporidium, Cyclospora*	**Completely automated multiplex nested PCR system** where all the steps are performed automatically by the system; giving result in about one hour. The FilmArray GI pouch has a rigid plastic component which contains reagents in freeze-dried form and a flexible plastic portion which is further divided into discrete segments (blisters) where all the steps from sample preparation to amplification and detection are carried out. The sample is inoculated in the pouch and then loaded into the BioFire system
BD MAX Enteric Parasite Panel	*Giardia lamblia* *Cryptosporidium* *Entamoeba histolytica*	**Multiplex qualitative PCR,** gives result in 4 hours, requires minimal handling. It automates sample lysis, DNA extraction, amplification, and detection of the amplified DNA sequence; using real-time PCR based on hydrolysis probe technique
Luminex (enteric panel)	11 diarrheal pathogens- virus, bacteria, and two parasites (*Cryptosporidium, Giardia*)	**Multiplex RT-PCR/PCR reaction:** The amplicons generated are added to a hybridization/detection reaction containing Luminex beads (coupled to sequences from Universal Array, streptavidin, R-phycoerythrin conjugate); which detect a specific microbial target by giving a specific intensity of fluorescence
APTIMA *Trichomonas vaginalis* Assay	*T. vaginalis,* accepted samples: endocervical swab, urine	Based on transcription-mediated amplification (TMA) and hybridization protection assay (HPA)
Affirm VPIII Microbial Identification Test	Detects 3 organisms causing vaginitis: *Candida, Gardnerella vaginalis,* and *T. vaginalis*	**DNA probe technology:** Employs a probe analysis card, using two probes for each organism—a capture probe and a color development probe. It gives result within 45 min

Note: These molecular tests are USA Food and Drug Administration (FDA) approved for use for parasitic diagnosis.

Table 15.11: Intradermal skin tests in parasitic diagnosis

Skin tests showing immediate hypersensitivity in	Showing delayed hypersensitivity in
Hydatid disease (Casoni's test)	Leishmaniasis (Montenegro test)
Filariasis	Trypanosomiasis
Schistosomiasis	Toxoplasmosis
Ascariasis	
Strongyloidiasis	
Trichinellosis (Bachman test)	

Table 15.12: Animal inoculation methods in parasitic diagnosis

Parasite tested	Animal used	Route of inoculation	Specimen inoculated	Method of demonstration	Observation after inoculation
Toxoplasma gondii	Mice and Rats	0.5 mL of material injected intra-peritoneally	Body fluid, blood, lymph node fluid or cerebrospinal fluid	Peritoneal fluid obtained after 7–10 days, stained with Romanowsky's stain	If animal survives after 6 months, the serum of the animal shows presence of antibodies
Leishmania donovani	Young hamsters (2–3 months old)	0.5–1 mL of material injected intraperitoneally	Aspirates or biopsy obtained from cutaneous ulcers, lymph nodes, spleen, liver or bone marrow	Splenic impression smears are prepared after 4–6 weeks, stained with Romanowsky's stain	Positive cases animal dies several days after the inoculation
Trypanosoma species	Mice and rats, guinea pigs	Intraperitoneal or in tail vein	Blood, lymph node aspirate or spinal fluid	Blood sample is collected after 2 weeks, smears are prepared and stained with Romanowsky's stain	Stained smear shows presence of the parasite
Trichinella spiralis	Rats	Feed orally	Infected muscle tissue	Rats are examined for *Trichinella spiralis* larvae in the muscle of the infected rat	Mainly, *Trichinella spiralis* larvae can be demonstrated in the diaphragm

CHAPTER 15 ◈ Laboratory Diagnosis of Parasitic Diseases

Table 15.13: Imaging methods in parasitic diagnosis

Disease	Imaging method used	Comments
Amoebic liver abscess	USG	Detects the location of abscess and its extrahepatic extension
Hydatid disease	X-ray, USG, CT scan and MRI	• **X-rays:** It is simple, inexpensive, yet useful technique to detect hepatomegaly and calcified cysts and cysts in lungs • **USG:** It is the imaging method of choice because of its low cost and high diagnostic accuracy. It detects both single and multiple cystic lesions, floating membrane (Water lily sign) and daughter cysts. It is also useful to monitor the response to treatment and for epidemiological studies • **CT scan:** It is superior to detect smaller cysts, calcified cysts, extrahepatic cysts and to differentiate from other cystic lesions. Also used as a prognostic marker • **MRI:** It has a higher contrast resolution, which makes cysts clearer. It can be used as an alternate to CT scan
Trichinella spiralis	X-ray	Detects calcified muscle cysts
Neurocysticercosis	CT scan and MRI	**Detects:** Number, location, size, of the cysts and extension and stage of the disease **CT scan:** For calcified cysts **MRI:** It is superior to CT scan, to detect extraparenchymal cysts, vesicular, necrotic lesions and noncystic lesions
Paragonimus westermani infection	X-ray, MRI and CT scan	**X-ray:** Pulmonary cysts **MRI and CT scan:** Locate extrapulmonary cysts (CNS)
Clonorchis and *Opisthorchis*	Cholangiography	Detects site of the lesion and obstruction of the biliary tract
Filariasis	USG	• Serpentine movement within the lymphatic vessels of scrotum (filarial dance sign) • Dilated and tortuous lymphatic vessels

Abbreviations: USG, ultrasonography; CT, computed tomography; MRI, magnetic resonance imaging; CNS, central nervous system.

EXPECTED QUESTIONS

I. Write short notes on:
  a. Culture methods in diagnostic parasitology.
  b. Stool concentration techniques.
  c. Blood concentration methods for microfilariae detection.
  d. Western blot in diagnostic parasitology.
  e. Use of Immunochromatographic tests in parasitic diagnosis.
  f. PCR in diagnostic parasitology.
  g. Use of ELISA in parasitic diagnosis.
  h. Xenodiagnostic techniques in diagnostic parasitology.
  i. Intradermal skin tests in parasitic diagnosis.
  j. Animal inoculation methods used in diagnostic parasitology.

II. Multiple choice questions (MCQs):

1. Advantages of saline mount are all, *except*:
   a. Useful in the detection of trophozoites and cysts of protozoa and eggs and larvae of helminths
   b. Nuclear details of cysts and helminthic eggs and larvae are better visualized
   c. Motility of trophozoites and larvae can be seen in acute infection
   d. Bile staining property can be appreciated

2. Flotation technique is useful for detection of:
   a. Fertilized eggs of *Ascaris lumbricoides*
   b. Larva of *Strongyloides*
   c. *Taenia* eggs
   d. Operculated eggs of trematodes

3. One of the statement is not correct for PVA (polyvinyl alcohol):
   a. Difficult to prepare
   b. Not good to preserve *Giardia* cyst
   c. Good for fecal immunoassay kits
   d. Contains mercury compounds

4. Boeck and Dr Bohlav's medium is used for the cultivation of:
   a. *Entameoba histolytica* b. *Leishmania donovani*
   c. Malaria parasite d. Hookworm

5. Which of the following medium is used for cultivation of malaria parasite:
   a. Diamond's (TYM) medium
   b. NNN medium
   c. Cysteine peptone liver maltose media
   d. RPMI 1640 medium

Answer
1. b 2. a 3. c 4. a 5. d

Medical Entomology

16 CHAPTER

CHAPTER OUTLINE

- Medical entomology
- Vector
- Class insecta
- Class arachnida
- Class crustacea
- Control of arthropods

MEDICAL ENTOMOLOGY

A study of the arthropods of medical importance is known as **medical entomology**. Arthropods act as important vectors in disease transmission of many parasitic diseases which are of human concern. Arthropods are invertebrates, consisting of a segmented body, several pairs of jointed legs, rigid exoskeleton, internal organs and body divided into head, thorax, and abdomen.

Phylum Arthropoda is divided into five classes, out of which Class Insecta, Class Arachnida, and Class Crustacea are of medical importance (Tables 16.1 and 16.2).

Ectoparasites inhabit the surface of the body of the host without penetrating into the tissues. They are important vectors transmitting the pathogenic microbes. The infection by these parasites is called as infestation. Examples include louse, fleas, mites, ticks etc. Some of these ectoparasites may penetrate into the host causing disease; examples include myasis, tungiasis and scabies (described later in this Chapter).

VECTOR

It is an arthropod that transmits infection. Transmission of infection to the host is by biting or by deposition of the infective material near the bite, on food or other objects. Biological transmission are of three types (see highlighted box).

Biological transmission
- **Propagative:** Only multiplication of the parasite takes place inside the vector, e.g. *Yersinia pestis* in rat fleas
- **Cyclodevelopmental:** Only development of the parasite takes place inside the vector, e.g. *Wuchereria bancrofti* in mosquitoes
- **Cyclopropagative:** Multiplication and development (both) takes place inside the vector, e.g. *Plasmodium* species in mosquitoes.

CLASS INSECTA

Mosquitoes

Anopheles, *Culex*, *Aedes* and *Mansonia* are the common mosquitoes which transmit infection to man.

Identification Features

Body of mosquito consists of three parts:
- ❖ **Head:** It is semi-globular, bears a pair of compound eyes, a long proboscis, a pair of palpi and a pair of antennae (bushy in males). The proboscis is used by the mosquito for biting during the feed
- ❖ **Thorax:** It is large and rounded. It bears a pair of wings dorsally and three pairs of legs ventrally
- ❖ **Abdomen:** It is long, narrow and has ten segments. The last two segments are modified to form external genitalia.

General identification features and diseases transmitted by *Anopheles*, *Culex* and *Aedes* mosquitoes are described in Tables 16.2 and 16.3.

Flies

Housefly

Musca domestica is the most common house frequenting fly. It is non-biting in nature. They act as mechanical vector for transmission of many diseases (see Fig. 16.1A).

Table 16.1: Classification of arthropods (Phylum Arthropoda)

Class	Common names
Insecta	Mosquitoes, black flies, sand flies, deer flies, house flies, tsetse flies, fleas, cockroaches, lice, bugs, wasps, etc.
Arachnida	Hard ticks, soft ticks, itch mites, chiggers, etc.
Myriapoda	Centipedes, millipedes, etc.
Pentastomida	Tongue worms, etc.
Crustacea	*Cyclops*, crabs, crayfish, etc.

Contd...

Table 16.2: Arthropods acting as vectors in transmission of medically important human diseases

Arthropods	Diseases transmitted		
	Parasitic	*Viral*	*Bacterial*
Mosquito	Malaria (*Anopheles*) Bancroftian filariasis (*Culex, Aedes* and *Anopheles*) Malayan filariasis (*Mansonia, Anopheles*)	Yellow fever (*Aedes*) Dengue fever (*Aedes*) Chikungunya (*Aedes*) Japanese encephalitis (*Culex*) Rift-Valley fever (*Aedes*) O'Nyong-Nyong (*Anopheles*) VEE, WEE and EEE (*Culex, Aedes*)	–
Sandfly	Kala-azar Oriental sore	Sandfly fever (Papatasi fever)	Oroya fever (Carrion's disease)
Tsetse fly	Sleeping sickness	–	–
Housefly (mechanical vector)	Amoebiasis Intestinal helminthiasis	Poliomyelitis Enterically transmitted hepatitis (hepatitis A and E)	Typhoid fever Paratyphoid fever Cholera Trachoma Yaws
Blackfly (*Simulium* species)	Onchocerciasis	–	–
Deer fly	Loiasis	–	–
Rat flea (*Xenopsylla cheopis*)	*Hymenolepis diminuta* and *Hymenolepis nana*	–	Bubonic plague Endemic typhus
Cockroach (mechanical vector)	Amoebiasis Helminthiasis	Hepatitis Poliomyelitis	Enteric pathogens
Reduviid bug	Chagas' disease	–	–
Louse	Ectoparasitic infection	–	Relapsing fever Epidemic typhus Trench fever
Hard tick	Babesiosis	Viral encephalitis Viral fever Viral hemorrhagic fever	Tularemia Tick typhus
Soft tick	–	–	Q-fever Relapsing fever
Trombiculid mite	–	–	Scrub typhus Rickettsial pox
Itch mite	Scabies	–	–
Cyclops	Dracunculiasis Diphyllobothriasis Gnathostomiasis	–	–
Crabs and crayfish	Paragonimiasis	–	–

Abbreviations: VEE, Venezuelanequine encephalitis; WEE, Western equine encephalitis; EEE, Eastern equine encephalitis

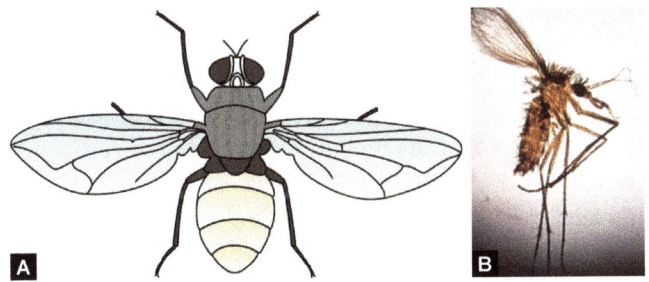

Figs 16.1A and B: (A) Housefly (schematic diagram); (B) Sandfly (real image)
Source: B—Public Health Image Library, ID# 6273/Centers for Disease Control and Prevention (CDC), Atlanta (*with permission*).

Identification features

- ❖ **Head:** It has a pair of compound eyes, a pair of antennae and a single proboscis on its head
- ❖ **Thorax:** Has pair of wings and three pairs of legs
- ❖ **Abdomen:** Segmented and shows dark and light markings.

Diseases transmitted by housefly—refer Table 16.2.

Sandfly

Identification features

Sandflies are light or dark brown flies, smaller than mosquitoes (Fig. 16.1B).

Table 16.3: Identification features of *Anopheles*, *Culex*, and *Aedes* mosquitoes

Identification features	Anopheles mosquito	Culex mosquito	Aedes mosquito
Body	Body is slender and rests with an angle to the surface	Body rests parallel to the surface	Head is slightly bent downward and body shows a hunch back at rest
Wings	Have dark spots	Unspotted	Unspotted and has white markings on legs and abdomen (hence named as tiger mosquito)
Hind legs	Held outstretched	Curled up over the back	Held curled upward
Proboscis and body	Proboscis and body is in same straight line	Proboscis and body at an angle to one another	Proboscis and body at an angle to one another
Maxillary palpi	Maxillary palpi are as long as proboscis (both sexes)	Maxillary palpi are shorter than proboscis (females)	Maxillary palpi are shorter than proboscis (females)
Tip of the abdomen	-	Blunt	Pointed
Biting time	Each species has specific peak biting hours and there are also variations in their preferences for biting indoors or outdoors	Midnight	Day time
Important species	A. culicifacies, A. fluviatilis, A. minimus, A. stephensi	C. fatigans, C. tritaeniorhynchus, C. tarsalis	A. aegypti A. albopictus
Vector for diseases	Malaria Encephalitis	Bancroftian filariasis West Nile fever Japanese encephalitis	Yellow fever Chikungunya fever Dengue Rift Valley fever Encephalitis
Schematic diagram and real images of *Anopheles*; *Culex* and *Aedes* mosquitoes	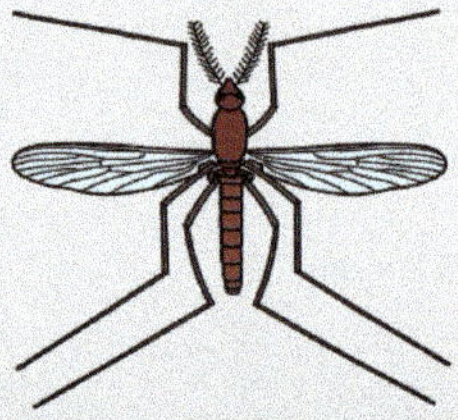 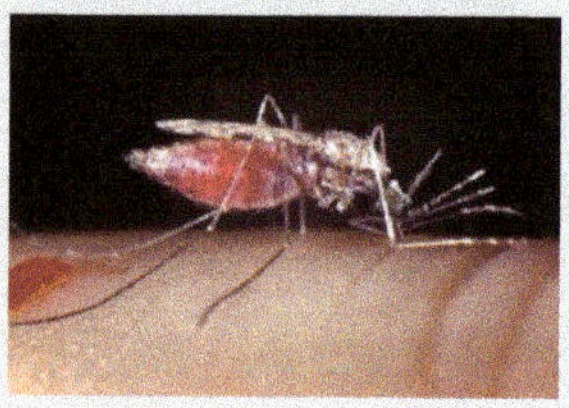	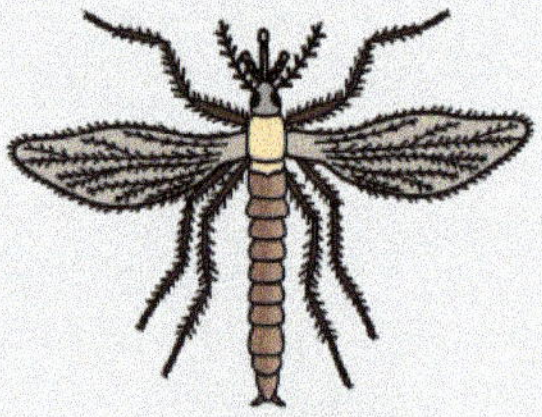 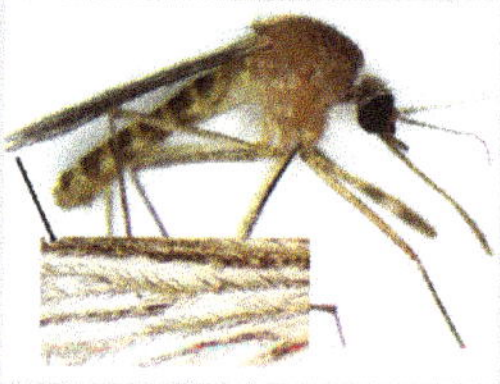	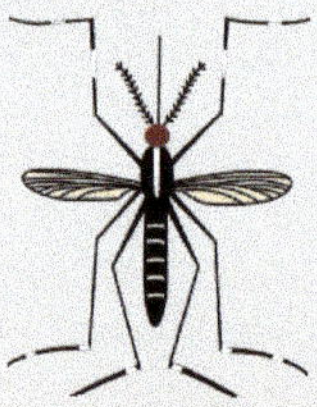 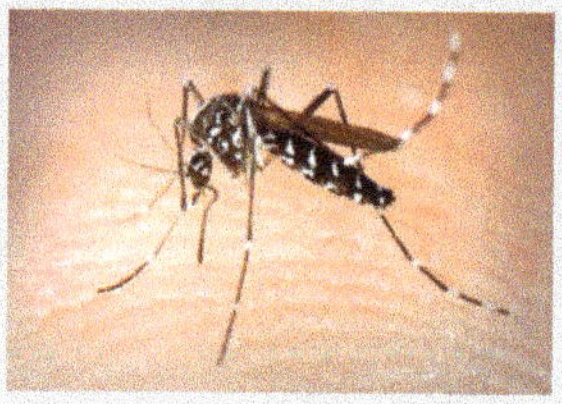

Source: DPDx Image Library, Centers for Disease Control and Prevention (CDC), Atlanta (*with permission*).

- Their body and wings are covered by dense hair
- Head contains pair of long, slender and hairy antennae, palpi and a proboscis
- Thorax contains pair of wings and three pairs of legs
- Abdomen has ten segments
- Though winged, they only hop about and do not fly
- The legs are longer as compared to the size of the body
- They bite during night and only females bite; the males live on fruit juices
- **Important species:** *Phlebotomus argentipes* (vector of kala-azar).

Diseases transmitted by sandfly—refer Table 16.2.

Tsetse Fly (Fig. 16.2A)

Tsetse flies belong to the genus *Glossina*, and family, Glossinidae. They are found only in tropical Africa.
- They are yellowish or dark brown, medium-sized flies
- They can be distinguished from other large biting insects by their forward pointing mouthparts
- They bite only in daytime
- They are biological vectors of trypanosomes; can transmit an infectious disease called as sleeping sickness.

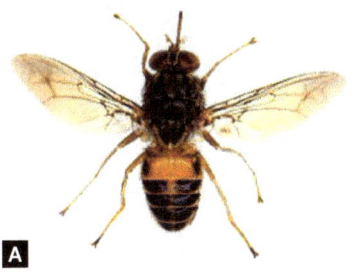 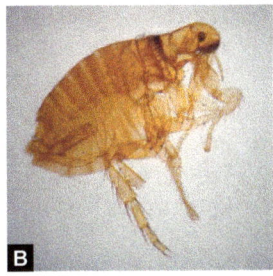 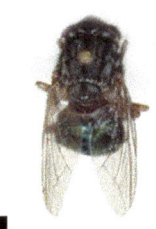 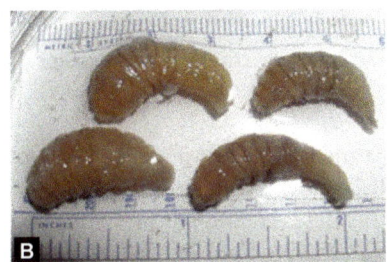

Figs 16.2A and B: (A) Tsetse fly (real image); (B) Male rat flea (mounted specimen)

Source: A—DPDx Image Library, Centers for Disease Control and Prevention (CDC), Atlanta (*with permission*); B— Head of Deptartment, Microbiology, Meenakshi Medical College, Chennai.

Figs 16.3A and B: *Dermatobia hominis:* (A) Adult and (B) larvae (maggots)

Source: A and B—DPDx Image Library, Centers for Disease Control and Prevention(CDC), Atlanta (*with permission*).

Blackfly

Blackfly (sometimes called as buffalo gnat) is a member of the family Simuliidae.

- They are usually small, black or gray in color, with short legs, and antennae
- *Simulium damnosum* and *S. neavei* are the important species
- It is the most widespread vector for river blindness.

Myiasis

Myiasis is an infestation on the host's body surface by the larval stage (known as **maggots**) of various flies of the order Diptera.

Types of myiasis

According to tissue viability, three types of myiasis have been described.

- **Specific myiasis:** These larvae attack only the living tissues of man and animals. Examples include *Dermatobia hominis* and members of Calliphorinae family such as *Cochliomyia, Auchmeromyia, Cordylobia, Sarcophaga,* etc.
- **Semispecific myiasis:** Here, the larvae breed on the bodies of dead animals and attach to dermal and subdermal area, and cavities. Examples include *Lucilia* species, *Calliphora* species
- **Accidental myiasis:** It is characterize by accidental and infrequent infections, transmitted by ingestion of food contaminated with larvae causing intestinal myiasis. They invade ears, nose, sinuses and urinary passage. Approximately 15 families can cause accidental myiasis.

Pathogenesis and life cycle

Adults of *Dermatobia hominis* are free-living flies. They capture blood sucking arthropods like mosquitoes and lay eggs on their body. When mosquito bites, eggs are deposited on host's bite wound, from where larvae emerge and penetrate the host tissue. The larvae reside in a subdermal cavity and develop into mature larvae which are dropped to the ground mainly during night or early morning. The larvae develop to pupa and then into adult forms in about 6 months and the cycle is repeated.

Geographic distribution

Myiasis is found worldwide. *Dermatobia* and *Cochliomyia* are Neotropical species, ranging from Mexico into South America. The *Auchmeromyia* and *Cordylobia anthropophaga* are distributed in South Africa. Myiasis is also reported from India.

Clinical presentation

Maggots can infest any organs or tissues accessible to oviposition of the fly. Pathological changes are due to larval penetration.

- **Cutaneous (skin) or mucocutaneous tissues** such as eyes, nose and ears: Furuncular myiasis is the most common presentation, mainly caused by *Dermatobia* and *Cordylobia*. It presents as papule or nodule with a central area that exudes serosanguinous or purulent fluid
- **Intestinal myiasis:** It occurs due to ingestion of food contaminated with eggs or larvae of flies. Few larvae may survive gastric acidity and temporarily lodge in intestinal crypts. Most infections are asymptomatic. Few develop symptoms such as abdominal pain, nausea, vomiting, anal pruritus and rectal bleeding. This is caused mainly by *Sarcophaga* species and *Fannia canicularis*
- Nosocomial transmission has been reported.

Laboratory diagnosis

The diagnosis of myiasis is made by the finding of fly larvae in tissue. Identification to the genus or species level involves comparing certain morphological structures on the larvae, including the anterior and posterior spiracles, chitinized mouthparts and cephalopharyngeal skeleton, abdominal spiracles and cuticular spines. PCR and RAPD (random amplified polymorphic DNA typing) can also be done for species identification.

Treatment

Definite treatment is by surgical removal of the larvae.

Tunga penetrans

Tungiasis is another ectoparasitic infestation, caused by *Tunga penetrans,* which is a small flea. It is seen in travelers returning from Latin America (largely Brazil) and Sub-Saharan Africa. The gravid females produce burrows on skins which ulcerate causing itching and irritation.

Flea

Rat Flea (Fig. 16.2B)

Identification features

Fleas are small, bilaterally compressed, wingless insects.
- Important species of rat fleas are *Xenopsylla cheopis* and *X. astia*
- Contains a hard chitinous exoskeleton and their body is covered by backward pointing spines
- **Head:** Conical and attached to the thorax without neck
- **Thorax:** Contains three segments and three pairs of legs; hind legs are well developed for jumping
- Abdomen is divided into ten segments. The male contains a coiled structure, the penis, and female contains a short, stumpy structure, the spermatheca, in the abdomen. The shape of spermatheca helps in distinguishing the species.

Diseases transmitted by rat flea—refer Table 16.2.

Louse (Fig. 16.4)

Identification features

Louse is a small wingless human ectoparasite.
- Human lice are of three types—(1) head lice (*Pediculus humanus capitis*), (2) body lice (*P. humanus corporis*) and (3) pubic or crab lice (*Pthirus pubis*)
- **Head:** Pointed in front and contains a pair of five jointed antennae. Mouth parts are adapted for blood sucking and they bite severely
- **Thorax:** Square-shaped, with three pairs of legs attached ventrally. The legs are provided with claws
- **Abdomen:** Elongated in shape and has nine segments.

The diseases transmitted by louse are:
- Epidemic typhus
- Trench fever
- Epidemic relapsing fever.

CLASS ARACHNIDA

Mites

Trombiculid Mite (Fig. 16.5A)

It contains four pairs of legs (first pair of legs is the largest).
- The body is not well demarcated into three parts (head, thorax and abdomen)
- Disease transmitted—scrub typhus.

Itch Mite/Sarcoptes scabei (Fig. 16.5B)

Scabies is caused by itch Mite or *Sarcoptes scabei*. It has four stages: egg, larva, nymph and adult. Transmission to man is through transfer of impregnated female mites during person to person and skin to skin contact.

Clinical manifestations

Initial infestation is asymptomatic for two months although the person can still transmit scabies during this time.

In case of reinfection, symptoms appear much earlier in 1-4 days.
- **Primary infection:** The mites burrow into the upper layer of the skin but never below the stratum corneum. Mites burrowing under the skin cause a **rash**, which is most frequently found on the hands, particularly the finger **web spaces;** wrist folds, elbow or knee; the penis; the breast; and/or the shoulder blades. **Severe itching** is the most common presentation, especially at night and over body surface, including areas where mites are undetectable

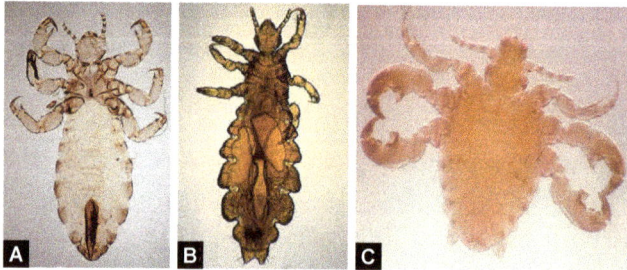

Figs 16.4A to C: Louse (mounted specimens) (A) Body louse; (B) Head louse; (C) Pubic louse (mounted specimen)

Source: DPDx Image Library, Centers for Disease Control and Prevention (CDC), Atlanta (*with permission*).

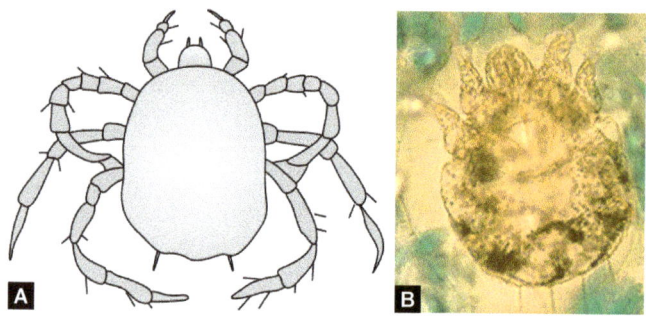

Figs 16.5A and B: (A) Trombiculid mite (schematic diagram); (B) *Sarcoptes scabiei* (Itch mite)

Source: B—DPDx Image Library, Centers for Disease Control and Prevention (CDC), Atlanta (with permission).

❖ **Crusted (Norwegian) scabies**: This is a severe form of scabies, seen among persons who are immunocompromised, elderly, or institutionalized. It is characterized by vesicles and formation of thick crusts over the skin, accompanied by abundant mites but only slight itching. Secondary bacterial infections are common.

Laboratory diagnosis

Suspicion of scabies is made based upon the appearance and distribution of the rash and the presence of burrows. It is confirmed by isolating the mites, ova or feces in a skin scraping at the burrows, especially on the finger webspace and wrist folds.

❖ **Skin scrapping:**
  - Scrapings are best performed at the end of the burrows in non-excoriated and non-inflamed areas using a sterile scalpel blade containing a drop of mineral oil. The mineral oil enhances the adherence of the mites to the blade and can then be transferred to a glass slide
  - An additional 1-2 drops of mineral oil can be added to the slide, followed by a coverslip for microscopic examination. Skin scrapings should be screened at 4× or 10× magnification and then evaluated at 40× magnification for confirmation.
❖ **Identification:** *S. scabies* is very small in size, just visible to naked eyes. Adult female mites measure 0.30–0.45 mm long; males are smaller at 0.20–0.24 mm long
  - Body is rounded above and flattened below
  - The body surface is covered with short bristles
  - It has two pairs of legs in front, and two pairs behind
  - The front legs have suckers at the end and the hind legs have long bristles.

Treatment

Scabies is treated with any of the following: (i) permethrin cream 5%, (ii) crotamiton lotion 10%, (iii) sulfur ointment 5%–10%, (iv) lindane lotion 1%, (v) oral ivermectin-two doses (200 μg/kg/dose), one week apart (vi) benzyl benzoate 25%, this is mainly for crusted scabies.

Ticks

Hard Tick (Ixodid Tick) (Fig. 16.6A)

Identification features

Hard tick has a hard, chitinous shield (scutum) covers the dorsum.
❖ Body cannot be distinctly separated into head, thorax and abdomen
❖ They have four pairs of legs, no antennae
❖ When viewed from above its head is visible
❖ They are dark/bright colored
❖ Both sexes suck blood and feed both day and night, cannot withstand starvation
❖ Medically important species:
  - *Haemaphysalis* species
  - *Amblyomma* species.

Diseases transmitted by hard tick—refer Table 16.2.

Soft Tick (Argasid Tick) (Fig. 16.6B)

Identification features

Ornithodoros species is a medically important soft tick
❖ Length of adult soft tick 5 mm
❖ They are oval in shape
❖ They have four pairs of short legs
❖ When viewed from above head is not visible
❖ They can survive without blood meals for long periods
❖ Both sexes suck blood
❖ They bite only at night time and their bite is very painful.

Diseases transmitted by soft tick—refer Table 16.2.

CLASS CRUSTACEA

Cyclops (Fig. 16.6C)

Identification Features

Cyclops are also called as **water fleas.**
❖ They measure less than 1mm in length and pear-shaped
❖ Their tail is forked

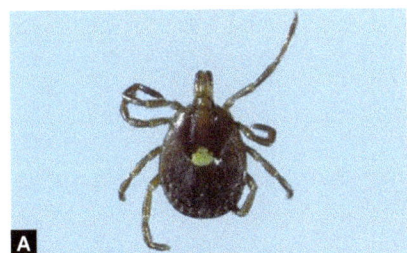
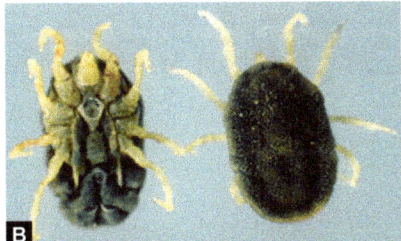
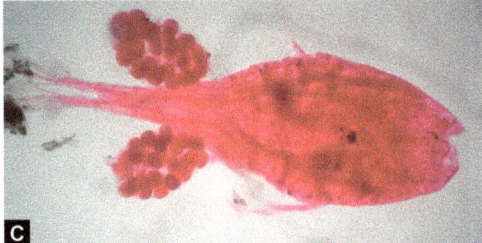

Figs 16.6A to C: (A) Female hard tick (*Amblyomma* species); (B) Dorsal and ventral view of soft tick; (C) Cyclops (mounted specimen)
Source: DPDx Image Library, Centers for Disease Control and Prevention (CDC), Atlanta (*with permission*).

- They have two pairs of antennae, five pairs of legs and a pigmented eye
- They swim in water with typical jerky movements.

Diseases transmitted by cyclops—refer Table 16.2.

CONTROL OF ARTHROPODS

Physical Control Methods

- Proper disposal of sewage, garbage, manure and elimination of stagnant water
- Use of door and window screens and bed nets.

Biological Control Methods

- Use of specific viruses, bacteria, protozoa, fungi which are pathogenic to various morphological forms of arthropods
- Use of Gambusia fish that feed on larvae of mosquitoes
- Barbell fish and Gambusia fish have been successfully used for control of cyclops.

Chemical Control

Insecticides can be used such as dichlorophenyl-trichloroethane (DDT), baygon and pyrethrum flowers, and arsenical compounds.

EXPECTED QUESTIONS

I. **Write short notes on:**
1. Role of mosquitoes in transmission of infectious diseases.
2. Role of ticks in transmission of infectious diseases.

II. **Multiple choice questions (MCQs):**
1. Mosquito acts as vector for transmission of all the parasitic infections, *except*:
   a. Malaria
   b. Bancroftian filariasis
   c. Malayan filariasis
   d. Leishmaniasis
2. House fly acts as mechanical vector for transmission of all the following infections, *except*:
   a. Amoebiasis
   b. Typhoid and paratyphoid fever
   c. Malaria
   d. Cholera
3. Rat flea acts as vector for transmission for which of the following parasitic infection:
   a. *Paragonimus westermani*
   b. *Hymenolepis diminuta*
   c. *Echinococcus granulosus*
   d. *Diphyllobothrium latum*
4. Hard tick acts as vector for transmission for which of the following parasitic infection:
   a. Babesiosis
   b. Diphyllobothriasis
   c. Dracunculiasis
   d. Leishmaniasis
5. Cyclops acts as vector for transmission for all the following parasitic infections, *except*:
   a. Diphyllobothriasis
   b. Dracunculiasis
   c. Gnathostomiasis
   d. Malaria

Answer
1. d 2. c 3. b 4. a 5. d

Appendix-1

CLINICAL SYNDROMES IN PARASITOLOGY (SYMPTOMATOLOGY)

Table A1.1: Symptomatology

Symptoms	Protozoa	Helminths		
		Cestodes	Trematodes	Nematodes
Diarrhea	Entamoeba histolytica Giardia lamblia (frothy stool) Cryptosporidium parvum Cyclospora cayetanensis Cystoisospora belli	Taenia solium Taenia saginata Taenia saginata asiatica	Fasciolopsis buski Clonorchis sinensis Paragonimus westermani Heterophyes heterophyes Metagonimus yokogawai Gastrodiscoides hominis	Trichinella spiralis Trichuris trichiura Strongyloides stercoralis Ancylostoma duodenale Necator americanus Capillaria philippinensis Trichostrongylus
Dysentery	Entamoeba histolytica Balantidium coli		Schistosoma japonicum Schistosoma mansoni	Trichuris trichiura
Anemia	Plasmodium species Babesia microti Leishmania donovani	Diphyllobothrium latum	Schistosoma haematobium	Ancylostoma duodenale Necator americanus Trichuris trichiura
Eye infection	Acanthamoeba species Trypanosoma cruzi Toxoplasma gondii Nosema species Encephalitozoon species Vittaforma corneae	Taenia solium Echinococcus granulosus		Onchocerca volvulus Toxocara Dirofilaria conjunctivae Loa loa
CNS infection	Entamoeba histolytica Naegleria fowleri Acanthamoeba species Balamuthia mandrillaris Plasmodium falciparum Toxoplasma gondii Trypanosoma brucei gambiense Trypanosoma brucei rhodesiense Trypanosoma cruzi Microsporidia	Taenia solium Spirometra Taenia multiceps Echinococcus granulosus Echinococcus multilocularis Echinococcus vogeli	Schistosoma japonicum Paragonimus westermani	Trichinella spiralis Angiostrongylus cantonensis Gnathostoma spinigerum Strongyloides stercoralis Toxocara canis Toxocara cati Loa loa
Malignancy			Schistosoma haematobium Clonorchis sinensis Opisthorchis viverrini	
skin and sub-cutaneous infections	Entamoeba histolytica (amoebiasis cutis) Leishmania species (cutaneous leishmaniasis and PKDL) Trypanosoma brucei Trypanosoma cruzi	Taenia solium (sc nodules) Multiceps multiceps (sc nodules)	Schistosoma (Cercarial dermatitis)	Agents of cutaneous larva migrans (creeping eruption) Hook worm (ground itch) Strongyloides stercoralis (larva currens) Onchocerca volvulus (Onchocercoma) Loa loa (Calabar swelling) Dracunculus medinensis (blisters) Mansonella streptocerca Mansonella ozzardi

Contd...

Contd...

Symptoms	Protozoa	Helminths		
		Cestodes	Trematodes	Nematodes
Opportunistic infections in AIDS patients	Toxoplasma gondii Cryptosporidium parvum Isospora belli Microsporidia Entamoeba histolytica Giardia lamblia Free- living amoebae Cyclospora cayetanensis Leishmania spp. (co-infection)			Strongyloides stercoralis (co-infection)

Abbreviations: CNS, central nervous system; SC, sub cutaneous; PKDL, Post Kala-azar dermal leishmaniasis; AIDS, accquired immuno deficiency syndrome.

Note: **Opportunistic parasitic diseases**—Immunocompromized hosts (e.g. HIV infected patients) are more prone to get a number of opportunistic parasitic infections. Both HIV and opportunistic parasites affect each other's pathogenesis.

Table A1.2: Common tropical parasitic diseases

food and water borne	Soil transmitted	Vector borne
Entamoeba histolytica	Ascaris lumbricoides	Plasmodium species
Giardia lamblia	Ancylostoma duodenale	Leishmania donovani
Cryptosporidium parvum	Ancylostoma braziliense	Wuchereria bancrofti
Cystoisospora belli	Ancylostoma caninum	Brugia malayi
Cyclospora cayetanensis	Trichuris trichiura	Onchocerca volvulus
	Strongyloides stercoralis	Trypanosoma brucei
		Trypanosoma cruzi

Appendix-2

RELATIVE SIZE OF MORPHOLOGICAL FORMS OF PARASITES

Table A2.1: Relative size of morphological forms of protozoa

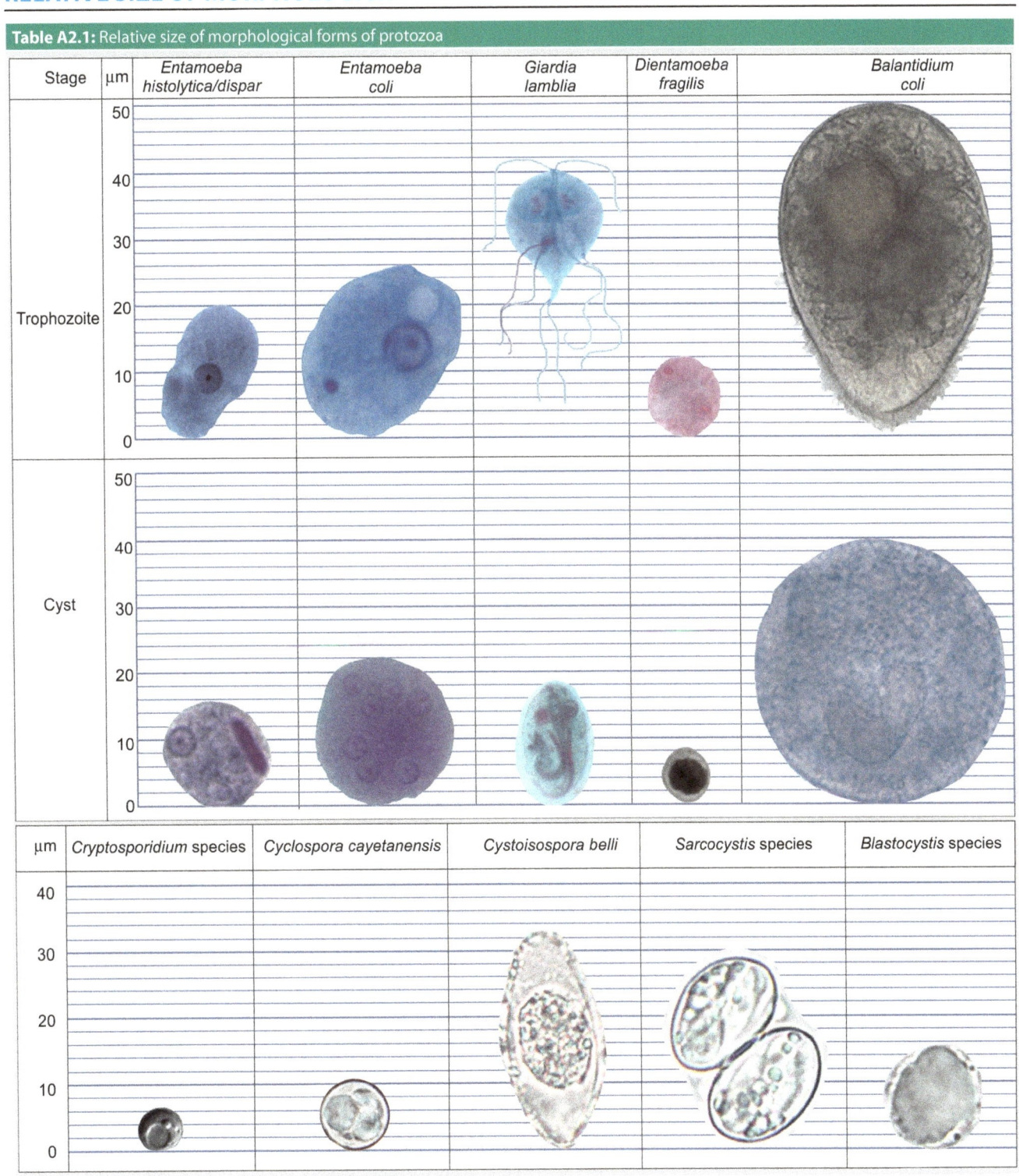

SECTION 4 ◆ Miscellaneous

Table A2.2: Relative size of morphological forms of helminths

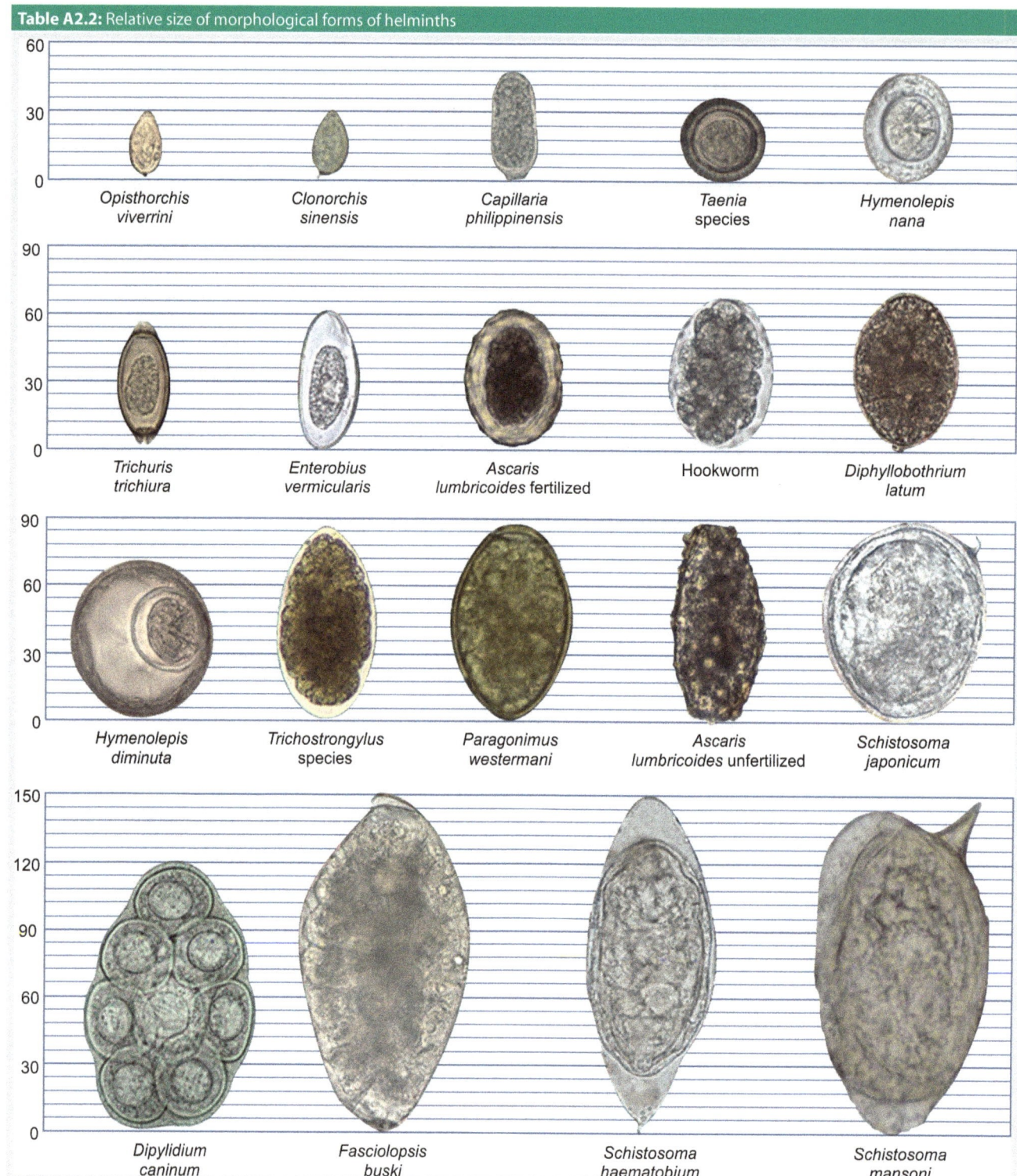

Index

Page numbers followed by *f* refer to figure and *t* refer to table.

A

Aberrant
  parasite 4
  sparganosis 132
Acanthopodia 32
Accidental parasite 3
Acid fast
  stain, modified 113, 238
  staining 104
Acquired immunity 79
Acute schistosomiasis 159
Adaptive immunity 7
Aedes 219
Agar plate
  culture 251
  technique 187, 192
Albendazole 10, 42, 110, 140, 179, 187, 218
Algid malaria 78
Amastigote form 51*f*, 63
Amoebapore 20
Amoebic
  dysentery 20
  keratitis 32
  liver abscess 22
  ulcer 21
Amoeboma 21, 22
Amoebostome 30
Amplifier host 4
Anchovy sauce pus 22*f*
Ancylostoma duodenale 182, 234
Angiostrongylus 201
Animal inoculation methods in parasitic diagnosis 256*t*
Anisakiasis 203
Anisakis simplex 203
Anopheles 72, 258
Antigenic
  mimicry 8
  shedding 8
Antimalarial drug resistance 86
Antiparasitic drugs 9
Armed tapeworm 126

B

Ascaris
  lumbricoides 192
  suum 196
Autofluorescence 107
Autoinfection 5, 103, 135, 180, 204
Axenic cultures 248
Axoneme 37, 51
Axostyle 42

B

Babesia 71, 90
  divergens 90
  microti 90
Bachman intradermal test 230
Bacillary dysentery 23*t*
Baermann funnel technique 187, 191, 251
Balamuth's medium 24, 249
Balamuthia mandrillaris 34
Balantidium coli 115
Bay sore 61
Baylisascaris procyonis 202
Benign malaria 75
Benzimidazole 26
Black water fever 78
Blastocystis hominis 118
Blood Concentration techniques 65
Blood flukes 154
Boeck and Dr Bohlav medium 257
Bradyzoites 94, 108
Brown-Brenn modification of Gram stain 113
Brugia
  malayi 219
  timori 220

C

Calabar swelling 220
Canal cells 127
Capillaria 175
  aerophila 205
  hepatica 205
  philippinensis 204*t*
Card agglutination test for trypanosomes 69
Casoni test 146
Cellophane tape method 181
Cercaria 123
Cercarial dermatitis 159, 161
Cerebral malaria 78
Cestodes 125
  morphology of 125
Chagas' disease 63
Chagoma 64
Chandler's index 183
Charcoal culture 251
Charcot Leyden crystals 196, 235
Chiclero ulcer 61
Chilomastix mesnili 46
Chinese liver fluke 164
Chloroquine 9, 26, 79, 87, 88
Cholangiocarcinoma 166
Chopra's antimony test 57
Chromatoid bodies 18
Chronic schistosomiasis 159
Cilia 117*f*
Cirrus 127
Clinical syndromes in parasitology 265
Clonorchis sinensis 164
Coccidian parasites 93
Coenurus 128
Colpitis macularis 43
Commensalism 4
Blood concentration techniques 65
Conjugation 116
Contracaecum species 203
Coproantigen 25, 254
Coracidium 127
Costa 42
Cryptosporidiosis 105
Cryptosporidium parvum 238
Culex 258
  quinquefasciatus 213
Culture techniques in parasitology 248

Cutaneous
　　larva migrans 190
　　leishmaniasis 59
Cyclophyllidean cestodes 125, 127f
Cyclops 129, 226
Cyclospora cayetanensis 105
Cysticercosis 133
Cysticercus
　　bovis 127f, 134
　　cellulosae 135
Cytocentrifugation 247

D

D'Antoni's iodine 236
DEC patch test 223
DEC provocation test 216
DelBrutto's diagnostic criteria 140t
Delhi boil, Aleppo boil and Baghdad button 59
Diamond's medium 25
Dientamoeba fragilis 47
Diethylcarbamazine (DEC) 11, 216, 221
Diffuse cutaneous leishmaniasis 57
Dilution egg counting method 242
Dioctophyme renale 206
Diphyllobothrium 124
Dipylidium caninum 125
Dirofilaria species 225
Disseminated strongyloidiasis 191
Dobeil's iodine 236
Dog tapeworm 142
Double pored tapeworm 150
Dracunculus medinensis 209

E

East African sleeping sickness 67
Echinococcus 142
　　granulosus 142
　　multilocularis 147
　　oligarthrus 147
　　vogeli 147
Echinostoma ilocanum 170
Egg counting methods 242, 243f
Encephalitozoon 111
Endolimax nana 29
Endoparasite 3
Enflagellation test 31
Entamoeba
　　coli 27, 36
　　dispar 27
　　gingivalis 28
　　hartmanni 27

　　histolytica 41, 117
　　　　minuta form of 19
　　moshkovskii 27
　　polecki 28
Enterobius vermicularis 179
Enterocytozoon 112
Enteromonas hominis 46
Entero-test 40
Enzyme linked immuno transfer blot 158
Eosinophilic meningitis 201
Epimastigote form 49
Espundia 61
Exflagellation 75

F

Facultative parasite 3
Falciparum malaria 77, 91t
Fasciola
　　gigantica 164
　　hepatica 162, 168t
Fasciolopsis buski 167
Fecal specimen, preservation of 241
Feces, examination of 233
Field's stain 246
Filarial dance sign 217
Filarial nematode 209, 210t
Filariasis control program 218
Filariasis
　　classical 215t
　　occult 215t
Fish tapeworm 128
Flame cells 127
Flea 262
Flies 258
Flotation techniques 240
Flukes 152
Forest yaws and uta 61
Formalin fixative method 242
Formol-ether sedimentation technique 240t
Free-living amoeba 29
Fulminant amoebic colitis 21

G

Gametocytes 87
Gametogony 74
Gastrodiscoides hominis 169, 169f
Geimsa stain 98f, 113
Giant
　　intestinal fluke 167
　　kidney worm 206
Giardia lamblia 37

Glossina 260
Glycogen mass 18
Gnathostoma species 203
Granuloma cutis 22
Granulomatous amoebic encephalitis 32
Ground itch 198

H

Hama-EITB 158
Hama-fast-ELISA 158
Hanging groin 223
Harada Mori filter paper tube method 190, 191
Hatching test 160
Hemoflagellates 49
Hemozoin pigment 74
Heterophyes heterophyes 169, 169f
Histidine rich protein 77
Hookworm 182
Host 3
Housefly 258
Human broad tapeworm 128
Hydatid cyst 127f, 143
Hydrogenosome 42
Hymenolepis
　　diminuta 150, 259
　　nana 148, 149f
Hyper-active malarial splenomegaly 78
Hyperinfection syndrome 190, 191
Hysterothylacium species 203

I

Imaging methods in parasitic diagnosis 257t
Immune evasion mechanisms of parasites 8t
Immunology of parasitic diseases 6
Incubation period 30
Innate immunity 6
Intermediate host 3
Intestinal
　　flukes 167
　　nematodes 174
　　sarcocystosis 109
　　taeniasis 133, 36
Intradermal skin tests in parasitic diagnosis 256t
Iodamoeba butschlii 29
Iodine mount 236
Iron-hematoxylin stain 238
Isoenzyme analysis 31
Isospora belli 106

Index

Itch mite 262
Ivermectin 11, 179, 196, 208, 223

J

James dots 76
Jaswant-Singh-Bhattacharya (JSB) stain 246
Jones' medium 249

K

Katayama fever 161
Kawamoto technique 82
Kerandel's sign 68
Kinetoplast 49
Kinyoun's cold method 238
Knott's concentration 247

L

Lagochilascaris minor 202
Large intestinal nematodes 177
Larva
    currens 198
    migrans 198
Lectin antigen 26
Leishman donovan (LD) bodies 55
Leishman's stain 246
Leishmania 50
    classification of 50
    donovani 51
    chagasi 62
    braziliensis complex 70
    mexicana complex 61*t*
    tropica 70
Leishmaniasis
    recidivans 59
    with HIV co-infection 54
Leishmanin test 57
Leishmanoma 53
Leopard skin 222
Liver flukes 162
Loa loa 220
Lobopodia 30
Loeffler's syndrome 195
Louse 262
Lugol'siodine 236
Lung fluke 170
Lutzomyia 50

M

Malabsorption 39
Malignant tertian malaria 77
Maltese cross form 90

Mansonella
    ozzardi 224
    perstans 224
    streptocerca 224
Maurer's dots 76
Mazzotti skin test 223
Megaloblastic anemia 131
Meglumine antimoniate 10
Mehlis' gland 126
Melarsoprol 70
Membrane filtration 247
Meningoencephalitis 64
Merthiolate-iodine formalin 242
Metagonimus yokogawai 170
Metronidazole 9, 26, 42, 45, 115
Meyers Kouwenaar syndrome 215
Microfilaria 210
Microfilariae of various filarial worms, comparison of 211*f*
Microfilarial periodicity 209
Microsporidium 16
Mites 262
Monoxenic culture 249
Montenegro test 57, 59, 62
Mosquito 213
Mott cells 69
Mucocutaneous leishmaniasis 50
Multiceps multiceps 141
Muscular sarcocystosis 109

N

Naegleria fowleri 29
Napier's aldehyde test 57
National Institute of Health media 24
Necator americanus 182, 183*f*, 234
Nelson's medium 24
Nematodes 174
    general properties of 124
Neoplasia 6
Neurocysticercosis 137
NIH swab 181, 234
NNN medium 56, 65, 250
Nonnutrient agar 31
Nosema 112
Nurse cells 229

O

Obligate parasite 3
Oesophagostomum 207
Onchocerca volvulus 221
Onchocercoma 222
Oocyst 75, 94

Opisthorchis
    felineus 167
    viverrini 166
Oriental lung fluke 170
Oriental sore 59
Oviparous 174
Ovoviviparous 174

P

Plasmodium 6
Paddy field dermatitis 162
Page's saline 250
Paragonimus westermani 131*t*
Parasite 3
Parasitism 4
Paratenic host 4, 130
Pentatrichomonas hominis 42
Pentavalent antimonial 58
Pernicious malaria 78
Petri dish/slant culture method 251, 251*f*
Phlebotomus 60, 260
Pin worm 179
Plasmodium knowlesi 79, 92
Pleistophora 112
Plerocercoid larva 129
Polyxenic culture 24, 249
Porrocaecum species 203
PKDL (post-kala azar dermal leishmaniasis) 54
Premunition or infection immunity or concomitant immunity or incomplete immunity 79
Prepatent period 74
Procercoid larva 130
Promastigote form 43, 51*f*
Protozoa, classification of 15
Pseudohookworm 205
Pseudoapolysis 129
Pseudophyllidean cestodes 126*f*, 128
Pseudoterranova species 203
PAIR (puncture, aspiration, injection and reaspiration) 9

Q

Quantitative buffy coat (QBC) examination 81, 83, 216
Quartan malarial nephropathy 78
Quinine 10, 78, 86, 87

R

Rapid diagnostic tests 83
Rat fleas 149, 262

Reduviid bug 63*f*, 254
Reservoir host 4
Retortamonas intestinalis 46
Ring form 73
River blindness 261
Robinson's medium 24, 249
Romana's sign 64, 64*f*
Romanowsky stains 245, 245*t*
Rostellum 126
RPMI 1640 medium 85, 250

S

Sabin-Feldman dye test 99
Saline mount 106*f*, 116, 134*f*
Sandfly 50
Sarcocyst 93
Sarcocystis 93
Sarcoptes scabei 262
Saturated salt flotation technique 241
Schaudinn's fluid 242
Schistosoma 5
   haematobium 5
   intercalatum 161
   japonicum 255
   mansoni 5
   mekongi 162
Schistosomula 156
Schizogony 73, 74, 111
Schneider's drosophila medium 56, 250
Schuffner's dots 76
Sedimentation technique 104, 240*f*
Septicemic malaria 78
Serine rich *E. histolytica* protein
   (SREHP) 25
Serpiginous tracks 186
Sheep liver fluke 162
Skin snips technique 223
Small intestinal nematodes 102
Somatic nematodes 209
Sowda 222
Sparganosis 132
Sparganum 127
Spirometra 132
Stallion's disease 62
Steatorrhea 39
Stichosome 177
Stoll's method 242
Strobila 126
Strongyloides
   fuelleborni 192

   stercoralis 5, 188, 251
Subcutaneous cysticercosis 137
Sulfadiazine 100
Swimmer's itch 159
Swollen belly syndrome 192
Symbiosis 4
Syngamy 116

T

Tachyzoite 93
Taenia 133
   multiceps 141
   saginata 134
     asiatica 141
   solium 135
Tapir nose 61
Ternidens deminutus 207
Thelazia species 208
Thick smear 65
Thin smear 65
Ticks 263
Tissue cyst 93
TORCH infection 97
Toxocariasis 199
Toxoplasma
   encephalitis 96
   gondii 93
Trachipleistophora 112
Trail sign 31
Transfusion malaria 78
Trematodes 152, 153
   classification of 152
Triage parasite panel 24*f*, 41
Triatoma infestans 63
Trichinella 227
Trichinellosis 227
Trichomonas 42
   tenax 45
   vaginalis 42
Trichostrongylus species 205
Trichrome stain 235
   modified 238
Trichuris trichiura 117
Tropical
   pulmonary eosinophilia 215
   splenomegaly syndrome 78
Tropical parasitic disease 154, 266*t*
Trypanosma 62
   equiperdum 62
   evansi 62

   lewisi 62
   brucei gambiense 62, 68*t*
   brucei rhodesiense 62, 68*t*
   cruzi 62
Trypanosomal chancre 68
Trypomastigote form 49, 63
Tsetse fly 260

U

Urogenital specimen, examination of 248

V

Variant
   surface protein 39
Visceral
   larva migrans 199
   leishmaniasis 53
Vitamin B_{12} deficiency 131
Vitelline gland 126
Vittaforma 112
Viviparous 174

W

Wakana disease 186
Wandering parasite 3
Water lily sign 146
Watsonius watsoni 169
Weingarten's syndrome 215
West African sleeping sickness 67
Western blot 139
Whiff test 45
Whipworm 177
Winter bottom's sign 68
Wright's stain 246
Wuchereria bancrofti 210

X

Xenodiagnosis 66

Y

Yager's liver infusion tryptose medium 65

Z

Ziemann's dots 76
Zinc sulphate flotation concentration
   technique 240
Zymodeme analysis 25

EU GSPR Authorised Reprsentative
Logos Europe, 9 rue Nicolas Poussin
1700, La Rochelle, France
Phone: +33 (0) 6 67 93 73 78
E-mail: contact@logoseurope.eu